D1710388

ECHOCARDIOGRAPHY IN PEDIATRIC HEART DISEASE

Echocardiography in Pediatric Heart Disease

A. REBECCA SNIDER, M.D.
Professor of Pediatrics and Communicable Diseases
C. S. Mott Children's Hospital
University of Michigan Medical Center
Ann Arbor, Michigan

GERALD A. SERWER, M.D.
Associate Professor of Pediatrics and Communicable
  Diseases
C. S. Mott Children's Hospital
University of Michigan Medical Center
Ann Arbor, Michigan

With illustrations by

RICHARD A. GERSONY, M.F.A.
Medical Illustration
Department of Surgery
University of Kentucky
Lexington, Kentucky

YEAR BOOK MEDICAL PUBLISHERS, INC.
Chicago • London • Boca Raton • Littleton, Mass.

1   2   3   4   5   6   7   8   9   0   K   R   94   93   92   91   90

Library of Congress Cataloging-in-Publication Data
Snider, A. Rebecca (Arleen Rebecca)
    Echocardiography in pediatric heart disease /
A. Rebecca Snider, Gerald A. Serwer.
        p.   cm.
    Includes bibliographical references.
    ISBN 0-8151-7850-6
    1. Echocardiography.   2. Heart—Diseases—Diagnosis.
    3. Pediatric cardiology.   I. Serwer, Gerald A. II. Title
        [DNLM: 1. Echocardiography.   2. Heart Diseases— diagnosis.
    3. Heart Diseases—in infancy & childhood.   WG 141.5.E2
    S672e]
    RJ423.5.U46S65   1990
    618.92′1207543—dc20   89-24768
    DNLM/DLC   CIP
    for Library of Congress

Sponsoring Editor: Richard H. Lampert
Associate Managing Editor, Manuscript Services:
    Deborah Thorp
Production Project Coordinator: Gayle Paprocki
Proofroom Supervisor: Barbara M. Kelly

PREFACE

Over the past decade, the noninvasive technique of echocardiography has assumed an increasingly important role in the diagnostic and therapeutic management of cardiac disease in children. M-mode echocardiography provided a method for the assessment of chamber size, wall thickness, and valve motion. The development of two-dimensional echocardiography provided a technique for the spatial anatomic display of cardiac structures and consequently led to more exact definition of cardiac anatomy, even in the more complex congenital heart defects. Recent technologic advances in equipment and image processing have allowed excellent visualization of cardiac structures—even in the fetus and small preterm infant. The more recent addition of Doppler ultrasonography to the two-dimensional echocardiographic examination has provided a technique for quantitation of valve gradients, cardiac output, and shunt size. The rapidly evolving body of knowledge and technology have created the need for a textbook of pediatric echocardiography—one that will provide the most current information on the noninvasive techniques and review the current applications of these techniques in the care of children with heart disease.

It was this environment of rapid expansion and new ideas that led us to write this book. The purposes of the book are twofold. First, this book was written to provide a complete and comprehensive educational textbook primarily for persons who already have a basic understanding of congenital heart disease and of the techniques of echocardiography. We have attempted to provide the in-depth treatment of the subject that is necessary for someone to learn pediatric echocardiography. In particular, we have written this textbook for pediatric cardiologists interested in echocardiography, pediatric cardiology fellows in training programs, adult echocardiographers, and echocardiography technologists who are performing pediatric examinations. Second, this book was written to provide a reference source that could be used in the daily practice of pediatric echocardiography. As a reference source, the book provides (1) an extensive list of references following each chapter, (2) quick access to the formulas and methods that are used to obtain quantitative information from the two-dimensional and Doppler echocardiograms, and (3) a guide to establishing the echocardiographic diagnosis, especially in unusual and very complex heart disease.

Most of the illustrations used in this book were obtained from echocardiographic examinations performed at C.S. Mott Children's Hospital, University of Michigan, Ann Arbor, over the past five years. The data shown in these figures has been validated by cardiac catheterization, surgery, and/or postmortem examination.

In Chapters 1 and 2, we have attempted to provide the reader with a thorough review of the current technology and instrumentation. These two chapters contain information of interest to the echocardiographer and lack excessive technical detail. Since most of the technical information is concentrated in Chapters 1 or 2, these chapters can be read immediately or the reader can begin with Chapter 3. However, it is our belief that the intelligent and appropriate use of the ultrasound technique requires this basic knowledge of physics and technology.

In Chapter 3, we have provided a detailed review of the normal cardiac anatomy. In order to understand the echocardiographic findings in complex congenital heart disease, one must have a thorough understanding of the spatial anatomic features of the normal heart. In this regard, the superb anatomic drawings by Richard A. Gersony illustrate not only the planar anatomy of the heart but also provide a three-dimensional view of cardiac spatial relationships. These anatomic drawings should provide an important reference for the beginning as well as the experienced echocardiographer. In addition, the usefulness of these drawings as an educational source is not limited to persons interested in echocardiography. We expect these illustrations to be important for medical students, house officers, or anyone learning basic cardiac anatomy.

Chapter 4 provides a very comprehensive review of the quantitative M-mode, two-dimensional, and Doppler techniques that are currently in use in the practice of clinical cardiology. Chapter 4 is by far the largest chapter in the book. Its size reflects the growth of echocardiography away from qualitative description and toward quantitative diagnosis. It is our hope that Chapter 4 will provide the reader with a thorough, comprehensive reference source for the formulas and methods used in obtaining quantitative information from the echocardiogram.

In Chapters 5 through 13, the echocardiographic features of most types of pediatric heart disease are reviewed. These chapters are designed to illustrate the clinical applications of echocardiography as well as to provide the reader with the information needed to recognize a specific condition. Finally, Chapter 14 represents our conceptual approach to the diagnosis of very complex congenital heart disease. This approach is based on a knowledge of cardiac anatomy as well as an understanding of how cardiac structures are identified on the two-dimensional echocardiogram. This final chapter illustrates the most sophisticated application of the basic principles of echocardiography that were presented in the first few chapters of the book.

A. REBECCA SNIDER, M.D.
GERALD A. SERWER, M.D.

ACKNOWLEDGMENTS

Throughout the course of preparing this text, we were encouraged and supported by many people, far too numerous to be listed individually here. We are deeply appreciative for this support and for the opportunity to work in such a uniquely rich academic environment. We would like to give special thanks, however, to a few key individuals without whose help this project could not have been completed. From the very beginning, this project was endorsed and enthusiastically supported by all of our colleagues in the Division of Pediatric Cardiology to whom we are very grateful. We are especially appreciative of the support and encouragement we received from our department chairman, Dr. Robert P. Kelch and our division chief, Dr. Amnon Rosenthal.

A very special note of thanks goes to the pediatric echocardiography technicians, Jane Peters and Lyne Merida-Asmus. Besides providing much of the material used in this text, they provided us with a constant daily source of strength, cheerfulness, and enthusiasm. We are indeed fortunate to work with two such highly skilled professional individuals whose technical abilities are matched only by their selflessness and dedication.

Another special note of thanks goes to Kathlene Chmielewski, CMA, who provided us with the editorial assistance necessary to prepare this textbook. We are deeply appreciative of the unfaltering energy and willingness with which she took on this monumental task. We are also grateful for the editorial assistance received from Robert Smith, our division manager, Sharon Badish, Kim LeVeque, and Shirley Adams.

A special thanks goes to all the pediatric cardiology fellows over the years whose love of learning and undying enthusiasm for echocardiography really inspired and motivated us to write this textbook. We are especially grateful to our current pediatric echocardiography fellow, Dr. Roger Vermilion, for contributing Chapters 1 and 2. We also wish to thank Gary Schwartz for his contribution to Chapter 2 on Doppler signal processing. The superb illustrations contained in Chapter 3 were contributed by Richard A. Gersony. We feel very privileged to be able to include such superior-quality illustrations in our textbook.

Finally, the greatest sacrifices of all were made by our families—our parents (Irma and Gifford Snider and Ora Serwer), spouses (Ric Hahn and Sheryl Serwer), and children (Brad, Valerie, Kathleen, James and Laura Serwer). Their tireless support and encouragement made this project possible. To them, we lovingly dedicate this book.

A. REBECCA SNIDER, M.D.
GERALD A. SERWER, M.D.

CONTENTS

COLOR PLATES

PLATE 1.
Doppler color-flow mapping examination from the parasternal short-axis view of a patient with pulmonary regurgitation (PR). The PR jet demonstrates the appearance of aliasing on the color Doppler system. Aliasing in color Doppler results in a color reversal. With a jet that is severely aliased, the jet will have a multilayered appearance with the highest velocities in the center. This accounts for the area of blue flow in the center. *AO* = aorta; *LA* = left atrium; *LT* = left; *PA* = pulmonary artery; *RA* = right atrium; *RT* = right; and *RV* = right ventricle.

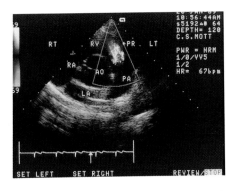

PLATE 2.
Color-flow mapping examination from the apical five-chamber view of a patient with severe subaortic stenosis. This figure illustrates the usefulness of the Doppler color-flow map for aligning the single-crystal Doppler beam parallel to flow in the jet.

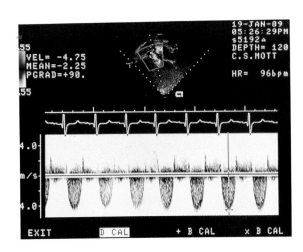

PLATE 3.
Color-flow Doppler examination from a normal patient. Apical four-chamber view shows ventricular diastolic inflow as a diffuse red color.

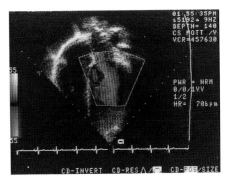

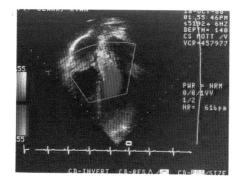

PLATE 4.
Color-flow Doppler examination from a normal patient. Apical four-chamber view shows systolic outflow as a blue color located primarily along the interventricular septum. The red color in the ascending aorta is caused by aliasing, which appears in color-flow Doppler as a color reversal.

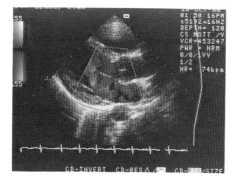

PLATE 5.
Color-flow Doppler examination from a normal patient. Low parasternal long-axis view shows left ventricular diastolic inflow as a diffuse red color.

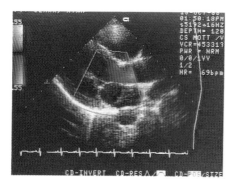

PLATE 6.
Color-flow Doppler examination from a normal patient. Low parasternal long-axis view shows left ventricular systolic outflow as a blue color.

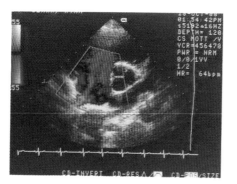

PLATE 7.
Color-flow Doppler examination from a normal patient. Parasternal short-axis view shows right ventricular diastolic filling as a red flow through the tricuspid valve toward the transducer in diastole. Note the low-velocity flow in the inferior vena cava, shown in red.

PLATE 8.
Color-flow Doppler examination from a normal patient. Parasternal short-axis view shows right ventricular systolic outflow as a blue color, indicating flow away from the transducer.

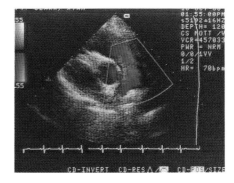

PLATE 9.
Doppler color-flow mapping in the parasternal four-chamber view from a patient with a large secundum atrial septal defect (ASD). The flow through the ASD appears as a red area because flow is directed toward the transducer. *LV* = left ventricle; *RA* = right atrium; and RV = right ventricle.

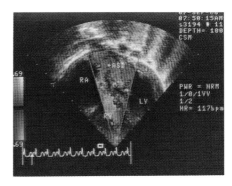

PLATE 10.
Subcostal four-chamber view from a patient with a secundum atrial septal defect (*upper jet*) and a primum atrial septal defect (*lower jet*). The jet flow through the atrial septal defect appears as a reddish-yellow flow area, indicating high-velocity, disturbed flow toward the transducer. *LA* = left atrium; *LT* = left; *LV* = left ventricle; *RA* = right atrium; *RT* = right; and RV = right ventricle.

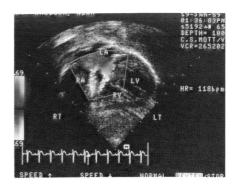

PLATE 11.
Parasternal long-axis view from a patient with a membranous ventricular septal defect (VSD). The high-velocity jet through the VSD is directed toward the transducer and is displayed primarily as an area of red-yellow flow. AO = aorta; LA = left atrium; LV = left ventricle; LVO = left ventricular outflow tract; RA = right atrium; and RV = right ventricle.

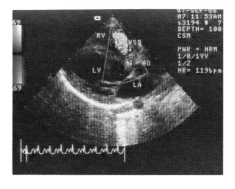

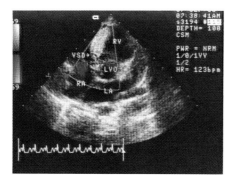

PLATE 12.
Parasternal short-axis view from the same patient shown in Plate 11.

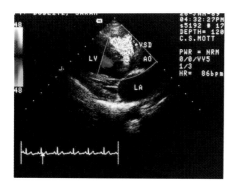

PLATE 13.
Parasternal long-axis view from a patient with a large membranous ventricular septal defect (VSD). The VSD is located superiorly in the ventricular septum just beneath the aortic (AO) valve. In this case, a mosaic of colors is present in the jet, indicating high-velocity disturbed flow. *LA* = left atrium; *LV* = left ventricle.

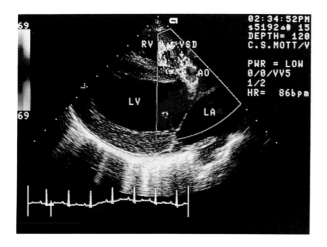

PLATE 14.
Parasternal long-axis view in systole from a patient with a large ventricular septal defect (VSD) and pulmonary vascular obstructive disease. In systole, the mosaic jet seen directed toward the transducer represents the left-to-right shunt through the VSD. AO = aorta; LA = left atrium.

PLATE 15.
Parasternal long-axis view in diastole from the patient shown in Plate 14 with a large ventricular septal defect (VSD) and pulmonary vascular obstructive disease. In diastole, the area of blue flow indicates the right-to-left shunt through the VSD from the right ventricle (RV) to the left ventricle (LV). This jet is blue because it is directed away from the transducer. AO = aorta; LA = left atrium.

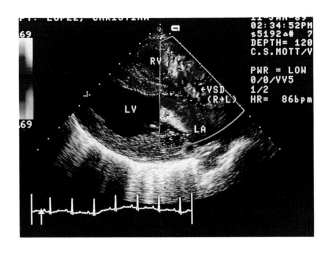

PLATE 16.
Parasternal long-axis view through the right ventricular (RV) inflow tract of a patient with an atrioventricular septal defect. The common atrioventricular valve is seen. In systole, two high-velocity jets are seen oriented away from the transducer (blue color). These jets represent regurgitation through the common atrioventricular valve, which has five leaflets; regurgitation can occur between any of these five leaflets. In this patient, regurgitation occurs at two distinct spots. *LA* = left atrium; *LV* = left ventricle; and *RA* = right atrium.

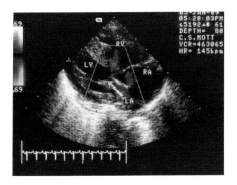

PLATE 17.
Apical four-chamber view from the same patient as in Plate 16. Again, two separate and distinct jets of atrioventricular valve regurgitation are seen. *LA* = left atrium; *LT* = left; *LV* = left ventricle; *RA* = right atrium; *RT* = right; and *RV* = right ventricle.

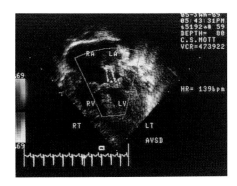

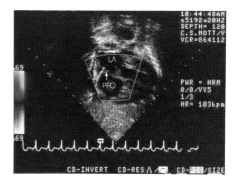

PLATE 18.

Doppler color-flow mapping examination in the subcostal four-chamber view from a patient with a patent foramen ovale (PFO) and left atrial (LA) hypertension. The jet flow across the PFO appears as a yellow mosaic flow, indicating high-velocity flow toward the transducer. Although this patient does not have a hypoplastic left heart, a PFO jet in the presence of LA hypertension appears the same regardless of etiology.

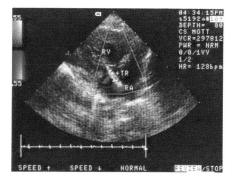

PLATE 19.

Doppler color-flow mapping in the parasternal long-axis view through the right ventricular (RV) inflow tract of a patient with critical pulmonary stenosis and tricuspid regurgitation (TR). The TR jet is displayed as an area of predominantly blue mosaic colors, indicating flow away from the transducer RA = right atrium.

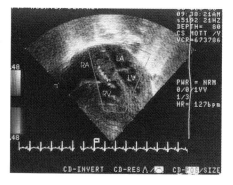

PLATE 20.

Apical four-chamber view from an infant with minimal tricuspid regurgitation, which appears as a predominantly blue flow area directed away from the transducer. RA = right atrium; RV = right ventricle; LA = left atrium; and LV = left ventricle.

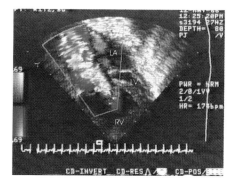

PLATE 21.

Color-flow mapping examination in the apical four-chamber view from an infant with Ebstein deformity of the tricuspid valve. The predominantly blue mosaic jet represents the tricuspid regurgitant flow from the right ventricle (RV), through the tricuspid valve to the right atrium and away from the transducer. The origin of this jet outlines the inferiorly displaced tricuspid valve leaflet. LA = left atrium; LV = left ventricle.

PLATE 22.
Parasternal short-axis view from a patient with Ebstein anomaly of the tricuspid valve and mild tricuspid regurgitation (TR). The tricuspid regurgitation jet has its origin more anterior than usual because of the displacement of the tricuspid valve. LA = left atrium; LT = left; LVO = left ventricular outflow tract; RA = right atrium; RT = right; and RV = right ventricle.

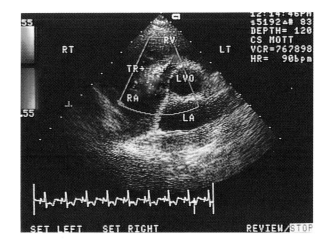

PLATE 23.
Doppler color-flow mapping examination from the apical four-chamber view of a patient with severe left lower pulmonary vein stenosis. The jet flow from the left lower pulmonary vein is displayed as a blue color, indicating flow away from the transducer. The color flow Doppler outlines the left lower pulmonary vein, which might otherwise be difficult to image directly because of its small size. LV = left ventricle; RA = right atrium; and RV = right ventricle.

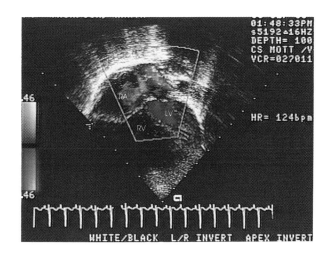

PLATE 24.
Doppler color-flow mapping examination in the apical four-chamber view from a patient with the membrane (MEMB) of cor triatriatum. A high-velocity jet is seen passing across the membrane. This jet is red and yellow, indicating high-velocity, disturbed flow directed toward the transducer. LV = left ventricle; RA = right atrium; and RV = right ventricle.

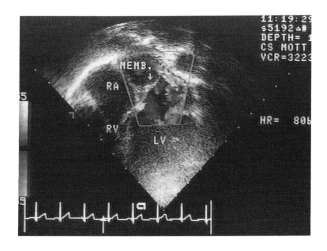

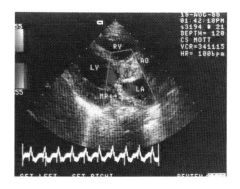

PLATE 25.
Doppler color-flow mapping examination in the parasternal long-axis view from a patient with mitral regurgitation (MR). The MR jet is seen directed away from the transducer, and thus is an area of blue mosaic flow. In addition, the MR jet is eccentric and layered along the left atrial (LA) posterior wall. This patient also has evidence of high-velocity disturbed flow in the ascending aorta (AO) as a result of aortic valve stenosis. LV = left ventricle; RV = right ventricle.

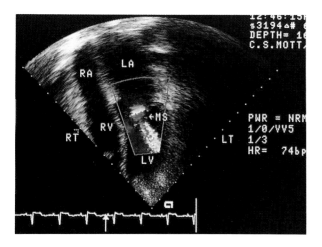

PLATE 26.
Apical four-chamber view from a patient with mitral stenosis (MS) caused by rheumatic fever. The blue flow area in the mitral valve funnel proximal to the tips of the mitral valve leaflets represents an area of high-velocity flow and color reversal or aliasing. This proximal acceleration of flow occurs because of a decrease in the effective flow area in that region. Distal to the tips of the mitral valve leaflets, an eccentric high-velocity jet with evidence of disturbed flow is seen. LA = left atrium; LV = left ventricular; RA = right atrium; and RV = right ventricle.

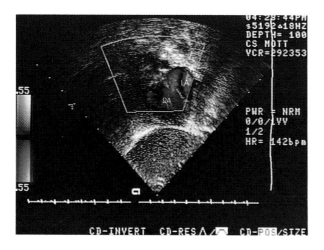

PLATE 27.
Doppler color-flow mapping of the atrial septum in an infant with critical pulmonary valve stenosis. In this view, a right-to-left atrial shunt is seen as an area of blue flow passing across the atrial septum. This indicates flow away from the transducer from the right atrium (RA) to the left atrium (LA).

PLATE 28.

Doppler color-flow mapping examination from the subcostal sagittal view of the right ventricle (RV) of a child with severe pulmonary valve stenosis. Systolic flow in the RV is directed away from the transducer and is therefore blue. Just proximal to the pulmonary valve (PV) in systole, a red flow area is seen. This area represents an area of increased flow velocity with aliasing or color reversal. Distal to the valve, a high-velocity mosaic jet of pulmonary stenosis (PS) is seen. LV = left ventricle.

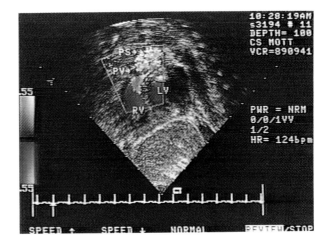

PLATE 29.

Color Doppler examination in a parasternal short-axis view from an infant with severe peripheral pulmonary stenosis (PPS) involving the right pulmonary artery. A high-velocity mosaic jet is seen in the right pulmonary artery, indicating disturbed high-velocity flow away from the transducer. AO = aorta; LT = left; PA = pulmonary artery; RA = right atrium; RT = right; and RV = right ventricle.

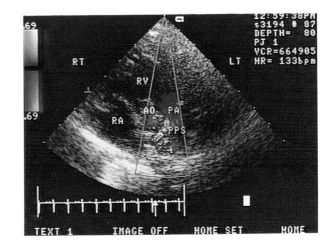

PLATE 30.

Color Doppler examination in diastole from the same patient as in Plate 30. The red flow area, seen adjacent to the mosaic jet of the peripheral pulmonary stenosis, indicates flow back toward the pulmonary valve in diastole. Diastolic back flow of blood is seen in patients with severe peripheral pulmonary stenosis. Care must be taken not to confuse the diastolic backflow for a patent ductus arteriosus.

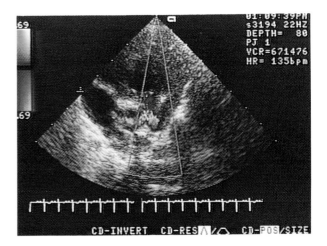

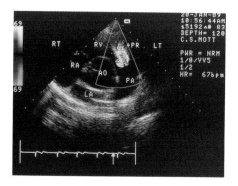

PLATE 31.
Color-flow Doppler examination in the parasternal short-axis view from a patient with Marfan syndrome and pulmonary regurgitation (PR). The PR jet is oriented toward the transducer and thus is displayed as a red flow area. The blue coloration in the center of the PR jet is a color reversal caused by aliasing. AO = aorta; LA = left atrium; LT = left; PA = pulmonary artery; RA = right atrium; RT = right; and RV = right ventricle.

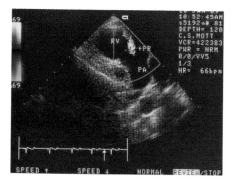

PLATE 32.
Color-flow Doppler in the parasternal long-axis view of the right ventricular outflow tract from the same patient as in Plate 32. In Plate 32, the PR jet is quite broad; in Plate 33, however, the PR jet is very narrow. This suggests that the regurgitant orifice is slit-like. PA = pulmonary artery; RV = right ventricle.

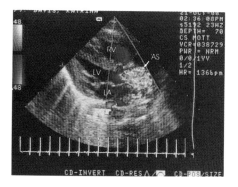

PLATE 33.
Color-flow Doppler examination in the parasternal long-axis view from a patient with aortic valvular stenosis (AS). The AS jet is seen as a high-velocity, mosaic flow area in the ascending aorta. LA = left atrium; LV = left ventricle; and RV = right ventricle.

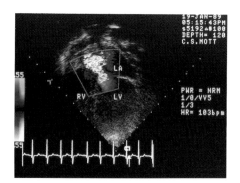

PLATE 34.
Color-flow mapping examination from the apical five-chamber view of a patient with discrete subvalvular aortic stenosis. The high-velocity mosaic jet, which begins in the left ventricle (LV) well below the aortic valve, confirms the presence of a subvalvular obstruction with a high-velocity jet proximal to the valve. LA = left atrium; RV = right ventricle.

PLATE 35.

Color-flow Doppler examination of the suprasternal notch from a patient with severe aortic insufficiency. The red flow area in the descending aorta in diastole indicates flow toward the transducer. This retrograde diastolic flow is caused by a runoff of blood from the aorta to the left ventricle through the insufficient aortic valve.

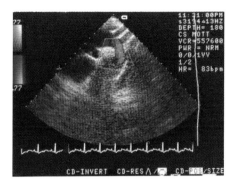

PLATE 36.

Color-flow mapping examination in the parasternal long-axis view from a patient with aortic regurgitation (AR). The AR jet is seen as a high-velocity, mosaic flow area color-coded primarily as blue (indicating flow away from the transducer). AO = aorta; LA = left atrium; LV = left ventricle; and RV = right ventricle.

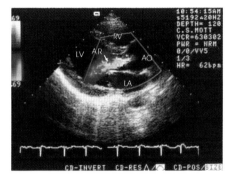

PLATE 37.

Doppler color-flow mapping examination from the parasternal short-axis view of an infant with a patent ductus arteriosus (PDA). The PDA jet appears as a high-velocity mosaic area with flow directed pre-dominantly toward the transducer. The high velocities in the PDA jet indicate a high pressure gradient between the descending aorta and the pulmonary artery. AO = aorta; LT = left; RA = right atrium; RT = right; and RV = right ventricle.

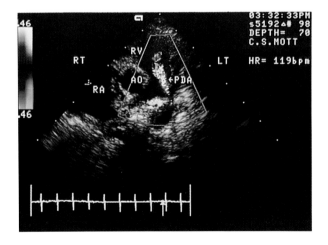

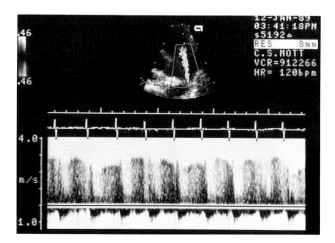

PLATE 38.

Color-flow Doppler examination from the same patient as in Plate 37. In the parasternal short-axis frame, the high-velocity jet through the patent ductus arteriosus is seen. The color Doppler display of the patent ductus arteriosus jet can be used to obtain proper alignment of the continuous-wave Doppler beam. The Doppler spectral tracing, *bottom,* shows a high-velocity continuous flow directed toward the transducer. The peak velocity of the jet is 3 m/sec, indicating a 36 mm pressure gradient between the descending aorta and pulmonary artery.

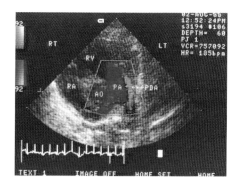

PLATE 39.

Color-flow mapping examination in the parasternal short-axis view from an infant with a patent ductus arteriosus (PDA) and pulmonary artery hypertension. In this case, the flow through the PDA is a red color, indicating flow from the descending aorta through the PDA toward the transducer. Flow velocity is relatively low (there is no aliasing or color reversals) because of the low pressure gradient between the descending aorta and pulmonary artery (PA) in this child with hypertension. Abbreviations: AO = aorta; LT = left; RA = right atrium; RT = right; and RV = right ventricle.

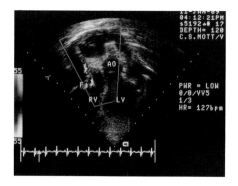

PLATE 40.

Color-flow Doppler examination in the apical five-chamber view from a patient with a coronary fistula (F) draining into the right ventricular (RV) outflow tract. To see the flow into the fistula, the plane of sound has been tilted far anteriorly. Flow through the fistula into the RV appears as a reddish-orange jet. The color-flow mapping examination is particularly useful for identifying the site of drainage of a coronary artery fistula. AO = aorta; LV = left ventricle.

PLATE 41.

Color Doppler examination in the suprasternal short-axis view in an infant with supracardiac total anomalous pulmonary venous return. The pulmonary veins can be seen joining inferiorly to form a pulmonary venous confluence (PVC). On the left, a left vertical vein (LVV) is seen arising from the PVC. Doppler signals from blood flow in the PVC and LVV are color-coded as red, indicating flow up the LVV toward the transducer. From the LVV, pulmonary venous return is to the innominate vein (IN) and right superior vena cava (SVC). Beneath this abnormal vascular connection, the transverse aorta (AO) is seen in cross-section and the right pulmonary artery (RPA) is seen in longitudinal section.

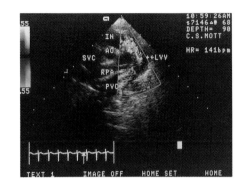

PLATE 42.

Parasternal long axis view from the same patient as in Figure 10–48. The high-velocity jet caused by right upper pulmonary vein stenosis is seen as a mosaic flow area.

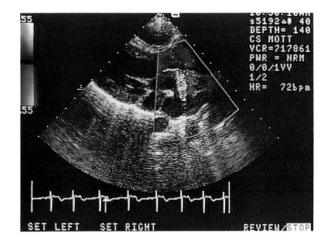

PLATE 43.

Color-flow mapping examination from the suprasternal long-axis view of a child with a coarctation of the descending aorta. The coarctation jet appears as an area of high-velocity mosaic flow in the descending aorta. The color-flow Doppler signals clearly outline the aortic arch in the area of the coarctation; thus, Doppler color-flow mapping is very useful for improved imaging of the flow area in the aortic arch.

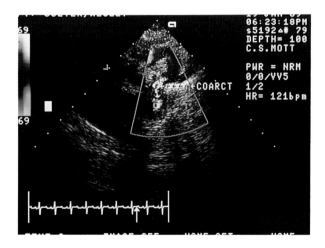

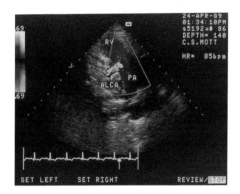

PLATE 44.

Color Doppler examination from a child with anomalous origin of the left main coronary artery from the pulmonary artery (PA). In this parasternal long-axis view of the right ventricular (RV) outflow tract, the anomalous left coronary artery (ALCA) can be seen arising from the PA. Flow in the ALCA is toward the PA and is therefore red.

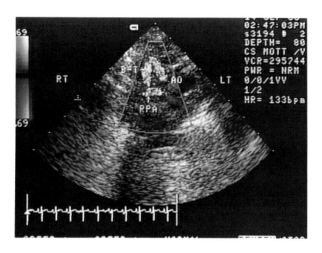

PLATE 45.

Color-flow mapping examination from the suprasternal short-axis view of an infant with a right Blalock-Taussig (BT) shunt. Flow in the shunt is displayed as a high-velocity, mosaic flow that in real time is continuous throughout systole and diastole. AO = aorta; LT = left; RPA = right pulmonary artery; and RT = right.

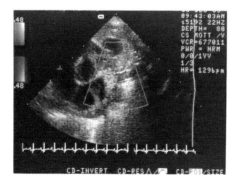

PLATE 46.

Color-flow mapping examination from the same patient as in Figure 13-2 and in the same view. The flow through the left Blalock-Taussig shunt is away from the transducer and therefore color-coded as blue. The flow in the left pulmonary artery is a mosaic, high-velocity, disturbed flow.

PLATE 47.

Subcostal sagittal view of the right ventricle (RV) from an infant who had recently undergone patch closure of a ventricular septal defect (VSD). On the color-flow Doppler examination, a large jet indicating flow toward the transducer is seen at the inferior margin of the VSD patch. This jet represents flow across the ventricular septum through a residual VSD. LV = left ventricle; PA = pulmonary artery.

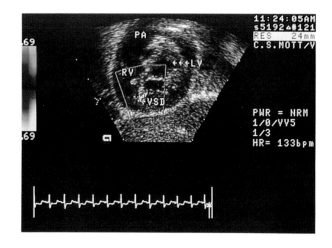

PLATE 48.

Apical four-chamber view from a patient who had recently undergone repair of a double-outlet right ventricle (RV). The color Doppler examination shows high-velocity disturbed flow originating from the area of the ventricular septum. This flow represents flow through a residual ventricular septal defect (VSD). A portion of the VSD jet passes from the left ventricle (LV) to the right ventricle, while another portion passes from the LV directly to the right atrium (RA). LA = left atrium.

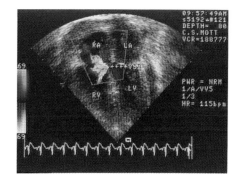

PLATE 49.

Color-flow Doppler examination from the parasternal view of a patient with a heterograft conduit between the left ventricle and pulmonary artery. The color-flow examination shows a high-velocity mosaic flow in the right pulmonary artery (RPA). This flow pattern indicates severe peripheral pulmonary stenosis at the distal insertion of the conduit into the RPA. RPA = right pulmonary artery.

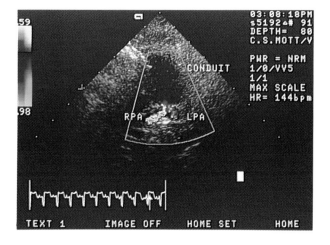

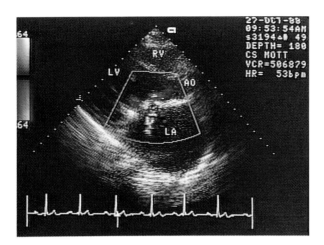

PLATE 50.
Parasternal long-axis view in systole from a patient with a Carpentier ring placed after repair of an atrioventricular septal defect because of severe mitral regurgitation. A mitral insufficiency jet can be seen originating between the Carpentier ring and the aortic (AO) root. This jet represents a perivalvular leak. LA = left atrium; LV = left venticule; and RV = right ventricle.

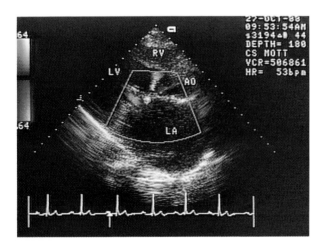

PLATE 51.
Parasternal long-axis view in diastole from the same patient shown in Plate 50. Several high-velocity jets directed toward the transducer (red flow areas) are seen, representing mitral stenosis. One jet is seen coming through the center of the Carpentier ring, while the other jet passes through the perivalvular orifice. LA = left atrium; LV = left ventricle; and RV = right ventricle.

Basic Physical Principles

Roger P. Vermilion, M.D.

PHYSICAL PRINCIPLES OF M-MODE AND TWO-DIMENSIONAL ECHOCARDIOGRAPHY

As medical ultrasound instrumentation has become more sophisticated, the need to understand the basic physical principles of ultrasound and its instrumentation has increased. A complete discussion of the physics and electronics of medical ultrasound instrumentation is beyond the scope of this text. The interested reader may wish to review a more comprehensive summary.[1,2] This chapter attempts to give an overview of basic concepts and emphasizes the points essential to the clinician who performs ultrasound studies so that he or she can more fully utilize the technology available. The second chapter discusses more specifically the instrumentation and reviews many of the concepts necessary for optimal utilization of available features.

Sound Waves

Sound is transmitted as a mechanical, longitudinal wave of regions of compression and rarefaction of the media through which it travels. Ultrasound refers to sound waves of frequencies higher than those audible to the human ear. This is generally defined as frequencies higher than 20,000 Hz (cycles per second). The speed of travel depends on the density and elastic properties of the media. The speed of transmission, the frequency, and wavelength of the wave are related by the following formula:

$$c = f \times w \tag{1}$$

where c = speed of sound in the media (m/sec); f = frequency of the wave (Hz); and w = wavelength (meters). In human tissue, this speed is relatively constant and is approximately 1,560 m/sec. The frequency range of use in medical applications is generally 2 to 10 MHz (MHz = megahertz, or 1,000,000 Hz), for reasons that will become apparent later. According to the preceding formula, the corresponding wavelengths are in the range of 0.8 to 0.16 mm. These wavelengths establish a fundamental limit to the resolution possible with a given transducer frequency, as points must be separated by more than one wavelength to be resolved.

Propagation of Sound Waves

The property that determines how sound is transmitted through a medium is the acoustic impedance. The acoustic impedance depends on the density and elasticity of the medium. As sound travels through a homogeneous medium, a portion of the energy is absorbed and the remainder is transmitted. The extent to which the sound is absorbed is determined by the acoustic impedance and the frequency of the sound wave. Absorption increases with frequency; therefore, a high-frequency ultrasound beam (i.e., 10 MHz) will not penetrate as far into tissue as a lower-frequency beam (such as 2.25 MHz). This limits the fre-

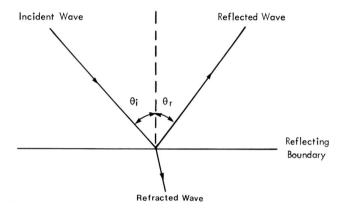

Incident Wave   Reflected Wave

θ_i θ_r

Reflecting
Boundary

Refracted Wave

FIG 1–1.
Diagram of the reflection of ultrasound waves.

quency of the transducer that may be used at a given depth (many other factors affect transducer selection and are discussed later).

When the ultrasound beam encounters an interface between two media of different acoustic density, some of the energy is reflected backward (the reflected wave) and some passes through the interface (the refracted wave) into the second medium (Fig 1–1). The relative degree of reflection vs. refraction is determined by the degree of mismatch between the acoustic impedance of the two media.

The degree of reflection vs. refraction also depends on the angle of incidence of the beam. This also influences the proportion of the reflected beam that returns in the direction of the transmitted beam. Given a truly flat interface, the reflected wave would return in the direction of the transmitted beam only if the interface were exactly perpendicular to the beam (just as a flashlight beam is reflected from a mirror). Biologic interfaces are irregular and the reflected wave is scattered in all directions from the interface. However, the intensity in any direction depends on the angle of incidence of the beam. Therefore, a very intensely reflective interface, when viewed from a perpendicular vantage point (such as the atrial septum from a subcostal four-chamber view), may be transparent when viewed from a vantage point nearly parallel to the interface (such as the same atrial septum viewed from the apical four-chamber view).

Image Production

Beginning with the M-mode display, ultrasound is used to produce images in the following way: The transducer is used to transmit and receive the sound impulses. The transducer crystal is capable of producing a short burst of sound at its natural frequency, aimed in the selected direction (equivalent to pointing a flashlight and briefly turning it on). For the purpose of this discussion, assume that the ultrasound beam is very narrow and without divergence, like a laser beam of light (later we will see that this is not the case). Unlike the light from the flashlight, however, the sound emitted requires a measurable length of

time to travel into the tissue and for the reflected waves to return. Because the speed of travel is known, the distance to any reflector is easily determined by the time required for its echo to reach the transducer (Fig 1–2). Many are familiar with the use of this principle in determining the distance to a lightning bolt by measuring the length of time between when lightning is seen and when thunder is heard. Each ultrasound pulse encounters many acoustic interfaces and, subsequently, a series of echoes return at intervals of time corresponding to their depths. In this way, each ultrasound pulse generates a line of information that corresponds to the structures encountered along the line of the ultrasound beam. For a typical M-mode display, these pulses are repeated 1,000 times per second or more (the pulse repetition frequency). On the M-mode graphic display (Fig 1–3), the line of information is plotted with the distance from the transducer displayed on the vertical or y axis. Along the horizontal or x axis, each line of information is plotted next to the previous line. Thus, the combination of depth information from the y axis and temporal information from the x axis provides a graphic display of the motion of the cardiac structures in real time (M-mode or motion-mode). The intensity of each returning echo determines the shade of gray of its corresponding dot on the M-mode recording.

This method yields excellent time resolution of moving structures, as the sampling rate (pulse repetition frequency) of 1,000/sec is much faster than the heart rate; thus there are many samples through each cardiac cycle. For example, even at a heart rate of 200 beats per minute, this technique provides 300 lines of information per heartbeat.

We will now review how a two-dimensional image can be constructed using multiple individual lines of information produced as discussed above. Each line of the image is produced as for an M-mode display. The transducer is then aimed at a slightly different angle and another line of information is formed. In this way, the entire image is produced one line at a time (Fig 1–4). A typical display will use 128 lines of information to produce one image, or frame. The process is then repeated, and multiple frames per second are constructed in real time. How fast this may be done depends on the depth of the field. The limiting factor is how much time must be allowed for the echoes

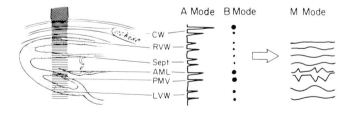

A Mode   B Mode   M Mode

CW
RVW
Sept
AML
PMV
LVW

FIG 1–2.
Diagram of the methods used to generate the M-mode echocardiogram. *CW* = chest wall; *RVW* = right ventricular wall; *Sept:* = septum; *AML* = anterior mitral leaflet; *PMV* = posterior mitral valve leaflet; and *LVW* = left ventricular wall.

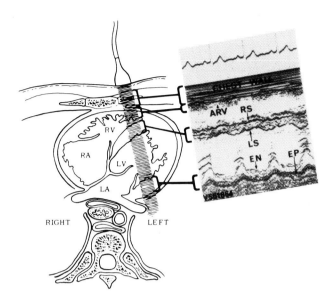

FIG 1–3.
Diagram and echocardiogram illustrating how echocardiography can obtain an ice pick or one-dimensional view of the heart through the right and left ventricles. *ARV* = anterior right ventricular wall; *RS* = right septum; *LS* = left septum; *EN* = posterior left ventricular endocardium; *EP* = posterior left ventricular epicardium; *RA* = right atrium; *RV* = right ventricle; *LV* = left ventricular; *LA* = left atrium. (From Feigenbaum H: *Echocardiography,* ed 3. Philadelphia, Lea & Febiger, 1981, p 13. Used by permission.)

from each pulse to return before redirecting the transducer. For typical depths in pediatric patients (5 to 15 cm), frame rates of 28 to 50 Hz may be achieved.

Image Quality

Before discussing Doppler echocardiography, a brief digression is necessary to discuss a number of basic concepts important to the quality of the resulting echocardiographic image. The quality of an image can be a somewhat elusive concept. For the purpose of this discussion, image quality will be divided into three component parts, as recently described by Maslak[3]: (1) detail resolution, or what is most often thought of as the dot resolution (i.e., a measure of how close together two points may be and still be resolved as two distinct dots); (2) contrast resolution, or the ability to distinguish differences in soft tissue density; and (3) uniformity of the image throughout the display. A variety of the artifacts that can interfere with proper interpretation of images will also be discussed, some of which relate to the equipment and some of which are inherent in the use of ultrasound for imaging.

Detail Resolution

Detail resolution refers to the ability to resolve small structures. This is often tested as the distance by which two dots must be separated before they can be distinguished as two dots rather than one. Detail resolution depends on many factors and is not the same in all directions.

Axial resolution refers to the dot width in the direction of the ultrasound beam. Lateral resolution refers to resolution in the direction perpendicular to the beam. Lateral resolution, discussed first, is inherently less than axial resolution.

The most important factor that affects lateral resolution is the width of the beam. Earlier, we assumed that the ultrasound beam was like a laser beam of light. Understanding the limits on lateral resolution requires a discussion of the beam profile, which is a means of describing the way in which the width of the ultrasound beam varies with distance (Fig 1–5). Because there is no discrete edge to the beam, it is necessary to make an arbitrary definition of beam width. Figure 1–5 shows the beam profile across a plane through the beam. The beam width is generally thought of as the width of the beam at the point where the signal intensity has decreased by 20 decibels (db). As labeled in the diagram, the narrowest region is the focal zone. The region between the transducer and the focal zone is referred to as the near field, while the region beyond the focal zone in which the beam diverges is the far field.

The image in the region beyond the focal zone (far field) is degraded rapidly with distance from the transducer (because of worsening lateral resolution). In the range of interest, several factors may be altered to improve lateral resolution (produce a narrower beam). The beam may be focused with an acoustic lens just as may be done with light waves. Theoretically, there is a limit on how narrow the beam can be focused. This limit depends on the trans-

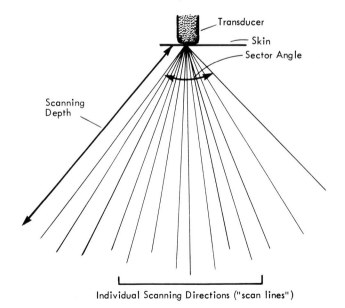

FIG 1–4.
Sector scanning pattern. (From Silverman NH, Snider AR: *Two-Dimensional Echocardiography in Congenital Heart Disease.* Norwalk, Conn, Appleton-Century-Crofts, 1982, p 3. Used by permission.)

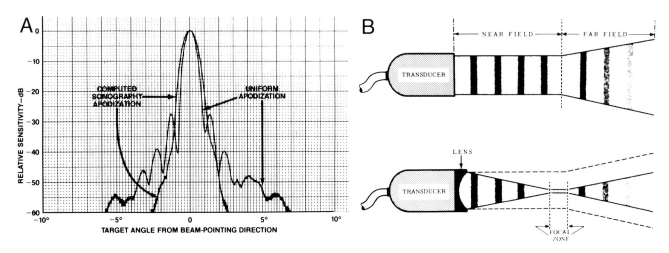

FIG 1–5.
A, effect of apodization on contrast resolution. Sector beam plot widens considerably at 50 dB with uniform apodization, resulting in poor resolution from low-level echoes. Computed sonography apodization shows excellent resolution at 50 dB. (From Maslak SH: Computed sonography, in Sanders RC, Hill MC (ed): *Ultrasound Annual 1985.* New York, Raven Press, 1985, p 13. Used by permission.) **B,** diagrams of the ultrasound beam emitted by an unfocused *(top)* and a focused *(bottom)* transducer. (From Feigenbaum H: *Echocardiography,* ed 3. Philadelphia, Lea & Febiger, 1981, p 7. Used by permission.)

ducer size and the frequency of the wave, and is expressed in the formula:

$$\text{Focal zone diameter} = \frac{(w)(x)}{d} \qquad (2)$$

where w is the wavelength of the sound wave, x is the distance to the point in question from the transducer, and d is the diameter of the transducer. Figure 1–6 plots this minimum beam width vs. distance for a transducer with a diameter of 1 cm and a frequency of 3.5 MHz.

It is apparent from this formula that, at least theoretically, the larger the transducer, the better the beam width at the focal zone and, consequently, the better the lateral resolution. While this is true in the far field image, practical considerations exist in the near field that result in an inability to focus as well in this region. Figure 1–7 shows the beam profile of two transducers of equal frequency but different diameters. Note the narrower minimum beam width and shallower angle of divergence in the far field for the larger transducer. However, these advantages come at the cost of a less well focused near field. In addition, when used in small windows such as the parasternal or apical views, the larger transducer may result in artifacts from ribs and other large reflectors. This will be discussed later. Therefore, a larger transducer gives the best far field for views such as the subcostal views and for use in larger patients. However, a smaller transducer will give better near-field images for views such as the parasternal views in small children.

The above formula also indicates that the possible beam width becomes narrower as the wavelength of sound decreases. Because wavelength and frequency are inversely related, this means that a higher-frequency transducer can

be more tightly focused than a lower-frequency transducer. In addition, the angle of divergence in the far field is lessened with higher-frequency transducers (decreased wavelength). This is apparent from the following formula, which relates the angle of divergence in the far field to the wavelength and transducer diameter:

$$\sin \Theta = 1.22 \; w/d \qquad (3)$$

where Θ is the angle of divergence. Unfortunately, as discussed above, the depth of penetration diminishes with frequency and limits the use of higher frequencies to very small children.

The factors that determine lateral resolution are now

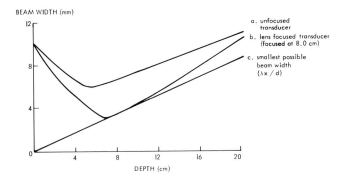

FIG 1–6.
Beam width: 1 cm transducer: 3.5 MHz. *A,* unfocused transducer; *B,* lens-focused transducer focused at 8 cm; and C, smallest possible beamwidth. (From Silverman NH, Snider AR: *Two-Dimensional Echocardiography in Congenital Heart Disease.* Norwalk, Appleton-Century-Crofts, 1982, p 7. Used by permission.)

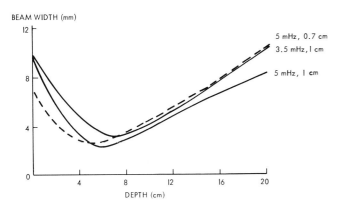

FIG 1–7.
Beam width for three different transducers. (From Silverman NH, Snider AR: *Two-Dimensional Echocardiography in Congenital Heart Disease*. Norwalk, Appleton-Century-Crofts, 1982, p 9. Used by permission.)

apparent. For two dots to be distinguished as separate points, they must be spaced farther apart than the beam width at that depth. Otherwise, both will appear to be on the same scan line. Therefore, lateral resolution parallels beam width and, consequently, the above discussion regarding beam width can be directly applied to lateral resolution. Bright objects are particularly affected, as the apparent beam width is wider for intense echoes. This is so because the beam does not have sharp edges and is particularly important for issues of contrast resolution. This will be discussed in the next section.

Axial resolution is independent of issues regarding the beam formation. Resolution along the axis of each scan line (depth) is determined only by timing of the echoes. Consequently, only factors that affect the ability to time the returning echoes precisely have any impact on the resolution in this direction. The principal determinant of depth resolution is the length of the sound pulse. In general, the sound pulse used for imaging contains approximately 5 cycles and therefore has a length that corresponds to about 5 wavelengths. For a 5 MHz transducer, this is about 1 mm in length. Thus, axial resolution is better than lateral resolution and does not depend on depth or transducer size.

Contrast Resolution

Contrast resolution refers to the ability to distinguish between differences in tissue density and the ability to resolve faint structures near bright reflectors. As with detail resolution, discussed above, axial resolution is better than lateral resolution. In addition, lateral resolution depends primarily on the beam width. However, for contrast resolution, the low-level signals are of greater relative importance. Therefore, the beam width at the 60 db level rather than the 20 db level is important. Generally, this beam width is considerably wider than the 20 db beam width (see Fig 1–5A). The newer technology of computer-controlled image production (computed sonography) allows considerable control over these low-level signals in order to optimize contrast resolution. Discussion of these meth-

ods is beyond the scope of this chapter. The user need not understand all these features and there is no user control over them in any currently available commercial system. These features may, however, considerably enhance the image and are important when comparing one system with another.

Uniformity of Image

Uniformity refers to the ability to maintain equivalent resolution throughout the field of view. With a mechanical sector scanner with a fixed focus transducer, considerable differences exist between the image in the area of best focus, the broadly smeared image in the far field, and the often fuzzy near-field region. The newer phased-array systems have improved uniformity considerably. This has been accomplished by a method of dynamic focusing during the receiving portion of the cycle. As the returning echoes are received, the focal zone is continually adjusted to match the distance that corresponds to that time interval. With this approach, the effective beam width is made much more uniform throughout a wide range of depths (Fig 1–8).

Artifacts

There are many potential sources of artifacts in ultrasound imaging that may complicate the interpretation of images. Because artifacts can be more easily understood and anticipated if the underlying reasons for their occurrence are known, several of the more common artifacts will be summarized in this section.

Dropout of parallel structures.—As discussed above, when structures are nearly parallel to the beam of ultrasound, very little of the sound energy is reflected back to the transducer. Therefore, structures with this orientation may be transparent to the ultrasound beam. For example, when viewed from the apex, the atrial septum runs nearly parallel to the direction of the ultrasound beam. Conse-

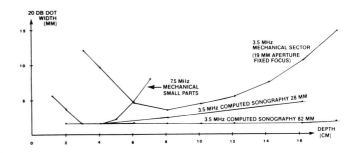

FIG 1–8.
Comparative beam plots for computed sonography transducers as well as for 3.5 and 7.5 MHz mechanical sector scanner transducers. Detail resolution (20 dB bandwidth) is virtually uniform for computed sonography transducers, while mechanical scanners exhibit highly nonuniform resolution. The 3.5 MHz mechanical scanner's resolution at 4 and 16 cm is two to four times worse than that of the computed sonography system. (From Maslak SH: Computed sonography, in Sanders RC, Hill MC (ed): *Ultrasound Annual 1985*. New York, Raven Press, 1985, p 9. Used by permission.)

quently, areas of dropout in the septum are frequently seen, which can make it difficult to distinguish real septal defects. However, if the septum is viewed from the subcostal region, it is nearly perpendicular to the beam and is easily viewed without evidence of dropout.

Shadowing by echo-dense structures.—Because generation of the image depends on the transmission of ultrasound through the media, any very dense region may produce a shadow that obscures the area behind it. For example, a prosthetic valve with very echo-dense prosthetic material can completely mask any view of the heart behind it. A mitral prosthesis viewed from the cardiac apex can make it impossible to see the left atrium behind it. Similarly, large catheters may cause shadows behind them that simulate septal defects.

Lateral spread of high-intensity echoes (side lobes).—As discussed in the preceding section, all images in the far field are spread laterally because of the width of the ultrasound beam. As the beam does not have discrete edges (i.e., the amplitude diminishes with distance from the center of the beam), very bright echoes will have considerable width. Because the normal-intensity echoes are not spread to the same degree, a bright structure near the edge of a vessel may appear to extend into the lumen of the normal vessel. For instance, because of this effect, a very bright region of the pericardium may appear to lie within the pulmonary artery if the pericardial reflection extends well beyond its actual boundary.

Instrument-related artifacts.—Many unusual shadows unrelated to the structures being visualized may be produced by noise produced within the system. A characteristic of these artifacts is their tendency to appear and disappear with changes in instrument settings, particularly depth.

PHYSICAL PRINCIPLES OF DOPPLER ULTRASOUND

The Doppler Effect

The Doppler principle states that the frequency of transmitted sound is altered when the source of the sound is moving. The frequency or pitch of the emitted sound remains constant; however, the audible transmitted pitch varies, becoming higher as the sound source approaches the receiver and becoming lower as the sound source moves away from it. The same effect occurs when the receiver is moving and the sound source is stationary. The change in frequency, first described in 1843 by the Austrian physicist Christian Johann Doppler, is called the Doppler shift in frequency or the Doppler frequency.

The Doppler principle applies to all types of waves in which the source and the receiver are moving relative to one another (e.g., light from a moving star, radar waves). In medical applications, an emitted ultrasound pulse strikes a moving region of blood, and the backscattered ultrasound

pulses are shifted in frequency compared with the emitted pulse. The shift in frequency is related to the velocity and direction of blood flow, as well as to other factors, such as the angle between the Doppler ultrasound beam and the blood flow and the speed of sound in tissue. The Doppler equation describes the mathematical relationship of all of these factors:

$$f_d = \frac{2\ (f_o)\ (V)\cos\Theta}{c} \qquad (4)$$

where f_d = the observed Doppler frequency shift, f_o = the transmitted frequency, c = the velocity of sound in human tissue at 37°C (approximately 1560 m/sec), V = blood flow velocity, and Θ = the intercept angle between the ultrasound beam and the blood flow. In the remainder of this section, each of these variables will be examined in more detail.

The observed Doppler frequency shift is usually in the magnitude of several kilohertz (KHz = 1,000 cycles/sec) and therefore produces an audible signal. The audible signal can be electronically processed and displayed graphically, thereby providing two outputs (audio signal and graphic display) from the Doppler examination. The Doppler signal consists of a spectrum of frequencies, rather than a single frequency. Most commonly, the Doppler-shifted frequencies undergo a fast Fourier transform (FFT) analysis, which transforms the original complex Doppler waveform into its frequency components and their corresponding amplitudes. The Doppler spectral tracing produced by the FFT analysis is graphically displayed, with frequency shift or velocity on the vertical axis, time on the horizontal axis, and amplitude or power as shades of gray. Doppler signals from blood flow toward the transducer are displayed above the baseline, and Doppler signals from blood flow away from the transducer are displayed below the baseline (Fig 1–9).

The variation in frequency distribution in normal blood flow is caused by factors such as (1) unequal distribution of flow velocity over the cross-sectional area of the vessel caused by viscous friction (flow velocity is lower near the vessel walls), (2) variations in red blood cell interspaces, and (3) divergence and nonuniformity of sound beams.[4] Despite these variations, when the blood flow through a cardiac chamber or peripheral vessel is laminar, the red blood cells are generally moving in parallel fashion and with similar velocities. In this situation, the Doppler frequency shifts are uniform and produce a tonal or musiclike sound on the audio output and a narrow frequency bandwidth on the graphic display. When blood flow is disturbed (as in turbulent flow), the red blood cells are moving in random directions and with varying velocities. In disturbed flow, the Doppler spectrum is composed of multiple, widely varying frequencies. The audio output is harsh or scratchy, and the graphic display has a wide-frequency bandwidth.[5, 6]

In Doppler flowmetry, the component of the flow velocity parallel to the ultrasound beam produces the Dop-

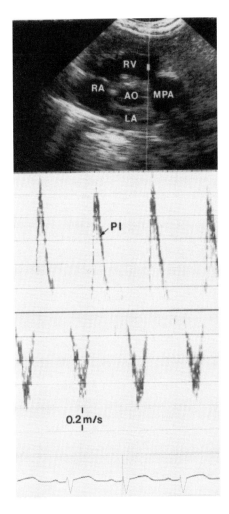

pler frequency shift occurs when the intercept angle Θ is 0 or 180° (where the cos Θ = 1). For intercept angles of less than 20°, the cos Θ is sufficiently close to 1 that it can be neglected in the calculation of velocity without introducing significant error. For example, by neglecting the intercept angle in the calculation the underestimation of the velocity is 6% at an angle of 20° (cos 20° = 0.94). For intercept angles exceeding 20°, the angle must be measured and the cos Θ included in the Doppler equation to minimize errors in the calculation of velocity. Several problems can occur in measuring Θ and cos Θ:

1. Even with the use of a two-dimensional echocardiographic display, Θ is difficult to measure accurately. From the two-dimensional echocardiographic image, Θ can be estimated in the x and y planes; however, it is never certain where the beam lies relative to the blood flow in the azimuthal or z plane.

2. The intercept angle Θ calculated from the two-dimensional image is the angle between the ultrasound beam and the vessel walls. The direction of blood flow in the vessel may not be parallel to the vessel walls. For example, with an eccentric stenotic aortic valve, the jet flow through the valve is usually directed toward the right border of the ascending aorta (from angiographic studies) rather than parallel to the walls of the ascending aorta. Color Doppler, with its ability to visualize the jet, has made it possible to align the Doppler beam with the jet rather than the vessel walls, although this can be quite difficult.

3. Because the cosine is a circular function, for angles between 30° and 60° small changes in angle can make a large difference in the estimated velocity.

FIG 1–9.
Example of a pulsed Doppler recording (*bottom*) from the parasternal short-axis view (*top*) of a patient with pulmonary insufficiency. The freeze-frame image on the top shows the position of the sample volume in the right ventricular (RV) outflow tract at the time of the Doppler recording. AO = aorta; LA = left atrium; MPA = main pulmonary artery; RA = right atrium.

pler frequency shifts. This component of the velocity vector is called the radial velocity and can be calculated from a reconstructed right-angle triangle to be equivalent to V cos Θ (Fig 1–10). This is the origin of the V cos Θ term in the Doppler equation.

The Doppler equation can be rearranged to solve for velocity, such that:

$$V = \frac{c\, f_d}{2f_o \cos \Theta} \tag{5}$$

C and f_o are constants and f_d can be measured with relative precision. Therefore, the principal source of error in the calculation of the flow velocity is in the determination of the intercept angle Θ between the ultrasound beam and the axis of flow. For a given velocity, the maximum Dop-

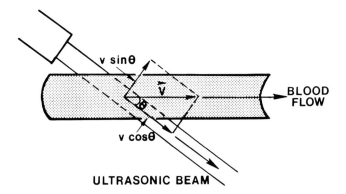

FIG 1–10.
The component of the velocity vector (V) parallel to the ultrasound beam gives rise to the Doppler shift in frequency. For a right-angle triangle, this component is called the radial velocity and is equal to V cos Θ (the angle between the ultrasound beam and the direction of blood flow in the vessel). (From Snider AR: Doppler echocardiography: Basic principles and clinical applications, in Buda AJ (ed): *Digital cardiac imaging*. The Hague, Martinus-Nijhoff, 1985, p 185. Used by permission.)

In clinical applications, the echocardiographer usually angles the ultrasound beam until the highest-pitched (most clear and tonelike) audio signal is found. When the highest-pitched signals are detected on the audio output of the Doppler, or when the highest velocities are recorded on the graphic display of the Doppler, the ultrasound beam can be assumed to be nearly parallel to the direction of jet flow, and no correction for intercept angle needs to be made. To obtain the best alignment between the Doppler beam and the jet flow, several different echocardiographic windows are usually attempted. Using this technique, it is only possible to underestimate the true velocity. Underestimation of the true flow velocity can occur if the intercept angle was actually significant (greater than 20°) when the examiner assumed that the angle was close to 0 and cos θ was close to unity. Overestimation or underestimation can occur unpredictably when angle correction is used to calculate the flow velocity. Because of the difficulties in measuring the intercept angle, most investigators do not use angle correction in the calculation of flow velocity.

Implementation

Three basic types of Doppler equipment have been developed for interrogating flow in the cardiac chambers and peripheral vessels. These are continuous-wave Doppler (CW), pulsed Doppler, and color-flow mapping. Historically, the first type of Doppler ultrasound system used was the continuous-wave Doppler system.

CW Doppler

The continuous-wave Doppler transducer has two crystals; one continuously transmits an ultrasound signal, while the other continuously receives backscattered ultrasound. Therefore, Doppler signals from all blood flow traversed by the ultrasound beam are received and displayed as a composite. With continuous-wave Doppler, there is no range resolution—it is not possible to sample flow velocity selectively from a known position within the heart. A major advantage of continuous-wave Doppler is that there is no limit to the maximum velocity that can be measured. Sampling theory holds that to detect or display a wave of a certain frequency moving in a certain direction, it is necessary to sample at twice that frequency at least. With continuous-wave Doppler, sampling is continuous, the sampling rate is infinite, and there is no limit to the ability to display very high frequency shifts.

Pulsed Doppler

In the range-gated pulsed Doppler system, a single ultrasound crystal alternately transmits and receives the ultrasound signal. Thus, a short burst of ultrasound is transmitted to a selected depth at a rate called the pulse repetition frequency (PRF). The backscattered signal is received with the same transducer. Doppler shifts in the returning signal can be analyzed from a time window that begins at a specified time after the emission of the ultra-sound burst. Because the velocity of ultrasound in human tissue is essentially constant, the time between the emission of the ultrasound burst and the time window (or range gate) determines the depth or range from the transducer at which the Doppler sampling occurs. The time window or analysis window is called the sample volume, which has a finite size—its width is the beam width and its length is determined by the length of time selected to listen for returning echoes. The lower limit on the sample volume length is the duration of the ultrasound pulse. Figure 1–9 is an example of a two-dimensional range-gated pulsed Doppler recording. The vessel being interrogated is imaged directly on the two-dimensional echocardiographic system. The Doppler cursor line, which indicates the direction of the Doppler ultrasound beam, is placed in the vessel being examined. The position of the range cell or sample volume along the cursor line is operator-controlled and is indicated on the display.

The principal advantage of pulsed Doppler is range resolution, or the ability to sample blood flow in a small, specific area whose location and depth can be varied. A disadvantage of pulsed Doppler, however, is that there are limits to the maximum frequency shifts that can be unambiguously displayed at any given depth. To avoid range ambiguity, the ultrasound pulse must travel down to the selected depth and back before the next pulse can enter the heart. Therefore, the PRF or sampling rate is limited at each depth. According to sampling theory, the maximum detectable frequency shift in one direction (without ambiguity) is only one-half the sampling rate, if the display is divided equally into both directions. At more shallow depths, the PRF and, therefore, the maximum detectable frequency, are higher than at deeper depths. The maximum detectable frequency is called the Nyquist limit and, if the display is divided into forward and reverse channels, is equivalent to ±PRF/2. For example, if the Doppler system has a PRF of 12,800 bursts per second at a depth of 5 cm, then the Nyquist limit at 5 cm is ±6,400 Hz (12,800/2) or ±6.4 KHz. If the depth setting is increased to 11 cm, the emitted pulse must travel twice as far before the next pulse can enter the heart; therefore, the PRF is approximately halved. If at 11 cm the PRF is 6,400 bursts per second, then the Nyquist limit at 11 cm is ±3,200 Hz (6,400/2) or ±3.2 KHz. The corresponding velocities that can be unambiguously displayed then depend on the frequency of the transducer used. Rearranging equation number 5 above, for a given Doppler shift the corresponding velocity is inversely proportional to the carrier frequency of the transducer. Therefore, a 2.5 MHz transducer may display velocities of twice the magnitude as a 5 MHz transducer at the same depth.

Two methods have been used to extend the Nyquist limit (increase the maximum velocity that can be displayed) on pulsed Doppler instruments: the zero-shift method and high pulse repetition frequency (HPRF). With the zero-shift display, the zero-flow line or baseline is shifted toward the top or bottom of the display so that more of the display can be used to examine flow in one of the directions

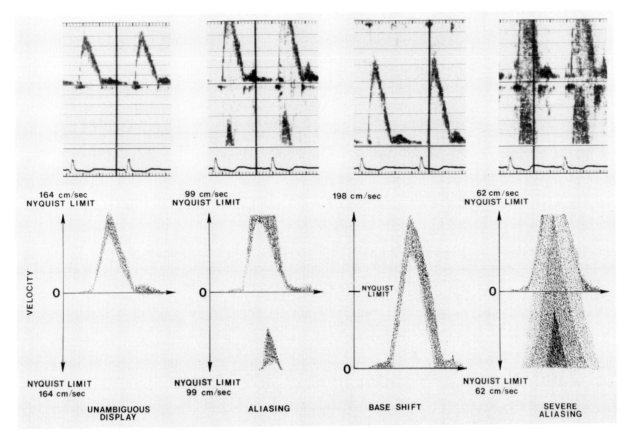

164 cm/sec
NYQUIST LIMIT

99 cm/sec
NYQUIST LIMIT

198 cm/sec

62 cm/sec
NYQUIST LIMIT

NYQUIST LIMIT
164 cm/sec

NYQUIST LIMIT
99 cm/sec

NYQUIST LIMIT
62 cm/sec

UNAMBIGUOUS
DISPLAY

ALIASING

BASE SHIFT

SEVERE
ALIASING

FIG 1–11.
Examples of aliasing in a pulsed Doppler ultrasound system. In the first frame (*far left*) the peak velocity of the Doppler signal does not exceed the Nyquist limit for that depth setting; therefore, the entire Doppler tracing is displayed unambiguously. In the second frame (*second from left*), the peak velocity of the Doppler tracing exceeds the Nyquist limit for that depth setting. The system cuts off the signal and displays it ambiguously in the opposite channel or direction. This is known as frequency aliasing, or wraparound. In the third frame (*second from right*), the depth setting and Nyquist limit are the same as in the second frame. This time, however, the zero flow line, or baseline, has been shifted to the bottom of the display so that the entire display is used to show flow in one direction only. With this baseline shift, the Doppler spectral tracing can be displayed unambiguously. In the fourth frame (*far right*), the Doppler spectral tracing wraps on itself several times so that signals are seen above and below the baseline. Severe aliasing can be difficult to distinguish from turbulence or disturbed flow.

(Fig 1–11). For example, if the baseline is moved to the bottom of the graphic display, the system can display Doppler frequency shifts toward the transducer from 0 up to the PRF (instead of ± PRF/2). With high pulse repetition frequency Doppler, the PRF is increased by sending each pulse before the preceding pulse has had time to return from the depth of interest. Therefore, because of the simultaneous transmission of more than one pulse within the patient, Doppler shifts are detected from more than one site or sample volume.

If a frequency shift occurs that exceeds the Nyquist limit, the equipment cuts off the true signal, electronically folds or wraps the signal around, and displays it ambiguously in the opposite direction (see Fig 1–11). This phenomenon is called frequency aliasing. Although the electronics of frequency detection are somewhat complex, the concept of aliasing can be easily understood by the analogy of observing a spinning wheel with a strobe light. The speed with which the wheel spins (revolutions per second) is equivalent to the frequency, and how often the strobe light is on (strobes per second) is equivalent to the PRF. Calculating the speed and direction of spin by the wheel's position at two successive strobes is equivalent to calculating the Doppler shift frequency. If the wheel has turned one-quarter turn between strobes, then the wheel is spinning at one-quarter the strobe frequency. However, it is necessary to know that the wheel is not spinning fast enough to have made more than one rotation. Otherwise, it might also have turned one and one-quarter turns and might be in exactly the same position when the strobe next turns on. In addition, it is not possible to distinguish between three-quarters of a turn in the opposite direction (or any multiple of turns plus three-quarters). This is the concept of aliasing: any multiple of turns plus one-quarter will appear to be the same as one-quarter of a turn. To be certain of the direction and speed of spin, it is necessary to know that sampling is being done at a rate of twice the time required to make one rotation (the sampling theorem referred to above). Analogously, to display a Doppler shift frequency (and corresponding velocity) unambiguously, the

PRF or sampling rate must be twice the maximum frequency in order to be detected.

Color Doppler

The most recent development in Doppler technology has been color-flow Doppler. With this technique, flow information is depicted in color superimposed over the two-dimensional image. In general, red is used to indicate flow toward the transducer (above the baseline in the graphic pulsed Doppler display) and blue is used to indicate flow away from the transducer (below the baseline in the graphic pulsed Doppler display). The intensity of the color indicates the magnitude of the *mean* velocity of flow. Flow information is obtained in the same manner as with the pulsed Doppler technique, with multiple sample volumes interrogated sequentially. The sequential gathering first of structural information and then of Doppler information requires different scan speeds, because the Doppler information requires much more time to generate. For this reason and others, it is not practical to perform color Doppler with mechanical scanners. A phased-array system is required, which allows random selection of scan lines with its electronically steered ultrasound beam.

Because of the tremendous quantity of information that exists in each color-flow image and the time required to gather it, many trade-offs are necessary to generate each color-flow image. Many sacrifices of information content must be made to achieve satisfactory temporal resolution (frame rate). Each image is generated by first producing a sector image in the usual fashion. To achieve greater speed, this image is sometimes made up of fewer scan lines than the usual image. The resulting coarser image can be smoothed with interpolating algorithms to fill in lost information. Although in the process some spatial information is lost, the image can be created significantly faster.

The structural information and the Doppler information are obtained from separate ultrasound pulses and can be acquired in any order, depending on the system design. The Doppler information requires much more time to acquire than the structural image, as each scan line must be sampled several times to obtain adequate flow information. Many compromises are necessary to produce a color image with sufficient speed to achieve an adequate frame rate. The simplest technique is to define a smaller sector within the image in which to calculate flow information. The maximum depth and width of this sector will determine the frame rate. The number of samples of each scan line can be altered to improve speed of acquisition; decreasing the number of samples, however, results in loss of frequency data. For color Doppler, no attempt is made to do an FFT to calculate complete spectral data. Instead, sufficient data are gathered to produce a reasonable estimate of the mean velocity and an estimate of the bandwidth of the returning frequencies, while using the minimum possible number of samples along each line. This is accomplished through a technique known as autocorrelation, which allows rapid estimation of the mean velocity without taking the time required for the usual FFT.

The estimate of bandwidth of the spectrum is referred to as variance. This can be displayed in many ways, the most common of which is to add a third color such as yellow to the color used to display flow. There is no standard in the industry on how to quantify the variance for display, but many approaches are in use. No quantification can be made from this display, although it can be useful to quickly detect areas of disturbed flow.

Color Doppler allows rapid display of a great deal of information. It is ideal for visualizing small disturbed jets and mapping jet orientation. However, color Doppler has many significant inherent limitations. First, the display depicts mean velocity and not peak velocity, which is more familiar. Because the accuracy of this estimate of the mean velocity has not been validated, no quantification is currently possible. However, it may prove possible to use this information in the quantification of flow, where mean velocity is the information required. Second, the Nyquist limit is restricted, as high pulse repetition frequency Doppler is not possible. Most disturbed jets in restricted orifices will exceed the Nyquist limit and result in aliasing. Consequently, the display is often ambiguous, as aliasing results in color reversals. Plate 1 shows the multiple layers of color that result from a pulmonary insufficiency jet of velocity greater than the Nyquist limit. There is aliasing of the central portion of the jet. Areas of disturbed flow may result in more complex patterns of aliasing.

REFERENCES

1. Wells PNT: *Biomedical Ultrasonics*. London, Academic Press, 1977.
2. Hatle L, Angelsen B: *Doppler Ultrasound in Cardiology: Physical Principles and Clinical Applications,* ed 2. Philadelphia, Lea & Febiger, 1985, pp 1–73.
3. Maslak SH: Computed sonography, in Sanders RC, Hill MC (eds): *Ultrasound Annual 1985.* New York, Raven Press, 1985.
4. Ried JM, Baker DW: Physics and electronics of the ultrasonic Doppler method, in Egerman H (ed): *Ultrasonic Medica.* Wein, 1971, p 109.
5. Pearlman AS, Stevenson JG, Baker DW: Doppler echocardiography: Applications, limitations, and future directions. *Am J Cardiol* 1980; 46:1256–1262.
6. Nishimura RA, Miller FA Jr, Callagan MJ, et al: Doppler echocardiography: Theory, instrumentation, technique, and application. *Mayo Clin Proc* 1985; 60:321–343.

Technology and Instrumentation

Roger P. Vermilion, M.D.

TECHNOLOGY AND INSTRUMENTATION OF M-MODE AND TWO-DIMENSIONAL ECHOCARDIOGRAPHY

This chapter provides a brief outline of the principal equipment features available for imaging and Doppler studies. The various techniques available and their appropriate selection will be reviewed. For each technique, the most frequently provided user controls and how they impact the structural or Doppler data will be discussed.

M-Mode Imaging

M-mode echocardiography is the oldest imaging technique. Early equipment used a standalone transducer with a single stationary crystal. Most recent equipment provides a steerable M-mode, which allows selection of an M-line from the two-dimensional image for subsequent M-mode display. The following controls are typically available:

Depth.—The depth may be set as desired to include as much in the recording as needed. Because the pulse repetition frequency is fixed, the depth setting in M-mode echocardiography does not affect the temporal resolution as it does in two-dimensional imaging.

Power.—The transmit power is set to obtain adequate penetration at the deepest depth required.

Gain.—Most systems allow control of both overall receiver gain and gain as a function of time (and therefore as a function of depth in the image). This depth-dependent gain control is required to compensate for the variable attenuation of the ultrasound signal with the distance traversed. It is important to adjust the gain controls to keep all signals within the dynamic range of the receiver. Signals of greater intensity create background noise and will decrease the receiver's sensitivity. Gain is usually controlled by either multiple slide levers that correspond to the gain at different depths, or by an adjustable ramp. In general, the multiple slide levers permit greater flexibility in gain settings and are easier to use. With either method, in order to avoid losing the lower-intensity signals, the gains should be adjusted as high as possible without causing saturation of the receiver by high intensity signals.

Log compression (or dynamic range).—Log compression is a means of changing the dynamic range of the returning signals. The dynamic range refers to the range of difference between the weakest and strongest signals (equivalent to the contrast of a corresponding visual image). Ultrasound equipment is capable of producing an output with greater dynamic range than can be displayed on current monitors. For this reason, M-mode echocardiograms with a wide range of signal intensity may be difficult to display without either saturating the brighter areas or losing the regions of lower intensity. The log compression feature allows control over the dynamic range of the signals being sent to the monitor, so that images with particularly high contrast can be compressed into a range that can be displayed without loss of information. It is often helpful to use decreased dynamic range in patients who are difficult to image and when there is excessive background noise. Images with little contrast, on the other hand, can be enhanced by increasing the dynamic range of the receiver. The dynamic range is usually expressed in decibels (db), and most current equipment will provide a dynamic range of approximately 20 to 60 db. Most two-dimensional imaging is effectively done with settings in the range of 40 to 55 db, which provides good tissue contrast without loss of information.

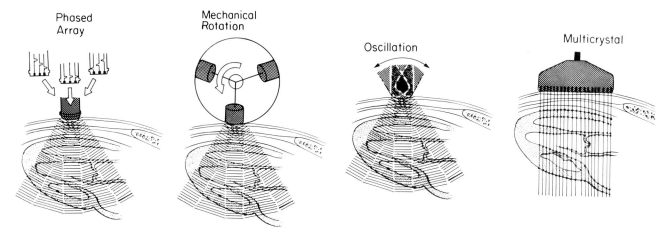

FIG 2–1.
Diagrammatic representation of some of the methods used to generate the two-dimensional echocardiogram.

Sweep speed.—Most systems allow control over the rate of sweep of the M-mode display. Fast sweep speeds make it easier to measure intervals, but at slow heart rates display very few cardiac cycles on any one screen.

Two-Dimensional Imaging

Types of Transducers

Three basic types of transducers are used for two-dimensional imaging: mechanical, phased-array, and linear-array (Fig 2–1). Mechanical and phased-array transducers produce a sector image, while linear-array transducers usually generate a rectangular image that is the width of the transducer.

Mechanical transducers use a crystal that is mechanically aimed for each scan line. Early systems used a single crystal that oscillated back and forth to generate each sweep across the arc of the image. Subsequently, transducers were produced that rotated continuously in one direction. In these transducers, three crystals are mounted at 120-degree increments around a center hub. As the unit rotates in one direction, each crystal is used in turn. These transducers avoid the problem with vibration inherent in oscillating transducers. However, neither approach allows *simultaneous* M-mode or Doppler information, as the transducer cannot be stopped without loss of the two-dimensional image. As the transducer turns, each successive pulse must be the next around the arc. Because Doppler ultrasound requires multiple pulses along the same line, it is not possible with a moving transducer. In addition, these transducers have a fixed focal zone. The annular-array is a newer form of mechanical transducer similar to the standard mechanical transducer; rather than a single crystal, however, the annular-array transducer has several circular crystals arranged concentrically. This arrangement allows improved (and dynamic) focusing of the transducer and therefore more uniform resolution throughout the image. With this type of mechanical transducer, one crystal of the array can be used to obtain M-mode and Doppler information, while the remaining crystals simultaneously obtain the two-dimensional image.

Recently developed phased-array transducers are made up of many independent transducer elements, each of which can be pulsed independently. Current systems use as many as 128 elements. The ultrasound beam is aimed not by moving the transducer but by electronically steering the beam through appropriate timing of the pulses from each element (Fig 2–2). Because the transducer remains stationary, scan lines can be selected at random. This allows simultaneous acquisition of Doppler and structural information, or, more accurately, rapidly sequential acquisition, because Doppler and structural information are obtained from different ultrasound pulses.

Linear-array transducers also use an array of many independent crystals aligned side by side. In the original linear-array transducers, each crystal was used as a separate transducer to create one line of the image directly under it. Movement of the transducer or steering of the beam was not necessary. A rectangular image the width of the transducer was created, and it was not possible to aim

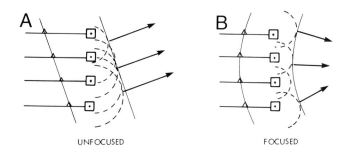

FIG 2–2.
Beam formations from phased away. **A,** unfocused, **B,** focused. (From Silverman NH, Snider AR: *Two-Dimensional Echocardiography in Congenital Heart Disease.* Norwalk, Conn, Appleton-Century-Crofts, 1982, p 5. Used by permission.)

the ultrasound beam away from the direction at right angles to the transducer surface. More recent linear array transducers have made use of the technology developed for the phased-array sector scanners. In these phased linear transducers, each line of information is generated from pulses created with a group of crystals. This makes it possible to focus the beam for enhanced resolution. In addition, electronic steering makes it possible to perform Doppler studies in directions other than at right angles to the transducer surface. Linear-array transducers are used primarily in peripheral vascular studies; these transducers provide superior near-field imaging as well as a wide field of view in the near field.

All of these types of transducers are currently available commercially. The mechanical scanners are the least expensive and are the simplest to use. With their decreased cost, however, comes much less versatility. As mentioned above, the standard mechanical transducers cannot be used for simultaneous imaging and Doppler and thus for color-flow imaging. Also, because the focal zone of the mechanical transducer is fixed (except with the annular array), it cannot match the uniformity of image attainable with a phased-array system. Because the mechanical transducers use motor-driven parts, they are more likely than the phased-array transducers to malfunction or require replacement. Although the phased-array systems are much more expensive they allow a great deal of versatility. With these systems, color-flow mapping, simultaneous imaging and pulsed or continuous-wave Doppler, and steerable pulsed or continuous-wave Doppler are all possible. In addition, the phased-array approach allows sophisticated computer control over the formation of the ultrasound beam. This provides improved focusing and more uniform resolution throughout the field of view.

Selection of Transducers

Proper transducer selection is critical for obtaining optimal structural information. In selecting a transducer, two factors must be considered—transducer size and frequency.

From the discussion in Chapter 1, it is apparent that the higher the frequency of the transducer the better the resolution of the image. However, the use of high frequencies is limited by the lack of adequate tissue penetration. Consequently, it is necessary to use the highest-frequency transducer that allows adequate penetration to the depth needed.

One exception to this rule is the use of high-frequency transducers with fixed focal zones. High-frequency transducers (>7 MHz) are generally intended for shallow depths and are designed with a shallow focal zone. For this reason they yield an inferior image to lower-frequency probes if they are used beyond their intended depth. For example, high-frequency transducers often provide adequate penetration for subcostal views in infants; in these cases, however, cardiac structures in the far field are well beyond the focal zone and thus are poorly resolved. The phased-array

systems avoid this problem by allowing control over the transmit focus.

Transducer size is the other important consideration in choosing the appropriate transducer for a particular study. From the discussion in Chapter 1, it is clear that the larger the transducer the better the resolution in the far field and focal zone. Therefore, for greater depths a larger transducer should be chosen. The near field may be less well focused, particularly with mechanical (single crystal) transducers. In addition, large transducers may not yield good images when the echocardiographic window is limited, such as in parasternal views in small children. In this situation, when the transducer is positioned over the ribs, reflections from the ribs produce many artifacts and background noise and a small transducer that fits between the ribs will provide a better image.

One other consideration unrelated to image quality is the ease with which the transducer can be positioned in the desired location. Large transducers, for instance, can be quite difficult to position appropriately in the suprasternal notch of a small child.

Equipment Controls

The following controls are generally available for manipulation of two-dimensional images:

Depth.—All systems allow adjustment of the depth of field viewed. The depth should be set at the minimum possible to still include the region of interest. An unnecessarily deep setting will decrease the frame rate and degrade temporal resolution.

Power, gain, and log compression (or dynamic range).—These should be set as discussed in the section on M-mode imaging.

Focal zone (or transmit focus).—The transmit focal zone is adjustable only on annular- and phased-array systems. The ultrasound beam width diverges beyond the focal zone. Therefore, for optimal resolution throughout the field of view, the focal zone should generally be set near the back of the area of interest. With single-crystal transducers it is important to keep in mind the focal zone of the transducer, as discussed above.

Preprocessing.—Preprocessing is a means of edge enhancement that accentuates the boundaries between tissue and blood-filled areas. For the most part, preprocessing creates aesthetic improvements in the image and should be adjusted according to the clinician's personal preferences in image appearance.

Persistence.—Persistence is a means of image enhancement by averaging sequential frames of the image and can be quite effective when imaging static structures (primarily in radiology). In general, however, persistence is not helpful in cardiac imaging because the rapid movement of the structures imaged creates blurring. Therefore, for cardiac imaging, persistence should be set for minimal averaging.

Postprocessing curves.—Postprocessing is the means by which the returning ultrasound signals are assigned to a gray-scale level after the detection and amplification steps are complete. Postprocessing is independent of previous stages, in which the signal is detected, amplified (gain), and expanded or compressed into the dynamic range desired (log compression). Most systems offer a choice of several standard curves, and some even permit the user to generate his or her own curve. While these curves alter the aesthetic appearance of the image, they do not alter the content of the information. These curves, therefore, are a matter of personal preference.

TECHNOLOGY AND INSTRUMENTATION OF DOPPLER ULTRASOUND

Three basic types of Doppler ultrasound technology are currently available: continuous-wave (CW) Doppler, pulsed Doppler, and color-flow Doppler. Each technique provides information complementary to the other techniques. Each of these three Doppler techniques will be described, including currently available features and the appropriate use of the controls. The various techniques will be compared and appropriate uses for each will be reviewed. An in-depth description of the technologies involved in processing the Doppler signals is given at the end of this chapter.

Continuous-Wave Doppler

Continuous-wave (CW) Doppler was first implemented using a single crystal transducer with no two-dimensional image (standalone transducer), and this approach still provides the best sensitivity. The newer phased-array systems, which allow a CW Doppler to be obtained using the same transducer that is used for imaging, provide simultaneous display of the two-dimensional image and CW Doppler information. A cursor line in the image indicates the direction of the CW Doppler beam. These systems combine the infinite frequency resolution (and thus, the velocity resolution) of CW Doppler with the anatomic orientation of a simultaneous image. With this approach, however, no range resolution is possible.

Transducer Selection
The transducer requirements for Doppler studies are somewhat different than for imaging, and may necessitate changing transducers between imaging and Doppler portions of the examination. Because of the relatively low-intensity signal that returns from blood, Doppler ultrasound requires much higher levels of power than two-dimensional imaging. Therefore, a lower-frequency transducer than would be used for imaging is often needed to obtain adequate penetration. For this reason, standalone

CW Doppler probes are generally between 2 MHz and 3 MHz. The only potential disadvantage of the low-frequency transducer is its relatively wide beam width, although this is usually an advantage in locating the jet flow when using a standalone probe without imaging capability. When transducers that combine steerable CW Doppler with two-dimensional imaging are used the higher-frequency CW Doppler may lack the necessary penetration and necessitate changing transducers for the Doppler study. The higher frequencies do, however, allow more precise focusing of the beam, which avoids detecting signals from flow outside the direction of interest.

Equipment Controls
The following controls are generally available for manipulation of the CW Doppler ultrasound display:

Power.—The transmit power can usually be left on the full power available. In occasional circumstances (particularly shallow depths) the receiver is saturated by returning signals of too great an intensity. This results in loss of sensitivity and can be avoided by decreasing the transmit power.

Gain.—In general, to provide the greatest sensitivity for low level signals, the gain should be adjusted upward until the background noise is just visible. This may necessitate a decrease in transmit power to avoid saturation by the signals of highest intensity.

Scale/baseline.—With CW Doppler, the scale setting has no impact on how the information is gathered, as it does with pulsed Doppler. Therefore, the scale and baseline may be set in whatever manner provides the most readable display.

Log compression or dynamic range.—As discussed in the section on two-dimensional imaging, log compression is a means of changing the dynamic range of the returning signals. Most Doppler studies are effectively done with a dynamic range of 25 to 30 db. Doppler studies with excessive background noise may be enhanced by decreasing the dynamic range.

Filters.—Filters are necessary to eliminate unwanted signals that arise primarily from wall motion. In general, these signals are of much higher intensity than the desired signals from blood flow, but of much lower frequency. For this reason, they may be suppressed by filters, known as high pass filters, that allow only high frequencies to get through. Most systems allow control over the frequency cutoff of these filters, and they should be set at as low a frequency as possible yet still avoid the excessive wall noise that may mask the desired signals. Unnecessarily high wall filter settings may result in loss of low frequency (and corresponding low velocity) information. Typical settings are between 200 and 800 Hz.

Focal zone.—The focal zone is adjustable only on phased-array systems, and should be set at the area of interest. This will maximize the signal strength from that region and minimize the spurious recording of unwanted surrounding flow signals.

Pulsed Doppler

The implementation of pulsed Doppler differs depending on the type of system used. With mechanical scanners, Doppler cannot be done simultaneously with imaging. In these systems, the Doppler sample volume is positioned while viewing the real time two-dimensional image. When the system is changed to Doppler mode, the image is frozen at the last frame. The sample volume can still be moved, if necessary, based on the frozen image. Phased-array scanners allow simultaneous pulsed Doppler and imaging. This simplifies positioning of the sample volume, since the imaging is still present in real time.

High pulse repetition frequency (HPRF) Doppler can be implemented on all types of systems to extend the velocity range. Most systems automatically change to HPRF when the velocity scale is changed to a range that requires HPRF. Because the maximum power that can be used is fixed, HPRF requires that the transmit power for each pulse be reduced.

Transducer Selection

As with CW Doppler, pulsed Doppler requires much more power than imaging. Consequently, lower-frequency transducers are needed for adequate penetration. In addition, the maximum velocity that can be displayed without aliasing depends on the transducer frequency, as discussed in Chapter 1. This, too, makes lower-frequency transducers preferable for pulsed Doppler. Their disadvantage, however, is decreased resolution in the two-dimensional image. Therefore, for pulsed Doppler, the lowest-frequency transducer that gives an image adequate to position the sample volume appropriately should be used.

Equipment Controls

The following controls are generally available for manipulation of the pulsed Doppler ultrasound display:

Power and gain.—These may be adjusted as outlined in the section on CW Doppler.

Scale/baseline.—Shift of the baseline allows the whole display to be used for either forward or reverse flow, which is useful if the flow is in only one direction. Shift of the baseline allows display of velocities of twice the magnitude without aliasing. The scale should be set no higher than necessary to display the desired flow velocities. A scale beyond the Nyquist limit results in changing to HPRF Doppler. Care must be taken to avoid confusion from spurious signals that arise from the additional sample volumes. HPRF Doppler may have insufficient power for adequate pene-

tration, if so, the scale must be kept below the Nyquist limit; or a change must be made to a lower-frequency transducer.

Log compression.—The log compression should be set as discussed previously under CW Doppler.

Gate size (or sample volume).—Choosing the appropriate gate, or sample volume, size involves many trade-offs. Increasing the sample volume size results in an increase in signal strength (summing more signal from more scatterers), a decrease in background noise, and decreased spatial resolution. Conversely, decreasing sample volume size decreases signal strength, increases noise, and improves spatial resolution. Because of the greater difficulty involved in keeping the sample volume away from wall structures, the larger sample volumes tend to suffer from greater interference from wall noise as well. In general, the smallest sample volume that results in an adequate signal-to-noise ratio should be used.

Filters.—The use of filters for pulsed Doppler is the same as that discussed for CW Doppler above.

Update.—This applies only to systems that allow simultaneous imaging and Doppler. The simultaneous mode results in a Doppler recording with reduced temporal resolution caused by the time required for generation of the two-dimensional image. Update mode changes to a mode in which the image is refreshed much less frequently than it is in real time. The result is a continuous Doppler trace with good temporal resolution and an updated image every few seconds. This compromise between a good quality Doppler trace and a simultaneous image allows accurate positioning of the sample volume.

Color-Flow Doppler

Color-flow Doppler is the most recent technique developed for evaluation of flow within the heart. As discussed above, this technique is possible only with phased-array or annular-array systems. Color Doppler provides the user with the most control over the processing features that significantly affect the information obtained. With color Doppler, therefore, it is particularly important to understand the fundamental concepts and the effects of user controls.

In general, commercial systems have adopted a uniform format for color Doppler displays. Red indicates flow toward the transducer, and blue indicates flow away from the transducer. The intensity of the color corresponds to an estimate of the mean velocity of the flow. Variance, an estimate of the bandwidth of the signal (corresponding to disturbed flow), is indicated by a third color (frequently yellow) that is added to the display. There are many variations on this basic format, and some systems provide a variety of color formats the user can select.

Transducer Selection

The combination of Doppler and simultaneous structural imaging results in trade-offs in selection of the appropriate transducer. As with other forms of Doppler ultrasound, decreasing frequency provides a higher Nyquist limit and improved penetration, while sacrificing resolution in the structural image. Unlike other forms of Doppler ultrasound, however, color Doppler provides spatial information, allowing mapping of jets, etc. Similar to structural imaging, decreased frequency of the transducer diminishes spatial resolution. In addition, since quantitative measurement of jet velocities cannot be made, it is not as important to achieve a display without aliasing of these high velocity flows. For these reasons, a higher-frequency transducer than might be optimal for other forms of Doppler ultrasound is often used for color Doppler studies, as long as adequate tissue penetration is obtained.

Equipment Controls

The following controls are generally available for manipulation of the color-flow Doppler display:

Power.—In general, the transmit power level may be left at the maximum. In some circumstances, however, particularly in very shallow depths, the power level may need to be decreased to avoid saturation of the receiver. Also, lower transmit power is recommended when color Doppler is used to examine the fetal heart.

Gain.—As for CW Doppler, the gain should be adjusted upward until the background noise is just visible as white noise in the color map. Although this adjustment will provide the greatest sensitivity for low-level signals, it may necessitate a decrease in transmit power to avoid saturation by the signals of highest intensity.

Scale.—In most instances, the scale should be set to the maximum available, depending on the Nyquist limit for the given transducer and the depth. However, in evaluating areas of relatively low-velocity flow, the scale may need to be lowered to allow display of these lower velocities that otherwise might be below the lower cutoff for display. The baseline may also be shifted in color. This is useful less often than it is with pulsed or CW Doppler, since most images will include flow in both directions.

Color sector size.—The calculation of color Doppler data takes a great deal of time. Therefore, the frame rate may be considerably improved by limiting the area for which color Doppler information is generated. Consequently, many systems allow selection of a small region of interest within the image for color Doppler display.

Pixel size.—Pixel size, which is equivalent to the sample volume size with pulsed Doppler, determines the number of individual pixels for which velocity information is calculated. Choosing larger pixels will increase the signal strength for each pixel, improve the signal-to-noise ratio, and allow a faster frame rate. However, these advantages come at the expense of diminished spatial resolution and the overall quality of the image.

Filters.—As in other forms of Doppler ultrasound, filters are used to separate low-frequency wall signals from flow information of much lower amplitude and higher frequency. This distinction is very important in color Doppler, since a determination must be made to display any given pixel as part of the structure (i.e., the wall) or to fill it in with color-flow information. Specific filtering techniques vary between systems. Different filter settings should be tried until the best compromise is reached between avoiding writing color over structural information and providing good fill-in of blood-filled spaces.

Focus.—For optimal spatial resolution of the color image, the focus should be set at the depth of interest within the color portion of the image rather than near the back of the structural image.

Comparison of Methods

The three types of Doppler ultrasound—CW, pulsed, and color-flow—provide complementary information, and each gives information the other does not. CW Doppler is the method of choice for evaluating high-velocity flows. Although there is no range resolution, the newer, steerable CW with a focused beam provides precise alignment of the beam. In most circumstances it is possible to assure measurement of the appropriate flow. Consequently, HPRF Doppler plays a much smaller role than it has previously.

Pulsed Doppler is the only way to precisely localize the velocity measurements essential for many calculations (volume flow calculations, for example). The measurable velocity is limited, but most situations in which precise localization is needed involve normal or near-normal flow velocities that fall within the Nyquist limit. In patients with serial obstruction, HPRF may be helpful in assessing at what level the velocity increases.

Color-flow Doppler currently does not permit quantitative velocity measurements. However, the color image provides spatial information about flows that is unavailable with the other techniques. This information is particularly valuable in assessing areas of disturbed flow. Color Doppler allows visualization of the orientation of the jet for subsequent alignment with the CW Doppler beam (Plate 2). This is very helpful for evaluating eccentric jets in which significant errors can be made because of poor alignment with the direction of peak velocity. In addition, color Doppler is useful for the spatial mapping of jets, although the significance of this mapping is questionable. Perhaps the most frequently used feature is the rapid screening for valvular insufficiency or stenosis, for which color Doppler is excellent.

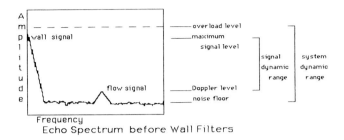

Echo Spectrum before Wall Filters

FIG 2–3.
Diagrammatic representation of the echo spectrum before the wall filters.

PROCESSING OF THE DOPPLER SIGNAL*

Like ultrasound pulse-echo imaging, echo-Doppler signal acquisition begins with insonification and echo reception. Beyond these similarities, however, the complexities of the Doppler flow signal dictate a radically different processing path.

Two major features of the ultrasound Doppler signal complicate the extraction of useful information, presenting significant challenges to both the clinician and the instrumentation designer. First, the desired flow signal represents only a small fraction of the signal energy returned to the transducer. This puts a severe burden on the system's dynamic range—its ability to handle a wide range of signal sizes without distortion. Second, the information desired is not directly represented in the signal, and must be decoded or detected before it can be used.

In order to get the Doppler information into a usable form, the signal is optimized and analyzed in a series of manipulations called signal processing. The mathematical basis for signal processing is beyond the scope of this discussion. A basic understanding of it is essential, however, because the variables the clinician must face require individual, situational optimization. The following sections develop a schematic description of Doppler signal processing and its related controls.

The Nature of the Doppler Signal

The Doppler flow signal is typically received by the transducer obscured by much larger echoes (Fig 2–3). The surrounding anatomy, typically vessel or chamber walls, will return 20 to 60 dB more (10× to 1,000×) signal than that reflected by the majority scatterers in blood—the red blood cells. This undesired echo is called the wall signal, or to borrow a term from the identical noise in Doppler radar, "clutter." The wall signal degrades and obscures the desired flow signal. The first goal, therefore, is to restrict our sample to only the echoes that come from the volume of interest. This sample volume may extend axially from

*This section was prepared by Gary A. Schwartz, principal engineer, Advanced Technology Laboratories.

1 to 20 mm, as in pulsed Doppler, or to 10 to 20 cm, as in continuous-wave (CW) Doppler.

The lack of range resolution in continuous-wave Doppler exacerbates the problems of dynamic range. Echoes from nearby targets will contribute substantial clutter. The same effect is present with high pulse repetition frequency (HPRF) Doppler when a close-in spurious sample volume includes echogenic targets. These techniques make severe demands on the system's dynamic range.

While the sample volume location is used to make spatial distinctions between the flow echo and the wall echo, the flow signal is further separated from the relatively slow-moving clutter by virtue of its higher Doppler shift frequency. As should be clear from the Doppler equation, the Doppler shift frequency for a given flow is relative to the ultrasound carrier frequency. In the case of pulsed Doppler, the transmitted ultrasound energy includes a wide range of frequencies. The Doppler effect on each of the component frequencies must be translated, or detected, to produce a signal that directly represents the flow signal.

Extracting the flow signal is not enough. A quantitative analysis requires that the signal be decomposed into its composite frequencies. The signal frequency indicates flow rate, and the frequency distribution can be used to indicate flow disturbances.

The Doppler Processing Chain

The elements of the Doppler signal processing are shown in block diagram form in Figure 2–4. The receiver amplifies the signal acquired by the transducer. The radio frequency (RF) gain sets the amplification factor. Not always labeled "RF gain," in some equipment it is controlled in a manner similar to the two-dimensional time gain compensation (TGC). In the case of single-dimensional Doppler acquisition with conventional pulsed or continuous-wave Doppler, no time gain compensation is needed; the gain, however, must be set to amplify the signal without distortion.

The receiver output is passed to the detector, which is responsible for synthesizing the sample volume in pulsed Doppler and converting the signal from the original RF form to a low-frequency audio signal. The wall filter provides the essential function of reducing the amplitude of wall echoes or clutter.

The audio channel continues with PRF filters that remove spurious copies or images of the Doppler spectrum that appear at multiples of the PRF or sampling rate. If as a result of inadequate filtering these images remain, they are heard as whistles in the audio output. Next comes the forward and reverse separation calculation that generates stereo sounds.

Spectral analysis attempts to do quantitatively what human ears do qualitatively—decompose the signal into its composite frequencies. The resulting spectrum is display processed into a gray-scale image, which is reviewed on a gray-scale video display.

Reception

Doppler signals place unique requirements on the receiver design. The most significant factors are the mutually dependent qualities of distortion, noise, sensitivity, bandwidth, and dynamic range.

The receiver's sensitivity determines the smallest signal that can be detected. In a classic receiver, the sensitivity is limited by the thermal noise inherent to the components used in the receiver. Ideally, this physical limit would determine the noise floor. Thermal noise has a wideband characteristic (composed of a wide range of frequencies) that becomes evident as hiss in the audio, or snow in the spectral display, that occurs as the RF gain is increased. Other noise sources may also be present, raising the noise floor and decreasing the sensitivity. Narrowband noise (restricted to a narrow range of frequencies), also called noise bands, can result from electromagnetic interference (EMI) produced by nearby electronic equipment, or from noise that originates in the ultrasound system itself.

The ideal setting for the RF gain is with the noise floor just visible or a faint background of noise present. This would optimize acquisition for the smallest receivable signal. In practice this is not always achieved, since the RF gain must be set to avoid overload (Fig 2–5). When a receiver begins to overload because of a signal that is too large for the gain setting, an unrecoverable distortion of the signal occurs. The distortion produces spurious signals, usually indistinguishable from noise. They result in a higher effective noise floor that obscures the desired signal and yields poorer sensitivity. This example is worth restating: An increase in receiver gain results in a decrease in sensitivity. A small signal that is not visible above the noise may be covered by distortion. Table 2–1 summarizes the relationships between the ultrasound system control

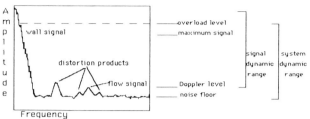

Echo Spectrum before Wall Filters, excessive gain

FIG 2–5.
Diagrammatic representation of the echo spectrum before the wall filters with excessive gain.

settings and the dependent quantities that determine sensitivity: signal, noise, clutter, and distortion levels.

Optimization

The Doppler flow signal must be extracted from the return signal. Originally coded as RF signals, in the process of detection or demodulation they are translated to much lower audio frequency signals.

The detector is also responsible for synthesis of the axial position and size of the sample volume. Detection and sample volume generation is of fundamental importance, since it affects many aspects of signal quality. The sample volume denotes the volume element over which the Doppler signal will be integrated, giving a summation of the targets within that volume. Its location is used to choose the flow site and exclude stationary targets. Even in the absence of obvious wall interference it is advisable to minimize wall echoes, as flow signals may be obscured.

A smaller sample volume size will help minimize wall noise by improving the spatial accuracy, but the price paid is an increase in the noise floor. A halving of the sample volume length can cause a noise increase of about 3 dB (a factor of 1.7). Conversely, larger sample volumes exhibit lower random noise levels but suffer from the worst wall noise interference.

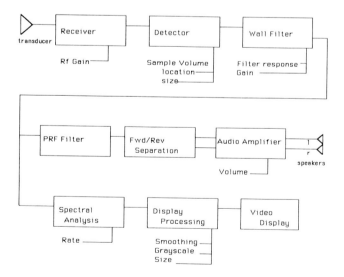

FIG 2–4.
Diagrammatic representation of the Doppler processing chain.

TABLE 2–1.

Effects of Gain, Sample Volume Size, and Wall Filter Setting on Signal Quality

	Clutter Level	Signal Level	Distortion Level	Sensitivity
Gain increase, no overload	+	+	0	+
Gain increase with overload	+	+	+ +	–
Sample volume size increase*	+	+	0	+
Wall filter increase†	–	0	0	0
Wall filter increase with overload†	–	0	–	+

*This assumes that the flow volume of interest is larger than the sample volume.
†This assumes that the wall filters reduce only clutter signal, leaving the flow signal unattenuated.

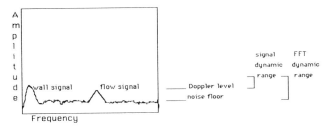

Echo Spectrum after Wall Filters

FIG 2–6.
Diagrammatic representation of the echo spectrum after the wall filters.

The sample volume size can be generated on reception in the traditional manner by simply summing the Doppler signals as they return from the desired range. An optimal approach uses another concept of radar theory, that of the matched filter. Here, the transmit burst length tracks the sample volume size and the sample volume summation is weighted to shape the response to the expected signal. The matched filter will improve the system's sensitivity by rejecting more noise and less of the desired signal.

It is important to note that the sample volume is a three-dimensional concept. Although typical ultrasound instrumentation quantifies the sample volume size by axial extent, the lateral dimension is also relevant. In fact, the sample volume usually thought of as a teardrop shape can vary from a flat disk to a cigar shape through various sample volume sizes and focal depths. The lateral extent is much more difficult to adjust, but as modern electronic beamforming techniques progress, more control will become available to the clinician.

The large dynamic range required is still a problem, however, because even under ideal conditions some wall signal will remain. Wall filters, also termed high-pass filters, selectively remove the lower-frequency signals in favor of the higher-frequency signals. Since the desired flow signals occupy the upper range of the total signal spectrum, this has the effect of improving the signal-to-noise ratio by reducing the wall noise. Even more significantly, since the wall noise is generally much larger than the flow signal, the total signal dynamic range is reduced as the lower-frequency wall noise is removed (Fig 2–6).

Wall filters are not ideal elements. Their nominal cutoff frequency is just that—a nominal value conventionally used to refer to a filter response. Generally, the cutoff frequency is stated at the frequency that is reduced by 3 dB (a 30% reduction). The filter response continues with further reductions at lower frequencies. Thus, it is not possible to say that the filter removes all signals below its cutoff. The truth of that assertion will vary with filter types and signal conditions. The logical step of making the filters as sharp as possible has other untoward side effects. The sharper the filter cutoff, the greater the distortion of the signal. This distortion, termed phase nonlinearity error, or pulse distortion, can result in a loss in time resolution. The typical appearance is of a smeared signal near the filter

cutoff frequency. While the wall filters are usually set to a cutoff much lower than the flow signals of interest, acquisition of low-velocity flow can be seriously affected. Under these conditions a different wall filter setting may move the smear out of the field of interest.

Instrumentation designs vary, some providing control of the post-wall filter gain, and some providing automatic gain adjustment. In both cases, the important point is that the ideal setting will be affected by the signal conditions and the wall filter response. For example, under conditions where wall returns cannot be avoided—even though the wall Doppler is not apparent in the display, having been removed by the wall filters—it still may overload the receiver. Under these conditions, the receiver gain should be decreased to avoid overload, the wall filter cutoff frequency should be increased to remove more of the wall energy, and the post-wall filter gain should be increased. The result is an improved flow signal with less noise and distortion.

The technological development that makes possible matched filter designs, flexible wall filters, and other powerful optimization techniques is digital signal processing (DSP). Digital techniques represent the signals as streams of numbers. In this context signal processing is implemented as mathematical operations. The advantages of this approach are many: elimination of manufacturing tolerance errors, easier modification and control of process characteristics, and perfect time and temperature stability.

Were it not for DSP techniques, simultaneous acquisition of Doppler data and two-dimensional image data would be feasible only with severe performance trade-offs. During simultaneous operation, the front end is shared between Doppler and two-dimensional image acquisition, typically spending most of the time with Doppler. During the short periods (5 to 50 msec) that two-dimensional data are acquired, the Doppler processing must synthesize audio and spectral data to fill the gap. Sometimes called a missing signal estimator, the data are synthesized based on the characteristics of the true data acquired before and after the gap. Because the actual data are missing over such a short duration, the synthesized data remove the discontinuity that otherwise would corrupt the data.

Analysis

The original ultrasound Doppler products had only an audio output, which limited the examination to a qualitative analysis by ear. While the first Doppler processors did not determine flow direction, in modern systems the optimized signal is processed to separate it into its composite forward and reverse flow signals. Stereo presentation of the information allows a rough determination of flow direction and velocity. In the early days of Doppler ultrasound, the analytical capabilities of the human ear and brain surpassed any reasonable alternative. Even in modern systems, the sensitivity of the audio channel usually exceeds that of the display. Flow signals are sometimes heard but not seen.

In cardiac Doppler applications, the measurement of

most interest is the flow velocity. This velocity information is coded in the echo as a frequency shift, or Doppler shift, from the original signal. If there were only one flow rate present in the sample volume, it would be possible simply to measure the period of the Doppler signal. This time-interval histogram method of Doppler flow quantification represented the state of the art until the early 1980s. As might be expected, the single flow rate assumption for the signal is not true enough under complex hemodynamic conditions.

A significant increase in technological capability was necessary for the next step—to use frequency-domain processing to analyze the signal. While the discrete Fourier transform (DFT, sometimes implemented as a fast Fourier transform, an FFT) is the classic tool for frequency-domain analysis, the requisite hardware was until recently too costly.

The Fourier transform analyzes the Doppler signal into its composite frequencies. The spectrum summarizes the signal amplitudes at a range of frequencies. The frequency represents the magnitude of the Doppler shift, and is a function of the velocity of the target. The amplitude indicates the number of targets and the efficiency of the echo. The transforms are typically run every 1 to 10 msec to try to keep up with the rapidly changing signal. These requirements—to know the component frequencies accurately and to respond to rapid changes—are mutually exclusive. The Fourier transform cannot avoid a fundamental trade-off between frequency resolution and signal bandwidth, or rate of change. As an increase in the transform frequency resolution is attempted, the time resolution is compromised. Because the signal is changing (the signal statistics are non-stationary) we are only evaluating spectral estimates. In general, more accurate frequency estimates mean poorer temporal resolution.

As signal processing techniques evolve, more sophisticated spectral estimators become available. The Chirp-Z transform requires more computational resources than the classic Fourier transform, but permits a more flexible trade-off between frequency resolution and observation time. Another class of spectral estimators commonly used for flow imaging removes the frequency resolution restriction entirely, but is only accurate for simple flow states.

Display

The display shows the Fourier transform results in time, giving a video, time-motion picture of the events of the flow. The choice of scroll rate affects the display quality in two ways. Generally because of the limits of display resolution, the transforms are performed more often than the display is updated. A faster scroll rate will improve the display time resolution. On the other hand, in most systems a slower display rate will improve the signal quality as successive transform results are averaged. This averaging reduces the random noise in the display, improving sensitivity.

Practical considerations limit the display dynamic range to about 20 to 25 dB. Even after the dynamic range reductions of the RF gain adjustment and wall filters, the dynamic range at the output of the transform can exceed 30 dB. In a manner identical to that used in imaging, the signal is compressed into the display restrictions by a gray-scale mapping function. Each flow amplitude is represented by a gray level. The choice of mapping function is not always available to the clinician. Some systems make do with only a display gain control, while some provide only a gray-scale select. As mentioned above with regard to the gain setting, the optimum gray-scale choice will depend on the signal conditions and the clinician's preference.

REFERENCES

1. Feigenbaum H: *Echocardiography*, ed 4. Philadelphia, Lea & Febiger, 1986.
2. Hatle L, Angelsen B: *Doppler Ultrasound in Cardiology: Physical Principles and Clinical Applications*, ed 2. Philadelphia, Lea & Febiger, 1985, pp 1–73.

The Normal Echocardiographic Examination

SPECIAL CONSIDERATIONS FOR THE PERFORMANCE OF THE PEDIATRIC ECHOCARDIOGRAPHIC EXAMINATION

A successful echocardiographic examination requires not only a thorough knowledge of spatial cardiac anatomy and congenital heart disease, but also an understanding of how best to approach the pediatric patient. In this section, some of the techniques that we have found useful in examining infants and children are discussed.

Introduction of the Child to the Echocardiography Laboratory

With all of its sophisticated instrumentation and technology, the echocardiography laboratory can be a frightening environment for the small child. How children are introduced to the laboratory can set the tone for their behavior during the examination; therefore, as soon as the child enters the laboratory, it is essential to dispel as many of his or her fears and anxieties as possible. For most children, a full explanation of the laboratory surroundings and the examination can quiet their fears and ensure their trust and co-operation.

We encourage the child's parents and family to enter the room and stay throughout the examination. Their presence reassures the child that the examination is not harmful; they are also reassured that the examination is not harmful or painful for the child. After we greet the child and the family, we introduce the child to the echocardiographic equipment by explaining that the equipment will be used to take a picture of the heart and also to listen to the heart. Many children are further reassured if they are allowed to hold the ultrasound transducer or touch the knobs on the machine before the procedure begins. Before

beginning the examination, we also explain the purposes of the electrodes and ultrasonic gel.

Often, a child's first reactions to the echocardiographic examination are greatly influenced by the room itself. The echocardiographic laboratory should be as cheerful and pleasant as possible. This can be accomplished by hanging pictures or posters that appeal to small children throughout the laboratory and by placing interesting objects in strategic positions in the room. For example, we have a musical mobile that hangs from the ceiling above the child's head. The mobile is an interesting object for the child to focus on during the suprasternal notch examination, and its music can be very soothing for young infants. We have also placed interesting toys, hats, and children's books on shelves throughout the room.

Special Equipment Needs

In our laboratory, the echocardiographic examination is performed with the child lying on a standard hospital bed. A hospital bed is preferable to an examination table for several reasons: (1) the head of the bed can be raised or lowered; (2) the height of the bed can be raised or lowered, making it easier for smaller children to get onto or off the bed; and (3) the side rails can be raised or lowered so that infants and small children cannot roll off the bed if the examiner has to leave the side of the bed for a moment. On the bed, we use a thick foam rubber mattress with a semicircular hole cut out of the left side to facilitate access to the cardiac apex. With the patient lying left side down and over the hole, the transducer can be placed in the hole and over the cardiac apex.[1] To maintain the body temperature of small infants during the examination, we place a rubber mattress warmer (Hamilton Aquamatic) with a rheostatic temperature control under the sheet in the area where the infant will be lying. The mattress warmer also makes the examination more comfortable for older children, who often have peripheral vasoconstriction because they are nervous and only partially clothed.

Electrodes can be applied to the child's right and left shoulders and to the right lower thorax so that the echocardiographic windows are freely accessible. In small infants, it may be preferable to apply the electrodes to the back over the right and left shoulders and left kidney. With this technique, the infant cannot pull on the wires and detach the electrodes, and the precordium is freely accessible for the examination. So that the infant or child is not made uncomfortable by the application of cold ultrasonic gel, we maintain the ultrasonic gel at a warm temperature, using a commercially available gel warmer.

In the pediatric echocardiography laboratory, patients range from infants to teens; therefore, a large variety of transducer sizes is needed to meet all the imaging requirements. For premature and newborn infants, a 7.5 MHz transducer is necessary for excellent near-field resolution and excellent lateral resolution. However, the ultrasound power of a 7.5 MHz transducer is low and its ability to penetrate to the far field is limited. As a result, in older infants and children, a 5 MHz transducer must be used to image cardiac structures. The 5 MHz transducers vary in their ability to penetrate and image posterior cardiac structures. This variation is related to many factors including type of technology (mechanical, phased-array, or annular-array), focal zone, power output, and even the patient's tissue characteristics. Therefore, for older infants and children, transducer selection is often a matter of trial and error. For optimal resolution, the highest frequency transducer should be tried first and, if penetration is inadequate, transducers of progressively lower frequency should be tried until the transducer with the best resolution and most adequate penetration is found. In pediatric echocardiography, it is not uncommon to use multiple transducers throughout the examination. For example, in an 8-year-old child, it might be possible to obtain the parasternal views with a 5 MHz transducer but also necessary to switch to a 3.5 MHz transducer to obtain the apical views and a 2.25 MHz transducer to obtain the pulsed Doppler examination.

It is essential that the child lie still and quiet during the examination so that accurate diagnostic information can be obtained. During the examination small infants can often be pacified with a bottle or a pacifier. If the pacifier is first dipped in raspberry syrup, the infant usually readily accepts it. Older children are rewarded for their cooperation during the examination by being allowed to select a sticker or small toy from a surprise box. Often, the anticipated reward is enough to keep a child quiet throughout the examination.

In spite of these techniques, it is often necessary to sedate an infant or young child in order to obtain accurate diagnostic information. In our laboratory, we use oral chloral hydrate in a dose of 75 to 100 mg/kg. The total dose should not exceed 1 gm. Chloral hydrate does not have the potential side effects (such as severe respiratory depression) of the barbiturates or morphine and is therefore ideally suited for use in the outpatient clinic. Gastrointestinal side effects do occasionally occur with chloral hydrate, and we have noted an increased frequency of vomiting when the child is given a bottle of milk immediately after administration of the drug.[1] Most children will fall asleep 15 to 20 minutes after they receive chloral hydrate and will remain asleep or drowsy for several hours. A few children, however, will have an idiosyncratic reaction to the drug and will exhibit drunken behavior sometimes for as long as an hour before they fall asleep. When the parents leave the echocardiography laboratory, we advise them to watch the child closely and not to offer nourishment until the child is fully awake and alert.

A thorough and careful echocardiographic examination is time-consuming and, in children with congenital heart disease, usually includes a lengthy two-dimensional echocardiographic examination for anatomic definition and a Doppler ultrasound examination for assessment of the hemodynamic severity of the defect. Young children often find it difficult to lie still and quiet for such a long period of time and will often become fretful and agitated just as the Doppler examination begins. Because the hemodynamic assessment of the severity of the defect is usually the most important part of the echocardiographic examination, we do not hesitate to sedate children in order to obtain the most accurate Doppler examination. If the heart rate and cardiac output during the Doppler examination are different than they are during cardiac catheterization, discrepancies will occur between the Doppler and the catheterization estimates of the severity of the defect. Stevenson and associates[2] have shown that in unsedated children Doppler estimates of the pressure gradient averaged 41.5% (range 3% to 275%) greater than pressure gradients measured in the same child sedated at cardiac catheterization. Because it is the sedated catheterization gradients that are currently used to make decisions on interventional therapy, the Doppler measurements should be obtained in the same physiologic state.

THE NORMAL TWO-DIMENSIONAL ECHOCARDIOGRAPHIC EXAMINATION

This section will describe the planes generated during a routine two-dimensional echocardiographic examination and the techniques used to obtain them. For each standard echocardiographic plane, the cardiac structures normally imaged in that plane will be discussed and illustrated.

Three basic planes can be used to examine the heart: (1) a long-axis plane that is parallel to the major axis of the left ventricle; (2) a short-axis plane that is perpendicular to the major axis of the left ventricle; and (3) a four-chamber plane that is a coronal plane through the cardiac apex (Fig 3–1, A). The anatomic reference for the echocardiographic planes is the major axis of the heart, not the major axis of the body; therefore, the echocardiographic planes do not correspond to the sagittal, horizontal, or

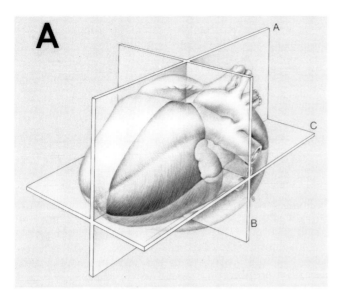
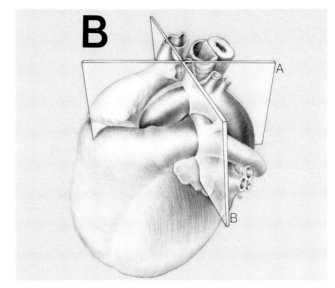

FIG 3–1.
A, diagram of the three basic cardiac planes. *Plane A* is a long-axis plane parallel to the major axis of the left ventricle, *plane B* is a short-axis plane perpendicular to the major axis of the left ventricle, and *plane C* is a coronal plane through the cardiac apex. **B,** diagram of the suprasternal notch planes. *Plane A* is a long-axis plane parallel to the major axis of the aortic arch; *plane B* is a short-axis plane perpendicular to the major axis of the aortic arch.

frontal body planes. Because the heart changes position in the thorax from birth to adulthood, the relationship between the echocardiographic and body planes also changes. For example, the heart of a fetus or newborn infant lies horizontally in the thorax, so that the echocardiographic long-axis plane is almost the same as a transverse-body plane. With growth, the cardiac apex swings downward and the adult heart is positioned more vertically in the thorax. In adults, the echocardiographic long-axis plane is nearly the same plane as a sagittal-body plane.

For imaging the great arteries and veins that enter and leave the heart, the anatomic reference for the echocardiographic planes is the major axis of the aortic arch. Thus, the long-axis plane is parallel to the major axis of the aortic arch; the short-axis plane is perpendicular to the major axis of the aortic arch (Fig 3–1, B).

Each echocardiographic plane represents not only a single static plane but rather a family of echocardiographic planes that can be obtained by aiming the plane of sound in different directions. For example, by tilting the transducer from right to left in the long-axis plane, a family of long-axis planes passing through the right ventricular inflow tract, the left ventricular inflow and outflow tracts, and the right ventricular outflow tract can be obtained. Similarly, the transducer can be tilted from a superior to an inferior direction to obtain a family of short-axis planes and from an anterior to a posterior direction to obtain a family of four-chamber planes. To understand the spatial relations of the family of long-axis planes and the family of four-chamber or coronal planes, it is helpful to think of the heart as composed of three major sections from right to left and three major sections from back to front. From right to left, the heart is composed of the right ventricular

inflow along the right heart border, the left ventricular inflow and outflow in the midsection of the heart, and the right ventricular outflow along the upper-left heart border. From back to front, the heart is composed of the inflow tracts of both ventricles in the posterior section, the left ventricular outflow tract in the midsection, and the right ventricular outflow tract in the most anterior section of the heart.

Because of limitations imposed by the air-filled lungs and bony thoracic structures, the echocardiographic planes can be obtained from only four areas of the body: (1) the parasternal area, a region adjacent to the sternum in the second, third, or fourth left intercostal spaces in which the anterior surface of the heart is not covered by lung tissue; (2) the cardiac apex; (3) the subcostal region; and (4) the suprasternal notch (Fig 3–2). In each location, two of the three basic echocardiographic planes can be obtained. The plane that is perpendicular to the direction of the sound beam as it exits the transducer cannot be imaged. In the parasternal area, for example, long- and short-axis planes can be obtained, but the plane of sound cannot be bent perpendicularly to image the coronal or four-chamber view.

Throughout this text, the orientation of the two-dimensional echocardiographic views is consistent with the recommendations of the American Society of Echocardiography.[3] Structures located closest to the transducer are displayed in the apex of the sector, while structures located most distant from the transducer are displayed in the widest portion of the sector. For the parasternal long-axis views, as the viewer faces the videoscreen, the patient's cranial structures are on the right side of the videoscreen and caudal structures are on the left side of the videoscreen. Similarly, for echocardiographic planes that have a right-left orientation, the patient's right-sided structures are displayed on the left side of the videoscreen and the left-sided structures are displayed on the right side of the videoscreen. For proper transducer and videoscreen orientation, most echocardiographic systems have an index mark on the transducer and a mark on the right or left side of the sector on the videoscreen. When the index mark on the transducer is located toward the patient's head or right side and the mark on the screen is located to the left of the sector as the viewer faces the screen, the orientation of the sector on the videoscreen will be as described above. The orientation of the sector on the videoscreen will also be correct if the reverse occurs—the index mark on the transducer is toward the patient's feet or left side and the mark on the screen is to the right of the sector as the viewer faces the screen. For echocardiographic views in which the plane of sound passes through the inferior or posterior portion of the heart and then through the superior or anterior portion of the heart (apical and subcostal views), it is highly recommended that the cardiac structures be displayed in a manner that corresponds to the anatomic position of the heart in the body rather than upside down on the videoscreen. Almost all current echocardiographic systems have an invert switch that allows the viewer to invert the sector on the screen, so that the superior and basal portion of the heart is located at the top of the videoscreen and the inferior or apical portion of the heart is located at the bottom. The use of an anatomically oriented display of the two-dimensional image is especially important in pediatric cardiology because it facilitates the understanding and interpretation of complex cardiac defects by displaying them in a manner familiar to everyone, including persons not acquainted with two-dimensional echocardiography.[4]

The Parasternal Views

For the parasternal views, the transducer is applied as closely as possible to the sternum in the second, third, or fourth left intercostal space.[5–8] It is possible to image the heart from the left parasternal area because the left lung lacks a middle lobe; therefore, no air-filled lung is located anterior to the heart in this region. The parasternal views are best obtained with the patient lying in the left lateral decubitus position, so that the left lung falls even farther away from the heart and the size of the parasternal echocardiographic window is increased. In patients with cardiomegaly or hyperinflated lungs, the heart is displaced downward and the parasternal window is usually located lower on the chest wall. The parasternal views can be ex-

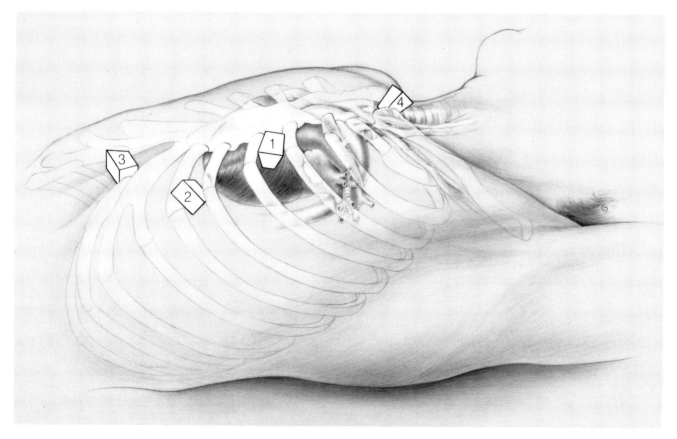

FIG 3–2.
Diagram depicting the four echocardiographic windows used to view the cardiac structures. Transducer *position 1* is the parasternal area, transducer *position 2* is the apical region, transducer *position 3* is the subcostal region, and transducer *position 4* is the suprasternal notch.

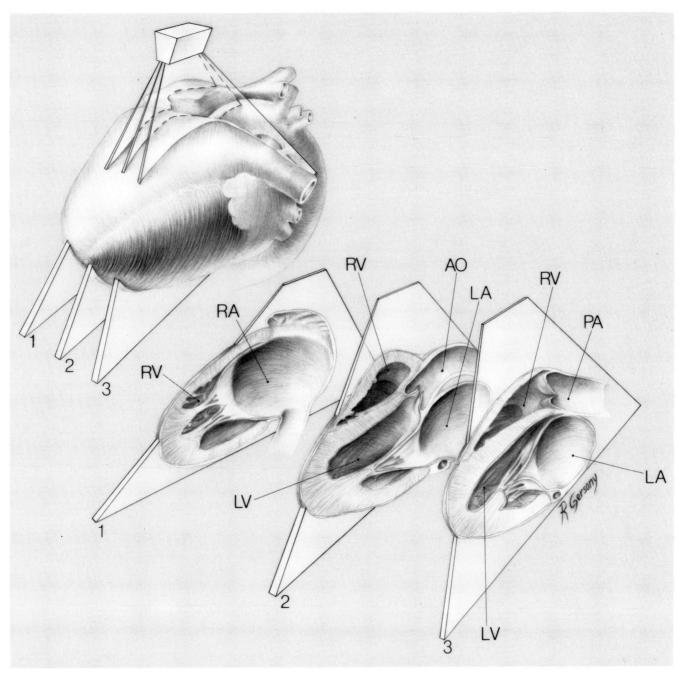

FIG 3–3.
Diagram of the family of parasternal long-axis views that can be obtained by applying the transducer to the parasternal location and tilting the plane of sound from right to left. *Plane 1* is a parasternal long-axis view through the right ventricular inflow tract, obtained by tilting the plane of sound toward the patient's right hip. *Plane 2* is the standard parasternal long-axis plane oriented along the major axis of the heart. *Plane 3* is a parasternal long-axis view obtained by tilting the plane of sound toward the patient's left shoulder. *AO* = aorta; *LA* = left atrium; *LV* = left ventricle; *PA* = pulmonary artery; *RA* = right atrium; and *RV* = right ventricle.

tremely difficult to obtain in patients with lung disease or in patients who are receiving assisted ventilation. It is apparent from Figure 3–1 that long- and short-axis planes can be obtained with the transducer positioned in the parasternal area; however, no four-chamber or coronal planes can be obtained from this location.

The Parasternal Long-Axis View

A family of parasternal long-axis views can be obtained by applying the transducer to the parasternal location and tilting the plane of sound from right to left (Fig 3–3). The standard parasternal long-axis view (Fig 3–3, plane 2) is obtained by orienting the plane of sound along the major axis of the heart, usually from the patient's left hip to the right shoulder. In this view (Fig 3–4), the echoes arising from the chest wall and right ventricular anterior wall occupy the apex of the sector. In infants and young children, echoes from the thymus can often be seen anterior to the right ventricular anterior wall. The next structure encountered in the sector is a portion of the right ventricular outflow tract. Next, echoes from the ventricular septum can be seen, continuous with echoes from the anterior aortic root. The inferior two-thirds of the ventricular septum is the trabecular ventricular septum, while the majority of the superior one-third of the ventricular septum in this view is the outlet or infundibular septum. In some patients, a small amount of the membranous portion of the ventricular septum is seen just beneath the aortic valve; however, the majority of the membranous ventricular septum is located to the right of this plane.

Because of the lack of a subaortic conus separating the aortic valve from the mitral valve, the inflow and outflow portions of the left ventricle can be visualized in the same long-axis plane. The situation is quite different for the right ventricle, where the inflow and outflow portions of the ventricle are separated by the subpulmonary conus and therefore are not visualized together in a single long-axis plane. Part of the sinus portion of the left ventricle can be imaged in the parasternal long-axis view. However, the cardiac apex usually cannot be imaged in this view for two reasons: (1) the plane is slightly medial to the ventricular apex, and (2) the 90° sector cannot incorporate the entire left ventricle. Posteriorly, the anterior and posterior leaflets of the mitral valve can be seen inserting by their chordae tendinae into the posteromedial papillary muscle. The anterior mitral valve leaflet is in fibrous continuity with the aortic valve and has its origin from the fibrous annulus superior to the origin of the posterior mitral valve leaflet. In the aortic root, the thin echoes that arise from the edges of the aortic valve leaflets can be seen. In systole, the aortic leaflets can be visualized in the open position close to the walls of the sinuses of Vaisalva. In diastole, the edges of the closed aortic valve can be seen in the center of the aortic root. Usually, the anterior or right coronary cusp and the posterior or noncoronary cusp of the aorta are seen in the standard parasternal long-axis view. In some patients, the ostium and a portion of the right main coronary artery can be seen arising from the anterior aortic root. In the normal heart, the aorta angles anteriorly as it exits the left ventricle.

Posteriorly, a portion of the left atrium is visualized behind the aortic root. The brightest echoes on the posterior surface of the left atrium and left ventricle arise from the fibrous pericardium. In some patients, pulmonary veins can be seen entering the left atrium, and a small coronary sinus can be seen in cross-section as a circular structure in the area of the atrioventricular groove and within the pericardial echo.[9] The descending thoracic aorta can be seen as an oval or circular structure behind the left atrium and outside of the pericardial echo.[10] That an oval or circular section of the descending aorta rather than a longitudinal section is visualized indicates how far the parasternal long-axis view is from the sagittal body plane.[11]

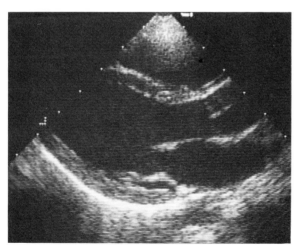 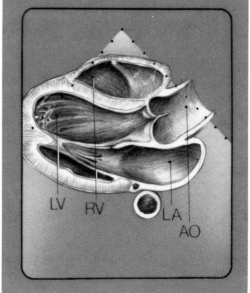

FIG 3–4.
Parasternal long-axis view of the left ventricle in a normal patient. This view provides imaging of the left ventricular inflow and outflow tracts simultaneously. Note the continuity between the ventricular septum and anterior aortic root and between the anterior mitral valve leaflet and posterior aortic root. AO = aorta; LA = left atrium; LV = left ventricle; and RV = right ventricle.

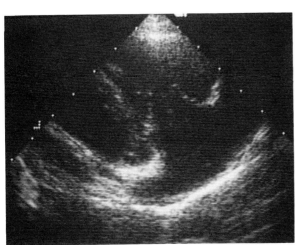 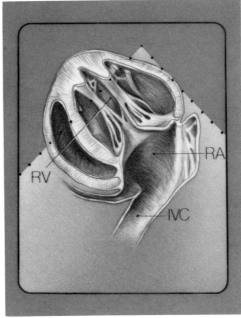

FIG 3–5.
Parasternal long-axis view through the right ventricular inflow tract in a normal patient. *IVC* = inferior vena cava; *RA* = right atrium; and *RV* = right ventricle.

If the parasternal long-axis view is correctly obtained, the septum and anterior aortic root will be aligned straight across the 90° sector. If the echoes arising from the anterior aortic root tilt downward toward the ventricular septum, the transducer is too high on the precordium; the transducer should be adjusted downward until the anterior aortic root and septal echoes are aligned. If the echoes from the ventricular septum are closer to the apex of the fan and run downward toward the anterior aortic root, the transducer is too low on the precordium and should be adjusted upward until the anterior aortic root and septal echoes are aligned.

If the transducer is angled from the standard parasternal long-axis view toward the patient's right hip, a parasternal long-axis view through the right ventricular inflow tract is obtained (Fig 3–3, plane 1). As the maneuver is performed, the plane of sound passes away from the aortic root and subaortic outlet ventricular septum through the area of the membranous septum, and toward the right atrium, tricuspid valve, and right ventricle. In the parasternal long-axis view of the right ventricular inflow tract (Fig 3–5), the anterior and septal leaflets of the tricuspid valve are visualized. A portion of the right atrium, the sinus or inflow portion of the right ventricle, and the right ventricular anterior and septal surfaces can be seen.

If the transducer is angled from the standard parasternal long-axis view toward the patient's left shoulder, a parasternal long-axis view through the right ventricular outflow tract is obtained (Fig 3–3, plane 3). As the sweep is performed, the plane of sound passes away from the

aortic root and subaortic outlet septum and through the area of the subpulmonic outlet septum, the outflow or infundibular portion of the right ventricle, the pulmonary valve, and the main pulmonary artery (Fig 3–6). As the plane of sound is angled between the aortic and pulmonic valves, it is often possible to image a considerable portion of the left main coronary artery in the left atrioventricular groove tissue and the left anterior descending coronary artery that courses down the surface of the ventricular septum (Fig 3–7). In some patients, bifurcation of the pulmonary artery into right and left pulmonary artery branches can be imaged in this plane.

The Parasternal Short-Axis View

The parasternal short-axis views are obtained by rotating the transducer 90° clockwise from the parasternal long-axis view.[12] With this transducer position, the plane of sound is usually oriented between the patient's right hip and left shoulder. A family of short-axis planes can be generated by tilting the transducer from the base of the heart superiorly to the cardiac apex inferiorly (Fig 3–8). At the base of the heart (Fig 3–9), the right ventricular anterior wall and a portion of the right ventricular outflow tract are seen in the anterior portion of the sector scan. The right atrium, the tricuspid valve, and a portion of the right ventricular inflow tract are seen on the left side of the videoscreen as the viewer faces the screen. The tricuspid valve leaflets seen in this view are the anterior and septal leaflets. In the center of the fan, the aortic valve is seen in cross-section as a circular structure. In diastole, the closed

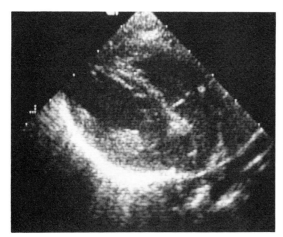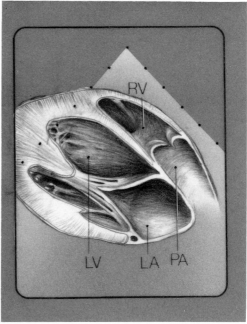

FIG 3–6.
Parasternal long-axis view through the right ventricular outflow tract in a normal patient. *LA* = left atrium; *LV* = left ventricle; *PA* = pulmonary artery; and *RV* = right ventricle.

aortic valve cusps form a Y pattern.[12] Because of the angle at which the aortic valve is situated in the heart, it is more common to visualize only two of the three diastolic closure lines simultaneously; therefore, a V pattern rather than a Y pattern is seen. The posterior commissure between the left and noncoronary cusps is oriented parallel to the plane of sound and is therefore difficult to image. The right coronary cusp is situated directly anteriorly between the septal leaflet of the tricuspid valve and the pulmonary valve. The left coronary cusp lies between the pulmonary valve and the left atrium, while the noncoronary or posterior cusp lies between the left atrium and tricuspid valve. The interatrial septum is situated perpendicular to the noncoronary cusp.

The pulmonary valve and the proximal portion of the main pulmonary artery can be seen to the left and anterior of the aortic valve. In the standard parasternal short-axis view at the base of the heart, the distal portion of the main pulmonary artery passes superiorly out of the imaging plane. Instead, the left atrial appendage is seen directly to the left of the aortic root. Care must be taken not to mistake the left atrial appendage for the main pulmonary artery or the mobile tip of the appendage for the pulmonary valve leaflets. Posterior to the aortic root, a portion of the left atrium can be seen.

With slight cranial and leftward angulation of the transducer from the standard parasternal short-axis view at the base of the heart, the distal main pulmonary artery branches can be visualized (Fig 3–10). This view can be obtained more easily if the transducer is repositioned in-

feriorly (about one intercostal space) and laterally on the chest wall. This maneuver places the right ventricular outflow tract directly beneath the transducer. The main pulmonary artery courses directly posteriorly. The left pulmonary artery continues as a posterior extension of the main pulmonary artery; only a short portion of the proximal left pulmonary artery is seen before it courses posteriorly and inferiorly out of the scan plane. The right pulmonary artery, however, arises from the main pulmo-

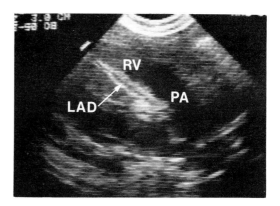

FIG 3–7.
Parasternal long-axis view through the right ventricular outflow tract. The left anterior descending (LAD) coronary artery is seen coursing down the surface of the ventricular septum. A small portion of the left main coronary artery is seen in the atrioventricular groove. *PA* = pulmonary artery; *RV* = right ventricle.

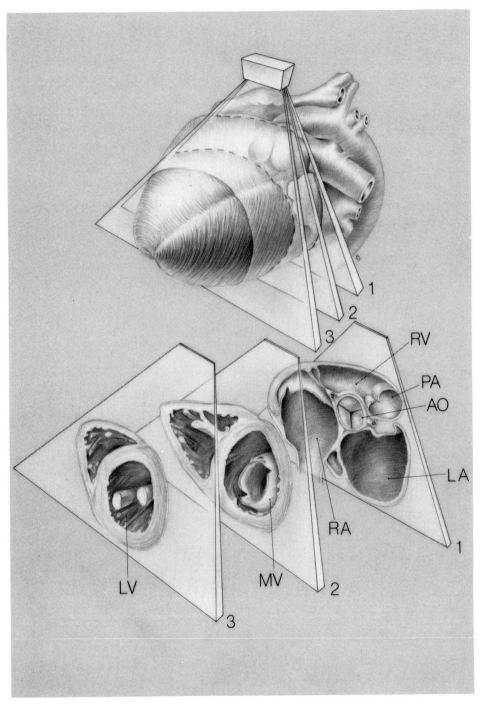

FIG 3–8.
Diagram of the family of parasternal short-axis views that can be generated by tilting the transducer from the base of the heart superiorly to the cardiac apex inferiorly. *Plane 1* is a parasternal short-axis view through the great vessels. *Plane 2* is a parasternal short-axis view at the level of the mitral valve leaflets. *Plane 3* is a parasternal short-axis view at the level of the left ventricular papillary muscles. *AO* = aorta; *LA* = left atrium; *LV* = left ventricle; *MV* = mitral valve; *PA* = pulmonary artery; *RA* = right atrium; and *RV* = right ventricle.

nary artery, then courses directly to the right behind the aortic root and superior to the roof of the left atrium. Thus, a considerable length of the right pulmonary artery can be seen in this view.

Both the right and left coronary arteries can be imaged from the parasternal short-axis view with slight changes in the direction of the plane of sound.[13, 14] In some patients, it is possible to image both the right and left coronary arteries simultaneously; it is easier, however, to image each

coronary artery separately. To visualize the right main coronary artery, the transducer is angled slightly cranially and rotated slightly clockwise so that the tricuspid valve leaflets are no longer seen. This maneuver images the plane in which the right main coronary artery exits the aorta and runs in the atrioventricular groove on the anterior surface of the right ventricle (Fig 3–11, A). With slightly more clockwise rotation of the transducer, the entire left main coronary artery can be seen in the left atrioventricular

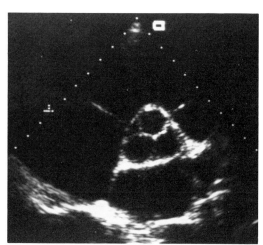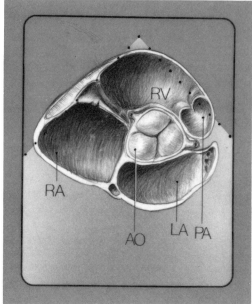

FIG 3–9.
Parasternal short-axis view at the base of the heart in a normal patient. The aorta (AO) is seen in cross-section in the middle of the plane. The right ventricular outflow tract courses from right to left anterior to the AO. The tricuspid valve is seen to the right of the AO and the pulmonary valve is seen to the left of the AO. LA = left atrium; PA = pulmonary artery; RA = right atrium; and RV = right ventricle.

groove, from its origin off the aortic root to its bifurcation into left anterior descending and left circumflex branches (Fig 3–11, B). Because the coronary arteries are imaged in the direction of the axial resolution of the equipment, they can be easily visualized even in newborn infants.

The standard parasternal short-axis view illustrates several important features of normal cardiac anatomy. First, the ascending aorta is aligned nearly parallel with the major axis of the left ventricle; however, the right ventricular outflow tract and main pulmonary artery course from right to left, anterior to the aortic root, so that the great arteries are wrapped around one another. In other words, in a short-axis view of the aortic root, the right ventricular outflow tract is seen in longitudinal section. The appearance of the aortic root and right ventricular outflow tract in the short axis view has been called the "circle-sausage" appearance.[12] Second, the parasternal short-axis view illustrates how the heart is composed of the right ventricular outflow tract anteriorly, the left ventricular outflow tract in the middle portion, and the atria posteriorly. Finally, the parasternal short-axis view shows how the heart is composed of the right ventricular inflow tract on the right heart border, the left ventricular outflow tract in the middle portion, and the right ventricular outflow tract on the left heart border. If the parasternal short-axis plane at the base of the heart is properly aligned, the movement of the tricuspid, aortic, and pulmonary valve leaflets can all be observed in one plane. If the tricuspid valve leaflet motion cannot be seen, the transducer should be rotated counterclockwise until the valve opening and closure can be observed.

From the parasternal short-axis view at the base of the heart, the transducer can be tilted caudally to image the left ventricular outflow tract just beneath the aortic valve. The left ventricular outflow tract is bordered anteriorly by the ventricular septum and posteriorly by the anterior mitral valve leaflet. The left atrium is seen posterior to the anterior mitral valve leaflet. The ventricular septum seen at this level includes the membranous septum, which is

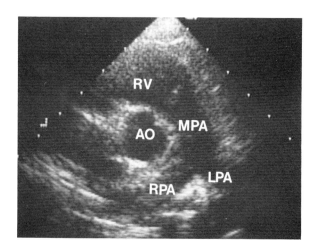

FIG 3–10.
Parasternal short-axis view at the base of the heart with the transducer tilted superiorly and leftward in order to visualize the bifurcation of the main pulmonary artery (MPA) into its two branches. AO = aorta; LPA = left pulmonary artery; RPA = right pulmonary artery; and RV = right ventricle.

A

B

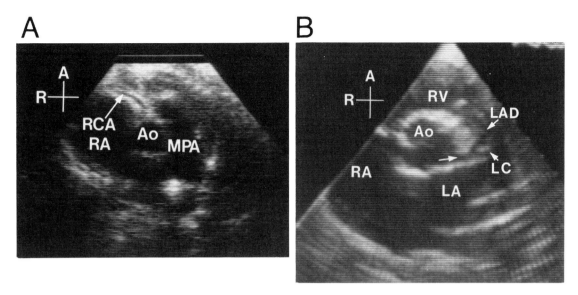

FIG 3–11.
A, parasternal short-axis view at the base of the heart, with the transducer rotated slightly clockwise to image the right coronary artery (*RCA*). *A* = anterior; *AO* = aorta; *MPA* = main pulmonary artery; *R* = right; and *RA* = right atrium. **B,** parasternal short-axis view at the base of the heart, with the transducer rotated even farther clockwise than in Figure 3–11A. This maneuver makes it possible to visualize the entire left main coronary artery (*arrow*) and its bifurcation into left anterior descending (*LAD*) and left circumflex (*LC*) branches. *A* = anterior; *AO* = aorta; *LA* = left atrium; *R* = right; *RA* = right atrium; and *RV* = right ventricle.

to the right and underneath the septal leaflet of the tricuspid valve. The remainder of the ventricular septum is the outlet septum, with the subaortic portion located directly anterior to the aortic valve and the subpulmonic portion located to the left, just proximal to the pulmonary valve. In this plane the coronary sinus can sometimes be seen in longitudinal section as it courses from left to right in the atrioventricular groove on the posterior surface of the heart.[9] The coronary sinus, especially when enlarged, should not be confused with a posterior pericardial effusion because it lies anterior to the pericardial echo.

With more caudal angulation, a parasternal short-axis view at the level of the mitral valve can be obtained (Fig 3–12). The anterior and posterior mitral valve leaflets have the appearance of a fish mouth as they open and close. The ventricular septum at this level is composed of the inlet septum to the right between the tricuspid and mitral valves and the trabecular septum anteriorly. With even more caudal angulation, short-axis views can be obtained through the papillary muscles and down to the cardiac apex. The ventricular septum in the parasternal short-axis view at the level of the papillary muscles consists of the muscular or trabecular septum (Fig 3–13). The anterolateral papillary muscle is located at the 4-o'clock position in the circular left ventricle, while the posteromedial papillary muscle is located at the 8-o'clock position. The apical portion of the right ventricle can be seen anterior and to the right. If the short-axis plane is aligned correctly, then the left ventricle will be circular in the cross-sectional views. If the left ventricle appears elongated or pear-shaped, then the transducer is located too high or too low on the precordium.

The Apical Views

For the apical views, the cardiac apex is palpated and the transducer is applied directly to the apical impulse.[15] The apical views are best obtained with the patient lying in the left lateral decubitus position, so that the cardiac apex is closer to the chest wall and the left lung falls downward away from the heart. If the apical impulse is located in the midaxillary line or farther posteriorly, then it may be difficult to position the transducer between the cardiac apex and the bed. This problem can be avoided by using a foam rubber mattress with a semicircular section cut out of the edge of the mattress. The patient lies on the bed with the cardiac apex positioned over the hole so that the transducer can then be applied to the cardiac apex and manipulated freely in all directions. From Figure 3–1 it is apparent that four-chamber and long-axis planes can be obtained from the apical window; however, no short-axis planes can be obtained from this location.

The Apical Four-Chamber View

A family of apical four-chamber views can be obtained by applying the transducer to the cardiac apex and tilting the plane of sound from posterior to anterior (Fig 3–14).[6, 7] The standard apical four-chamber view is obtained by orienting the plane of sound in a nearly coronal body plane through both ventricles and both atria (Fig 3–14, plane 2). For the beginning echocardiographer, this view is often the most difficult to obtain. If the transducer is correctly aligned, the apex of the left ventricle is seen in the apex of the fan (Fig 3–15). All four cardiac chambers, mitral and tricuspid valves, and both atrial and ventricular septa are visualized.

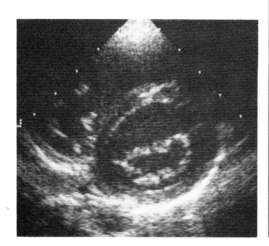 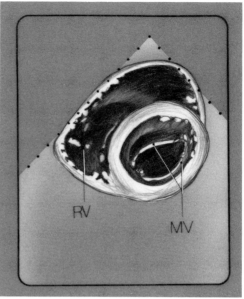

FIG 3–12.
Parasternal short-axis view at the level of the mitral valve in a normal patient. The anterior and posterior mitral valve leaflets have the appearance of a fish mouth in the open position. *MV* = mitral valve; *RV* = right ventricle.

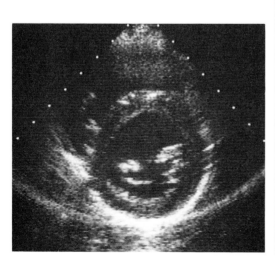 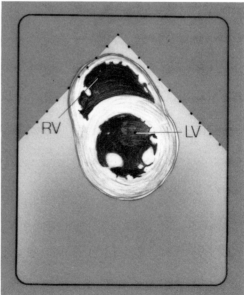

FIG 3–13.
Parasternal short-axis view at the level of the left ventricular papillary muscles. The anterolateral papillary muscle is located at the 4-o'clock position in the circular left ventricle (*LV*), while the posteromedial papillary muscle is located at the 8-o'clock position. *RV* = right ventricle.

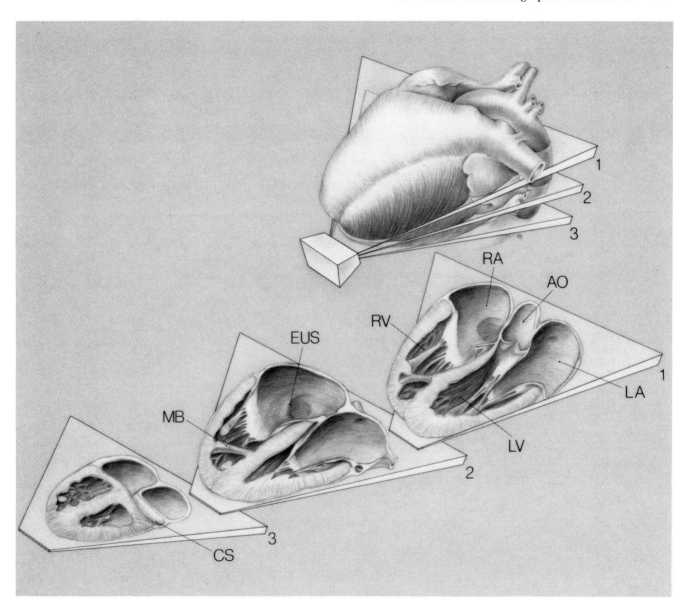

FIG 3–14.
Diagram of the apical four-chamber views that can be obtained by applying the transducer to the cardiac apex and tilting the plane of sound from anterior to posterior. *Plane 1* is an apical four-chamber view that passes through the left ventricle (LV), LV outflow tract, and ascending aorta (AO). *Plane 2* is a standard apical four-chamber view showing all four cardiac chambers simultaneously. *Plane 3* is an apical view with the plane of sound tilted posteriorly in order to image the coronary sinus (CS) in the atrioventricular groove. *LA* = left atrium; *MB* = moderator band; *RA* = right atrium; and *RV* = right ventricle.

If a portion of the right ventricle is visualized in the apex of the fan, the transducer is positioned too medially on the chest and should be moved laterally over the left ventricular apex. If both ventricles are visualized but only a small portion of the atria is seen, the transducer is tilted too caudally and should be tilted cranially to image both atria completely. If the mitral valve leaflets can be seen well but the tricuspid valve leaflet motion is seen poorly, the transducer is rotated too far counterclockwise and should be rotated clockwise to visualize the right atrium, the right ventricle, and the tricuspid valve leaflets completely. Obtaining a perfectly aligned apical four-chamber view is difficult and requires practice. Several good reasons exist for giving such meticulous attention to the correct alignment of this view: (1) if the transducer is not positioned directly over the cardiac apex, pathologic conditions involving the apex will not be detected, especially because no other plane is as useful for imaging this area; (2) incorrect transducer placement can lead to mistakes in evaluating the relative sizes of the two atria and two ventricles; and (3) incorrect transducer placement can cause mistakes in evaluating the relative positions of the two atrioventricular valves.

Because all four cardiac chambers and both the atrial and ventricular septa are visualized simultaneously in the apical four-chamber view, this view is especially useful for determining atrial situs and the atrioventricular connections. The morphology of each cardiac chamber is largely determined by the characteristics of its septal surface,[16] which usually can be determined completely from the apical four-chamber view. The morphologic right atrium is characterized by an atrial septal surface that receives the insertion of the eustachian valve. The eustachian valve, a remnant of one of the fetal cardiac valves, originates at the ostium of the inferior vena cava, runs along the floor of the right atrium, and terminates with a tendinous insertion into the primum atrial septum as part of the inferior limbic system of the fossa ovalis. This structure can often be seen in the apical four-chamber view as a thin membrane that crosses the body of the right atrium obliquely and inserts into the lower portion of the atrial septum just distal to the fossa ovalis.[17] In some patients, the eustachian valve is large and redundant and moves with a whiplike motion in the body of the right atrium. The eustachian valve can even prolapse into the tricuspid valve funnel. A prominent eustachian valve should not be mistaken for a right atrial thrombus or mass.

The morphologic left atrium is characterized by the flap valve of the foramen ovale on its atrial septal surface. In the four-chamber view of the fetal heart the flap valve of the foramen ovale is usually visualized as a membranous structure that protrudes into the body of the left atrium.

In some newborn infants, the flap valve of the foramen ovale can be seen moving back and forth in the area of the foramen ovale. However, in most patients, this structure cannot be imaged separately from the atrial septum. In this view, a right and left pulmonary vein can usually be seen draining into the left atrium.

The septal surface of the morphologic right ventricle is characterized as (1) being heavily trabeculated, (2) having muscle bundles (septal-parietal muscle bundles) that course from the septum to the parietal free wall of the right ventricle, and (3) receiving tendinous insertions of the atrioventricular valve. All of these features are easily visualized in the apical four-chamber view, making it ideal for identifying the morphologic right ventricle. In addition, the morphologic right ventricle has an atrioventricular valve (the tricuspid valve), which is situated slightly closer to the cardiac apex than the mitral valve. The sinus and trabeculated portions of the right ventricle are imaged in the apical four-chamber view. In the sinus portion of the right ventricle, the anterior and septal leaflets of the tricuspid valve and the insertions of the septal leaflet into the ventricular septum are seen. In the trabeculated portion, coarse septal-parietal muscle bundles are imaged. The largest of these muscle bundles is usually the moderator band. The right ventricular wall seen in this view is the anterior right ventricular wall.

The septal surface of the morphologic left ventricle is smooth, has no septal-parietal muscle bundles, and receives no tendinous insertions from the mitral valve. The

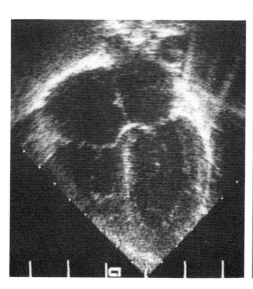
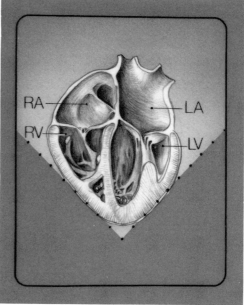

FIG 3–15.
Apical four-chamber view in a normal patient. This view visualizes all four cardiac chambers, the atrial septum, and ventricular septum simultaneously. In the normal heart, the right ventricle (RV) has an atrioventricular valve (tricuspid valve) that is closer to the cardiac apex than the mitral valve. The right ventricle also has heavy septal-parietal free wall muscle bundles. The left ventricle (LV) has an atrioventricular valve (the mitral valve) that is farther from the cardiac apex. The septal surface of the left ventricle is smooth. Note the drainage of the pulmonary veins to the left atrium (LA). *RA* = right atrium.

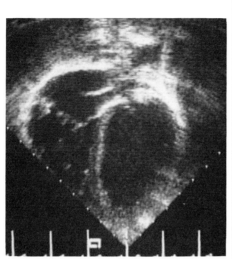
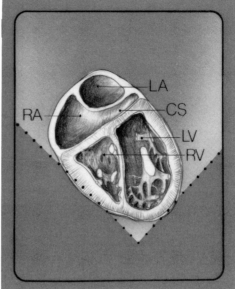

FIG 3–16.
Apical four-chamber view with the plane of sound tilted posteriorly to image the posterior surface of the heart. In this view, the coronary sinus (CS) can be seen coursing from left to right in the atrioventricular groove. *LA* = left atrium; *LV* = left ventricle; *RA* = right atrium; and *RV* = right ventricle.

morphologic left ventricle has an atrioventricular valve (the mitral valve), which is situated farther from the cardiac apex than the tricuspid valve. The anterior (medial) and posterior (lateral) leaflets of the mitral valve and the papillary muscles of the mitral valve can be imaged in this view. The sinus and trabeculated portions of the left ventricle and the lateral left ventricular wall are imaged in the apical four-chamber view.

A large portion of the atrial and ventricular septa are imaged in the apical four-chamber view. The lower one-third of the atrial septum adjacent to the atrioventricular valves is the area where primum atrial septal defects occur. The middle portion of the atrial septum is occupied by the fossa ovalis and is the area where secundum atrial septal defects occur. Frequently, echocardiographic dropout occurs in this portion of the atrial septum because it is thin and aligned parallel to the plane of sound. The posterior and superior portion of the atrial septum is the area where sinus venosus defects occur. Several portions of the ventricular septum can be imaged in the apical four-chamber view: (1) the inferior two-thirds of the ventricular septum, which in this view is the muscular or trabecular septum, (2) the upper one-third of the ventricular septum between the atrioventricular valves, which is the inlet septum, and (3) the ventricular septum above the tricuspid valve and below the mitral valve, which is the supratricuspid portion of the membranous septum (pars atrioventricularis). In some patients, the atrial and ventricular septa can be imaged more clearly by moving the transducer medially so that these structures are more perpendicular to the plane of sound. With this new transducer position, a parasternal

four-chamber view, with the right ventricle in the apex of the fan, is obtained.

In some patients, the coronary sinus can be seen in cross-section near the lateral wall of the left atrium in the atrioventricular groove.[9] The descending aorta can sometimes be identified as a circular structure posterolateral to the left atrium.[18]

With posterior angulation of the transducer, an apical four-chamber view corresponding to plane 3 in Figure 3–14 is obtained.[6] As the transducer is tilted posteriorly, the mitral and tricuspid valve leaflets and most of the ventricular cavities are no longer imaged. Instead, the plane of sound passes through the coronary sinus as it courses from left to right on the posterior surface of the heart in the atrioventricular groove (Fig 3–16). The ostium of the coronary sinus can often be imaged in the right atrium. During the sweep of the transducer, posterior portions of the right main coronary artery and the left circumflex coronary artery can be seen in the atrioventricular groove.

With anterior angulation of the transducer from the apical four-chamber view, the aortic root can be seen arising from the left ventricle.[6] This plane, which has been called the apical five-chamber view, is analogous to plane 1 in Figure 3–14. As the plane of sound is tilted anteriorly, the tricuspid valve and right ventricular inflow tract are no longer seen, and the left ventricular outflow tract, aortic valve, and a portion of the ascending aorta come into view (Fig 3–17). Often, an anterior portion of the right main coronary artery, the left main coronary artery, and an anterior portion of the left circumflex coronary artery are seen in this projection. The left atrial appendage can be seen

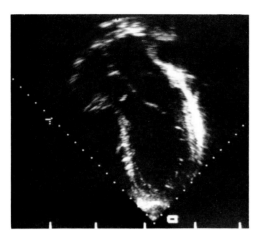
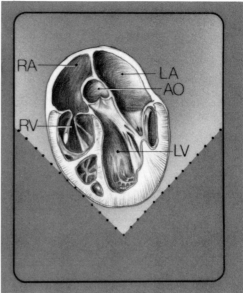

FIG 3–17.
Apical four-chamber view with the plane of sound tilted anteriorly to visualize the left ventricular outflow tract and ascending aorta (AO). This view has been called the apical five-chamber view. *LA* = left atrium; *LV* = left ventricle; *RA* = right atrium; and *RV* = right ventricle.

along the left lateral border of the heart. In some patients, it is possible to tilt the transducer even more anteriorly without losing contact with the chest wall and to visualize the right ventricular outflow tract and pulmonary valve from the apical position.

The Apical Long-Axis View

The apical long-axis view is obtained by rotating the transducer 90° counterclockwise from the apical four-chamber view (Fig 3–18).[6, 15] The plane of sound passes through the mitral valve, the cardiac apex, and the aortic valve, and thus is aligned along the major axis of the left ventricle (Fig 3–19). The inferior two-thirds of the ventricular septum seen in this view is the trabecular septum, while the superior one-third consists of the subaortic outlet septum and a small portion of the membranous septum.

Like the parasternal long-axis view, the apical long-axis view provides a plane for imaging the left atrium, anterior and posterior mitral valve leaflets, the left ventricular outflow tract, the right and noncoronary aortic valve leaflets, and a portion of the ascending aorta. Unlike the parasternal long-axis view, however, the apical long-axis view passes directly through the cardiac apex, places the left ventricular outflow tract and aortic valve perpendicular to the plane of sound, and images the superior border of the left atrium more clearly. The apical long-axis and four-chamber views are orthogonal planes obtained by 90° rotation around the major axis of the left ventricle and are, therefore, ideally suited for use in biplane left ventricular volume analysis.

With slight lateral angulation of the transducer from the standard apical long-axis view, an echocardiographic plane that passes through only the left atrium, the mitral valve, and the left ventricle can be obtained. This view has been called the apical two-chamber view.

The Subcostal Views

For the subcostal views, the transducer is placed in the abdomen just below the xyphoid process of the sternum and is tilted cranially and caudally to image supradiaphragmatic and infradiaphragmatic cardiovascular structures.[19, 20] The subcostal views are best obtained with the patient lying supine on the bed. In older patients, flexion of the legs at the knees and hips can reduce the tension of the abdominal muscles and increase the ease of obtaining the subcostal images. Also, in older patients in whom the heart can be quite distant from the transducer, subcostal imaging can be improved by having patients hold their breath at deep inspiration. This maneuver lowers the diaphragm, brings the heart closer to the transducer, and improves the penetration of the sound beam.

It is important to be aware of several problems that can occur during the subcostal examination. First, in small infants, if the transducer is pressed too deeply into the abdomen it is possible to interfere with respiration. This can be a particular problem in the examination of premature infants who are receiving assisted ventilation. In these infants, vigorous application of the transducer can impair diaphragmatic motion and lung inflation and result in a fall in transcutaneous oxygen tension. Second, in small infants, if the transducer is pressed too deeply in the abdomen it is possible to occlude the inferior vena cava, diminish systemic venous return, and decrease cardiac output. Third, in many patients the abdomen is tender and vigorous transducer application can cause the patient considerable discomfort. This problem frequently arises in postoperative patients and patients with ascites or distended livers. In these situations, alternative transducer positions away from the tender area (i.e., the surgical incision or liver edge) should be attempted.

As seen in Figure 3–1, coronal planes and short-axis planes can be obtained with the transducer positioned in the subcostal region; however, the true long-axis planes cannot be obtained from this location. As will be discussed below, the outflow tracts of the left and right ventricles can be imaged in the subcostal coronal planes. For this reason, some investigators have referred to these planes as the subcostal long-axis views.[19]

The Subcostal View of the Abdomen

A considerable length of the descending aorta and in-

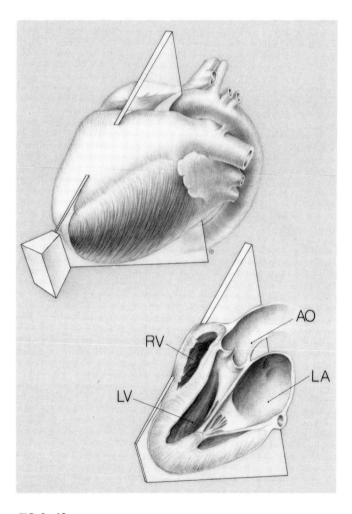

FIG 3–18.
Diagram of the apical long-axis view. This view is obtained by rotating the transducer 90° counterclockwise from the apical four-chamber view. *AO* = aorta; *LA* = left atrium; *LV* = left ventricle; and *RV* = right ventricle.

ferior vena cava can be imaged by placing the transducer in the subcostal region in a sagittal body plane. The transducer is slowly tilted toward the patient's left side until the vertebral column and descending aorta are visualized (Fig 3–20). The descending aorta is easily recognized by its prominent arterial pulsations. Usually, the celiac and superior mesenteric arteries can be visualized as the first and second major arterial branches off the descending abdominal aorta. If the transducer is tilted cranially toward the heart, a considerable length of the descending thoracic aorta can be visualized above the diaphragm and behind the left atrium. Frequently, an area of echocardiographic dropout can be seen anterior to the superior portion of the descending abdominal aorta. This space is formed by the posterior insertion of the left hemidiaphragm and the left costophrenic angle and should not be mistaken for another abdominal vessel or for pleural or abdominal fluid.

From the sagittal view of the descending abdominal aorta, the transducer can be tilted slowly toward the patient's right side to visualize the inferior vena cava (Fig 3–20). The pulsations of the inferior vena cava are more subtle than the descending aorta pulsations and do not correspond to ventricular systole. To visualize the inferior vena cava-right atrial junction, the transducer must often be tilted anteriorly and rotated slightly clockwise because of the angle at which the inferior vena cava passes through the liver and joins the heart. Usually, several prominent hepatic veins can be seen joining the inferior vena cava; however, in normal patients, no other large vascular structures are imaged when the transducer is swept from the descending aorta view to the view of the inferior vena cava.

A cross-sectional view of the inferior vena cava and descending aorta can be obtained by placing the transducer in the subcostal space in a transverse body plane and tilting the transducer caudally until the vertebral body is seen in cross-section (Fig 3–20). In this view, the descending aorta is normally visualized in the left paravertebral gutter; the inferior vena cava is seen to the right of the spine and slightly anterior to the descending aorta. This view not only makes it possible to visualize the positions of the aorta and inferior vena cava in the abdomen but also makes it possible to diagnose pleural effusions and assess diaphragmatic motion. The motion of both sides of the posterior portion of the diaphragm can be observed as the patient breathes quietly; in this way, phrenic nerve palsies can be detected. Also, with the patient lying supine, pleural effusions will layer along the posterior costophrenic angles and can be detected in this view. As the transducer is tilted cranially from the standard cross-sectional view of the abdomen, the liver can be seen on the patient's right and the stomach bubble can be imaged on the patient's left. The more anterior portions of the diaphragm can be imaged by this maneuver, making it possible to detect diaphragmatic hernias and eventrations.

The Subcostal Coronal View

A family of subcostal coronal or four-chamber views can be obtained by applying the transducer to the subcostal

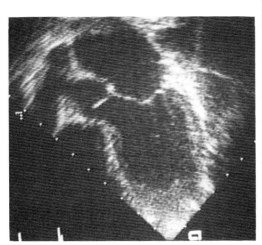
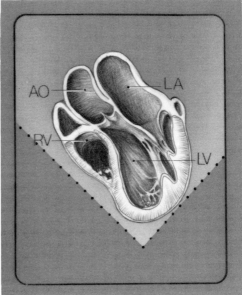

FIG 3–19.
Apical long-axis view in a normal patient. This view provides simultaneous imaging of the left ventricular inflow and outflow tracts. *AO* = aorta; *LA* = left atrium; *LV* = left ventricle; and *RV* = right ventricle.

region and tilting the plane of sound from posterior to anterior (Fig 3–21). For the coronal views, the plane of sound is oriented between the patient's right and left side; the transducer is pressed into the abdomen underneath and nearly parallel to the sternum. The most posterior angulation of the transducer (Fig 3–21, plane 1) provides a coronal section through posterior portions of both atria and the posterior atrioventricular groove. In this plane, it is often possible to image the eustachian valve of the inferior vena cava in the right atrium and the right and left pulmonary veins that join the left atrium (Fig 3–22). If the plane is positioned posterior to the atrioventricular valve funnels, the coronary sinus can be seen as it courses from left to right in the posterior atrioventricular groove. Care should be taken not to mistake the ostium of the coronary sinus for an atrial septal defect. A considerable amount of the posterior interatrial septum can be imaged in this view.

With slight anterior angulation from plane 1, the standard subcostal four-chamber view can be obtained (see Fig 3–21, plane 2). This view, like the apical four-chamber view, is extremely useful for identifying the morphologic characteristics of each cardiac chamber and, consequently, for determining atrial situs and atrioventricular connections (Fig 3–23). The morphology of each cardiac chamber is largely determined by the characteristics of the septal surface.[16] The morphologic right atrium is characterized by having an atrial septal surface that receives the insertion of the eustachian valve. In this view, the eustachian valve is seen crossing the floor of the right atrium from its origin at the orifice of the inferior vena cava to its insertion in the inferior limbic system of the fossa ovalis. The morphologic left atrium is characterized by the flap valve of

the foramen ovale on its atrial septal surface. In the fetus in utero and in some newborn infants, the flap valve of the foramen ovale can be seen to prolapse into the left atrial cavity. In most patients, however, this structure cannot be imaged separately from the atrial septum. In this view, a right and left pulmonary vein can usually be seen draining into the left atrium.

The interatrial septum is visualized especially well in the subcostal view because it is perpendicular to the plane of sound and imaged in the direction of the axial resolution of the equipment. In general, the subcostal four-chamber view is more useful than the apical four-chamber view for detecting atrial septal defects because it contains less artificial echo dropout in the region of the thin fossa ovalis. The portions of the atrial septum imaged in the subcostal four-chamber view include the superior-posterior portion, where sinus venosus defects occur, the middle portion, where secundum atrial septal defects occur, and the inferior portion adjacent to the atrioventricular valves, where primum atrial septal defects occur.

The morphologic right ventricle is characterized by a septal surface that has coarse trabeculations, that receives tendinous insertions from the atrioventricular valve, and that has muscle bundles coursing from the septum to the parietal free wall. The largest of the septal-parietal muscle bundles is usually located near the right ventricular apex and is called the moderator band. In addition, the morphologic right ventricle has an atrioventricular valve (the tricuspid valve) situated slightly closer to the cardiac apex than is the mitral valve. The subcostal four-chamber view, like the apical four-chamber view, allows visualization of the sinus and trabeculated portions of the right ventricle.

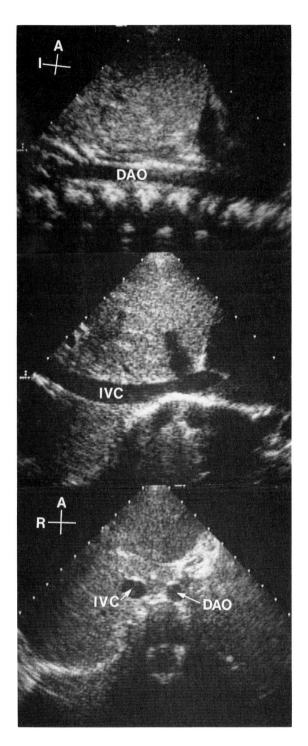

FIG 3–20.
Subcostal views of the abdominal vessels. The *top frame* is a sagittal view of the descending aorta (DAO). Celiac and superior mesenteric arteries can be visualized as the first and second major arterial branches off the DAO. In the *middle frame*, the inferior vena cava (IVC) is seen in sagittal section. The *bottom frame* shows a cross-section of both vessels in the abdomen. The DAO lies to the left of the spine, while the IVC is situated to the right. *A* = anterior; *I* = inferior; and *R* = right.

In the sinus portion, the septal and anterior leaflets of the tricuspid valve and the insertions of the septal leaflet into the ventricular septum are seen. In the trabeculated portion, coarse septal-parietal muscle bundles are visible. The right ventricular wall seen in this view is the diaphragmatic surface of the right ventricle.

The septal surface of the morphologic left ventricle is smooth, devoid of tendinous insertions from the mitral valve, and also devoid of septal-parietal muscle bundles. Its atrioventricular valve (the mitral valve) is situated farther from the cardiac apex than the tricuspid valve. The anterior (medial) and posterior (lateral) leaflets and the papillary muscles of the mitral valve can be imaged in this view. The sinus and trabeculated portions of the left ventricle and the posterolateral left ventricular wall are imaged in the subcostal four-chamber view.

Several portions of the ventricular septum are imaged in the subcostal four-chamber view: (1) the inferior two-thirds of the septum, which in this view is the muscular or trabecular septum; (2) the upper one-third of the septum between the atrioventricular valves, which is the inlet septum; and (3) the septum above the tricuspid valve and below the mitral valve, which is the pars atrioventricularis of the membranous septum.

In the subcostal four-chamber view, as in its apical counterpart, the coronary sinus can frequently be seen in cross-section along the lateral wall of the left atrium in the atrioventricular groove.[9] The descending aorta can often be visualized in cross-section as a circular structure posterolateral to the left atrium.

With anterior angulation of the transducer from the subcostal four-chamber view, the left ventricular outflow tract can be imaged (see Fig 3–21, plane 3). This view has been called the subcostal long-axis view of the left ventricle because it images the entire length of the left ventricular outflow tract. However, it is important to note that this plane is really analogous to the apical five-chamber view and is in reality 90° orthogonal to the true apical long-axis view. In the subcostal view of the left ventricular outflow tract (Fig 3–24), the mitral valve and inflow portion of the left ventricle can no longer be seen. Instead, the trabeculated and outflow portions of the left ventricle, the aortic valve, and a variable portion of the ascending aorta and aortic arch are visualized. Imaging of the aortic arch can be enhanced by rotating the transducer 10° to 15° clockwise from the standard subcostal coronal plane position. Usually, the left main coronary artery and its bifurcation into circumflex and anterior descending coronary artery branches can be seen in the left atrioventricular groove tissue. Along the left side of the ascending aorta, the main pulmonary artery and the left atrial appendage can be visualized. With posterior-anterior tilting of the transducer, the entire length of the right pulmonary artery can be seen coursing posterior to the ascending aorta from its origin from the main pulmonary artery to the hilum of the right lung. Along the right side of the ascending aorta, the superior vena cava and its junction with the right atrium can be visualized. In addition, the right atrium, the tricuspid

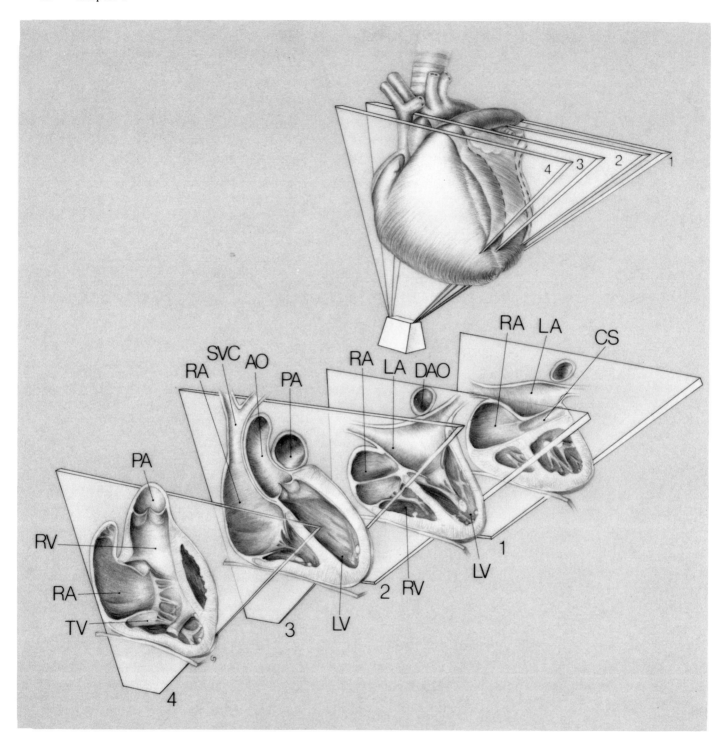

FIG 3–21.
Diagram of the subcostal coronal, or four-chamber, views that can be obtained by applying the transducer to the subcostal region and tilting the plane of sound from posterior to anterior. *Plane 1* is a posterior subcostal coronal view through the coronary sinus (CS). *Plane 2* is a subcostal four-chamber view in which all four cardiac chambers can be imaged simultaneously. *Plane 3* is a subcostal coronal view of the left ventricular outflow tract. *Plane 4* is a subcostal coronal view of the right ventricular outflow tract. The subcostal views are particularly useful for determining the atrioventricular and ventriculoarterial connections. *AO* = aorta; *DAO* = descending aorta; *LA* = left atrium; *LV* = left ventricle; *PA* = pulmonary artery; *RA* = right atrium; *RV* = right ventricle; *SVC* = superior vena cava; and *TV* = tricuspid valve.

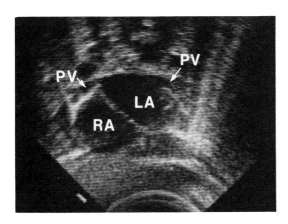

FIG 3–22.
Subcostal four-chamber view with the plane of sound tilted far posteriorly to image the pulmonary veins (PV) as they enter the left atrium (LA). *RA* = right atrium.

valve, and a portion of the right ventricular inflow can be imaged. The ventricular septum imaged in this view includes the trabecular septum (lower two-thirds), the subaortic outlet septum (upper one-third), and a small portion of the membranous septum (subaortic and to the right).

With even more anterior angulation of the transducer, the left ventricular outflow tract is no longer seen and the right ventricle and right ventricular outflow tract come into view (see Fig 3–21, plane 4). In this view, as the plane is tilted anteriorly, the tricuspid valve and the sinus portion of the right ventricle are seen. As the plane is tilted even farther anteriorly, the trabeculated and outflow portions of

the right ventricle, the pulmonary valve, and a portion of the main pulmonary artery are imaged (Fig 3–25). The trabeculated and outflow portions of the right ventricle are separated by a horseshoe-shaped group of muscle bundles that make up the crista supraventricularis. The septal and parietal muscle bundles of the crista are cut in cross-section by the imaging plane and lie along the right and left borders of the outflow tract beneath the pulmonary valve. These muscle bundles are not obvious in the subcostal views of normal patients; however, in many forms of congenital heart disease the muscle bundles of the infundibulum are hypertrophied and are easily seen.

The structures visualized in the family of subcostal coronal planes underscore several important points of cardiac anatomy. First, as the plane of sound is tilted from a posterior to an anterior position, it is clear that the posterior portion of the heart consists of the atria and both ventricular inflows, the middle portion of the heart is largely occupied by the left ventricle and the left ventricular outflow tract, and the anterior portion of the heart is mostly occupied by the right ventricular outflow tract. Second, the transducer sweep from the left ventricular to the right ventricular outflow tract views shows how in the normal heart the ventricular outflow tracts and the great arteries are wrapped around one another. From the subcostal views, it is possible to see that the left ventricular outflow tract and ascending aorta are pointed toward the patient's right shoulder (see Fig 3–24). The right ventricular outflow tract, on the other hand, crosses from right to left in front of the left ventricular outflow tract; therefore, the right ventricular outflow tract and the main pulmonary artery are pointed toward the patient's left shoulder. These complex spatial

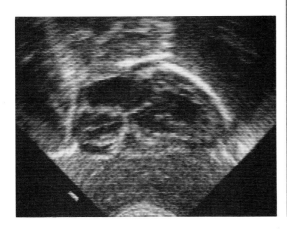

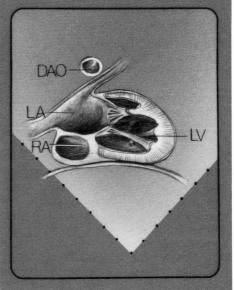

FIG 3–23.
Subcostal four-chamber view in a normal patient. This view is particularly useful for determining atrioventricular connections. *DAO* = descending aorta; *LA* = left atrium; *LV* = left ventricle; and *RA* = right atrium.

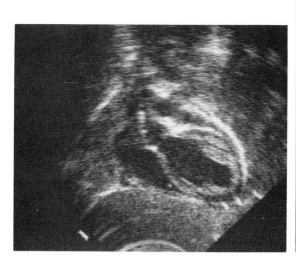 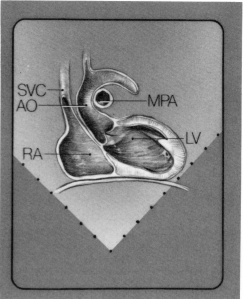

FIG 3–24.
Subcostal four-chamber view tilted anteriorly to image the left ventricular outflow tract. *AO* = aorta; *LV* = left ventricle; *MPA* = main pulmonary artery; *RA* = right atrium; and *SVC* = superior vena cava.

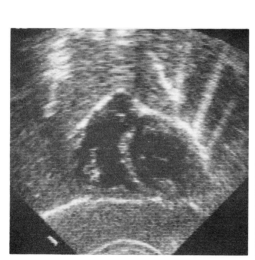 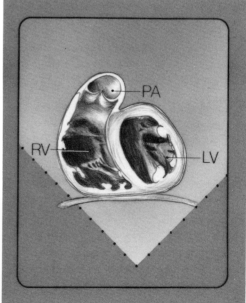

FIG 3–25.
Subcostal coronal view of the right ventricular outflow tract in a normal patient. This view is obtained by tilting the plane far anteriorly. *LV* = left ventricle; *PA* = pulmonary artery; and *RV* = right ventricle.

relations reflect the inversion of the ostium bulbi that occurred during early embryonic life.[16]

The Subcostal Short-Axis View

The subcostal short-axis views are obtained by rotating the transducer 90° clockwise from the subcostal four-chamber views. A family of subcostal short-axis views can be obtained by tilting the plane of sound from right to left (Fig 3–26). If the plane of sound is tilted to the patient's extreme right, an echocardiographic view corresponding to plane 1 on Figure 3–26 is obtained. In this view, the superior and inferior venae cavae and their junctions with the right atrium are imaged in a longitudinal section (Fig 3–27). The right atrial appendage is imaged anteriorly and a portion of the left atrium is imaged posteriorly. The posterior portion of the interatrial septum is seen in this view. In addition, the right pulmonary artery is seen in cross-section behind the superior vena cava and above the roof of the left atrium. The azygous vein can often be seen entering the posterior aspect of the superior vena cava superior to the right pulmonary artery. In this view, with slow and careful tilting of the transducer from right to left, the pulmonary veins can often be seen entering the left atrium.

By angling the transducer from plane 1 in Figure 3–26 toward the patient's vertebral bodies, plane 2 in Figure 3–26 can be obtained. Generation of this plane makes it possible to image the aortic arch but may require slight adjustments in the degree of transducer rotation (Fig 3–28). If imaging is optimal, the entire aortic arch including the vessels to the head and neck and the descending thoracic aorta can be visualized. Underneath the aortic arch, the right pulmonary artery can be seen in cross-section. Below the aorta, the right and left atria and the interatrial septum are imaged.

With slightly more leftward angulation of the transducer, a view similar to the parasternal short-axis view is obtained. In this view, the aortic valve is seen in cross-section and a portion of the anterior mitral valve leaflet is also seen. Anteriorly, a cross-sectional view of the right ventricle at the level of the tricuspid valve is imaged. The septum between the aortic and tricuspid valves is the membranous ventricular septum. Posteriorly, a portion of the left atrium is visualized and, often, with careful left-to-right angulation of the transducer, entry of the left pulmonary veins into the left atrium, is seen.

With extreme leftward angulation of the transducer, a subcostal short-axis view corresponding to plane 3 on Figure 3–26 is obtained (Fig 3–29). This plane closely resembles the lateral cineangiographic projection. In this view, the entire right ventricular outflow tract, the pulmonary valve, the main pulmonary artery, and occasionally, the left pulmonary artery are seen (Fig 3–30). Posteriorly, a portion of the left ventricle and the mitral valve apparatus are imaged. The ventricular septum seen in this view is the outlet septum superiorly and the midmuscular septum inferiorly.

The last subcostal short-axis view (see plane 4, Fig 3–26) is obtained by tilting the transducer even more leftward and slightly inferiorly. This plane provides a cross-sectional view of the left ventricle at the level of the mitral valve papillary muscles (Fig 3–31). The anterolateral and posteromedial papillary muscles are imaged at 1-o'clock and 5-o'clock positions in the circular left ventricle. The ventricular septum seen in this view is entirely the trabecular septum. The apical portion of the right ventricle is seen to the right.

The Suprasternal Views

For the suprasternal views, the transducer is placed in the suprasternal notch and aligned as closely parallel as possible with the sternum. In order to gain access to the suprasternal notch, the patient is positioned supine, with a pillow placed beneath the shoulders to extend the neck without producing tension on the sternocleidomastoid muscles. The patient's head is turned to the left or right so that the chin does not prevent adequate placement of the transducer in the suprasternal notch. In infants, it may be easier for a parent or assistant to extend the child's neck by placing a hand beneath the infant's scapulae and gently lifting the back. In newborns, it is often possible to image the entire aortic arch from the manubrium sternum; this structure is cartilaginous and allows transmission of ultrasound. When examining infants who are intubated and receiving assisted ventilation, imaging of the aortic arch from the manubrium sternum is safer for the patient because it is not necessary to extend the infant's neck and risk extubation. With older children, it is helpful to place pictures or other objects of interest on the wall above or behind the bed to focus the child's attention elsewhere during the examination. As illustrated in Figure 3–1, B, the aortic arch can be imaged in long- and short-axis planes.

The Suprasternal Long-Axis View

To obtain the suprasternal long-axis view, the transducer is placed in the suprasternal notch with the plane of sound oriented between the right nipple and the left scapular tip (Fig 3–32, plane 1).[21–23] In this view, the ascending, transverse, and descending thoracic aorta is visualized (Fig 3–33). The first, and usually the largest, branch that arises from the aortic arch is the innominate artery. Its bifurcation into right subclavian and right common carotid arteries can often be seen by rotating or tilting the transducer slightly in this plane. The second and third arterial branches off the aortic arch are the left common carotid and left subclavian arteries. Anterior to the innominate artery and superior to the transverse aorta, the left innominate vein is seen in cross-section as it courses from left to right to join in forming the superior vena cava. In some patients, the entire ascending aorta and the aortic valve leaflets can be seen in the suprasternal long-axis view.

Beneath the aortic arch, the right pulmonary artery and the right main stem bronchus are seen in cross-section. The right bronchus is densely echo-reflective because it is

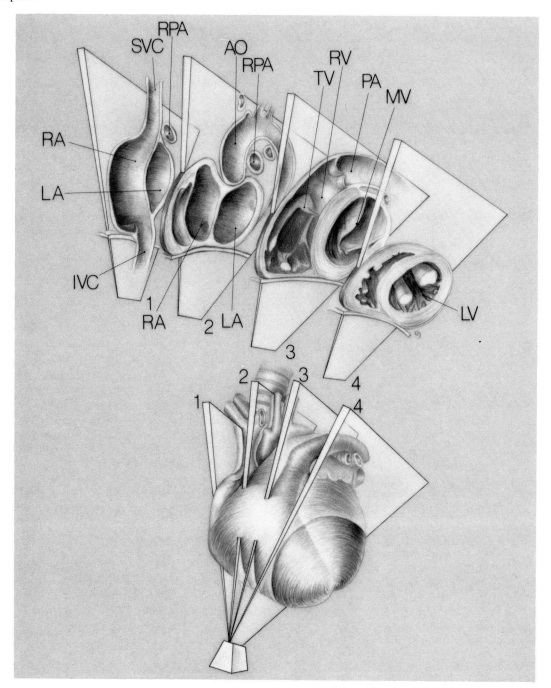

FIG 3–26.

Diagram of the subcostal short-axis or sagittal views that can be obtained by rotating the transducer 90° clockwise from the subcostal coronal views. A family of subcostal short-axis views can be obtained by tilting the plane of sound from right to left. *Plane 1*, obtained by tilting the plane of sound to the patient's extreme right, demonstrates the entrance of the superior vena cava (SVC) and inferior vena cava (IVC) into the right atrium (RA). *Plane 2*, obtained by tilting the plane slightly leftward, demonstrates the entire aortic arch. *Plane 3* is obtained by tilting the plane even more leftward and shows a sagittal view of the right ventricular outflow tract. *Plane 4* is obtained by tilting the plane of sound to the patient's far left. In this plane, a cross-section of the left ventricle (LV) is obtained. *AO* = aorta; *LA* = left atrium; *MV* = mitral valve; *PA* = pulmonary artery; *RPA* = right pulmonary artery; *RV* = right ventricle; and *TV* = tricuspid valve.

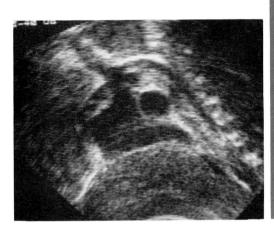 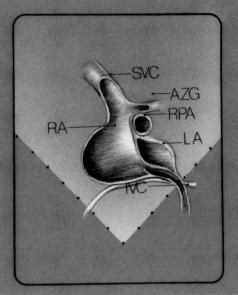

FIG 3–27.
Subcostal short-axis view through the junctions of the superior vena cava (SVC) and inferior vena cava (IVC) with the right atrium (RA). *AZG* = azygous vein; *LA* = left atrium; and *RPA* = right pulmonary artery.

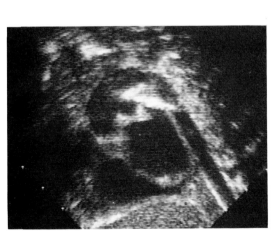 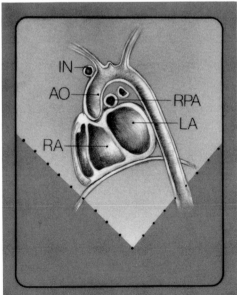

FIG 3–28.
Subcostal short-axis view through the aortic arch. This view allows imaging of the entire ascending and descending aorta (AO). *IN* = innominate vein; *LA* = left atrium; *RA* = right atrium; and *RPA* = right pulmonary artery.

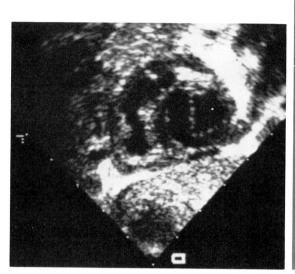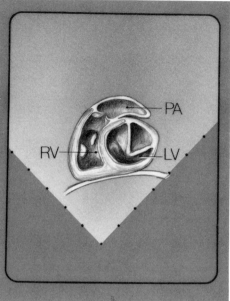

FIG 3–29.
Subcostal short-axis view through the right ventricular outflow tract in a normal patient. This view corresponds to the lateral cineangiographic projection and allows visualization of the entire right ventricular outflow tract, pulmonary valve, and main pulmonary artery (PA). *LV* = left ventricle; *RV* = right ventricle.

filled with air. It is an eparterial bronchus and therefore is located above the right pulmonary artery and below the transverse aortic arch.

If the plane of sound is tilted toward the patient's left, the right pulmonary artery disappears and the main and left pulmonary arteries come into view (see Fig 3–32, plane 2). In this projection, the main and left pulmonary arteries are sectioned tangentially and resemble a comma (Fig 3–34). The main pulmonary artery is the circular portion of the comma, and the left pulmonary artery is its tail. The left pulmonary artery lies alongside the descending aorta; therefore, the plane in which the left pulmonary artery is imaged does not usually include the ascending aorta. Because the left bronchus is a hyparterial structure, no air-filled bronchus is seen interposed between the left pulmonary artery and the aorta.

By tilting the transducer to the right from the standard suprasternal long-axis view, it is possible to image the air-filled trachea and its cartilaginous rings (Fig 3–35). The trachea is in the same plane as the ascending aorta. In the case of the normal left aortic arch, the transverse aorta arches to the left of the trachea; therefore, to visualize the entire aortic arch, the plane of sound must be tilted away from the trachea toward the patient's left side. This maneuver, in fact, is a method for diagnosing a left aortic arch. In a patient with a right aortic arch, the aorta ascends, arches, and descends to the right of the trachea. Therefore, in the case of a right aortic arch, the plane of sound is tilted away from the trachea toward the patient's right side to image the entire aortic arch. If the transducer is placed in

the standard plane in the suprasternal notch and a long-axis view of the aortic arch cannot be found, the presence of a right aortic arch should be suspected. The transducer should then be rotated 60° to 90° counterclockwise until the aortic arch is fully visualized. The usual plane of a right aortic arch is oriented slightly rightward and between the right nipple and the right scapular tip.[23–25]

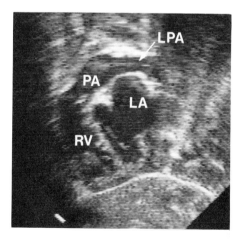

FIG 3–30.
Subcostal short-axis view from a normal patient, demonstrating visualization of a long length of the left pulmonary artery (LPA). *LA* = left atrium; *PA* = pulmonary artery; and *RV* = right ventricle.

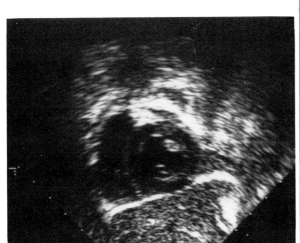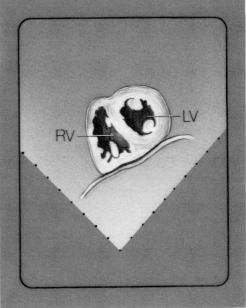

FIG 3–31.
Subcostal short-axis view of the left ventricle (LV) at the level of the papillary muscles in a normal patient. *RV* = right ventricle.

The Suprasternal Short-Axis View

To visualize the suprasternal short-axis views, the transducer is placed in the suprasternal notch and aligned parallel with the sternum. The plane of sound is oriented in a body frontal plane.[23] By tilting the transducer from anterior to posterior, a family of suprasternal short-axis views can be generated (Fig 3–36). To visualize the suprasternal short-axis views, it may be necessary to press the transducer posteriorly in the suprasternal notch so that the plane of sound is parallel and posterior to the bony sternum.

In the standard suprasternal short-axis view, the transverse aorta is visualized in cross-section as an anterior circular structure (Fig 3–37). Superior to the transverse aorta, the left innominate vein can be seen in longitudinal section, coursing from left to right. On the right side of the transverse aorta, the left innominate vein joins the right innominate vein to form the superior vena cava. A short segment of the superior vena cava is imaged alongside the transverse aorta before it passes anteriorly out of the imaging plane. Inferior to the transverse aorta, the entire right pulmonary artery is seen in longitudinal section from its origin from the main pulmonary artery on the patient's left to its termination in the hilum of the lung on the patient's right. Usually, the right upper lobe branch can be seen arising from the right pulmonary artery just proximal to its termination in the right lung. Beneath the right pulmonary artery, the left atrium is imaged in frontal section. If in this view penetration of the sound beam is good, the pulmonary veins can be seen entering the left atrium. With

anterior and posterior angulation, the origins of the head and neck vessels from the aortic arch can be seen.

If the plane of sound is tilted anteriorly, a suprasternal short-axis view through the ascending aorta can be obtained (see Fig 3–36, plane 1). In this view, it is often possible to image the entire ascending aorta from the valve leaflets to the origin of the head and neck vessels (Fig 3–38). To the left of the aorta, the main pulmonary artery is seen in cross-section. To the right of the aorta, the superior vena cava and its junction with the right atrium are visualized.

In infants and young children, an excellent view of the main pulmonary artery and its bifurcation into the two pulmonary artery branches can be obtained from the manubrium sternum (Fig 3–39). To generate this view, the transducer is first placed in the suprasternal notch in the standard short-axis plane. The transducer is then gradually moved inferiorly onto the manubrium sternum and tilted superiorly until the entire pulmonary artery bifurcation is imaged.

THE NORMAL M-MODE ECHOCARDIOGRAPHIC EXAMINATION

With the marriage of M-mode and two-dimensional ultrasound systems, the performance of the M-mode echocardiographic examination using a standalone M-mode instrument has been virtually abandoned. Now, M-mode echocardiograms are usually generated from the two-dimensional ultrasound system with the imaging plane used to guide placement of the M-mode ultrasound beam. Thus, an M-mode echocardiogram of any cardiac structure can be obtained from any cardiac plane simply by obtaining a two-dimensional echocardiographic image and positioning a cursor line on the image through the structure to be interrogated. The use of a two-dimensional image for operator guidance and orientation has greatly increased the ease and rapidity of obtaining the M-mode echocardiogram.

M-Mode Echocardiogram of the Right and Left Ventricles

M-mode echocardiograms of the right and left ventricles can be generated from many different two-dimensional echocardiographic planes; however, prior to the development of two-dimensional echocardiography, the first M-mode examination of the right and left ventricles was obtained from a location corresponding to the parasternal long-axis view.[26-33] Both the parasternal long- and short-axis views can be used to generate conventional M-mode

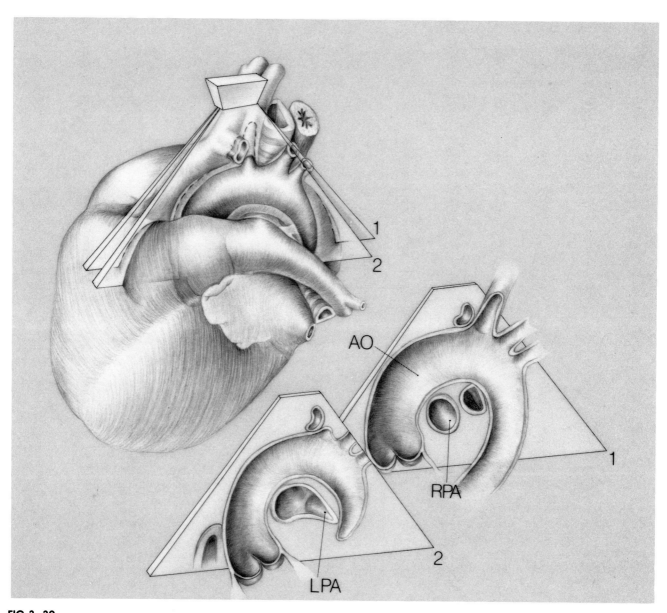

FIG 3–32.
Diagram of the suprasternal long-axis planes. *Plane 1* is a long-axis view through the entire aortic arch. *Plane 2* is a long-axis view obtained by tilting the plane slightly leftward to visualize more of the descending aorta and left pulmonary artery (LPA). *AO* = aorta; *RPA* = right pulmonary artery.

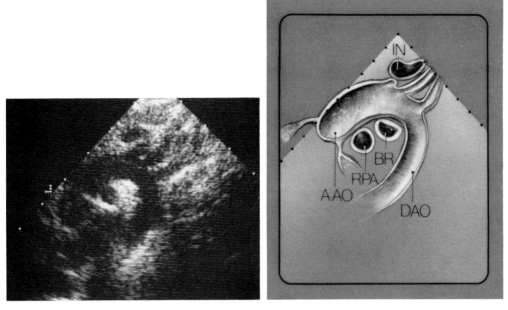

FIG 3–33.
Suprasternal long-axis view of the entire aortic arch from a normal patient. *AAO* = ascending aorta; *BR* = right mainstem bronchus; *DAO* = descending aorta; *IN* = innominate vein; and *RPA* = right pulmonary artery.

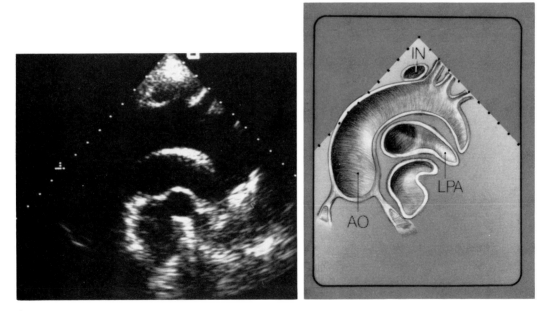

FIG 3–34.
Suprasternal long-axis view with the plane of sound tilted to visualize the left pulmonary artery (LPA). *AO* = aorta, *IN* = innominate vein.

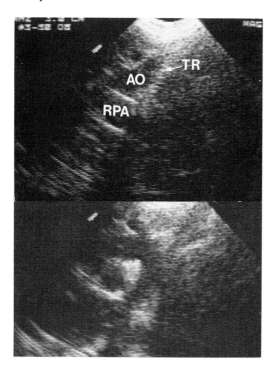

FIG 3–35.
Suprasternal long-axis views from a normal patient with a left-sided aortic arch. In the *top frame*, the cartilaginous rings of the trachea (TR) are visualized alongside the ascending aorta (AO). In the *bottom frame*, the plane of sound is tilted toward the patient's left side and the entire aortic arch can be seen. This maneuver demonstrates that the aortic arch is located to the left of the trachea. *RPA* = right pulmonary artery.

echocardiograms of the right and left ventricles. With the parasternal short-axis view, the operator has the advantage of being certain that the ultrasound beam is directly perpendicular to the septum and the left ventricular posterior wall and through the center of the left ventricular cavity. This allows more accurate and reproducible measurements of the left ventricular walls and cavity than is possible from the parasternal long-axis view, where the left ventricular walls can be sectioned tangentially by the plane of sound or the plane of sound may not pass through the largest minor-axis dimension of the ventricle.

Using either the parasternal long- or short-axis view, a continuous M-mode echocardiographic recording of the cardiac structures from the level of the papillary muscles of the left ventricle to the level of the aortic valve can be obtained (Fig 3–40).[26–33] In the parasternal long-axis view, this recording is obtained by moving the cursor line from the left ventricular apex on the left side of the sector to the aortic root on the right side of the sector. In the parasternal short-axis view, this recording is obtained by leaving the M-mode cursor line stationary through the center of the left ventricle while the transducer is tilted superiorly until the aortic root is imaged.

At the level of the papillary muscles (Fig 3–41), the

ultrasound beam first traverses the chest wall, which appears at the top of the M-mode recording as a series of dense linear echoes. Next, the echoes that arise from the anterior wall of the right ventricle are seen. With high-frequency transducers and good near-field resolution, it is possible to distinguish echoes that arise from the epicardial and endocardial surfaces of the right ventricular anterior wall. This structure moves posteriorly during ventricular systole. The next structure seen on the M-mode echocardiogram is an echo-free space that represents the cavity of the apical portion of the right ventricle. After traversing the right ventricular cavity, the ultrasound beam traverses the interventricular septum. Echoes can be seen arising from the right and left ventricular surfaces of the septum. The normal septum moves posteriorly with ventricular systole. Often, echoes arising from papillary muscles or muscle bundles in the right ventricle are seen just anterior to the right ventricular surface of the septum. These echoes can be difficult to distinguish from the echoes that arise from the septal surface, and care must be taken not to overestimate the thickness of the ventricular septum. Posterior to the ventricular septum, the left ventricular cavity, another echo-free space, is encountered. Finally, the ultrasound beam traverses the left ventricular posterior wall and the posterior pericardium. The pericardial echo is generally the densest echo on the recording. In normal patients, echoes that arise from the epicardial surface of the left ventricular posterior wall cannot be distinguished from the pericardial echoes in diastole. In some patients in systole, a slight separation, visible as an echo-free space, can be seen between these two structures. The left ventricular endocardial echo is usually identified as the echo with the greatest amplitude of motion and the fastest rate of motion. In normal patients, the left ventricular posterior wall moves anteriorly in systole.

As the ultrasound beam is aimed more superiorly (see Fig 3–40), echoes that arise from the papillary muscles and chordae tendinae are encountered. In some patients, it may be difficult to distinguish these echoes from the echoes that arise from the left ventricular endocardium. In general, the chordal echoes have a lower amplitude and slower rate of motion than the true endocardial echoes. With more superior tilting, echoes arising from the posterior leaflet of the mitral valve are seen in the cavity of the left ventricle. As the sweep continues, echoes arising from the anterior leaflet of the mitral valve are seen. The anterior mitral valve leaflet has a complex pattern of motion that reflects events during diastolic filling.[34–37] The posterior mitral valve leaflet motion is a virtual mirror image of the motion of the anterior mitral valve leaflet. The motion of the normal mitral valve is illustrated in Figure 3–40. The point at which the mitral valve opens and mitral leaflet separation occurs in the beginning of diastole has been labeled the D point of the mitral valve. The valve opens with a rapid motion in early diastole and reaches its peak opening position during rapid ventricular filling at the E point. Following rapid filling, the valve begins to reclose fairly rapidly and

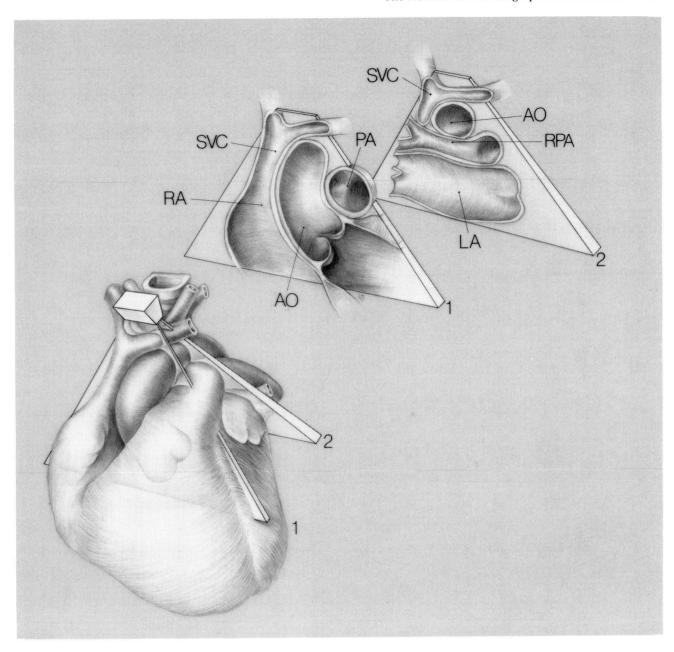

FIG 3–36.
Diagram of the suprasternal short-axis views obtained by placing the transducer in a frontal body plane in the suprasternal notch and tilting the transducer from anterior to posterior. *Plane 1* is obtained by tilting the transducer far anteriorly to image the entire ascending aorta (AO). *Plane 2* is obtained by tilting the transducer posteriorly to image the right pulmonary artery (RPA) and left atrium (LA). *PA* = pulmonary artery; *RA* = right atrium; and *SVC* = superior vena cava.

reaches a partially closed position labeled the F point. Following atrial systole, the valve reopens and reaches a maximum reopening at the A point. Following the A point, the valve rapidly begins to close and leaflet coaptation occurs at the C point. In some patients, a small forward motion occurs on the mitral valve echo between the A and C points. This point has been termed the B point and is caused by ventricular systole. After the C point, a single echo arising from the closed anterior and posterior mitral valve leaflets is seen throughout systole from the C to D points. This echo has a slight anterior motion in the left ventricle during systole, thought to be caused by the anterior motion of the mitral annulus during systole.

As the ultrasound beam is tilted more anteriorly, echoes that arise from the posterior mitral valve leaflet are no longer seen. At this level, the cavity anterior to the anterior

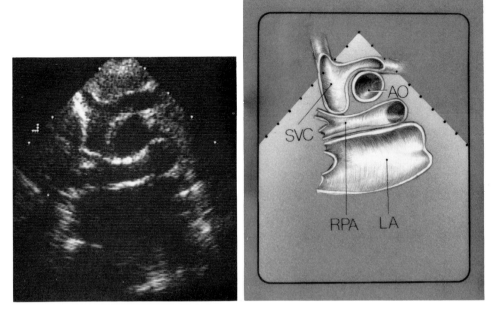

FIG 3–37.
Standard suprasternal short-axis view in a normal patient. In this view, a long section of the right pulmonary artery (RPA) can be seen.
AO = aorta; LA = left atrium; and SVC = superior vena cava.

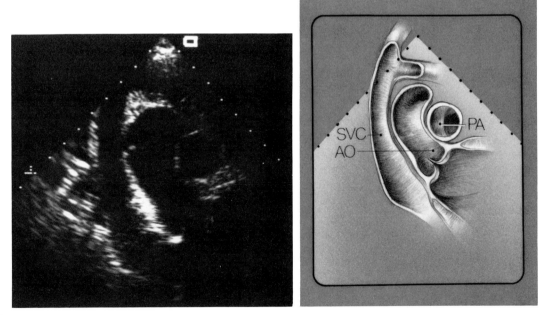

FIG 3–38.
Suprasternal short-axis view of the ascending aorta (AO) in a normal patient. A long section of the superior vena cava (SVC) and its junction with the right atrium can be seen along the right side of the AO. PA = pulmonary artery.

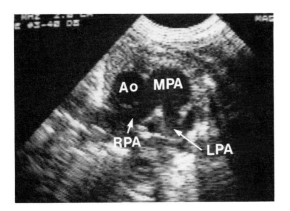

FIG 3–39.
A short-axis view obtained from the manubrium sternum of a normal patient. In this view, the entire main pulmonary artery (MPA) and its bifurcation into right and left pulmonary artery branches (RPA, LPA) can be seen. This view is particularly useful for determining if the pulmonary artery branches are continuous with one another and for diagnosing pulmonary artery stenosis.

mitral valve leaflet is the left ventricular outflow tract, and the cavity posterior to the anterior mitral valve leaflet is the inferior portion of the left atrium. Posteriorly, the left ventricular posterior wall echoes are no longer seen; in their place, the left atrial wall echoes can be seen. As the beam is tilted more anteriorly, the echoes from the ventricular septum are continuous with the echoes of the anterior aortic root, and the echoes of the anterior mitral valve leaflet are continuous with the echoes of the posterior aortic root. At the level of the aortic valve, the right ventricular

cavity is seen anteriorly. The aortic root occupies the middle of the recording, and the left atrial cavity is seen posteriorly. The echoes that arise from the aortic root move anteriorly in systole and posteriorly in diastole. The posterior aortic root echo really represents the echoes that arise from both the posterior aortic wall and the anterior wall of the left atrium. In the normal patient, virtually no perceptible motion of the left atrial posterior wall is seen at the level of the aortic root. Most of the change in the left atrial volume that occurs throughout the cardiac cycle is caused by displacement of the posterior wall of the aorta and, as a consequence, motion of the left atrial anterior wall.[38, 39] Left atrial posterior wall motion is more pronounced at the level of the atrioventricular junction, where anterior motion occurs during ventricular diastole, which mirrors the anterior mitral valve leaflet motion.[40]

From the parasternal long-axis view of the right ventricle, or from the parasternal short-axis view, it is possible to obtain an M-mode echocardiogram of the right atrium and tricuspid valve. Tricuspid valve motion is identical to mitral valve motion and is labeled in the same way (Fig 3–42).

M-Mode Echocardiogram of the Aortic and Pulmonic Valves

From the parasternal short-axis view, the M-mode cursor line can be positioned through the aortic or the pulmonic valve so that valve leaflet motion can be recorded (Fig 3–43).[41–43] Throughout diastole, a single echo can be seen arising from the closed semilunar valve leaflets. This

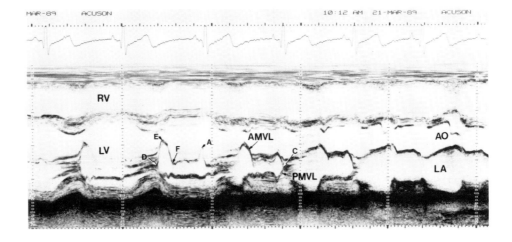

FIG 3–40.
Normal M-mode echocardiographic recording from the level of the mitral valve chordae to the level of the aortic valve. This M-mode echocardiogram shows the right ventricle (RV) anteriorly and the left ventricle (LV) posteriorly. Note that the echoes that arise from the ventricular septum are continuous with the anterior aortic (AO) root. Similarly, the echoes that arise from the anterior mitral valve leaflet (AMVL) are continuous with the posterior aortic root. The left atrium (LA) is seen behind the AO. The motion of the normal AMVL has been labelled. Mitral leaflet separation occurs at the beginning of diastole at the point labelled *D*. The valve reaches its peak opening position at the *E* point. Following rapid filling, the valve begins to reclose fairly rapidly and reaches a partially closed position, labelled *F*. Following atrial systole, the valve reopens and reaches a maximum reopening at the *A* point. Following the A point, the valve rapidly begins to close and leaflet coaptation occurs at the *C* point. The motion of the posterior mitral valve leaflet (PMVL) mirrors that of the AMVL.

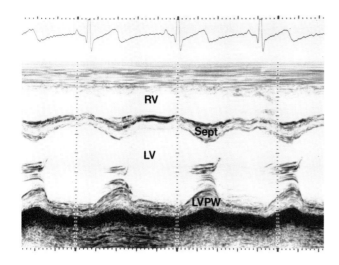

FIG 3–41.
Normal M-mode echocardiographic recording at the level of the papillary muscles of the left ventricle (LV). The right ventricle (RV) is seen anteriorly. Between the RV and LV, the echoes that arise from the ventricular septum (Sept) are seen. Far posteriorly, echoes arising from the endocardial and epicardial surfaces of the left ventricular posterior wall (LVPW) are seen.

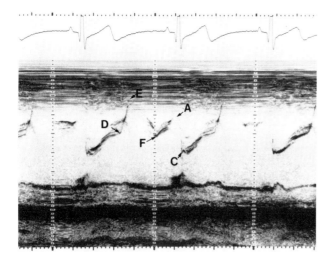

FIG 3–42.
M-mode echocardiogram of a normal tricuspid valve. Tricuspid valve motion is nearly identical to mitral valve motion and is labeled as it is in Figure 3–40.

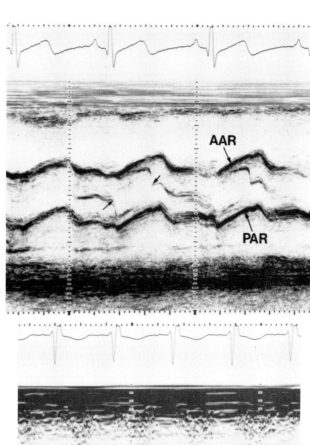

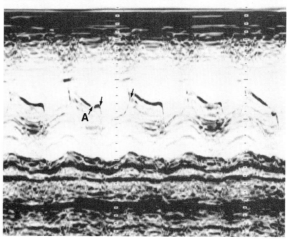

FIG 3–43.
M-mode echocardiographic recordings of the normal aortic (*top*) and pulmonary (*bottom*) valves. Throughout diastole, a single echo can be seen arising from the closed semilunar valve leaflets. At the end of diastole, the valve leaflets move rapidly to the open position and remain open throughout systole. At the end of systole, the leaflets close very rapidly. The *arrows* indicate the opening and closure of the semilunar valve leaflets. A = the A-wave of the pulmonary valve echo caused by right atrial contraction; AAR = anterior aortic root; and PAR = posterior aortic root.

echo has a gradual posterior motion throughout diastole. Following atrial systole, a posterior indentation can be seen on the echo that arises from the closed semilunar valve. This indentation is caused by pressure transmitted to the closed semilunar valve during the atrial filling phase of ventricular diastole. Because the pulmonary artery diastolic pressure is low, this identation, called the A wave,

is more pronounced on the pulmonary valve echo than on the aortic valve echo. Also, because right atrial and right ventricular filling are influenced by respiration, the size of the A wave of the pulmonary valve varies considerably throughout the respiratory cycle.[40]

Following the A wave at the end of diastole, the valve leaflets move rapidly to the open position and remain open throughout systole. At the end of systole, the leaflets close rapidly. If two leaflets of the valve are crossed by the ultrasound beam, the echocardiogram of the valve resembles a box throughout systole.[40] Frequently, only one leaflet of the valve can be seen; however, the opening and closure points of the valve in systole can usually still be identified because of the rapid motion that the valve makes at these time points.

THE NORMAL DOPPLER EXAMINATION

Pulsed and continuous-wave Doppler echocardiography can be performed using a standalone Doppler transducer or a transducer that combines two-dimensional imaging and Doppler ultrasound. In the combined systems, the imaging plane is used to guide placement of the Doppler ultrasound beam. Most cardiac structures can be examined with Doppler echocardiography from multiple transducer positions and multiple imaging planes; however, usually only one or two transducer positions will allow the Doppler beam to be aligned parallel with blood flow in the structure being interrogated. As noted in Chapter 1, if the intercept angle between the Doppler beam and red blood cell flow is greater than 20 degrees, a correction for intercept angle should be made by dividing the Doppler frequency shifts by the cosine of the intercept angle. Because of the difficulties of measuring the intercept angle, discussed in Chapter 1, we do not recommend the use of angle-corrected Doppler velocities. In this section, techniques for performing the normal Doppler examination will be reviewed, and only those approaches that allow the Doppler recording to be obtained without the need for angle correction will be discussed.

Superior and Inferior Venae Cavae

Superior vena caval flow velocity can be recorded from the suprasternal notch or from the subcostal position. These recordings are easily accomplished without imaging by simply directing the Doppler beam lateral to the ascending aorta (toward the patient's right side). From the suprasternal notch, flow in the superior vena cava is directed away from the transducer (below the baseline); from the subcostal approach, flow is toward the transducer (above the baseline). Inferior vena caval flow is usually best recorded from a subcostal position (especially the subcostal sagittal view of the venae cavae). From this position, flow in the inferior vena cava is directed away from the transducer (below the baseline).

Blood flow in the caval veins is continuous, with one peak in systole and one peak in early diastole before atrial contraction (Fig 3–44). Increases in forward flow can be seen with inspiration. Flow reversals (of short duration and very low peak velocities) can be recorded in early diastole before the second peak and with atrial contraction.

Peak flow velocities in the venae cavae range from 0.5

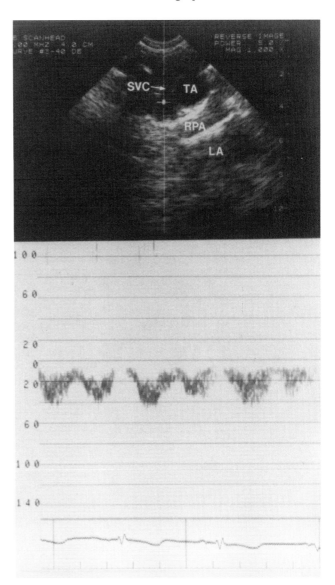

FIG 3–44.
Doppler recording from the superior vena cava (SVC) of a normal patient. The freeze-frame image (*top*) of the suprasternal short-axis view shows the position of the sample volume at the time of the Doppler recording. The Doppler spectral recording (*bottom*) shows normal forward flow away from the transducer and below the baseline. This flow is continuous, with one peak in systole and one peak in diastole before atrial contraction. LA = left atrium; RPA = right pulmonary artery; and TA = transverse aorta. (From Snider AR: Doppler echocardiography in congenital heart disease, in Berger M (ed): *Doppler Echocardiography in Heart Disease.* New York, Marcel Dekker, Inc, 1987, p 216. Used by permission.)

to 1.5 m/sec but can reach as high as 2 m/sec during deep inspiration. Flow velocities are usually higher in infants and small children than in adults. The highest velocity usually occurs during systole. With rapid heart rates, only one peak is seen, and forward flow is continuous.[44]

Tricuspid Valve Inflow

Tricuspid valve flow velocities are best recorded from a parasternal short-axis view or an apical four-chamber view. In these views, forward flow across the tricuspid valve is directed toward the transducer and therefore is displayed above the baseline. The tricuspid valve velocity profile closely resembles a tricuspid valve M-mode echo, with forward flow peak velocities occurring during rapid ventricular filling (peak E velocity) and atrial contraction (peak A velocity) (Fig 3–45). The lowest values for the peak E and A velocities are recorded with the sample volume positioned just on the atrial side of the tricuspid annulus. As the sample volume is advanced through the valve, the

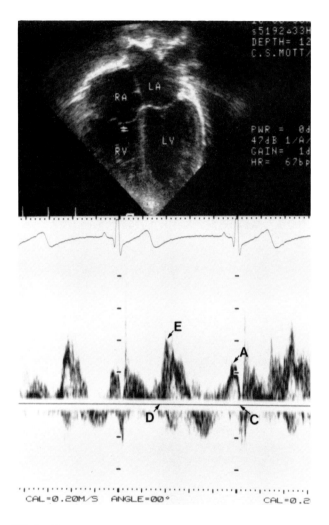

FIG 3–45.
Doppler recording from the tricuspid valve of a normal patient. The freeze-frame image (*top*) of the apical four-chamber view shows the position of the sample volume at the time of the Doppler recording. The Doppler spectral recording (*bottom*) shows normal forward flow toward the transducer and above the baseline at rapid ventricular filling (*E*) and with atrial contraction (*A*). The tricuspid valve opens at the beginning of diastole at the point labelled *D* and closes at the point labelled *C*.

peak E and A velocities increase (probably because the effective flow area decreases) and the valve leaflet motion can be recorded as a high-amplitude, high-velocity signal. The highest values for peak E and peak A velocity are usually recorded near the tips of the valve leaflets.

In general, tricuspid valve peak E velocity is higher than the tricuspid valve peak A velocity and lower than the mitral peak E velocity. In normal adults, the tricuspid peak E velocity is 0.5 m/sec (range 0.3 to 0.7 m/sec). In normal children, the peak E velocity is 0.6 m/sec (range 0.4 to 0.8 m/sec),[44, 45] the peak A velocity is 0.4 m/sec (range 0.2 to 0.6 m/sec), and the E/A velocity ratio is 1.6 (range 0.6 to 2.6). In normal patients, there is no flow across the tricuspid valve in systole.

Although the tricuspid peak E velocity is higher than the tricuspid peak A velocity in most normal subjects, there is one important exception. In the normal fetus and newborn infant, the tricuspid valve peak A velocity is larger than the tricuspid valve peak E velocity.[46, 47] The higher peak A velocity in the fetus and newborn infant indicates a greater reliance on the atrial contribution to right ventricular filling, probably as a result of right ventricular hypertrophy. In one study of normal fetuses from 20 to 40 weeks gestation, the tricuspid valve peak E velocity was 0.37 ± 0.08 m/sec, peak A velocity was 0.52 ± 0.07 m/sec, and the tricuspid velocity time integral was 5.9 ± 1.3 cm.[46] At each gestation, tricuspid valve peak E, peak A, and velocity time integral were higher than for the mitral valve (probably reflecting increased flow across the tricuspid valve in utero). The E/A velocity ratio for the tricuspid valve increased from 0.52 at 20 weeks to 0.84 at 40 weeks.

The tricuspid valve Doppler tracing shows a much greater variation in velocity with respiration than does the mitral valve Doppler tracing. With inspiration, tricuspid peak E and peak A velocities increase, and there is usually flow throughout diastole. In normal children (ages 1.5 to 11 years), the tricuspid peak E velocity increases by 26% from expiration to inspiration, the tricuspid peak A velocity increases by 18%, and the E/A velocity ratio remains unchanged. The percentages of the total Doppler area that occur during the first third of diastole, under the E wave, and under the A wave also remain unchanged with inspiration (see Chapter 4).[48]

Right Ventricular Outflow and Main Pulmonary Artery

The right ventricular outflow and pulmonary artery velocities are best recorded from the left parasternal or subcostal position. If the parasternal short-axis view is used, it may be necessary to place the transducer one or two intercostal spaces below the standard parasternal position. From this location, the transducer can be tilted very superiorly to align the Doppler beam with blood flow from the right ventricle. If the subcostal views are used, the transducer must be aimed anteriorly until the Doppler beam is parallel with the sternum and pointed slightly leftward.

On the Doppler graphic display, the right ventricular

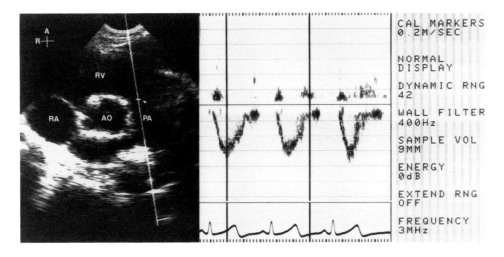

FIG 3–46.
Doppler recording from the pulmonary artery (PA) of a normal child from the parasternal short-axis view. The freeze-frame image (*left*) shows the position of the sample volume (*arrow*) in the PA just distal to the pulmonary valve at the time of the Doppler recording. The Doppler spectral recording (*right*) shows normal flow in systole below the baseline and away from the transducer. The peak velocity of the systolic flow is about 0.7 m/sec. A small amount of retrograde flow is recorded in early diastole and is caused by movement of the column of blood back down to the closed pulmonary valve. A = anterior; AO = aorta; R = right; RA = right atrium; and RV = right ventricle. (From Snider AR: Doppler echocardiography in congenital heart disease, in Berger M (ed): *Doppler Echocardiography in Heart Disease*. New York, Marcel Dekker, Inc, 1987, p 215. Used by permission.)

outflow velocity appears as a negative waveform (flow is away from the transducer) in systole. As the sample volume is moved from the right ventricular outflow tract through the pulmonary valve, pulmonary valve opening and closure are seen. When the sample volume is moved farther distally into the main pulmonary artery, the velocity patterns are similar to those in the right ventricular outflow tract; however, the peak velocity is slightly higher and the time from the onset of flow to the peak velocity (acceleration time) is shorter.[49] On the main pulmonary artery Doppler (Fig 3–46), the initial downward deflection usually has a narrow bandwidth up to the peak velocity. Spectral broadening occurs following the peak velocity. At end-systole, the velocity returns to zero and remains close to zero throughout diastole. Occasionally, a small amount of retrograde flow can be recorded in early diastole. This retrograde flow is caused by movement of the column of blood back down to the closed pulmonary valve. Also, in young children especially, a small, forward-flow velocity can often be recorded in late diastole and is caused by right atrial contraction.[45]

Normal values for pulmonary artery peak velocities in children have been reported to be slightly higher than those in adults (children = 0.9 m/sec, range 0.7 to 1.1; adults = 0.75 m/sec, range 0.6 to 0.9).[44] A recent study of normal pulmonary artery peak velocities has shown some age-related differences. In 28 newborns, peak pulmonary velocities (0.68 ± 0.09 m/sec) were significantly lower than those in older children (0.80 ± 0.12 m/sec).[45]

Pulmonary Veins

Velocities in the pulmonary veins can be recorded from several transducer locations; the best alignment with flow, however, is usually obtained from an apical or subcostal position. As in the caval veins, flow in the pulmonary veins is nearly continuous. Unlike in the caval veins, however, the peak velocity occurs during diastole before atrial contraction. Short periods of flow reversal can often be seen at the beginning of diastole and after atrial contraction.[44]

Mitral Valve Inflow

Maximal velocities through the mitral valve are usually best recorded from the apical four-chamber view. In this view, forward flow across the mitral valve is directed toward the transducer and is therefore displayed above the baseline. Like the tricuspid valve, the mitral valve velocity profile closely resembles a mitral valve M-mode recording (Fig 3–47). Forward flow occurs during rapid ventricular filling (peak E velocity) and during atrial contraction (peak A velocity). The lowest values for the peak E and A velocities are recorded with the sample volume positioned just on the left atrial side of the mitral annulus. As the sample volume is advanced through the valve, the peak E and A velocities increase (because of a decrease in the effective flow area) and the valve opening and closure can be recorded. The highest values for peak E and peak A velocity are recorded near the tips of the mitral leaflets.

Usually, the mitral peak E velocity is higher. Following the peak E velocity, the diastolic flow velocities decline rapidly toward zero flow, then increase again during the smaller peak A velocity. Normally, mitral valve flow velocities exceed tricuspid valve flow velocities. In normal adults, mitral peak E velocity is 0.6 to 0.68 m/sec, peak A velocity is 0.38 to 0.48 m/sec, and E/A velocity ratio is 1.7 ± 0.4 to 2.5 ± 0.9.[50–53] In normal children we have examined, peak E velocity is 0.91 ± 0.11 m/sec, peak A velocity is 0.49 ± 0.08 m/sec, and E/A velocity ratio is 1.9 ± 0.4.[48, 54]

In most normal subjects, the mitral valve peak E ve-

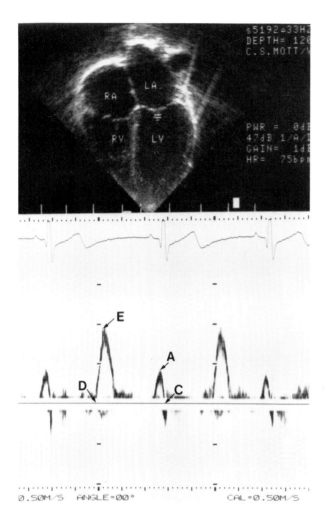

FIG 3–47.
Doppler spectral recording from the mitral valve of a normal patient. The freeze-frame image (*top*) of the apical four-chamber view shows the position of the sample volume at the time of the Doppler recording. The Doppler spectral recording (*bottom*) shows normal forward flow toward the transducer and above the baseline at rapid ventricular filling (*E*) and during atrial contraction (*A*). The opening of the mitral valve leaflets occurs at the beginning of diastole (*D*) and the closure of the leaflets is labelled *C*.

locity is higher than the mitral valve peak A velocity, although there are several age-related exceptions. In the fetus and newborn infant and in elderly adults, mitral peak A velocity is normally higher than the peak E velocity.[46, 47, 52] The higher peak A velocity in the normal fetus and newborn infant indicate a greater reliance on the atrial contribution to left ventricular filling. This may be caused by decreased compliance of the neonatal left ventricular myocardium, possibly as a result of its higher water content and myofiber disarray. In one study of fetuses from 20 to 40 weeks gestation, the mitral peak E velocity was 0.33 ± 0.06 m/sec, peak A was 0.45 ± 0.07 m/sec, and the velocity time integral was 5.3 ± 1.1 cm.[46] The E/A velocity ratio for the mitral valve increased from 0.63 at 20 weeks to 0.83 at 40 weeks. At each gestational age, mitral valve peak E, peak A, and velocity time integral were lower than for the tricuspid valve (probably reflecting less flow in utero across the mitral valve); however, the E/A ratios of the two valves were similar throughout gestation, indicating equivalent diastolic ventricular function.[46]

With respiration, the mitral valve Doppler tracing shows less variability than does the tricuspid valve Doppler tracing. With inspiration in normal adults, the mitral peak E velocity decreases by 9% and peak A velocity remains unchanged.[55] In normal children (ages 1.5 to 11 years), mitral peak E velocity decreases by 8% from expiration to inspiration, mitral peak A velocity remains unchanged, and the E/A velocity ratio decreases by 14%.[48]

Left Ventricular Outflow and Ascending and Descending Aorta

The left ventricular outflow tract velocity is best recorded from an apical four-chamber view with the transducer tilted anteriorly to image the ascending aorta. From this position, the left ventricular outflow velocity appears as a negative waveform (flow is away from the transducer) in systole. The peak velocity is normally 1.0 m/sec (range 0.7 to 1.2 m/sec) in children.[44] As the sample volume is advanced through the aortic annulus, valve leaflet motion can be detected. At this point, the velocity profile changes slightly. The peak velocity occurs earlier and is slightly higher. With further advancement of the sample volume, the ascending aorta Doppler can be recorded (Fig 3–48).

Ascending aortic flow velocities can be recorded from the suprasternal notch, cardiac apex, or a high right parasternal location. In normal subjects, higher velocities can often be recorded from the suprasternal notch using the small, static Doppler transducer.[44] To record flow in the ascending aorta from the suprasternal notch, the transducer is tilted anteriorly and slightly rightward. For the descending aorta Doppler recording, the transducer is tilted posteriorly and slightly leftward. From the suprasternal and high right parasternal locations, systolic flow in the ascending aorta is directed toward the transducer (above the baseline), while from the apical location, ascending aorta flow is directed away from the transducer (below the baseline).

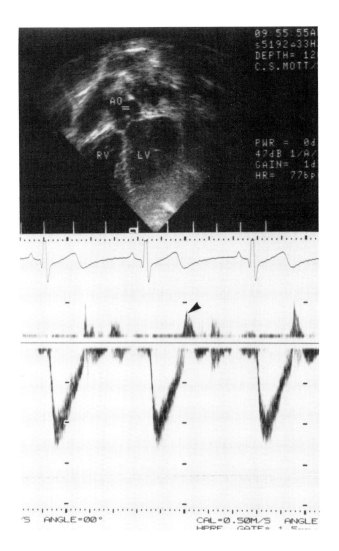

FIG 3–48.
Doppler recording from the ascending aorta (AO) of a normal child. The freeze-frame image (*top*) of the apical five-chamber view shows the position of the sample volume at the time of the Doppler recording. The Doppler spectral recording (*bottom*) shows normal forward flow away from the transducer and below the baseline throughout systole. A small amount of retrograde flow (*arrow*) is recorded in early diastole and is caused by movement of the column of blood back down to the closed aortic valve. *LV* = left ventricle; *RV* = right ventricle.

In the ascending aorta, the initial systolic deflection is abrupt, reaches the peak velocity early, and has a narrow bandwidth. After the peak velocity, spectral broadening occurs and the downslope reaches the zero flow line rather rapidly. A short period of flow reversal is usually recorded in early diastole and represents movement of the column of blood back toward the closed aortic valve. Compared with the normal pulmonary artery velocity profile, the aortic velocities are higher, have a more rapid rate of acceleration to the peak velocity, and have a shorter time interval from the onset of flow to the peak velocity. Maximal aortic

flow velocity in children (1.5 m/sec, range 1.2 to 1.8 m/sec) is higher than it is in adults (1.35 m/sec, range 1.0 to 1.7).[44] In a recent study, no differences were noted between ascending aortic velocities in newborns (0.89 ± 0.13 m/sec) and older children (0.90 ± 0.16 m/sec).[45]

Descending aortic flow velocities can best be recorded from the suprasternal notch. From this location, the velocity profile is similar to that recorded for the ascending aorta, but flow is directed away from the transducer (Fig 3–49). Normal values for descending aortic flow velocities recorded from the suprasternal notch of children have been reported to be 0.88 m/sec (range 0.51 to 1.04 m/sec).[45]

The Normal Color-Flow Doppler Examination

On the color Doppler instrument, the detected Doppler frequency shifts are assigned colors based on their direction and magnitude. In most systems, Doppler frequency shifts arising from blood flow toward the transducer are color-coded as red, and Doppler frequency shifts arising from blood flow away from the transducer are color-coded as blue. The velocity is proportional to the brightness of the color, and most systems have 16 or more gradations of each color. The degree of variance or turbulence is calculated and color-coded as yellow or green; these colors, when mixed with red or blue, produce a mosaic of colors. Color-coding demonstrates three aspects of intracardiac flow: direction of flow, velocity of flow, and turbulence.

With the transducer at the cardiac apex or in a low parasternal position, left ventricular diastolic inflow normally appears as a diffuse red color and systolic outflow appears as a blue color located primarily along the interventricular septum (Plates 3 to 8). To perform the examination, the echocardiographer first obtains a conventional two-dimensional echocardiographic image. The color Doppler is then activated, and color-flow information is superimposed on the two-dimensional image. Several factors are important when performing the color Doppler examination. First, anatomical imaging is most effective when the echocardiographic targets are perpendicular to the ultrasound beam; flow detection by Doppler examination, on the other hand, is most effective when the echocardiographic targets (red blood cells) are parallel to the ultrasound beam. Therefore, transducer positions that provide the best images of the cardiac structures are usually not optimal positions for obtaining the Doppler color-flow information. It is necessary to move the transducer into multiple positions and planes for optimal visualization of the Doppler color-flow map. Second, several black areas appear in the normal Doppler color-flow map. The black areas occur where (1) no Doppler frequency shifts are detected because in that area flow is perpendicular to the ultrasound beam or because there is no flow in that area, (2) the flow velocity is below the minimal threshold for recording a flow velocity (this threshold is 20 to 30 cm/sec in most instruments, e.g., around the cardiac apex), and (3) the black area is too distant from the transducer for adequate ultrasound penetration (e.g., left atrium). Third, because on most instruments the Nyquist limit is low (60 to 80 cm/sec) at the depth settings necessary to image most patients, aliasing will occur at normal outflow velocities. This accounts for the mosaic pattern seen in the left ventricular outflow tract in systole in the normal patient in Plate 6.

From the parasternal short-axis view at the base of the heart, right ventricular diastolic inflow is seen on the right as a red color; right ventricular systolic outflow is seen on the left as a blue color. From the subcostal positions, flow in the normal superior vena cava is of low velocity and directed towards the transducer (red). On the other hand, inferior vena cava flow is directed away from the transducer and is therefore blue. As in the apical and parasternal views, ventricular diastolic inflow is seen as a diffuse red color and ventricular systolic outflow is seen as a blue color, often with mild aliasing just proximal to the semilunar valve. In the suprasternal views, systolic flow in the ascending aorta is directed toward the transducer and is therefore red. Systolic flow in the descending aorta is away from the transducer and is blue. Superior vena caval flow is blue because it is directed away from the transducer.

On the Doppler color-flow examination, more low-velocity flow information (i.e., in the atria, the pulmonary veins, or the systemic veins) can be displayed by setting the wall filters at their lowest cutoff value or by decreasing the velocity scale (or pulse repetition frequency) of the color Doppler display. On the Doppler color flow examination, areas of mosaic flow can be caused by the presence of high velocity, disturbed flow, or can be caused by aliasing of normal flow. These two conditions can be distinguished by increasing the Nyquist limit of the color Doppler

system (i.e., increasing the velocity scale or shifting the baseline) to display the flow unambiguously. If these maneuvers allow the flow to be displayed as a single color, the mosaic colors represent aliasing of normal flow signals. If the mosiac flow pattern is not altered by these maneuvers, it most likely represents an area of high velocity, disturbed flow. This conclusion can be confirmed by examination of the mosaic flow area with pulsed or continuous-wave Doppler techniques.

Valvular Insufficiency in Normal Subjects

Using pulsed and color-flow Doppler techniques, recent investigators have reported variable incidences of valvular regurgitation in apparently healthy subjects. One study of 20 normal individuals found tricuspid regurgitation in 95%, pulmonary regurgitation in 35%, mitral regurgitation in 10%, and aortic regurgitation in 0%.[56] Another study using pulsed Doppler echocardiography showed prevalence rates for valvular insufficiency to be 92% for the pulmonary valve, 44% for the tricuspid valve, 40% for the mitral valve, and 33% for the aortic valve.[57] Using color-flow mapping, Yoshida and colleagues found that the incidence of valvular regurgitation in normal subjects was related to age.[58] For the mitral valve, the prevalence of insufficiency was 38% to 45% in all age groups. Aortic insufficiency was found in none of the normal subjects (whose ages were from 6 to 49 years old). For the right heart valves, the prevalence of valvular regurgitation decreased with advancing age. For example, tricuspid regurgitation was found in 78% of subjects aged 6 to 9 years old

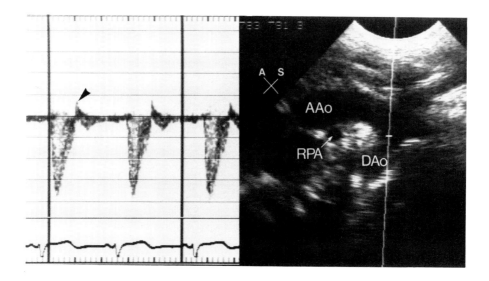

FIG 3–49.
Doppler recording from the descending aorta (DAO) of a normal patient. The freeze-frame image (*right*) shows the position of the sample volume in the DAO at the time of the Doppler spectral recording. The Doppler tracing (*left*) shows normal forward flow in systole away from the transducer and below the baseline. In diastole, a small amount of retrograde flow (*arrow*) is seen above the baseline. This short period of flow reversal represents movement of the column of blood back toward the closed aortic valve. A = anterior; AAO = ascending aorta; RPA = right pulmonary artery; and S = superior. (From Snider AR: Doppler echocardiography: Basic principles and clinical applications, in Buda A (ed): *Digital Cardiac Imaging*. The Hague, Martinus-Nijhoff, 1985, p 187. Used by permission.)

and 15% of subjects aged 40 to 49 years old. Pulmonary regurgitation occurred in 88% of children and 28% of middle-aged adults. It is postulated that the higher prevalence of right heart-valve regurgitation in younger persons is caused by superior ultrasound penetration in these subjects. With advancing age, ultrasound penetration becomes poorer and small amounts of physiologic regurgitation become more difficult to detect.[58] Also, the overall incidence of physiologic valvular regurgitation is higher in studies using color-flow mapping than in those using conventional pulsed Doppler techniques. Because many regurgitant jets in normal subjects are localized or extremely eccentric, failure to position the sample volume of the pulsed Doppler in the jet can lead to false negative results.

For normal or physiologic valvular regurgitation, the regurgitant flow signals are localized to the vicinity of the valve closure, and the regurgitant jet area measured from the color Doppler examination is much smaller than that seen in patients with organic valvular regurgitation. The diagnosis of abnormal valvular regurgitation requires a larger regurgitant jet area and the presence of elevated intravascular pressures, dilated valve annulus, or structural abnormality of the valve itself. In addition, physiologic valvular regurgitation can be distinguished from Doppler ghosting or other low-velocity signals by requiring that the regurgitation peak velocity approximate that expected for the normal Bernoulli-predicted pressure gradients between the affected chambers.[59] This velocity is 1.2 to 1.5 m/sec for right heart valves. For left heart valves, the peak velocity often cannot be measured accurately because the tiny regurgitant orifice leads to a spray rather than a discrete jet. Artifacts caused by the motion of valves or wall structures can be difficult to distinguish with certainty from physiologic valvular regurgitation. In general, these artifacts are limited in time and have a sharp, high-pitched audio signal.[57]

THE NORMAL CONTRAST ECHOCARDIOGRAPHIC EXAMINATION

In the late 1960s, Gramiak and Shah first described the echocardiographic contrast effect produced by the injection of indocyanine green dye during cardiac catheterization.[1, 60] Using injections of this dye, dextrose water, saline, or the patient's own blood, subsequent investigators used contrast echocardiography to (1) verify structures on the echocardiogram, (2) detect intracardiac shunts, (3) visualize intracardiac flow patterns, and (4) evaluate complex congenital malformations.[61–67] In many of these circumstances, pulsed and color-flow Doppler techniques have replaced the need for contrast echocardiography. However, there are still some echocardiographic examinations in which contrast injections are necessary to obtain complete diagnostic information.

In this section, we will review the techniques for performing the contrast echocardiogram and provide examples of the more common clinical applications of this technique. Throughout the remaining chapters, the results of contrast echocardiographic examinations in specific cardiac defects will be included in situations where this technique is especially useful.

Basic Principles of Contrast Echocardiography

It is believed that tiny gas bubbles suspended in the contrast agent act as specular reflectors of ultrasound and produce contrast echoes. It has been suggested that these microbubbles form by cavitation at the needle tip during forceful injections or that they are caused by the injection of small amounts of gas trapped in the injecting apparatus.[68, 69] The studies of Meltzer and Popp suggest that microbubbles ranging in diameter from 10 to 100 μm are present in the injectant and are the source of the contrast effect.[70]

The cloud of echoes produced by the contrast injection follows the downstream flow of blood. Microbubbles giving rise to the contrast effect are completely filtered by the systemic and pulmonary capillary beds. Therefore, contrast echoes will not appear in the left heart following a systemic venous injection unless an intracardiac or intrapulmonary right-to-left shunt is present. Also, contrast echoes will not appear in the right heart following a left heart injection unless an intracardiac left-to-right shunt is present.[1]

Techniques for Performing Contrast Echocardiography

Peripheral venous contrast echocardiography can be performed using the superficial veins of the scalp, arms, or legs. In our laboratory, a 23- or 25-gauge needle is placed in the vein and connected by a stopcock to two small syringes filled with saline. Vigorous shaking of the vial of saline prior to filling the syringes enhances the contrast effect (probably by increasing the amount of microbubbles in the solution). For the contrast injection, 0.5 to 3 cc of saline are rapidly injected from the first syringe with a force similar to that of a good hand angiogram, followed by a similar injection from the second syringe. For the newborn infant, a contrast echocardiogram can be performed with as little as 1 cc of saline. In older patients, the contrast effect can be enhanced by squeezing or elevating the arm after the contrast injection to free microbubbles that adhere to the vessel endothelium. In patients old enough to cooperate, the contrast effect can be enhanced by injecting both syringes of saline while the patient performs a Valsalva maneuver and observing the echocardiogram during the release phase of the maneuver.[1]

Clinical Applications of Contrast Echocardiography

Detection of Right-to-Left Shunts

Peripheral venous contrast echocardiography is especially useful for the detection of right-to-left shunts. The appearance of contrast echoes in the left heart following a peripheral venous injection indicates a right-to-left shunt, either intracardiac or intrapulmonary. With intrapulmonary right-to-left shunts, contrast echoes are delayed three to four cardiac cycles before their appearance in the left atrium.[71] With intracardiac right-to-left shunts, contrast echoes appear in the left heart on the same or subsequent cardiac cycle. Contrast echocardiography is extremely sensitive and can be used to detect intracardiac right-to-left shunts as small as 5% of systemic blood flow.[62, 66]

The apical four-chamber view, which images all four cardiac chambers and the atrial and ventricular septa simultaneously, is especially useful for localization of the site of an intracardiac shunt. In patients with atrial right-to-left shunts, contrast echoes appear first in the right atrium, then cross the interatrial septum into the left atrium during rapid ventricular filling and at the onset of ventricular diastole. Contrast echoes then enter the right and left ventricles nearly simultaneously by passing through the atrioventricular valve orifices in diastole (Fig 3–50).[62, 63] Atrial right-to-left shunting can be observed in infants with primary pulmonary hypertension, patients with Ebstein anomaly of the tricuspid valve, patients with baffle leaks after the Mustard operation, and children with congenital heart disease and obligatory right-to-left atrial shunting (i.e., total anomalous pulmonary venous return). Also, most simple atrial septal defects exhibit bidirectional shunting because of the right-to-left pressure gradient present with the onset of ventricular contraction.[72] Contrast echocardiography is extremely sensitive and can detect this interatrial right-to-left shunt even when systemic arterial saturations are normal and standard dye curves show no right-to-left shunting.[62] The detection of the right-to-left shunt in a simple atrial septal defect can be enhanced by having the patient perform a Valsalva maneuver during the contrast injection.

In patients with ventricular right-to-left shunts, contrast echoes appear first in the right atrium and right ventricle and then pass into the left ventricle. The right-to-left ventricular shunt commences with the onset of the isovolumic relaxation phase of ventricular diastole (Fig 3–51).[62, 63, 67] Right-to-left ventricular shunts occur in patients with tetralogy of Fallot, double-outlet right ventricle, pulmonary atresia with a ventricular septal defect, and truncus arteriosus. Also, in isolated ventricular septal defects in which the right ventricular pressure is increased to approximately 50% or more of the left ventricular pressure, right-to-left shunting occurs because of asynchronous changes in pressure of the two ventricles.[63, 65, 67, 73] In small ventricular septal defects, right ventricular pressure does not exceed left ventricular pressure in early diastole and no right-to-left shunt occurs. In ventricular septal defects with moderately elevated right ventricular pressure, the right-to-left shunt occurs only in early diastole. In ventricular septal defects with near-systemic right ventricular pressure, the right-to-left shunt persists throughout the duration of diastole.[73] In some large, nonrestrictive ventricular septal defects, right-to-left shunting also occurs in late ventricular systole, and blood flows directly from the right ventricle into the aorta in systole.

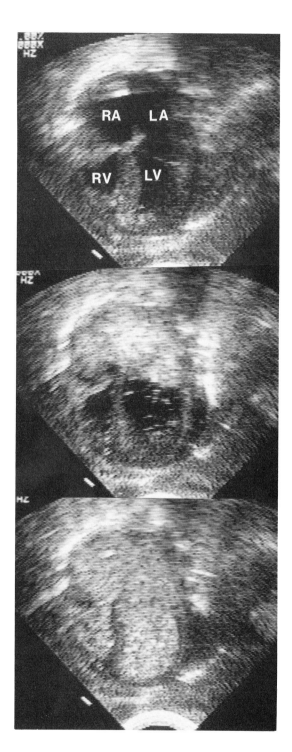

FIG 3–50.
Apical four-chamber views from a patient with Ebstein anomaly of the tricuspid valve who was postoperative tricuspid valve annuloplasty. The *top frame* shows the apical four-chamber view before injection of a contrast agent into a peripheral vein. In the *second frame,* contrast echoes are seen filling the right atrium (RA) and left atrium (LA). This indicates a right-to-left atrial shunt. In the *bottom frame,* contrast echoes are seen filling both the right ventricle (RV) and the left ventricle (LV) because of forward flow during diastole.

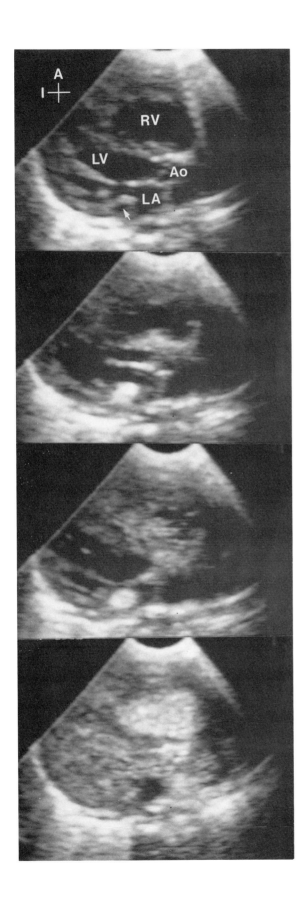

FIG 3–51.
Left arm vein contrast injection in the parasternal long-axis view in a patient with persistent left superior vena cava draining to the coronary sinus and a large ventricular septal defect. The *top frame* shows the long-axis view before injection of the contrast agent. The coronary sinus (*arrow*) was enlarged, suggesting the possibility of a persistent left superior vena cava draining to the coronary sinus. The *second frame* was obtained immediately after injection of contrast into a left arm vein. Contrast echoes, seen first filling the coronary sinus, confirm the presence of a left superior vena cava draining to the coronary sinus. In the *third frame,* contrast echoes are seen filling the right ventricle (RV) because of forward flow from the coronary sinus to the right atrium to the RV. In the *fourth frame,* contrast echoes are seen filling the left ventricle (LV) and the aorta (AO) because of a right-to-left shunt through a ventricular septal defect. *A* = anterior; *I* = inferior; and *LA* = left atrium.

Structure Identification

Contrast echocardiography has been especially useful in verifying normal and abnormal anatomic structures seen during the two-dimensional echocardiographic examination.

For example, Figure 3–51 shows a large structure lying in the area of the atrioventricular groove. This structure probably represents an abnormal coronary sinus, possibly enlarged because of a connection to a persistent left superior vena cava. Echoes from a contrast injection in a left-arm vein first opacify the structure thought to be the coronary sinus and then appear in the right atrium and right ventricle. Thus, the existence of a persistent left superior vena cava draining to the coronary sinus is verified.[1]

Definition of Flow Patterns

After a contrast injection, microbubbles follow the downstream passage of blood and allow the identification of specific flow patterns in certain complex congenital heart defects. In this way, contrast echocardiography adds important physiologic flow information to the anatomic information already obtained from the two-dimensional echocardiogram. For example, in patients with situs ambiguus, right- and left-arm-vein injections can be used to define systemic venous flow patterns. In patients with d-transposition of the great arteries who have undergone an intra-atrial baffle procedure, contrast echocardiography can be used to detect the abnormal systemic venous flow patterns associated with superior vena caval obstruction (see Chapter 6).[1]

Detection of Left-to-Right Shunts

Left-to-right shunts can be diagnosed at cardiac catheterization and in the immediate postoperative period (in patients with a left atrial line) by contrast injections made in the left heart. Some types of left-to-right shunt can also be detected during peripheral venous contrast echocardiography. During contrast injections in patients with an atrial septal defect, non-contrast-containing blood passes across the atrial septum and washes contrast-containing blood out of the right atrium. This left-to-right atrial shunt produces a negative contrast effect in the right atrium.[74]

Left-to-right shunting through a patent ductus arteriosus can be detected by contrast injections into an umbilical artery catheter positioned in the descending thoracic aorta.[64]

Spontaneous Microcavitations

During the two-dimensional echocardiographic examination in some patients who do not have an indwelling venous line, spontaneous contrast echoes can be seen passing through the systemic veins and the right heart. Spontaneous microcavitations are seen most often in patients with impaired forward flow in the right heart or in those with hemodynamically significant pericardial effusions or severe congestive heart failure. Spontaneous microcavitations have been seen in the inferior vena cava and hepatic veins of infants with necrotizing enterocolitis. Similarly, spontaneous microcavitations have been seen in the left heart, especially in patients who have prosthetic valves. The origin and significance of spontaneous microcavitations is not always clear.[1]

THE FETAL ECHOCARDIOGRAPHIC EXAMINATION

The newest area of echocardiography is the study of the fetal heart in utero. With improvements in image resolution, visualization of the fetal heart is now possible. The original description of visualization of the human fetus in utero was by Winsberg in 1972.[75] However, image quality was poor and only M-mode examinations without two-dimensional guidance were possible. It is only recently that two-dimensional image resolution has become sufficient to permit true diagnostic studies to be performed. The cardiologist is now able to extend care of the child with cardiac disease to the fetus, permitting in utero diagnosis of cardiovascular disease and in some situations providing in utero therapy for certain disease states. Use of echocardiography to study the fetus in utero also expands our knowledge of human fetal cardiac physiology. Such knowledge expands the frontiers of in utero cardiovascular therapy—medical and, eventually, surgical.

This chapter will discuss not only the technique of performing a fetal study, but also the unique diagnostic information—structural and functional—that can be obtained. This provides an opportunity to correlate anatomic, hemodynamic, and electrophysiologic information. Fetal echocardiography makes it possible to assess the effects of abnormal anatomic states upon fetal cardiovascular hemodynamics and abnormal dysrhythmic states upon in utero hemodynamics, and, thus assess the need for therapeutic intervention and the type of intervention necessary.

Indications for a Fetal Study

The incidence of congenital heart disease in the general population is low, usually estimated at approximately 8 in 1,000 live births. Because there remains some question about the effect of ultrasonic energy upon the fetus, as will be discussed later, routine examination of all fetuses is not warranted. Fetal studies should be restricted to those situations where certain indications are present, including:

1. The presence of extracardiac anomalies.
2. Evidence of abnormal fetal growth.
3. Evidence for fetal distress.
4. The presence of chromosomal anomalies.
5. The presence of fetal cardiac dysrhythmias.
6. The presence of certain maternal diseases.
7. Parents with a history of previous children with heart disease.

Extracardiac Anomalies

The frequency of structural cardiac defects in the presence of various other anomalies is variable, depending upon the organ system involved. The incidence can range from as low as 2% to 5% when central nervous system malformations are present to as high as 50% when there are anomalies of the renal system.[76] However, even when the lesser-associated organ systems are involved, the incidence of cardiac defects is still increased significantly enough over the incidence in the general population that fetal echocardiography is warranted.

In addition, the examiner should be aware of certain extracardiac anomalies that have a high association with specific forms of congenital cardiac defects. While a complete discussion of such associations is beyond the scope of this book, certain common associations should be mentioned. The most common is that of omphalocele and either a ventricular septal defect or tetralogy of Fallot. The incidence can range from 10% if the caudal fold is involved to nearly 100% if the cephalic fold is involved.[76]

Another common association is that between abnormalities of splenic formation (asplenia or polysplenia) and atrioventricular septal defects. In the presence of asplenia, right atrial isomerism may also be present, and abnormalities of pulmonary flow and pulmonary venous drainage may exist. In the presence of polysplenia, left atrial isomerism may exist with an associated increase in systemic venous anomalies. In addition, there also tends to be an increased incidence of dysrhythmias presumed to be caused by altered sinoatrial node development.

Abnormal Fetal Growth and Fetal Distress

Although the incidence of cardiac defects is lower in fetuses with abnormal growth or fetal distress, this group remains extremely important because of the necessity for prompt therapeutic intervention. The fetus may demonstrate difficulty coping with the cause of the poor growth or the reason for the distress and, in most cases, requires assistance. Care must be taken not to assume that there is no cardiac problem. Specifically, diseases such as tachydysrhythmias can cause such problems but may not be present at the time of the examination.[77, 78] In these situations, repeat studies may be indicated.

Chromosomal Anomalies

Whenever a chromosomal anomaly is detected by amniocentesis, fetal echocardiography is indicated, as the association with congenital heart disease is high.[79] The incidence is variable with differing anomalies, yet is significant in all. The most likely cardiac defect differs with the chromosomal anomaly present, and the examiner must be aware of the defect most likely to be present for a given chromosomal aberration. The most well known is trisomy 21, which is associated with atrioventricular septal defects, isolated ventricular septal defects, and tetralogy of Fallot.

Conversely, fetuses in whom structural cardiac defects are found are felt to be at increased risk for having chromosomal defects. Some centers recommend karyotyping whenever cardiac defects are found. This is controversial, however.[76]

Fetal Cardiac Dysrhythmias

One of the more common reasons for referral of fetuses for an echocardiogram is the presence of an irregular heart rhythm. With a few exceptions, most dysrhythmias are not associated with structural defects. However, many defects can cause dysrhythmias, particularly when there is significant chamber dilatation.

Another major association that must be considered is that of l-transposition of the great arteries and congenital complete heart block. All fetuses found to have heart block should be carefully examined for evidence of this defect as well as for evidence of tricuspid valve abnormalities.

Fetuses presenting with supraventricular tachycardias also warrant close inspection of the atrioventricular junction, as there is a well-known association of such dysrhythmias with lesions such as Ebstein anomaly of the tricuspid valve and l-transposition of the great arteries.

Maternal Illnesses

The association of specific maternal illnesses and the known teratogenic effect of certain drugs and chemical agents is well documented. Mothers with illnesses such as diabetes mellitus, connective tissue disorders, seizure disorders requiring chronic medication, and exposure to agents known to induce anomalies all warrant study.[76]

Prior Child With Cardiac Disease

In most centers, this is the most common indication for fetal echocardiography. While the increased risk of congenital cardiac disease in fetuses with first order relatives who have congenital heart disease is low, there is a significant increase in the risk over the general population. More importantly, parents' anxiety about whether or not they will have a second child with heart disease may be very high. For this reason, fetal echocardiography is routinely offered to all parents with prior children having congenital heart disease.[79]

Examination Technique

Equipment

Because the structures to be examined are small, all efforts must be made to maximize resolution. Newer equipment with better focusing techniques is mandatory. Higher-frequency transducers are also advantageous, although they do have limitations. Depth penetration is limited with the higher frequencies, and the operator must choose the highest-frequency transducer that affords the needed penetration. Most studies are performed with a 5 MHz transducer, although in older fetuses or obese mothers a 3 MHz transducer may be necessary. Focal depth must also be carefully chosen to include the fetal heart within the focal zone. Thus, to perform fetal studies on fetuses of a wide range of gestational age, a wide variety of transducers must be available.[80]

Exam Technique

A systematic uniform method must be followed.[81, 82]

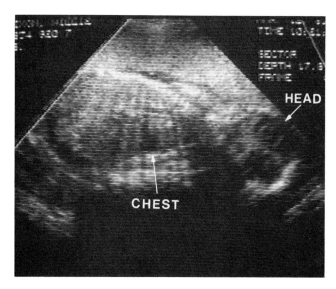

FIG 3–52.
Coronal plane through the head and thorax of a normal fetus in utero. This plane is particularly useful for determining the fetal lie.

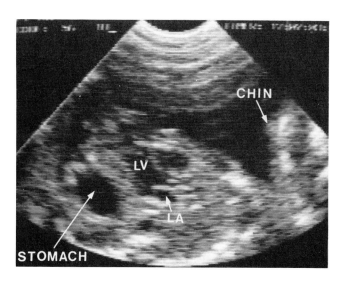

FIG 3–53.
Sagittal body plane through the head and thorax of a normal fetus. In this view, the left ventricle (LV) can be seen lying adjacent to the stomach bubble. *LA* = left atrium.

All studies begin with a wide-angle format to permit the determination of fetal orientation. The fetus is imaged en face, with the scan plane passing through the fetus from side to side (Fig 3–52). In this view, the fetal spine and thoracic and abdominal cavities are seen, providing the ventral-dorsal and cephalad-caudal relationships of the fetus. From this position, angulation of the scan plane toward the ventral surface permits visualization of the liver within the abdomen and the heart within the thorax (Fig 3–53). The presence or absence of ascites and pericardial effusion is easily determined in this view (Fig 3–54).

The heart is then centered in the plane and the inflow portion of the heart is visualized. This four-chamber view of the heart permits examination of the atrioventricular valves, atrial septum, and inlet portion of the ventricular septum (Fig 3–55). Most importantly, the septum primum is seen moving within the left atrium because of flow across the foramen ovale. As the septum primum is always within the left atrium, it serves as a marker for the left atrium, even when there is atrioventricular discordance. Next, the tricuspid and mitral valves can be distinguished, as the mitral valve attaches to the crux of the heart slightly more

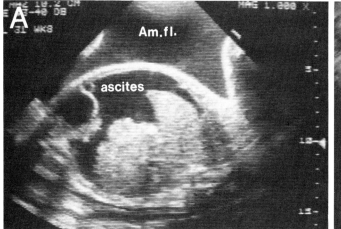

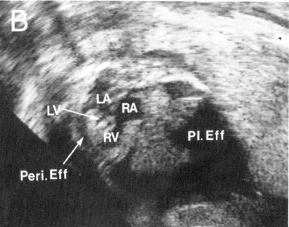

FIG 3–54.
A, sagittal body plane from a fetus with severe hydrops fetalis. There is polyhydramnios and severe fetal ascites. The liver and intestines can be seen outlined by the ascitic fluid. *Amfl* = amniotic fluid. **B,** four-chamber view from a fetus with hypoplastic left ventricle (LV) and severe hydrops fetalis. Both pleural and pericardial effusions are present. *EFF* = effusion; *LA* = left atrium; *PERI* = pericardial; *PL* = pleural; *RA* = right atrium; and *RV* = right ventricle.

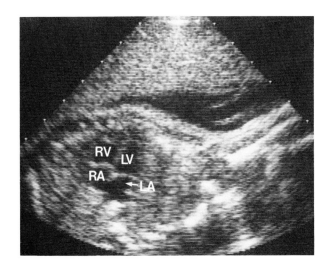

FIG 3–55.
Four-chamber view from a normal fetus. Note the pulmonary veins draining to the left atrium (LA). The left ventricle (LV) has a smooth septal surface and an atrioventricular valve farther from the cardiac apex. The right ventricle (RV) has a moderator band and an atrioventricular valve closer to the cardiac apex. *RA* = right atrium.

cephalad than does the tricuspid valve (see Fig 3–55). Because the mitral valve is always within the morphologic left ventricle, atrioventricular concordance or discordance can be determined. Finally, abnormalities of the atrioventricular junction resulting in atrioventricular septal defects can be evaluated. The four-chamber view is the single most useful view of the fetal heart. Although it does not allow detection of all defects, it does allow determination of the more serious defects. Before other areas of the heart can be examined, a good four-chamber view is mandatory.

From the four-chamber view, progressive angulation of the scan plane in a ventral direction results in imaging the outlet portion of the heart, beginning with the left ventricular outflow region (Fig 3–56). The aorta is seen to arise from the left ventricle. Its identity as the aorta is confirmed by following its course and imaging the origin of the arch vessels (Fig 3–57). The ascending aorta and arch vessels are easily seen by following the aortic arch as it arcs cephalad to the heart. The transition between the proximal arch and the descending aorta may be small, as the flow through this region is low. It may be difficult to distinguish a normal small transverse arch and a true coarctation. Total interruption of the aorta, however, can usually be distinguished.

Ventral angulation from the view showing the left ventricular outflow tract results in imaging the right ventricular outflow tract and the pulmonary artery (Fig 3–58). The main pulmonary artery can be seen connecting to the ductus arteriosus that joins the descending aorta. At this point the scan plane can be rotated 90 degrees to image the great vessels in short axis at the base of the heart (Fig 3–59). This affords some evaluation of the branch pulmonary arteries. However, as the blood flow through them is small, these vessels are small and difficult to visualize.

The systemic veins should be imaged next. Entrance of the hepatic veins and the inferior vena cava into the right atrium can be imaged by visualizing the inlet portion of the heart with the scan plane passing through the liver. Also at this time, the position of the liver and stomach should be determined to define abdominal situs. If the abdominal and thoracic situs are discordant, the chance of systemic venous anomalies is high. This can be quickly determined by noting whether or not the cardiac apex points

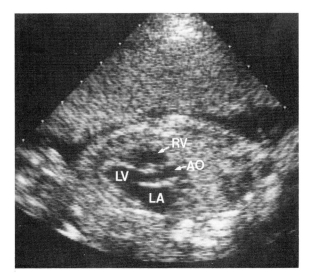

FIG 3–56.
Long-axis view of the left ventricle from a normal fetus. *AO* = aorta; *LA* = left atrium; *LV* = left ventricle; and *RV* = right ventricle.

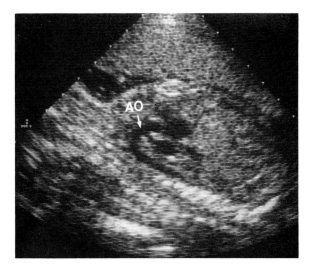

FIG 3–57.
Sagittal body plane from a normal fetus. In this view, the entire aortic (AO) arch and a considerable length of the descending AO can be visualized. The small circular structure underneath the arch is the right pulmonary artery.

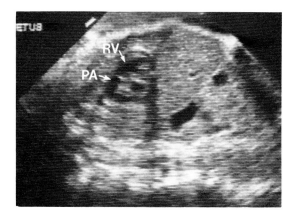

FIG 3–58.
View of the right ventricular (RV) outflow tract from a normal fetus. The entire RV and the main pulmonary artery (PA) can be seen.

toward the stomach or liver, or if the liver appears to occupy a midline position.

Using this sequential approach, all regions of the fetal heart can be imaged. However, patience is required, as most fetuses exhibit a significant amount of motion, especially in early gestation. While there are no air-containing structures to limit access, fetal limbs can often overlie the thorax, causing shadowing and making it impossible to image the heart. The examiner must try many positions on the maternal abdomen to find the one that is optimal. Changes in maternal position can also be helpful. Most women are more comfortable lying on their left side, and this should be tried first.

Using this approach, fetuses as young as 16 to 17 weeks can be studied. The average examination lasts 30 to 45 minutes but is generally tolerated well by the mother. The examiner must be extremely meticulous to make certain that omissions do not occur.

Because of the small size of the structures being examined, limitations do exist. Small defects, such as a small ventricular septal defect, can easily be overlooked; however, this usually is of no clinical significance. Pulmonary veins can also be difficult to image. Thus, anomalies of pulmonary venous drainage are one of the major cardiac lesions not likely to be imaged reliably. Finally, pathologic defects of the atrial septum are also difficult to image if they exist in the region of the foramen ovale. Conversely, defects of the ostium primum type are easily seen.

M-Mode Quantitation of Fetal Cardiac Structures

Initial studies of the fetal heart by Winsberg contained M-mode measurements of cardiac dimensions.[75] However, the unknown orientation of the ultrasound beam to the fetal heart introduced significant variability into these measurements. To perform a reproducible M-mode examination, the orientation of the beam relative to the fetal cardiac structures must be uniform from study to study, and the timing of the measurement within the cardiac cycle

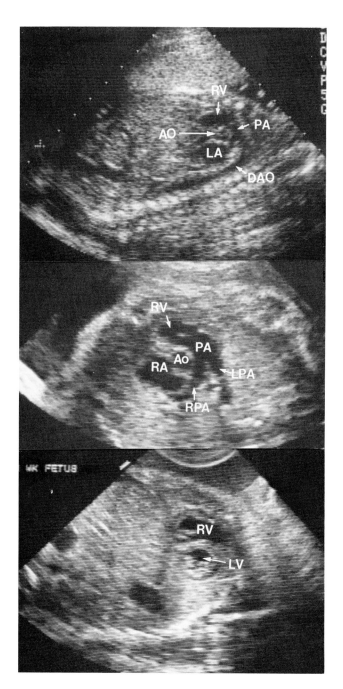

FIG 3–59.
Short-axis views from a normal fetus. The *top frame* is a short-axis view at the base of the heart. The aorta (AO) can be seen in cross-section. The right ventricular (RV) outflow tract can be seen coursing from right to left in front of the AO. The pulmonary artery (PA) can be seen to the left of the AO. It is also possible to see the arch created by the communication between the PA and descending aorta (DAO) with the patent ductus arteriosus. It is important not to mistake the ductus arch for the true aortic arch. In the *middle frame,* the plane of sound has been tilted anteriorly to visualize the PA bifurcation. In the *bottom frame,* the plane of sound has been tilted toward the chordae to obtain a short-axis view of the ventricles. *LA* = left atrium; *LPA* = left pulmonary artery; *LV* = left ventricle; *RA* = right atrium; and *RPA* = right pulmonary artery.

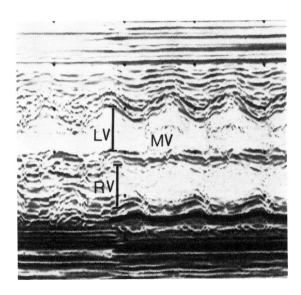

FIG 3–60.
M-mode echocardiogram obtained by passing the cursor through both ventricles in the four-chamber view. This M-mode echocardiogram is used to measure the minor-axis dimensions of the ventricles. *LV* = left ventricle; *MV* = mitral valve; and *RV* = right ventricle.

must be the same. To address these problems, the two-dimensional reference image is used to position the M-mode beam, and all measurements are taken from the M-mode trace. Because the sampling rate is much slower, measurements taken from the two-dimensional image directly do not provide the same temporal or spatial resolution. The two-dimensional image is recorded at 30 frames/sec, providing only 12 to 15 frames/cardiac cycle rather than the 1,000 samples/sec of the standard M-mode tracing, or 420 to 500 samples/cardiac cycle. DeVore has pointed out the difficulty of using measurements taken from the two-dimensional reference image.[83]

To measure the ventricular minor-axis dimensions, the two-dimensional image of the four-chamber view described above is obtained. The M-mode cursor line is then positioned pependicular to the ventricular septum just at the tips of the atrioventricular valve leaflets (Fig 3–60). Measurements of both the right and left ventricular minor-axis dimensions are taken at their maximal and minimal values, presumably representative of end-diastole and end-systole. The M-mode cursor line can then be oriented through the two atria perpendicular to the atrial septum for measurement of the right and left atria at their maximal dimensions. Finally, the left ventricular outflow tract is imaged so that the aortic valve leaflets are seen. The cursor line is positioned perpendicular to the aortic wall through the valve leaflets.The aortic root dimension is measured at this point. These measurements are similar to those obtained postnatally; however, there are marked differences. The ventricular dimensions are measured in the inlet portion of the heart rather than in the outlet portion. In the fetus, the atrial dimensions are measured in a lateral direction rather than in an anteroposterior direction, as in

the usual exam. Finally, some authors have reported the biventricular outer-to-outer dimension.[84]

Numerous studies have reported normal dimensions at various gestational ages.[84–90] All have shown a linear increase in left ventricular and right ventricular dimension with increasing gestational age. The same is true for the atria and aortic root. The ratio of the right ventricular to left ventricular dimension, however, remains constant at approximately 1. This measurement is particularly useful, as it is possible to quickly decide if one chamber is either abnormally large or small. Yet if both chambers are equally dilated, the ratio will remain normal even in the presence of abnormal chamber sizes.

Hemodynamic Flow Studies Across Fetal Cardiac Valves

Use of Doppler techniques to evaluate flow through the fetal heart has been the subject of significant investigation. Evaluation of flow in the great vessels,[47, 91] the umbilical vessels,[92, 93] and through the atrioventricular valves[94] have all been studied. Use of such studies to evaluate normal as well as altered flow states has been useful. Nevertheless, Doppler studies require a significant increase in the amount of energy delivered to the fetus. Until the safety of such energy levels is shown, the use of Doppler techniques should be limited to those situations in which the information provided is clinically important. Diagnosis of semilunar valve obstruction and regurgitation is performed identically to the method used in routine Doppler studies. The sample volume is positioned within the vessel being studied at as near an angle of zero degrees as possible. Flow patterns in both the aorta and pulmonary artery can be obtained.

Diagnosis of atrioventricular valve obstruction and/or regurgitation is similar to routinely used methods, as will be discussed in subsequent chapters. A careful search for valve regurgitation is necessary when a dysrhythmia is present, as will be discussed later, or when ascites is seen (i.e., tricuspid regurgitation may produce ascites). Changes in diastolic compliance of the ventricles with increasing gestational age have also been studied.[94] The degree of filling that occurs in early diastole vs. that following atrial systole changes with increasing gestational age. Younger fetuses possess a ventricle that is stiffer and in which more filling occurs during atrial systole than do older fetuses. With increasing gestational age, the area under the early diastolic velocity profile increases. Failure to show this normal progression should raise the question of an altered myocardial state.

Evaluation of flow in the umbilical vessels has been used to assess placental vascular impedance, with conclusions being drawn as to placental function (Fig 3–61). Altered umbilical artery flow patterns have been shown in placental insufficiency states.[92] Normally, flow in the umbilical arteries is phasic yet continuous, as the placenta affords a low impedance circuit. Flow velocities in the normal fetus never fall to zero, even in late diastole. When it is noted that flow has reached zero, an abnormal rise in placental impedance must be suspected. This has been associated with placental dysfunction.

Signs of Congestive Heart Failure

The criteria for assessing the presence or absence of in utero heart failure differ from those used postnatally. Late signs include the development of ascites, pleural effusions, pericardial effusions, and scalp edema.[77] In addition, fetal motion is diminished. However, the examiner must carefully assess the fetus for signs of early heart failure. This can be difficult, as there are no specific indicators. Progressive chamber dilatation is often useful, as are changes in diastolic filling, especially when either structural defects or dysrhythmias exist. It is also necessary to keep in mind that because of the altered physiologic state of the fetus compared to the infant, different lesions are more susceptible to the development of in utero heart failure. Lesions that restrict flow from the right heart, such as a restrictive foramen ovale or Ebstein anomaly of the tricuspid valve, are particularly prone to produce heart failure. Also, atrioventricular valve regurgitation, particularly tricuspid regurgitation, may result in heart failure.

Fetal Dysrhythmias

Use of echocardiography for the diagnosis of cardiac dysrhythmias is unique to the fetus.[95–98] The difficulty in obtaining noninvasive fetal electrocardiograms makes the use of echocardiographic techniques advantageous. Although the presence of a dysrhythmia can often be suspected from auscultation, diagnosis of the exact nature and effect of the dysrhythmia upon the fetus cannot be determined from the clinical examination.

Diagnosis of dysrhythmia can be done using either M-mode or Doppler recordings. In most situations, M-mode

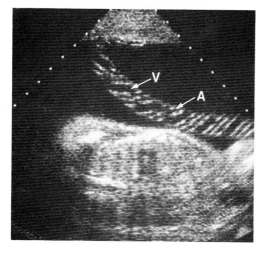

FIG 3–61.
Normal umbilical cord, which consists of one large umbilical vein and two small umbilical arteries wrapped around one another in a spiral. *A* = umbilical artery; *V* = umbilical vein.

recordings are diagnostic, obviating the need for Doppler studies with their attendant higher energy levels. Rhythm diagnosis is performed by passing the M-mode cursor line through the fetal heart so that both the ventricular and the atrial walls are traversed; in this way, motion of both the atria and the ventricles can be recorded simultaneously (Fig 3–62). A foreshortened long-axis view most often accomplishes this best. From such a recording, the atrial rate, the ventricular rate, and the relationship between the atrial and ventricular contractions can be determined in the same way an electrocardiogram can be analyzed. Questions that must be asked and answered are:

1. What is the atrial rate?
2. What is the ventricular rate?
3. Is there any relationship between atrial and ventricular contractions?
4. Is the rhythm regular or irregular?

Bradydysrhythmias

Slow fetal heart rates are often the reason for referral for an echocardiogram. The most common cause is complete heart block; this must be distinguished from sinus bradycardia, which has a much worse prognosis. Sinus bradycardias, defined as a rate below 100/min, are uncommon; when they occur, however, they usually indicate fetal compromise. In their presence, careful inspection of the anatomy is necessary as well as evaluation for signs of in utero heart failure. The heart rate in an older fetus is normally somewhat slower but should remain above 100/min. Sinus pauses can also occur but are much less ominous. Pauses up to 1 second can be seen especially in the fetus near term and are not necessarily associated with fetal compromise.

Complete heart block, manifest as a slow ventricular rate with a *faster* atrial rate (Fig 3–63), can be noted at any stage of gestation but is not necessarily present from the time of conception. We have seen several fetuses with a prior documented heart rate in the normal range. While no formal studies have been done, limited experience indicates that heart block often becomes manifest after 20 weeks. The fetus must be observed for the development of heart block when predisposing factors are present. The presence of maternal collagen vascular disease, for instance, is a well known predisposing factor.[99] This does not have to take the form of overt clinical disease in the mother but may be present only as a positive serologic test. In addition, complete heart block can be associated with certain structural diseases in the fetus, such as *l*-transposition of the great arteries and any anomaly of the tricuspid valve.

The fetus may or may not be adversely affected by the slow heart rate. In general, fetuses with complete heart block exhibit heart rates greater than 70/min and fetuses with slower heart rates have a higher incidence of in utero heart failure. The presence of associated structural disease predisposes the fetus to a higher risk of congestive heart failure. Other maternal diseases such as diabetes also place the fetus at a higher risk.

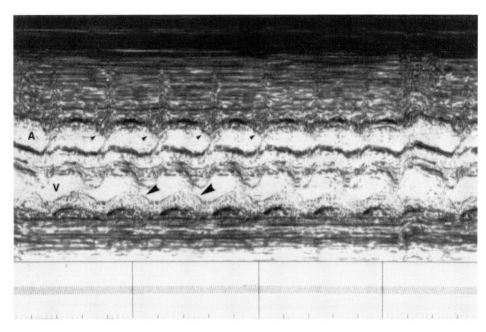

FIG 3–62.
M-mode echocardiogram from a fetus in normal sinus rhythm. Atrial (A) contractions are denoted by the *small arrows* and ventricular (V) contractions by the *large arrows.*

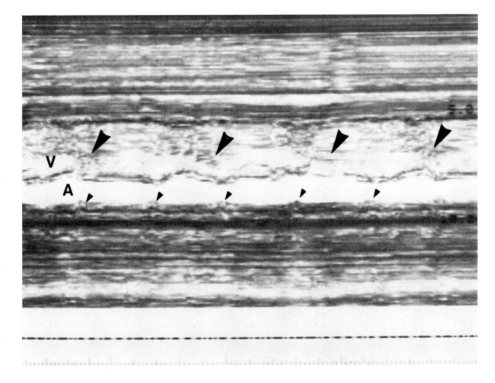

FIG 3–63.
M-mode echocardiogram from a fetus with complete heart block. Atrial (A) contractions are denoted by the *small arrows* and ventricular (V) contractions by the *large arrows.*

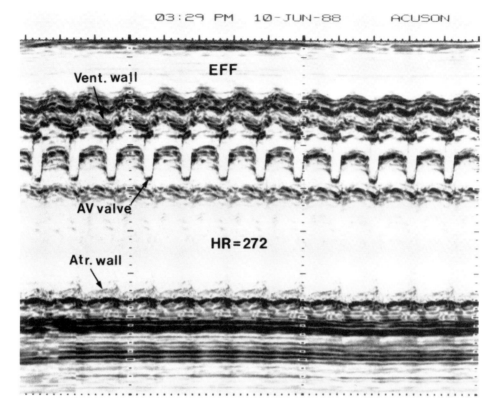

03:29 PM   10-JUN-88   ACUSON

EFF

Vent. wall

AV valve

HR = 272

Atr. wall

FIG 3–64.
M-mode echocardiogram from a fetus with supraventricular tachycardia and a heart rate of 272 beats per minute. There is 1:1 conduction from the atrium to the ventricle. *ATR* = atrial; *AV* = atrioventricular; *EFF* = effusion; and *Vent* = ventricular.

Fetuses with heart block should be monitored closely with repeat echocardiograms for the development of congestive heart failure. Currently, there is no proven in utero therapy, and premature delivery must be considered when signs of significant heart failure develop. The consequences of a premature birth must be weighed against the possibility of in utero fetal death. If multiple risk factors are present, this possibility may be high.

Tachydysrhythmias

Dysrhythmias with a rapid fetal heart rate in excess of 200/min are the most common pathologic dysrhythmias (Fig 3–64). The tachydysrhythmias that have been recognized in utero include supraventricular tachycardia, atrial flutter, and ventricular tachycardia. Of these, supraventricular tachycardia is the most common and can be recognized as a fetal heart rate in excess of 200/min with 1:1 atrioventricular conduction. While supraventricular tachycardia is usually not associated with structural disease, a careful inspection of the heart is needed, as the hemodynamic effects tend to be worse in those fetuses with cardiac defects. Also, when anomalies of the tricuspid valve are present, the presence of Wolff-Parkinson-White syndrome is more likely and may have some influence upon the form of therapy used. Finally, the examiner should make some effort to determine if the tachycardia is incessant or inter-

mittent. The intermittent form tends to have less serious hemodynamic effects. Again, the fetus must be examined for signs of heart failure, and frequent serial examinations are indicated to determine whether or not heart failure is present.

Atrial flutter can be recognized by a more rapid atrial rate and usually by the presence of a slower heart rate (Fig 3–65). In our experience, the atrial rate is usually greater than 400/min, which distinguishes atrial flutter from supraventricular tachycardia with associated atrioventricular block. Although atrial flutter is usually not associated with structural disease, structural anomalies must be excluded. The presence or absence of heart failure depends not only upon the ventricular rate but also upon the degree of effect of the dysrhythmia on ventricular filling. More chaotic atrial rhythms tend to have a more pronounced effect. It is unknown if this is caused entirely by altered filling in a less compliant ventricle or if other factors contribute.

Ventricular tachycardia can be difficult to recognize. The diagnostic feature is atrioventricular dissociation with the ventricular rate faster than the atrial rate (Fig 3–66). In general, the ventricular rate is 160 to 200/min, although it can be quite variable. When retrograde conduction is present, resulting in 1:1 atrioventricular conduction, the diagnosis of ventricular tachycardia can only be inferred. One clue is the presence of variability in the fetal heart

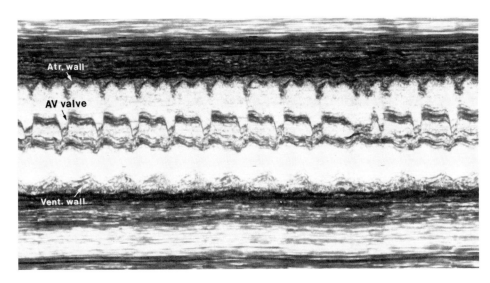

FIG 3–65.
M-mode echocardiogram from a fetus with atrial flutter. The atrial rate is 400 beats per minute and greater, and the ventricular rate is 200 beats per minute. *ATR* = atrial; *AV* = atrioventricular; and *Vent* = ventricular.

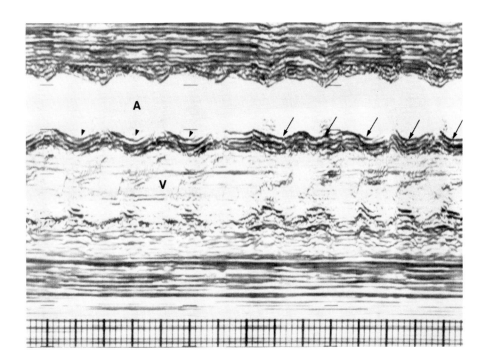

FIG 3–66.
M-mode echocardiogram from a fetus with intermittent ventricular tachycardia. When the fetus is in ventricular tachycardia (*large arrows*), the ventricular (V) rate exceeds the atrial (A) rate. When the fetus is in sinus rhythm (*small arrows*) the rates of the ventricular and atrial contractions are the same.

rate. In the presence of ventricular tachycardia, the fetal heart rate is quite stable with loss of the normal variability. This is particularly true in late gestation and can be detected as a lack of heart rate variability on a nonstress test. Ventricular function must be assessed because of the association of ventricular tachycardia and viral myocarditis. The effects of this dysrhythmia upon cardiac hemodynamics are quite variable. In our limited experience, the presence of atrioventricular synchrony leads to less compromise. Thus, even if the dysrhythmia cannot be completely stopped, slowing it enough to restore atrioventricular synchrony can lead to significant improvement.

Effects of Ultrasonic Energy on the Fetus

Even though ultrasound has been used for many years to evaluate the fetus in utero, the possibility of adverse effects on the fetus remains in question. With the advent of Doppler echocardiography and the higher energy levels it delivers to the fetus, this question has become even more important. Studies in animal fetuses have shown an effect of ultrasonic energy. In dogs, the fetal abdominal temperature was raised in proportion to the time and intensity of the sound energy applied to the fetal thorax.[100] If significant elevation of the fetal core temperature occurs, deleterious effects might result. Heart rate increases, but no known permanent injury has been documented. Energy delivered in these animal experiments has exceeded that delivered by most commercial instruments; nevertheless, care must be exercised to keep to a minimum the amount of energy delivered to the fetus. For this reason, examinations should be as short as possible, consistent with performing an adequate study, and Doppler studies should be performed only when the information to be gained cannot be acquired by other means. Power levels should also be minimized as much as possible.

Future Trends

As new technologic advances are made in the field, they will be applied to the study of the fetus. Color Doppler flow mapping is one such recent advance. Preliminary work has shown the possibility of using such a technique to study the spatial orientation of fetal flow patterns.[101, 102] However, resolution remains low in such small structures and the efficacy of the technique remains in question, given the increased energy required. Until the precise effects of ultrasonic energy upon the fetus are known, it is necessary to be prudent in applying techniques that deliver more energy but provide no more information than can be obtained with techniques that deliver lower energy.

Currently, the major clinical use of fetal echocardiography is in identifying structural anomalies in the fetus, with assessment of their hemodynamic effects and the diagnosis and management of fetal dysrhythmias. Of equal importance is the ability of this technique to provide direct assessment and study of human fetal cardiovascular hemodynamics. To date, all studies of fetal hemodynamics have been based upon experimental animal models. Fetal echocardiography will change this because it will allow better and earlier diagnosis of cardiac disease (both structural and functional) and will permit earlier intervention and a better outcome for the fetus with cardiac disease.

REFERENCES

1. Silverman NH, Snider AR: *Two-Dimensional Echocardiography in Congenital Heart Disease.* Norwalk, Appleton-Century-Crofts, 1982, pp 16–18, 47–66.
2. Stevenson JG, Kawabori I, French JW: Critical importance of sedation when measuring pressure gradients by Doppler (abstract). *Circulation* 1984; 70 (suppl 2):363.
3. Henry WL, DeMaria A, Gramiak R, et al: Report of the American Society of Echocardiography Committee on Nomenclature and Standards in Two-Dimensional Echocardiography. *Circulation* 1980; 62:212–217.
4. Van Mill GJ, Moulaert AJ, Harinck E: *Atlas of Two-Dimensional Echocardiography in Congenital Cardiac Defects.* Boston, Martinus-Nijhoff Publishers, 1985, pp 1–23.
5. Tanaka M, Neyazaki T, Koska S, et al: Ultrasonic evaluation of anatomical abnormalities of heart in congenital and acquired heart diseases. *Br Heart J* 1971; 33:686–698.
6. Tajik AJ, Seward JB, Hagler DJ, et al: Two-dimensional real-time ultrasonic imaging of the heart and great vessels: Technique, image orientation, structure identification and validation. *Mayo Clin Proc* 1978; 53:271–303.
7. Seward JB, Tajik AJ: Two-dimensional echocardiography. *Med Clin North Am* 1980; 64:177–203.
8. Sahn DJ: Real-time two-dimensional echocardiography. *J Pediatr* 1981; 99:175–185.
9. Snider AR, Ports TA, Silverman NH: Venous anomalies of the coronary sinus. Detection by M-mode, two-dimensional and contrast echocardiography. *Circulation* 1979; 60:721–727.
10. Mintz GS, Kotler MN, Segal BL, et al: Two-dimensional echocardiographic recognition of the descending thoracic aorta. *Am J Cardiol* 1979; 44:232–238.
11. Silverman NH, Snider AR: *Two-Dimensional Echocardiography in Congenital Heart Disease.* Norwalk, Conn, Appleton-Century-Crofts, 1982, p 23.
12. Henry WL, Maron BJ, Griffith JM: Cross-sectional echocardiography in the diagnosis of congenital heart disease. *Circulation* 1977; 56:267–273.
13. Weyman AE, Feigenbaum H, Dillon JC, et al: Noninvasive visualization of the left main coronary artery by cross-sectional echocardiography. *Circulation* 1976; 54:169–174.
14. Fisher EA, Sepehri B, Lendrum B, et al: Two-dimensional echocardiographic visualization of the left coronary artery in anomalous origin of the left coronary artery from the pulmonary artery: Pre- and postoperative studies. *Circulation* 1981; 63:698–704.

15. Silverman NH, Schiller NB: Apex echocardiography. A two-dimensional technique for evaluation of congenital heart disease. *Circulation* 1978; 57:503–511.

16. Goor DA, Lillehei CW: *Congenital Malformations of the Heart.* New York, Grune and Stratton, 1975, pp 1–37, 38–102.

17. Limacher MC, Gutgesell HP, Vick GW, et al: Echocardiographic anatomy of the eustachian valve. *Am J Cardiol* 1986; 57:363–365.

18. Seward JB, Tajik AJ: Non-invasive visualization of the entire thoracic aorta: A new application of wide-angle two-dimensional sector echocardiographic technique. *Am J Cardiol* 1979; 43:387.

19. Bierman FZ, Williams RG: Subxyphoid two-dimensional imaging of the interatrial septum in infants and neonates with congenital heart disease. *Circulation* 1979; 60:80–90.

20. Lange LW, Sahn DJ, Allen HD, et al: Subxyphoid cross-sectional echocardiography in infants and children with congenital heart disease. *Circulation* 1979; 59:513–524.

21. Allen HD, Goldberg SJ, Sahn DJ, et al: Suprasternal notch echocardiography: Assessment of its clinical utility in pediatric cardiology. *Circulation* 1977; 55:605–612.

22. Sahn DJ, Allen HD, McDonald G, et al: Real-time cross-sectional echocardiographic diagnosis of coarctation of the aorta: A prospective study of echocardiographic-angiographic correlations. *Circulation* 1977; 56:762–769.

23. Snider AR, Silverman NH: Suprasternal notch echocardiography: A two-dimensional technique for evaluating congenital heart disease. *Circulation* 1981; 63:165–173.

24. Huhta JC, Gutgesell HP, Latson LA, et al: Two-dimensional echocardiographic assessment of the aorta in infants and children with congenital heart disease. *Circulation* 1984; 70:417–424.

25. Shrivastava S, Berry JM, Einzig S, et al: Parasternal cross-sectional echocardiographic determination of aortic arch situs: A new approach. *Am J Cardiol* 1985; 55:1236–1238.

26. Lundstrom N, Edler I: Ultrasound cardiography in infants and children. *Acta Paediatr Scand* 1971; 60:117–128.

27. Gramiak R, Shah PM: Cardiac ultrasonography: A review of current applications. *Radiol Clin North Am* 1971; 9:469–490.

28. Solinger R, Elbl F, Minhas K: Echocardiography in the normal neonate. *Circulation* 1973; 47:108–118.

29. Meyer RA, Kaplan S: Noninvasive techniques in pediatric cardiovascular disease. *Prog Cardiovasc Dis* 1973; 15:341–367.

30. Solinger R, Elbl F, Minhas K: Deductive echocardiographic analysis in infants with congenital heart disease. *Circulation* 1974; 50:1072–1096.

31. Sahn DJ, Allen HD, Goldberg SJ, et al: Pediatric echocardiography: A review of its clinical utility. *J Pediatr* 1975; 87:335–352.

32. Meyer RA: Echocardiography in congenital heart disease. *Semin Roentgenol* 1975; 10:277–290.

33. Popp RL: Echocardiographic assessment of cardiac disease. *Circulation* 1976; 54:538–552.

34. Zaky A, Grabhorn L, Feigenbaum H: Movement of the mitral ring: A study of ultrasound cardiology. *Cardiovasc Res* 1967; 1:121–131.

35. Zaky A, Nasser WK, Feigenbaum H: Study of mitral valve action recorded by reflected ultrasound and its application in the diagnosis of mitral stenosis. *Circulation* 1968; 37:789–799.

36. Rubenstein JJ, Pohost GM, Dinsmore RE, et al: The echocardiographic determination of mitral valve opening and closure: Correlation with hemodynamic studies in man. *Circulation* 1975; 51:98–103.

37. Laiken SL, Johnson AD, Bhargava V, et al: Instantaneous transmitral blood flow and anterior mitral leaflet motion in man. *Circulation* 1979; 59:476–482.

38. Strunk BL, Fitzgerald JW, Lipton M, et al: The posterior aortic wall echocardiogram: Its relation to left atrial volume change. *Circulation* 1976; 54:744–750.

39. Akgun G, Layton C: Aortic root and left atrial wall motion: An echocardiographic study. *Br Heart J* 1977; 39:1082–1087.

40. Feigenbaum H: *Echocardiography.* Philadelphia, Lea & Febiger, 1981, pp 63, 179, 212.

41. Gramiak R, Shah PM: Echocardiography of the normal and diseased aortic valve. *Radiology* 1970; 96:1–8.

42. Gramiak R, Nanda NC, Shah PM: Echocardiographic detection of pulmonary valve. *Radiology* 1972; 102:153–157.

43. Weyman AE, Dillon JC, Feigenbaum H, et al: Echocardiographic patterns of pulmonary valve motion in valvular pulmonary stenosis. *Am J Cardiol* 1974; 34:644–651.

44. Hatle L, Angelsen B: *Doppler Ultrasound in Cardiology: Physical Principles and Clinical Applications,* ed 2. Philadelphia, Lea & Febiger, 1985, pp 74–96.

45. Grenadier E, Lima CO, Allen HD, et al: Normal intracardiac and great vessel Doppler flow velocities in infants and children. *J Am Coll Cardiol* 1984; 4:343–350.

46. Kenny JF, Plappert T, Doubilet P, et al: Changes in intracardiac blood flow velocities and right and left ventricular stroke volumes with gestational age in the normal human fetus: A prospective Doppler echocardiographic study. *Circulation* 1986: 74:1208–1216.

47. Huhta JC, Strasburger JF, Carpenter RJ, et al: Pulsed Doppler fetal echocardiography. *J Clin Ultrasound* 1985; 13:247–254.

48. Riggs TW, Snider AR: Respiratory influence on right and left ventricular diastolic filling in normal children. *J Am Coll Cardiol* 1989; 13:205A.

49. Shaffer EM, Snider AR, Serwer GA, et al: Effect of sampling site on Doppler-derived right ventricular systolic time intervals. *Circulation* 1987; 76 (suppl 4):173.

50. Wind BE, Snider AR, Buda AG, et al: Pulsed Doppler assessment of left ventricular diastolic filling in patients with coronary artery disease before and immediately after coronary angioplasty. *Am J Cardiol* 1987; 59:1041–1046.

51. Spirito P, Maron BJ, Bellotti P, et al: Noninvasive

assessment of left ventricular diastolic function: Comparative analysis of pulsed Doppler ultrasound and digitized M-mode echocardiography. *Am J Cardiol* 1986; 58:837–843.

52. Miyatake K, Okamoto M, Kinoshita N, et al: Augmentation of atrial contribution to left ventricular inflow with aging as assessed by intracardiac Doppler flowmetry. *Am J Cardiol* 1984; 53:586–589.

53. Fujii J, Yazaki Y, Sawada H, et al: Noninvasive assessment of left and right ventricular filling in myocardial infarction with a two-dimensional Doppler echocardiographic method. *J Am Coll Cardiol* 1985; 5:1155–1160.

54. Snider AR, Gidding SS, Rocchini AP, et al: Doppler evaluation of left ventricular diastolic filling in children with systemic hypertension. *Am J Cardiol* 1985; 56:921–926.

55. Dabestani A, Takenaka K, Allen B, et al: Effects of spontaneous respiration of diastolic left ventricular filling assessed by pulsed Doppler echocardiography. *Am J Cardiol* 1988; 61:1356–1358.

56. Yock PG, Schnittger I, Popp RL: Is continuous wave Doppler too sensitive in diagnosing pathologic valvular regurgitation? *Circulation* 1984; 70(supp. 1):381.

57. Kostucki W, Vandenbossche J-L, Friart A, et al: Pulsed Doppler regurgitant flow patterns of normal valves. *Am J Cardiol* 1986; 58:309–313.

58. Yoshida K, Yoshikawa J, Shakudo M, et al: Color Doppler evaluation of valvular regurgitation in normal subjects. *Circulation* 1988; 78:840–847.

59. Sahn DJ, Maciel BC: Physiological valvular regurgitation. Doppler echocardiography and the potential for iatrogenic heart disease. *Circulation* 1988; 78:1075–1077.

60. Gramiak R, Shah PM; Echocardiography of the aortic root. *Invest Radiol* 1968; 3:356–366.

61. Gramiak R, Shah, PM, Kramer DH: Ultrasound cardiography: Contrast studies in anatomy and function. *Radiology* 1969; 2:939–948.

62. Seward JB, Tajik AJ, Spangler JG, et al: Echocardiographic contrast studies: Initial experience. *Mayo Clin Proc* 1975; 50:163–192.

63. Valdes-Cruz LM, Pieroni DR, Roland J-MA, et al: Echocardiographic detection of intracardiac right-to-left shunts following peripheral vein injections. *Circulation* 1976; 54:558–562.

64. Sahn DJ, Allen HD, George W, et al: The utility of contrast echocardiographic techniques in the care of critically ill infants with cardiac and pulmonary disease. *Circulation* 1977; 56:959–968.

65. Seward JB, Tajik AJ, Hagler DJ, et al: Peripheral venous contrast echocardiography. *Am J Cardiol* 1977; 39:202–212.

66. Pieroni DR, Varghese J, Freedom RM, et al: The sensitivity of contrast echocardiography in detecting intracardiac shunts. *Cathet Cardiovasc Diagn* 1979; 5:19–29.

67. Serruys PW, VanDenBrand M, Hugenholtz PG, et al: Intracardiac right-to-left shunts demonstrated by two-dimensional echocardiography after peripheral vein injection. *Br Heart J* 1979; 42:429–437.

68. Kremkau FW, Gramiak R, Carstensen EL, et al: Ul-

trasonic detection of cavitation at catheter tips. *Am J Roentgen* 1970; 110:177–183.

69. Barrera JG, Fulkerson PK, Rittgers SE, et al: The nature of contrast echocardiographic targets. *Circulation* 1978; 57–58(suppl 2):233.

70. Meltzer RS, Tickner EG, Sahines TP, et al: The source of ultrasound contrast effect. *J Clin Ultrasound* 1980; 8:121–127.

71. Shub C, Tajik AJ, Seward JB, et al: Detecting intrapulmonary right-to-left shunt with contrast echocardiography: Observations in a patient with diffuse pulmonary arteriovenous fistulas. *Mayo Clin Proc* 1976; 51:81–84.

72. Fraker TD Jr, Harris PJ, Behar VS, et al: Detection and exclusion of interatrial shunts by two-dimensional echocardiography and peripheral venous injection. *Circulation* 1979; 59:379–384.

73. Serwer GA, Armstrong BE, Anderson PAW, et al: Use of contrast echocardiography for evaluation of right ventricular hemodynamics in the presence of ventricular septal defects. *Circulation* 1978; 58:327–337.

74. Weyman AE, Wann LS, Caldwell RL, et al: Negative contrast echocardiography: A new method for detecting left-to-right shunts. *Circulation* 1979; 59:498–505.

75. Winsberg F: Echocardiography of the fetal and newborn heart. *Invest Radiol* 1972; 3:152–158.

76. Copel JA, Pilu G, Kleinman CS: Congenital heart disease and extracardiac anomalies: Associations and indications for fetal echocardiography. *Am J Obstet Gynecol* 1986; 541:1121–1132.

77. Kleinman CS, Donnertein RV, DeVore GR: Fetal echocardiography for evaluation of in utero congestive cardiac failure: A technique for study of nonimmune hydrops. *N Eng J Med* 1982; 306:568–575.

78. DeVore GR, Donnerstein RL, Kleinman CS, et al: Fetal echocardiography. II. The diagnosis and significance of a pericardial effusion in the fetus using real-time-directed M-mode ultrasound. *Am J Obstet Gynecol* 1982; 144:693–700.

79. Nora JJ, Nora AH: The evolution of specific genetic and environmental counseling in congenital heart diseases. *Circulation* 1978; 57:205–213.

80. Sahn DJ: Resolution and display requirements for ultrasound/Doppler evaluation of the heart in children, infants and unborn human fetus. *J Am Coll Cardiol* 1985; 5(suppl 1):12s–19s.

81. Cyr DR, Guntheroth WG, Mack LA, et al: A systematic approach to fetal echocardiography using real-time/two-dimensional sonography. *J Ultrasound Med* 1986; 5:343–350.

82. Silverman NH, Golbus MS: Echocardiographic techniques for assessing normal and abnormal fetal cardiac anatomy. *J Am Coll Cardiol* 1985; 5(suppl 1):20s–29s.

83. DeVore GR, Platt LD: The random measurement of the transverse diameter of the fetal heart: A potential source of error. *J Ultrasound Med* 1985; 4:335–341.

84. DeVore GR, Siassi B, Platt LD: Fetal echocardiography. IV. M-mode assessment of ventricular size and contractility during the second and third trimesters

of pregnancy in the normal fetus. *Am J Obstet Gynecol* 1984; 150:981–988.

85. DeVore GR, Donnerstein RL, Kleinman CS, et al: Fetal echocardiography I. Normal anatomy as determined by real-time-directed M-mode ultrasound. *Am J Obstet Gynecol* 1982; 144:249–260.

86. St. John Sutton MG, Gewitz MH, Shah B, et al: Quantitative assessment of growth and function of the cardiac chambers in the normal human fetus: A prospective longitudinal echocardiographic study. *Circulation* 1984; 69:645–654.

87. Azancot A, Caudell TP, Allen HD, et al: Analysis of ventricular shape by echocardiography in normal fetuses, newborns, and infants. *Circulation* 1983; 68:1201–1211.

88. Allen LD, Joseph MC, Boyd EGCA, et al: M-mode echocardiography in the developing human fetus. *Br Heart J* 1982; 47:573–583.

89. DeVore GR, Siassi B, Platt LD: Fetal Echocardiography. V. M-mode measurements of the aortic root and aortic valve in second and third trimester normal human fetuses. *Am J Obstet Gynecol* 1985; 152:543–550.

90. Shime J, Gresser CD, Rakowski H: Quantitative two-dimensional echocardiographic assessment of fetal growth. *Am J Obstet Gynecol* 1986; 154:294–300.

91. Maulik D, Nanda NC, Saini VD: Fetal Doppler echocardiography: Methods and characterization of normal and abnormal hemodynamics. *Am J Cardiol* 1984; 53:572–578.

92. Schulman H, Fleischer A, Stern W, et al: Umbilical velocity wave ratios in human pregnancy. *Am J Obstet Gynecol* 1984; 148:985–990.

93. Chen HY, Lu CC, Cheng YT, et al: Antenatal measurement of fetal umbilical venous flow by pulsed Doppler and B-mode ultrasonography. *J Ultrasound Med* 1986; 5:319–321.

94. Reed KL, Sahn DJ, Scagnelli S, et al: Doppler echocardiographic studies of diastolic function in the human fetal heart: Changes during gestation. *J Am Coll Cardiol* 1986; 8:391–395.

95. Kleinman CS, Copel JA, Weinstein EM, et al: Treatment of fetal supraventricular tachyarrhythmias. *J Clin Ultrasound* 1985; 13:265–273.

96. Allen LD, Anderson RH, Sullivan ID, et al: Evaluation of fetal arrhythmias by echocardiography. *Br Heart J* 1983; 50:240–245.

97. Kleinman CS, Hobbins JC, Jaffe CC, et al: Echocardiographic studies of the human fetus: Prenatal diagnosis of congenital heart disease and cardiac dysrhythmias. *Pediatrics* 1980; 65:1059–1067.

98. Silverman NH, Enderlein MA, Stanger P, et al: Recognition of fetal arrhythmias by echocardiography. *J Clin Ultrasound* 1985; 13:255–263.

99. McCue CM, Mantakas ME, Tinglestad JB, et al: Congenital heart block in newborns of mothers with connective tissue disease. *Circulation* 1977; 56:82–89.

100. Gross DR, Williams AR, Mann CW, et al: Thermal and heart rate response to ultrasonic exposure in the second and third trimester dog fetus. *J Ultrasound Med* 1986; 5:507–513.

101. Maulik D, Nanda NC, Hsiung, MC, et al: Doppler color flow mapping of the fetal heart. *Angiology* 1986; 37:628–632.

102. Reed KL, Meijboom EJ, Sahn DJ, et al: Cardiac Doppler flow velocities in human fetuses. *Circulation* 1986; 73:41–46.

Methods for Obtaining Quantitative Information From the Echocardiographic Examination

The widespread use of M-mode and two-dimensional echocardiography as diagnostic techniques resulted from their ability to differentiate cardiac structures from blood-filled cavities without the need to inject a contrast agent. Because of this capability, M-mode and two-dimensional echocardiography were initially used to provide qualitative information on cardiac spatial anatomy. With these techniques, no direct information on blood flow is obtained; therefore, quantitative assessment of the severity of a cardiac defect is limited to observation of secondary hemodynamic consequences of the defect such as cardiac wall hypertrophy, chamber dilatation, or changes in the rates of valve or wall motion. The introduction of Doppler echocardiography provided a technique for obtaining direct information on blood flow and, thus, direct assessment of the hemodynamic severity of cardiac defects. Currently, the combination of quantitative information obtained from the M-mode, two-dimensional, and Doppler echocardiographic examinations makes it possible to determine precisely the hemodynamic severity of most cardiac defects.

During the past few years, many different quantitative echocardiographic techniques have been developed and described. Many of these methods and formulae are only of historic interest and have been replaced by newer, more accurate techniques for noninvasive quantification of the severity of the cardiac defect. The purpose of this chapter is to review the measurement and quantitation techniques currently in common use in clinical echocardiography laboratories. Those techniques that are of historic value and have been replaced by newer methods or are seldom used will not be discussed in this chapter.

QUANTITATIVE M-MODE ECHOCARDIOGRAPHY

M-mode echocardiography provides a technique for the indirect assessment of the severity of the cardiac disease by measurement of the secondary hemodynamic consequences of the disease (i.e., wall hypertrophy, chamber dilatation). Because of its rapid sampling rates and ease of quantitation, M-mode echocardiography is particularly suitable for evaluating rapid events in the heart such as rates of change in wall motion, cavity dimensions, and valve motions. The higher temporal resolution of M-mode echocardiography compared with two-dimensional echocardiography (several thousand pulses per second for M-mode echocardiography vs. 30 frames or less per second for two-dimensional echocardiography) makes M-mode echocardiography the preferred technique for measuring cardiac dimensions at precise times in the cardiac cycle.

Measurement of Cardiac Structural Dimensions

The medical literature contains several excellent reports of M-mode echocardiographic measurements of cardiac dimensions in normal subjects from birth to adulthood.[1-5] These studies show that throughout childhood cardiac chamber dimensions and wall thicknesses are related to changes in weight, height, and body surface area. Figure 4–1 is a graphic representation of the M-mode echocardiographic measurements of cardiac structures in normal children, as reported by Roge and colleagues.[4] These graphs show the 90% tolerance limits of the normal data and can be used to predict with 90% certainty if a mea-

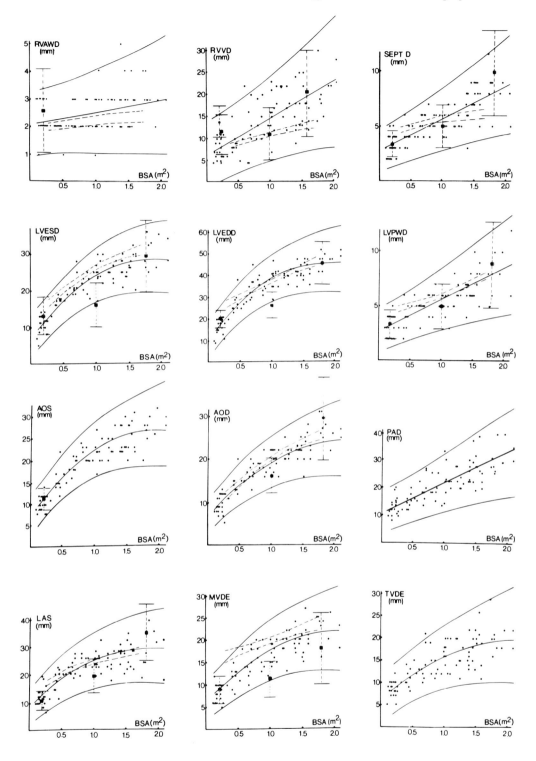

FIG 4–1.
Echocardiographic dimensions from 93 normal children without heart disease, plotted against the body surface area (BSA). The data points for each variable are shown by dots. The 90% tolerance lines are shown by heavy continuous lines. *RVAWD* = right ventricular anterior wall thickness in diastole; *RVDD* = right ventricular end-diastolic dimension; *SEPT D* = septal thickness at end-diastole; *LVESD* = left ventricular end-systolic dimension; *LVEDD* = left ventricular end-diastolic dimension; *LVPWD* = left ventricular posterior wall thickness at end-diastole; *AOS* = aortic diameter in systole; *AOD* = aortic diameter in diastole; *PAD* = pulmonary artery diameter; *LAS* = left atrial dimension in systole; *MVDE* = anterior mitral valve leaflet excursion; and *TVDE* = anterior tricuspid valve leaflet excursion. (From Roge CLL, Silverman NH, Hart PA, et al: *Circulation* 1978; 57:288. Used by permission.)

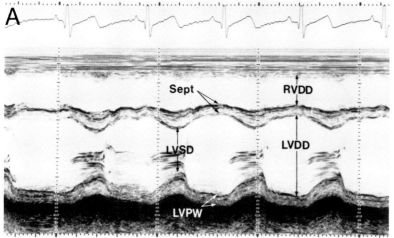
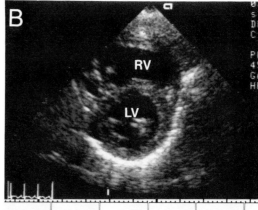
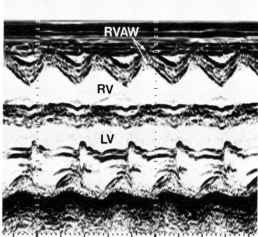

FIG 4–2.

A, M-mode echocardiogram of the left ventricle at the level of the posterior mitral valve leaflet showing the methods used to measure the ventricular chamber dimensions and wall thickness. Measurements are made from leading edge to leading edge at end-systole and end-diastole. *LVDD* = left ventricular dimension at end-diastole; *LVSD* = left ventricular dimension at end-systole; *LVPW* = left ventricular posterior wall thickness measured at end-diastole; *RVDD* = right ventricular dimension at end-diastole; and *SEPT* = septal thickness at end-diastole. **B,** M-mode echocardiogram *(bottom)* through the right ventricle (RV) and left ventricle (LV), demonstrating the technique used to measure the right ventricular anterior wall (RVAW) thickness in diastole. The freeze-frame image *(top)* shows the position of the M-mode cursor line at the time of the M-mode recording. The RVAW is measured at end-diastole from leading edge to leading edge. To make this measurement accurately, a clear recording of the RVAW epicardial and endocardial surfaces is necessary.

surement is normal or abnormal. The normal data are displayed as a function of body surface area; however, the data correlate just as strongly with mathematical functions of height and weight. Graphic displays of regression equations that use body surface area are particularly useful, because so many hemodynamic measurements in children are expressed in relation to body surface area. In infants, it is probably more useful to relate normal echocardiographic dimensions to body weight because a large change in body weight (i.e., from 2 to 4 kg) results in only minimal changes in body surface area.[4]

The normal M-mode echocardiographic measurements were obtained from echocardiograms recorded using stand-alone M-mode echocardiographic systems. Currently, most echocardiography laboratories use M-mode echocardiographic tracings derived from the two-dimensional echocardiogram. Measurements from derived M-mode echocardiograms have correlated well with those obtained from independent M-mode echocardiograms.[6] The derived M-mode echocardiograms are usually generated from the parasternal long- or short-axis views. Visualization of the right ventricular anterior wall can be optimized by placing the

transducer in a high left parasternal position, as close as possible to the sternal border. The M-mode cursor line is positioned perpendicular to the major axis of the left ventricle at the level of the posterior mitral valve leaflet (Fig 4–2). In infants under one year of age, the mitral valve leaflets extend farther toward the cardiac apex; therefore, in these children ventricular dimensions should be measured at the point of maximal excursion of both mitral valve leaflets.[2] M-mode echocardiographic measurements are made according to the recommendations of the Committee on M-mode Standardization of the American Society of Echocardiography.[7] Wall thickness and cavity dimensions are measured from the leading edge of the anterior echo to the leading edge of the posterior echo. Measurements are made at end-diastole at the onset of the QRS complex and at end-systole where the septum and left ventricular posterior wall are in closest approximation. The aortic root and left atrium are measured with the cursor line positioned at the level of the aortic valve leaflets in the parasternal long- or short-axis views (Fig 4–3).

In addition to wall thickness, total left ventricular mass can be calculated from M-mode echocardiographic measurements.[8, 9] Devereux and Reichek[8] compared eight different echocardiographic methods of measuring left ventricular mass to anatomic measurements of left ventricular mass. The best estimate of left ventricular mass was obtained using a formula derived from the assumption that the left ventricle is a prolate ellipsoid with minor radii that are one-half the major radii (cube formula) and using a measurement technique known as the Penn convention. In this method, the thickness of the endocardial echoes is excluded from measurements of the ventricular septum and posterior wall and included in the measurement of left ventricular diastolic dimension. Using these techniques, left ventricular mass is estimated as:

Anatomic LVM =
    1.04 ([LVID + PWT + IVST]^3 − [LVID]^3) − 13.6 gm

where LVM = left ventricular mass
         LVID = left ventricular internal dimension in diastole
         PWT = posterior wall thickness in diastole
         IVST = interventricular septal thickness in diastole

Using this formula, excellent correlation was found between anatomic and echocardiographic measurements of left ventricular mass (correlation coefficient = 0.96, standard deviation = 29.1 gm).

An alternative to the Penn measurement convention is M-mode measurement with the American Society of Echocardiography convention[7] (leading edge to leading edge), which can be used in the following cube formula to estimate left ventricular mass:

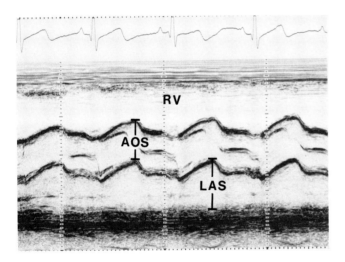

FIG 4–3.
M-mode echocardiogram of the aorta (AO) at the level of the valve leaflets demonstrating the techniques used to measure the aortic and left atrial dimensions. Measurements are made from leading edge to leading edge. *LAS* = left atrial dimension in systole; *AOS* = aortic diameter in systole; and *RV* = right ventricle.

ASE − cube LV mass =
    1.04 ([LVID + PWT + IVST]^3 − LVID]^3)

ASE − cube left ventricular mass correlated well with necropsy left ventricular mass (correlation coefficient = 0.90, standard deviation = 47 gm); however, this echocardiographic technique tended to overestimate necropsy values.[10] ASE − cube left ventricular mass measurements can be corrected to reflect necropsy left ventricular mass from the following equation:[10]

LVM = 0.80 (ASE − cube LV mass) + 0.6 gm

Values for left ventricular mass should be indexed for body surface area and compared to sex-specific normal data. In adults, indexed left ventricular mass of more than 134 gm/m^2 in men and more than 110 gm/m^2 in women indicated left ventricular hypertrophy.[9] In a recent study, echocardiographically determined left ventricular mass was measured in normal patients (6 to 23 years old) and indexed to height and body surface area. In male patients, left ventricular mass of more than 184.9 gm, 99.8 gm/m, or 103 gm/m^2 indicated left ventricular hypertrophy.[11] In female patients, the comparable values were 130.2 gm, 81.0 gm/m, or 84.2 gm/m^2.

Measurement of Valve Motion

Because of its rapid sampling rate, M-mode echocardiography is ideally suited for measuring the rate and extent of valve motion, as well as for timing the opening and closure of the valve leaflets.

Figure 4–4 shows a normal mitral valve M-mode echocardiogram and the conventional labelling used to describe various points on the echocardiogram. The D point represents the onset of valve opening. The E point is the point of maximum excursion of the valve during rapid ventricular filling. The F point is the nadir of initial diastolic closure. During atrial systole, the valve reopens and reaches a maximum excursion at the A point. Following the A point, the valve begins to close with atrial relaxation and reaches the completely closed state at the C point. A slight interruption in the rate of closure may occur between the A and C points as a result of ventricular systole. When present, this point is called the B point.[12]

From the mitral and tricuspid valve M-mode echocardiograms, the extent of valve opening (the D to E excursion measured as the vertical distance between these two points) and the rate of initial diastolic closure (the E to F slope) can be measured. Normal values for mitral and tricuspid valve D to E excursion and E to F slope are available from birth to adulthood (see Figure 4–1).[3–5] D to E excursion and E to F slope have been shown to be reduced in patients with ventricular inflow obstruction and in patients with ventricular dysfunction.

Figure 4–5 shows a normal aortic valve M-mode echocardiogram and the labeling used to describe this echocardiogram. Before the introduction of two-dimensional

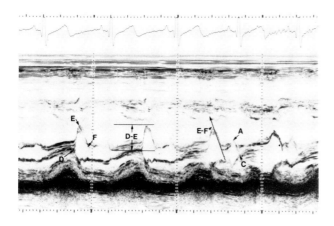

FIG 4–4.
M-mode echocardiogram of the left ventricle at the level of the anterior mitral valve leaflet. The conventional labelling used to describe the various points on the anterior mitral valve leaflet are displayed. The *D point* represents the onset of valve opening. The *E point* is the point of maximum excursion of the valve during rapid ventricular filling. The *F point* is the nadir of initial diastolic closure. During atrial systole, the valve reopens and reaches a maximum excursion at the *A point*. Following the A point, the valve reaches a completely closed state at the *C point*. The extent of valve opening, the D to E excursion, is measured as the vertical distance between the *D and E points*. The rate of initial diastolic closure, the E to F slope, is measured as the slope of a straight line drawn from the *E to F points*.

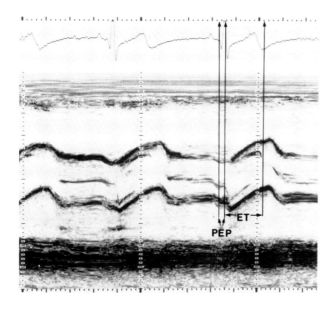

FIG 4–5.
M-mode echocardiogram of the aortic root at the level of the valve leaflets demonstrating techniques for measuring the systolic time intervals. The pre-ejection period (PEP) is measured from the Q-wave on the electrocardiogram to the onset of valve opening; the ejection time (ET) is measured from the onset of valve opening to the time of valve closure.

TABLE 4–1.
Equations for Heart Rate-Corrected Time Intervals

$LVET_c$	=	$LVET + 1.6 \, (HR)$*
$LVPEP_c$	=	$LVPEP + 0.4 \, (HR)$†
$RVET_c$	=	$RVET + 1.09 \, (HR) - 2.59 \, (\text{age in yrs})$‡
$RVPEP_c$	=	$RVPEP + 0.37 \, (HR)$‡

*Equation from Weissler AM, Harris LC, White GD: Left-ventricular ejection time index in man. *J Appl Physiol* 1963; 18:919-923.
†Equation from Weissler AM, Harris WS, Schoenfeld CD: Systolic time intervals in heart failure in man. *Circulation* 1968; 37:149-159.
‡Equation from Riggs T, Hirschfeld S, Borkat G, et al: Assessment of the pulmonary vascular bed by echocardiographic right ventricular systolic time intervals. *Circulation* 1978; 57:939-947.

HR = heart rate (beats/min); LVET = left ventricular ejection time; $LVET_c$ = heart rate-corrected left ventricular ejection time; LVPEP = left ventricular pre-ejection period; $LVPEP_c$ = heart rate-corrected left ventricular pre-ejection period; RVET = right ventricular ejection time; $RVET_c$ = heart rate-corrected right ventricular ejection time; RVPEP = right ventricular pre-ejection period; and $RVPEP_c$ = heart rate-corrected right ventricular pre-ejection period.

and Doppler echocardiography, measurements taken from the M-mode echocardiograms of the semilunar valves (i.e., the depth of the A wave, eccentricity index, etc.) were used to indicate certain disease states; these measurements have been replaced by more accurate two-dimensional and Doppler techniques and are no longer in routine use. However, the aortic and pulmonary valve M-mode echocardiograms are still useful for measuring left and right ventricular systolic time intervals. Thus, the pre-ejection period (PEP) is measured from the Q wave on the electrocardiogram to the onset of valve opening, and the ejection time (ET) is measured from the onset of valve opening to the time of valve closure.[13] The systolic time intervals vary with heart rate; therefore, to compare systolic time intervals in patients with different heart rates, it is necessary to correct the time intervals for heart rate using regression equations such as those described by Weissler et al.[14] and Riggs et al.[15] or to use a ratio of time intervals (PEP/ET).[16] Regression equations for heart rate-corrected time intervals are listed in Table 4–1.

The normal value for the heart-rate corrected left ventricular ejection time is 395 ± 13 msec for adult males and 415 ± 11 msec for adult females.[14] Left ventricular ejection time values for normal children under 13 years old are shorter and show no sex differences. Normal values for a child of a given age and heart rate can be calculated according to the formula:[17]

$$LVET \, (\text{msec}) = 0.35 \, (\text{age in months}) - 1.35 \, (\text{heart rate}) + 337$$

The normal value for the heart rate-corrected left ventricular pre-ejection period is 131 ± 13 msec in adults.[18] In children under 13 years old, the pre-ejection period varies with age and is shorter than the adult normal value.[17]

The ratio of left ventricular PEP/ET has been reported to be unrelated to heart rate or age. Reported normal values are 0.35 in adults and 0.32 in children.[19] In patients with left ventricular systolic failure, the left ventricular PEP is prolonged and the left ventricular ET is shortened; therefore, the left ventricular PEP/ET is increased.[20] In patients with aortic stenosis, the left ventricular PEP is shortened, the ET is prolonged, and the left ventricular PEP/ET is decreased.

The normal value for the heart rate-corrected right ventricular pre-ejection time in children is 109 ±11 msec. Right ventricular ejection time in children varies with both heart rate and age. The normal heart rate-corrected right ventricular ejection time is 373 ±21 msec. In children, right ventricular PEP/ET ratio does not correlate with heart rate or age. Normal values for this ratio have been shown to range from 0.17 to 0.33.[15]

Several investigators have reported correlations between right ventricular systolic time intervals and pulmonary artery pressure and resistance. With pulmonary hypertension, right ventricular PEP lengthens, ET shortens, and PEP/ET increases. Strong correlations have been demonstrated between right ventricular PEP/ET and pulmonary artery diastolic pressure measured at cardiac catheterization.[15, 16] Likewise, good correlations have been reported between pulmonary vascular resistance and the right ventricular PEP/ET ratio.[21] On the other hand, the right ventricular PEP/ET ratio and systolic time intervals vary with heart rate, ventricular loading conditions, ventricular inotropic state, and pharmacologic state of the patient.[22] The relationships between right ventricular systolic time intervals and pulmonary artery pressure or resistance predict a wide range of pulmonary artery diastolic pressure for any given value of PEP/ET. For these reasons, right ventricular systolic time intervals should not be used alone to evaluate the hemodynamic status of the patient's pulmonary vascular bed. When abnormal, however, these time intervals and the PEP/ET ratio provide supportive evidence for a diagnosis of pulmonary hypertension.

Measurements of Ventricular Function

Ventricular Systolic Function

Several different types of indexes of left ventricular systolic performance can be derived from the M-mode echocardiogram. One of the simplest and most widely used M-mode indexes of left ventricular function is the percent change in left ventricular diameter that occurs with systole or the shortening fraction. The shortening fraction is calculated using the equation:

$$\%SF = \frac{LVDD - LVSD}{LVDD} \times 100$$

where LVDD = left ventricular end-diastolic dimension
 LVSD = left ventricular end-systolic dimension
 SF = shortening fraction

The shortening fraction, an ejection phase index of ventricular performance, has a normal mean value of 36%

with a range of 28% to 44%.[2] This index is independent of age and heart rate, but dependent on ventricular preload and afterload. The shortening fraction readily distinguishes children with congestive cardiomyopathy (mean shortening fraction 16±7%) from normal children. In children with left ventricular volume overload, the shortening fraction increases with increasing volume loading.[23, 24] Once left ventricular failure occurs, the shortening fraction returns to normal or less than normal. In children with increased left ventricular afterload (i.e., severe aortic stenosis), the shortening fraction is increased; however, superimposed congestive heart failure causes a marked decrease in the shortening fraction.[25]

The extent of shortening of the left ventricular posterior wall is another M-mode index of contractility. The increase in thickness that occurs with contraction is usually expressed as a percentage of the end-diastolic wall thickness and is called the thickening fraction. The average thickening fraction in normal subjects is 60%; however, the range of normal values is large (30% to 100%), making this a much less useful index of myocardial dysfunction. Decreased posterior wall thickening occurs in patients with congestive cardiomyopathy, muscular dystrophy, and thalassemia.[26]

Besides the extent of shortening, the rate of shortening of the left ventricle can be calculated as an index of systolic function. *Peak* and *mean* rates of shortening of the left ventricle can be calculated by dividing the change in dimension by the change in time. Peak rates of ventricular shortening are calculated from computer-assisted analysis of digitized tracings of the left ventricular endocardium. This technique will be discussed in detail in a later section. One commonly used measurement of the mean rate of shortening is the mean velocity of circumferential fiber shortening, normalized for end-diastolic dimension (mean Vcf). Mean Vcf is calculated from the formula:

$$Mean\ Vcf = \frac{LVDD - LVSD}{LVDD \times LVET}$$

where LVDD = left ventricular end-diastolic dimension
 LVSD = left ventricular end-systolic dimension
 LVET = left ventricular ejection time

Left ventricular ejection time is usually measured from the aortic valve M-mode echocardiogram. Normal values for the mean Vcf are 1.5±0.04 circumferences/sec for premature and newborn infants and 1.3±0.03 circ/sec for 2- to 10-year old children.[27, 28] The gradual decrease in the normal values for mean Vcf throughout childhood to adulthood reflects the dependence of this ratio on heart rate and afterload. A heart rate-corrected mean Vcf (mean Vcf$_c$) can be calculated using a rate-corrected ejection time (LVET$_c$). Thus:

$$Mean\ Vcf_c = \frac{LVDD - LVSD}{LVDD \times LVETc}$$

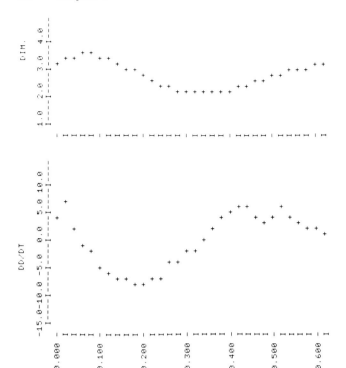

FIG 4–6.
Computer printouts of a digitized tracing of the left ventricular endocardial surfaces. The top graph displays the absolute value of the left ventricular minor axis dimension (DIM) with respect to time. The bottom graph displays the rate of change of this dimension with respect to time (dD/dt). From the bottom graph, the peak rate of shortening and the peak rate of relaxation of the ventricle can be determined.

where

$$LVET_c = \frac{LVET}{\sqrt{R - R \text{ interval}}}$$

The normal value for the heart rate-corrected mean Vcf is 0.98 ±0.07 circ/sec.[29]

In infants with left ventricular volume overload, mean Vcf is usually significantly larger than normal. The increased mean Vcf is probably caused by an increase in left ventricular end-diastolic dimension, as well as by augmented ventricular shortening. Thus, a normal mean Vcf in a patient with significant left ventricular volume overload (i.e., with ventricular septal defect, patent ductus arteriosus, or aortic or mitral insufficiency) suggests abnormal myocardial function. Children with minimal left ventricular volume overload (i.e., with small shunts or mild valvular insufficiency) often have near-normal values for mean Vcf.[28] In patients with cardiomyopathy, mean Vcf is significantly lower than normal. The decrease in mean Vcf relates directly to the severity of the disease.[26, 28]

Besides the mean rate of shortening, the peak rates of change in left ventricular cavity dimensions or posterior

wall thickness can be calculated using computer analysis of digitized tracings of the left ventricular endocardial or posterior wall surfaces. Using a digitizing tablet and desktop computer, the M-mode echocardiogram is digitized by tracing the endocardial echoes of the septum and the posterior wall over several cardiac cycles.[30, 31] From the digitized tracings, a computer printout of the absolute values of the left ventricular minor axis dimension and the rate of change of this dimension with respect to time (dD/dt) is available, usually at 3 to 5 msec intervals (Fig 4–6).

The peak rate of shortening (peak dD/dt) correlates well with catheterization measurements of peak dP/dt;[31] however, this index is dependent on heart rate and left ventricular dimension.[32] The peak rate of shortening can be normalized to left ventricular size by dividing this index by the left ventricular diastolic dimension

$$(\frac{1}{D} \times \frac{dD}{dt}).$$

The normalized peak rate of shortening is known as the peak Vcf. Either end-diastolic or instantaneous diastolic dimension can be used to normalize the peak rate of shortening.[30–32] The resultant peak Vcf values are nearly the same, regardless of which diastolic dimension is used.[32] Table 4–2 lists values for peak shortening rates of the left and right ventricles of normal infants and children.[32–36]

Digitized tracings of the endocardial and epicardial surfaces of the cardiac walls can be used to calculate peak rates of wall thickening or thinning with respect to time.[30, 31, 34, 37] As with the cavity dimensions, the peak rates of wall thickening or thinning can be normalized to instantaneous wall thickness. Table 4–3 lists values for peak rates of thickening and thinning of the cardiac walls in normal infants.[34] As the level from which the M-mode echocardiogram is obtained changes, regional nonuniformity of wall dynamics is found in normal infants and children. From the base to the apex of the ventricle, the extent of left ventricular posterior wall thickening in systole increases, the peak rate of posterior wall thinning increases, and the peak rate of posterior wall thickening does not change. Thus, when examining wall dynamics, the exact level of the M-mode echocardiogram is crucial.[38]

The digitized M-mode echocardiographic technique requires a very high quality M-mode recording of the left ventricle just below the level of the anterior mitral valve leaflet. Use of an expanded scale and rapid paper speed (100 mm/sec) for recording the M-mode echocardiogram will increase the accuracy and reproducibility of the digitized tracings. The variability of the normal data shown in Tables 4–2 and 4–3 shows that this technique is very observer-dependent; however, when special attention is given to optimizing the technical quality of the digitized tracings, interobserver, intraobserver, and beat-to-beat variability can be kept to acceptably low levels.[35]

The distance from the E point of the mitral valve to the most posterior excursion of the ventricular septum— E point-septal separation—can be used to assess left ventricular function (Fig 4–7). E point-septal separation is less

TABLE 4–2.

Rates of Dimension Change in Systole in Normal Children*

Source	No. of Patients	Patient Ages	LV PSR	LV Peak Vcf	RV Peak Vcf
Upton and Gibson[33]	—	Adult	9.6 ± 1.4	2.3 ± 0.4	—
St. John Sutton et al.[34]	50	1–3 days	—	3.8 ± 1.0	3.6 ± 1.0
Friedman and Sahn[35]	52	6 mo–18 yr	9.6 ± 0.3	—	—
Kugler et al.[32]	62	1–17 yr	7.1 ± 2.0	2.1 ± 0.5	—
Hofstetter et al.[36]	60	3.6 days	—	4.6 ± 1.5	4.1 ± 2.2

*Data are expressed as mean ± SD. LV = left ventricular; RV = right ventricular; PSR = peak shortening rate (cm/sec); Vcf = velocity of circumferential fiber shortening (circ/sec).

TABLE 4–3.

Wall Dynamics in Normal Children*†

	% Change in Thickness	Normalized Peak Thickening Rate (sec⁻¹)	Normalized Peak Thinning Rate (sec⁻¹)
RVAW	127 ± 38	5.5 ± 1.7	7.9 ± 2.2
Sept	95 ± 40	6.0 ± 2.1	5.6 ± 2.2
LVPW	130 ± 50	5.4 ± 1.3	8.0 ± 2.2

*From St. John Sutton MS, Hagler DJ, Tajik AJ, et al: Cardiac function in the normal newborn. Additional information by computer analysis of the M-mode echocardiogram. *Circulation* 1978; 57:1198–1204. Used with permission.
†LVPW = left ventricular posterior wall; RVAW = right ventricular anterior wall; and Sept = septum.

than 4 mm in normal adults and is inversely related to ejection fraction in patients with coronary artery disease.[39] Although this index cannot be used to assess left ventricular function in the presence of cardiac diseases that alter mitral valve motion (i.e., aortic insufficiency and mitral stenosis), it has been shown to be a valid indicator of ventricular performance even in the presence of abnormal or reversed septal motion. Thus, E point-septal separation has an advantage over shortening fraction, which has limited usefulness in the presence of abnormal septal motion.[40, 41]

In 105 normal children, aged 1 day to 15 years old, E point-septal separation was 2.5 ± 1.7 mm. E point-septal separation can be normalized to ventricular size by dividing the E point-septal separation by the left ventricular end-diastolic dimension (EPSS/EDD). In normal children, EPSS/EDD was 0.08 ± 0.06.[42] In children with left ventricular volume overload (ventricular septal defect, patent ductus arteriosus), E point-septal separation and EPSS/EDD were similar to those of normal subjects. However, in children with congestive cardiomyopathy, E point-septal separation and EPSS/EDD were significantly increased to 16.5 ± 5.1 mm and 0.39 ± 0.09 respectively.[42] Thus, the E point-septal separation is a simple and accurate method of separating normal from abnormal left ventricular function.

Left ventricular systolic function is determined by a complex interaction of four variables: myocardial contractile state, end-diastolic myocardial length, afterload, and left ventricular mass.[43] Ejection-phase indexes such as ejection fraction, shortening fraction, and mean velocity of circumferential fiber shortening can be used to identify left ventricular pump dysfunction; these indexes, however, provide no information about the relative role of each of the above four variables in causing the pump dysfunction. Noninvasive techniques for measuring end-diastolic myocardial length (preload) and left ventricular mass have been described above. Noninvasive techniques for quantitation of afterload and contractility will be reviewed below.

Left ventricular systolic pressure and systemic vascular resistance are commonly used measurements of afterload. However, end-systolic pressure is determined by many additional variables such as stroke volume, vascular resistance, and ejection rate. Likewise, systemic vascular resistance is a mathematically derived number used to express the relationship between peripheral pressure and flow and is therefore not a true physical load seen by the left ventricle. The best measurement of the true left ventricular afterload is the systolic wall tension. To permit comparisons between hearts of different wall thicknesses and diameters, systolic wall tension is expressed as tension per unit of cross-sectional area of myocardium or wall stress.

Meridional wall stress is defined as the force per unit area acting at the equatorial plane of the ventricle in the direction of the apex-to-base axis. Meridional wall stress is independent of the long-axis length of the left ventricle and can be calculated using a formula initially validated with angiographic techniques[44] and later validated with echocardiography[43]:

$$\text{Wall stress (g/cm}^2) = \frac{0.334\ P \times LVID}{LVPW\ (1 + LVPW/LVID)}$$

where   P   = left ventricular pressure (mm Hg)
        LVID = left ventricular minor axis dimension (cm)
        LVPW = left ventricular posterior wall thickness (cm)

Circumferential wall stress is the force per unit area acting along the circumference of the left ventricle at its minor axis and, theoretically, relates more closely to the mean velocity of circumferential fiber shortening. The formula for circumferential wall stress was first validated with angiography[45] and later with echocardiographic techniques[46]:

$$\text{Wall stress (g/cm}^2) = \frac{1.35\ Pr\ (1 - [2r^2/L^2])}{LVPW}$$

where   P   = left ventricular pressure (mm Hg)
        r   = left ventricular minor axis dimension divided by 2 (cm)
        LVPW = left ventricular posterior wall thickness
        L   = long axis of the left ventricle (cm)

The long-axis length (L) of the left ventricle can be mea-

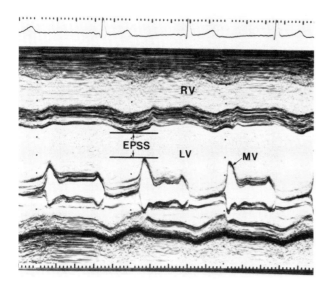

FIG 4–7.
M-mode echocardiogram of the left ventricle (LV) at the level of the anterior mitral valve leaflets (MV) demonstrating the technique used to measure the E point-septal separation (EPSS). The EPSS is measured from the maximum excursion of the MV in early diastole to the most posterior excursion of the septum. *RV* = right ventricle.

sured from the two-dimensional echocardiogram or can be assumed to be equal to twice the minor-axis dimension.

Values for meridional wall stress are usually nearly twice those for circumferential wall stress, and the two techniques correlate closely with one another.[47–49] Since meridional wall stress does not require measurement of the long-axis length of the left ventricle, this simpler calculation has become the preferred echocardiographic index of left ventricular afterload.

Left ventricular wall stress varies continuously throughout systole, so that the instantaneous left ventricular afterload is constantly changing.[43] Thus, peak systolic wall stress is the *largest* of all the instantaneous values for the wall stress throughout ejection, while mean systolic wall stress is the *average* of all the instantaneous values for the wall stress throughout systole.[50] End-systolic wall stress is calculated using left ventricular pressure and dimensions measured at end-systole. Controversy still remains about which wall stress measurement is the best index of left ventricular afterload. Recent studies suggest that peak systolic wall stress is a determinant of the degree of left ventricular hypertrophy, while mean systolic stress is a determinant of myocardial oxygen requirements.[44, 51, 52] It is important to note that peak wall stress usually occurs toward the end of the first one-third of systole and, therefore, does not occur at the time of peak left ventricular pressure (which usually occurs near midsystole).[46]

Isolated heart studies have shown that ejection ends when instantaneous myocardial force reaches the isometric value for the myocardial length.[43, 53, 54] End-systolic wall stress, therefore, is the afterload that limits ejection. For a given contractile state, only a decrease in end-systolic wall stress can result in an increased emptying of the ventricle. Since end-systolic wall stress represents the limiting factor in fiber shortening, it is the most relevant measurement of wall stress when ventricular function is assessed.[29, 43] End-systolic wall stress can be determined from M-mode measurements taken at the time of minimum left ventricular dimension and the arterial blood pressure. In one simple approach that has been validated against invasive measurements, the cuff systolic arterial pressure is used along with the M-mode measurements to calculate end-systolic wall stress.[43] This simple approach is successful because cuff systolic blood pressure is closely related to end-systolic micromanometer left ventricular pressure, except in cases of severe mitral regurgitation. In severe mitral regurgitation, left ventricular pressure decreases in late systole, and therefore cuff systolic arterial pressure is significantly higher than true left ventricular end-systolic pressure. Using the cuff systolic arterial pressure, end-systolic meridional wall stress was 64.8 ± 19.5 gm/cm² in normal adults.[43]

In another approach, the carotid pulse tracing is calibrated to the cuff arterial blood pressure and an estimate of dicrotic notch pressure is made.[55] Dicrotic notch pressure is then used to calculate end-systolic wall stress. The problems with this approach include difficulty in recording a clear dicrotic notch (especially in patients with aortic insufficiency) and underestimation of end-systolic micromanometer left ventricular pressure.[43]

In another approach, carotid pulse tracings are calibrated using an automated blood pressure monitoring device. Systolic pressure is assigned to the peak and diastolic pressure is assigned to the nadir of the tracing. End-systolic pressure is estimated by linear interpolation either to the aortic closing component of the second heart sound on a simultaneously recorded phonocardiogram or to the incisura on the carotid pulse tracing.[29, 56, 57] Using this technique, end-systolic meridional wall stress was reported to be 51 ± 9 gm/cm² in one study of 68 normal patients (3 to 70 years old)[29] and 43 ± 3 gm/cm² in another study of 24 children (2 to 22.5 years old).[49] In infants in whom the carotid artery pulse tracing can be technically difficult to record, an indirect axillary pulse tracing calibrated to an automated blood pressure monitoring device may be used.[58] With this approach, the end-systolic meridional wall stress was 37 ± 10 gm/cm² in 30 infants (1 day to 48 months old).[58]

Several studies have shown that the end-systolic force-length relationship can be used to characterize myocardial contractility.[52–54] This relationship can be examined noninvasively using left ventricular end-systolic pressure or wall stress as the force measurement and left ventricular end-systolic dimension or volume as the length measurement. Borow and colleagues devised a noninvasive technique for describing this relationship from simultaneous recordings of the M-mode echocardiogram of the left ventricle, carotid pulse tracing, and the phonocardiogram.[56, 59] The carotid pulse tracing was calibrated by simultaneous recording of the arm blood pressure, as noted above. The left ventricular end-systolic dimension and pressure were measured either at the time of the dicrotic notch or at the time of the aortic closure component of the second heart sound on the phonocardiogram. Pressure-dimension relations were studied at rest and following infusion of methoxamine and dobutamine to alter ventricular loading conditions. The left ventricular end-systolic pressure-dimension relationship was found to be independent of preload, to incorporate afterload, and to vary with contractile state. In all cases the curves describing this relation were linear and the slope of the curve was highly sensitive to changes in inotropic state, becoming steeper with positive inotropic intervention. Further, the slope of the noninvasively determined end-systolic pressure-volume relationship using cubed M-mode dimensions to approximate volumes correlated closely with the slope determined at catheterization using measured pressures and angiographic volumes.

Although these pressure-dimension relationships are useful clinically, to be determined accurately they require manipulation of afterload conditions. To describe a load-independent index of contractility, Colan and colleagues investigated the relationship between left ventricular end-systolic meridional wall stress and the rate-corrected mean velocity of circumferential fiber shortening.[29] A linear, inverse relationship was found between wall stress and rate-

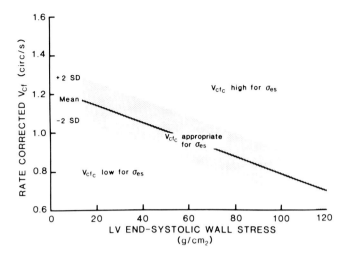

FIG 4–8.
Graphic display of the relationship between the rate-corrected velocity of circumferential fiber shortening (Vcf) and the left ventricular (LV) end-systolic wall stress. This relationship is a sensitive indicator of contractile state that is independent of preload and is normalized for heart rate. For any given wall stress, a normal range of rate-corrected Vcf can be defined. Using this graph, it is possible to distinguish a reduced Vcf caused by excessive afterload from a reduced fiber shortening caused by depressed contractility. (From Colan SD, Borow KM, Newmann A: *J Am Coll Cardiol* 1984; 4:722. Used by permission.)

corrected velocity of circumferential fiber shortening. The relationship was a sensitive indicator of contractile state that was independent of preload and was normalized for heart rate. This index can be determined noninvasively without manipulating loading conditions, and a normal range of values can be established. Figure 4–8, from their paper, illustrates the clinical utility of the stress shortening relationship. For any given wall stress, a normal range of rate-corrected velocity of circumferential fiber shortening can be defined. Using this graph, it is possible to distinguish a reduced velocity of circumferential fiber shortening caused by excessive afterload from a reduced fiber shortening caused by depressed contractility. Because both wall stress and velocity of circumferential fiber shortening are normalized for cardiac size, the relationship applies to all age groups.

Ventricular Diastolic Function

Several different types of indexes of left ventricular diastolic function can be derived from the M-mode echocardiogram. The diastolic indexes include diastolic time intervals that reflect the time course of relaxation, peak and mean filling rates of the left ventricle, and the percentage of total filling that occurs in the various phases of diastole. In general, these indexes are measured from a digitized tracing of the left ventricular endocardium using the techniques described above. A simultaneously recorded phonocardiogram is useful for determining the end of systole (at the aortic closure component of the second heart sound).

The different diastolic time intervals that have been used to describe the time course of ventricular relaxation include:[60, 61]

1. Isovolumic relaxation time, measured from the first high-frequency deflection of the aortic closure sound to the initial separation or D point of the mitral valve leaflets.
2. Relaxation time index, measured from the minimum left ventricular systolic dimension to the D point of the mitral valve.
3. Protodiastole, measured from the minimum left ventricular systolic dimension to the aortic closure sound.
4. Total relaxation time, measured from the minimum left ventricular systolic dimension to the point when the change in left ventricular minor-axis dimension with respect to time (dD/dt) decreases to 50% of its peak value. This latter point corresponds roughly to the transition between the rapid- and slow-filling phases of diastole.
5. Time to peak filling rate, measured from minimum left-ventricular systolic dimension to peak dD/dt.
6. Rapid filling period, calculated as total relaxation time minus (isovolumic relaxation time + protodiastole).

Normal values for the diastolic time intervals are given in Table 4–4. In general, the use of time intervals to assess left ventricular diastolic function is limited by their dependence on cardiac cycle length as well as by ventricular loading conditions and systolic function. As cardiac cycle length decreases, passive relaxation occupies an increasing proportion of diastole. The only time interval that is independent of cardiac cycle length is the isovolumic relaxation time.[61] This time period is directly related to the duration of the left ventricular-left atrial pressure gradient during isovolumic relaxation. Thus, in patients with normal filling pressures and impaired left ventricular relaxation (decreased filling rate), the isovolumic relaxation time is prolonged. In patients with high filling pressures and impaired ventricular compliance, the isovolumic relaxation time is shortened.

The peak filling rate of the left ventricle is another index of diastolic function that can be measured from the digitized M-mode echocardiogram. This index is the peak rate of increase in left ventricular dimension (dD/dt) in early diastole. Like the peak rate of shortening, the peak

rate of lengthening can be normalized so that values for different-sized ventricles can be compared. Techniques for obtaining a normalized peak rate of lengthening (dD/dt/D) include division of dD/dt by the maximum diastolic dimension, the instantaneous diastolic dimension, and the fractional shortening.[30–36, 61–63] Like the diastolic time intervals, the usefulness of the peak rate of lengthening is limited by its dependence on ventricular loading conditions and systolic function.[61] Normal values for the peak rate of relaxation are listed in Table 4–5.

From the digitized M-mode echocardiogram, the percentage of total left ventricular filling that occurs in the different phases of diastole can be determined.[64] For these measurements, diastole is divided into the following four phases:

1. Isovolumic relaxation, the time between minimum left ventricular systolic dimension and mitral valve opening.
2. Rapid filling phase, the time from mitral valve opening to the time when the normalized lengthening rate decreases to 50% of its peak value.
3. Slow filling phase, the time from the end of the rapid filling phase to the point where the lengthening caused by atrial contraction reaches half its maximum value.
4. Atrial contraction, the time from the end of the slow filling phase to the peak of the R wave of the next cardiac cycle.

In normal adults, the percentage of the total increase in left ventricular diastolic dimension that occurs during the rapid filling phase is 62 ±10%. The dimensional increase in the slow filling period is 22 ±9%, and the dimensional increase during atrial contraction is 16 ± 10%. No significant increase in dimension occurs during isovolumic relaxation. Hanrath and colleagues[64] found a shift in left ventricular filling toward the end of diastole in patients with impaired relaxation caused by left ventricular hypertrophy. Patients with systemic hypertension and aortic valve stenosis had a decreased percentage of total change in left ventricular diastolic dimension during the rapid filling phase and an increased percentage of total filling during atrial contraction. As a result, the total left ventricular diastolic filling was normal. Patients with hypertrophic cardiomyopathy also had a decreased percentage of left ventricular filling occurring during the rapid filling phase but lacked a compensatory increase in filling during atrial contraction. As a result, total left ventricular diastolic filling was reduced in these patients. These studies demonstrate how measurements of the percentage of filling of the left ventricle in the different phases of diastole can be useful in assessing ventricular relaxation properties.

QUANTITATIVE TWO-DIMENSIONAL ECHOCARDIOGRAPHY

Two-dimensional echocardiography provides a tech-

TABLE 4–4.

M-Mode Diastolic Time Intervals in Normal Subjects*

	Children[†]	Adults[‡]
Ages (yr)	3–18	18–61
Isovolumic relaxation time	35 ± 10	62 ± 14
Total relaxation time	180 ± 40	201 ± 30
Time to peak filling rate	120 ± 40	152 ± 24
Rapid filling period	100 ± 20	110 ± 36

*Data are expressed as mean ± SD; time intervals are in msec.
†Data collected in 34 children at the University of Michigan.
‡Data from Bahler RC, Vrobel TR, Martin P: The relation of heart rate and shortening fraction to echocardiographic indexes of left ventricular relaxation in normal subjects. *J Am Coll Cardiol* 1983; 2:926-933.

TABLE 4-5.
M-Mode Echo Relaxation Rates in Normal Patients*

Source	Number Patients	Patient Ages	LV Peak dD/dt	LV Peak dD/dt/D	RV Peak dD/dt	RV Peak dD/dt/D
St. John Sutton et al.[34]	50	1–3 days	7.7 ± 1.9	3.8 ± 1.0	3.7 ± 1.1	3.6 ± 1.0
Hofstetter et al.[36]	60	3–6 days	—	6.3 ± 3.1	—	4.3 ± 2.1
Kugler et al.[32]	62	1–17 yr	8.5 ± 3.5	—	—	—
St. John Sutton et al.[63]	20	19–63 yr	14.5 ± 2.3	2.7 ± 0.4	—	—
Bahler et al.[61]	28	18–61 yr	15.2 ± 3.6	3.1 ± 0.8	—	—
Fifer et al.[62]	48	4–75 yr	16.2 ± 4.8	10.3 ± 3.0	—	—

*Data are expressed as mean ± SD. dD/dt = rate of change in diastolic dimension with respect to time; dD/dt/D = normalized rate of change in diastolic dimension with respect to time; LV = left ventricle; RV = right ventricle. dD/dt was normalized by dividing by end-diastolic dimension in reference 61, fractional shortening in reference 62, and instantaneous diastolic dimension in references 34, 36, 32, and 63.

nique for the spatial display of cardiac structures and thus allows visualization of a larger area of the heart at one time than does M-mode echocardiography. When regional abnormalities of wall motion are present, two-dimensional echocardiography provides the most accurate assessment of ventricular function. The ability to visualize the entire contour of the ventricle at one time makes two-dimensional echocardiography the preferred technique for quantitation of ventricular volume and ejection fraction. One limitation of two-dimensional echocardiography is that sampling rates are slow (30 frames per second for two-dimensional echocardiography vs. several thousand pulses per second for M-mode echocardiography). For measurement of cardiac dimensions at precise times in the cardiac cycle (especially at fast heart rates), M-mode echocardiography provides better temporal resolution and is the preferred technique.

Measurement of Cardiac Structural Dimensions

Even though M-mode echocardiography is the preferred technique for measurement of chamber dimension and wall thickness, situations occur in which it may be necessary to measure chamber size using two-dimensional echocardiography. For example, in some patients it may not be possible to image the standard parasternal views used to obtain the M-mode dimension measurements. Similarly, using M-mode echocardiography, it may not be possible to image a structure in a standardized view suitable for measurement (i.e., the size of the mitral or tricuspid annulus). In these circumstances, the two-dimensional echocardiogram can be used to measure the dimensions of the cardiac chambers, the sizes of the valve annuli, and the diameter of the aorta and pulmonary arteries.[65–67] The measurement error caused by the limited temporal resolution of two-dimensional echocardiography is small in comparison to the size of the chamber being measured. If a cardiac wall thickness is measured, the measurement error is large compared with the size of the wall being measured; therefore, measurement of cardiac wall thicknesses from the two-dimensional echocardiogram is not recommended.

Normal values are available for cardiac chamber dimensions measured from the two-dimensional echocardiogram in adults.[65, 68, 69] Similar normal data for cardiac chamber dimensions from infancy to adulthood are not yet available. In one study of 35 normal adults,[65] the major- and minor-axis dimensions of the cardiac chambers were measured using the techniques shown in Figure 4–9. The

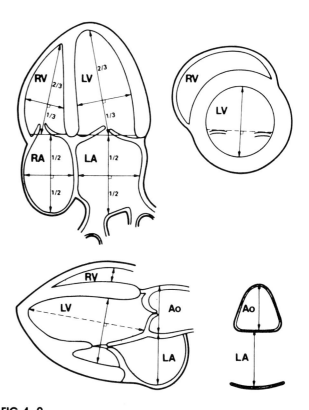

FIG 4-9.
Diagrammatic representation of the methods used to measure cardiac chamber dimensions from the two-dimensional echocardiogram of 35 normal adults. *AO* = aorta; *LA* = left atrium; *LV* = left ventricle; *RA* = right atrium; and *RV* = right ventricle. (From Schnittger I, Gordon EP, Fitzgerald PJ, et al: *J Am Coll Cardiol* 1983; 2:935. Used by permission.)

TABLE 4–6.
Cardiac Chamber Dimensions by Two-Dimensional Echocardiography*

View	Mean (cm)	Normal† Range (cm)	Indexed Normal Range (cm/m²)
Apical four-chamber			
LVed major	8.6	6.9–10.3	4.1–5.7
LVed minor	4.7	3.3–6.1	2.2–3.1
LVes minor	2.8	1.9–3.7	1.3–2.0
LV% FS	38.0	27.0–50.0	—
RV major	8.0	6.5–9.5	3.8–5.3
RV minor	3.3	2.2–4.4	1.0–2.8
LA major	5.1	4.1–6.1	2.3–3.5
LA minor	3.5	2.8–4.3	1.6–2.4
RA major	4.5	3.5–5.5	2.0–3.1
RA minor	3.7	2.5–4.9	1.7–2.5
Parasternal Long-Axis			
LVed	4.8	3.5–6.0	2.3–3.1
LVes	3.1	2.1–4.0	1.4–2.1
%FS	36.0	25.0–46.0	—
RV	2.8	1.9–3.8	1.2–2.0
LA	3.6	2.7–4.5	1.6–2.4
AO	2.9	2.2–3.6	1.4–2.0
Parasternal Short-Axis Aorta			
LA	3.6	2.6–4.5	1.6–2.4
AO	3.0	2.3–3.7	1.6–2.4
Chordae			
LVed	4.8	3.5–6.2	2.3–3.2
LVes	3.2	2.3–4.0	1.5–2.2
LV%FS	34.0	27.0–42.0	—
Papillary Muscles			
LVed	4.7	3.5–5.8	2.2–3.1
LVes	3.1	2.2–4.0	1.4–2.2
LV%FS	34.0	25.0–43.0	—

*Data from Schnittger I, Gordon EP, Fitzgerald PJ, et al: Standardized intracardiac measurements of two-dimensional echocardiography. *J Am Coll Cardiol* 1983; 2:934-938.
†Normal (NL) range = mean ± 2 standard deviations. AO = aorta; FS = fractional shortening; LA = left atrium; LVed = left ventricle at end-diastole; LVes = left ventricle at end-systole; RA = right atrium; and RV = right ventricle.

major axis of the ventricle was defined as the maximum length of the chamber. At a distance of one-third the length of the major axis from the atrioventricular valve plane, the minor axis was measured perpendicular to the major axis. Normal values using this method are given in Table 4–6. In another study of 50 normal adults,[12] the minor-axis dimension was measured at the tips of the mitral valve rather than at a point one-third of the long axis from the base. In this method, normal data differed slightly.

Normal values have been reported for mitral and tricuspid valve annulus diameter measured from the two-dimensional echocardiogram in normal children.[70] In one study, annulus diameters were measured in 103 children whose ages ranged from 1 day to 15 years old and whose body surface areas ranged from 0.2 to 1.4 m². The normal values for the anteroposterior diameter of the mitral valve (measured as the largest dimension during the cardiac cycle from a parasternal long-axis view) are shown in Figure 4–10. Lateral dimensions of the mitral and tricuspid annuli

were measured from the apical and subcostal four-chamber views and the view that gave the largest diameter was used to generate the normal values shown in Figure 4–11.

Normal values have also been reported for aortic and pulmonary artery sizes measured from the two-dimensional echocardiograms of patients from infancy to adulthood.[66] In this study, the aorta and pulmonary arteries were measured in 110 normal children whose ages ranged from 1 day to 18 years old and whose body surface areas ranged from < 0.25 to > 1.50 m². Measurements were made using the techniques shown in Figure 4–12. The normal values for the aortic and pulmonary artery sizes throughout childhood are shown in Figures 4–13 and 4–14. In almost all cases, the change in great vessel diameters throughout childhood was a function of the square root of the body surface area. In all cases, vessel diameters measured at end-systole exceeded those measured at end-diastole and, for vessels seen in cross-section, axial measurements exceeded lateral measurements of the same vessel. This study also

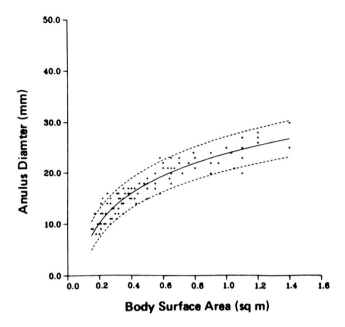

FIG 4–10.
Normal values for the anteroposterior diameter of the mitral valve, measured as the largest dimension during the cardiac cycle from a parasternal long-axis view. (From King DH, Smith EO, Huhta JC, et al: *Am J Cardiol* 1985; 55:788. Used by permission.)

showed that the parasternal short-axis view was particularly ill-suited for measuring the main and right pulmonary artery diameters because of the amount of cardiac motion apparent in this plane and also because the longitudinal orientation of the pulmonary arteries in this view can lead to an underestimation of maximum vessel diameter. Measurements of the right pulmonary artery diameter from the suprasternal long- and short-axis views correlated closely with normal values for this vessel measured at angiography.

Measurements of Cardiac Chamber Volumes

Left Ventricular Volumes and Ejection Fraction

Because the heart can be viewed from several planes and because contraction of a larger area of the heart can be viewed at one time, two-dimensional echocardiography provides a more accurate estimate of chamber volume than does M-mode echocardiography.[71, 72] Left ventricular volumes and ejection fraction measured with two-dimensional echocardiography have correlated well with those measured with cineangiography in children and adults.[71–74] To maximize the accuracy of two-dimensional echocardiographic volume analysis, several technical factors must be considered:

Resolution.—Endocardial definition is greatly influ-

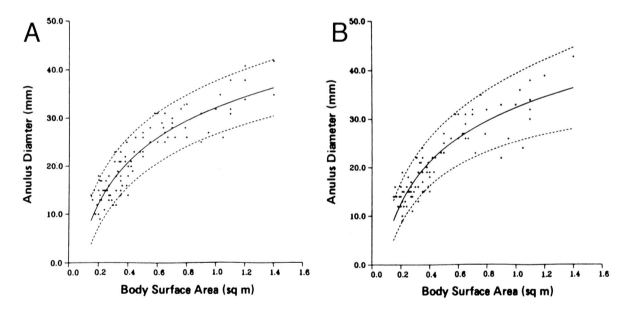

FIG 4–11.
A, normal values for the lateral dimensions of the mitral annulus measured from the apical and subcostal four-chamber views. The view that gave the largest diameter was used to generate the normal values. **B,** normal values for the lateral dimension of the tricuspid annulus measured from the apical and subcostal four-chamber views. The view that gave the largest diameter was used to generate the normal values. (From King DH, Smith EO, Huhta JC, et al: *Am J Cardiol* 1985; 55:788. Used by permission.)

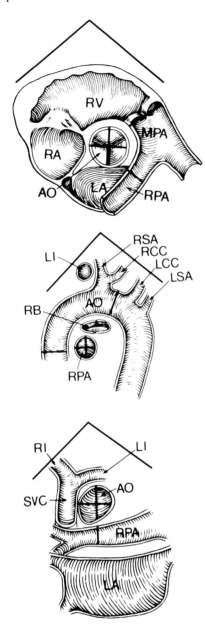

FIG 4–12.
The three echocardiographic views and techniques used to measure the aorta (AO), main pulmonary artery (MPA), right pulmonary artery (RPA), and left pulmonary artery (LPA) in 110 normal children from infancy to adulthood. The *heavy black lines* show the positions used in each view to make the measurements. *LA* = left atrium; *LCC* = left common carotid artery; *LI* = left innominate vein; *LSA* = left subclavian artery; *RA* = right atrium; *RB* = right bronchus; *RCC* = right common carotid artery; *RI* = right innominate vein; *RSA* = right subclavian artery; *RV* = right ventricle; and *SVC* = superior vena cava. (From Snider AR, Enderlein MA, Teitel DF, et al: *Am J Cardiol* 1984; 53:219. Used by permission.)

enced by the axial and lateral resolution of the ultrasound system. For optimal lateral resolution, the highest-frequency transducer that provides adequate penetration should be used. The focal point of the transducer should be as close to the center of the ventricle as possible.

Gain setting.—Gain settings should be optimized in order to image the endocardial targets clearly. Too much gain will cause blooming of the endocardial echoes; too little gain will cause echocardiographic dropout along the endocardial surfaces.

Depth setting.—The depth setting of the displayed image can influence the precision of the measurements. For example, if the left ventricle is imaged in a magnified presentation, the information being analyzed contains more pixels. The more pixels, the less error in the digitizing process. Also, at shallower depths (magnified images), the frame rate of the ultrasound equipment is higher. With faster frame rates, end-diastolic and end-systolic images can be obtained more precisely.

Calibration.—In the ultrasound system, a given distance in the vertical direction may not be displayed the same in the horizontal direction. The ratio of the vertical to horizontal display lengths of a known distance is called the aspect ratio. If images are recorded on videotape and analyzed at an off-line computer and video monitor, the off-line measurements must be corrected for the difference in the vertical and horizontal display formats. The correction is made using the aspect ratio, which can be calculated by imaging targets in a phantom that are a known distance apart in the vertical and horizontal directions. The distance between the targets as they are displayed by the ultrasound system is then measured and compared to the true distance between the targets for both vertical and horizontal directions. In addition to the aspect ratio calibration, the off-line analysis system must also be calibrated for the depth setting at which the recording was made. For on-line measurements, calibration by the user is not necessary because the equipment contains an internal calibration.

Video recordings.—Videotape recorders contain analog information so that nearly 50% of the video information will be lost on a video freeze frame. This loss of video information can be prevented by tracing digital images, which can be obtained in several ways: (1) by measuring images on line at the time of the study, (2) by saving images in digital format on high-density diskettes rather than in analog format on videotape, or (3) by digitizing the video frames before analysis rather than by measuring directly from the tape.

Frame selection.—Ventricular volumes are computed

at end-diastole and end-systole. The end-diastolic frame is chosen as the frame that shows initial coaptation of the mitral valve leaflets or the frame in which the QRS complex first appears. The end-systolic frame is chosen as the frame that precedes initial early diastolic mitral valve opening or the frame with the smallest ventricular dimension (if the mitral valve is not clearly seen).

Tracing techniques.—Tracing of the endocardial echoes should be along the black/white tissue-blood pool interface on the video monitor (Fig 4–15). When endocardial drop-out is present, the tracing should be extrapolated across the gap; however, tracings should terminate at the limits of the sector and segments that leave the imaging plane should not be fabricated. The tracing should cut across the base of the papillary muscles and thus exclude them from the traced outline of the ventricle.

Left ventricular volumes have been calculated using several different methods. In several early studies, volumes were calculated from parasternal short-axis and apical long-

ASCENDING AORTA – SUPRASTERNAL LONG AXIS

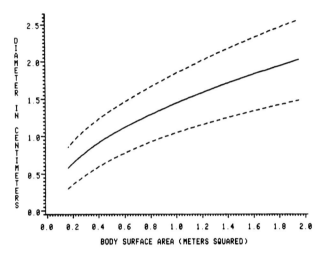

ASCENDING AORTA – PARASTERNAL SHORT AXIS

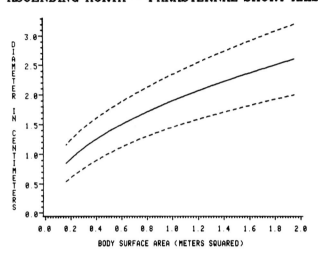

TRANSVERSE AORTA – SUPRASTERNAL LONG AXIS

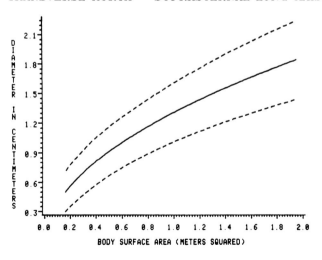

TRANSVERSE AORTA – SUPRASTERNAL SHORT AXIS

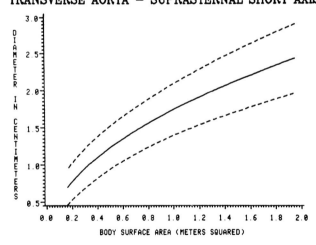

FIG 4–13.
Relations between measurements of the ascending and transverse aorta in different echocardiographic views and the body surface area in 110 normal children. Where possible, the measurements for these graphs were made in diastole and in an axial direction. The dashed lines are the tolerance limits weighted for body surface area for prediction of normal values for 80% of the future population with 50% confidence. (From Snider AR, Enderlein MA, Teitel DF, et al: *Am J Cardiol* 1984; 53:220. Used by permission.)

RIGHT PULMONARY ARTERY – SUPRASTERNAL LONG AXIS

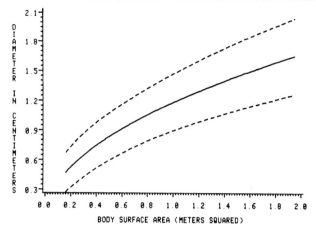

RIGHT PULMONARY ARTERY – PARASTERNAL SHORT AXIS

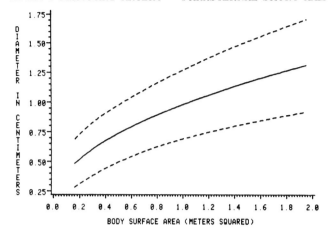

RIGHT PULMONARY ARTERY – SUPRASTERNAL SHORT AXIS

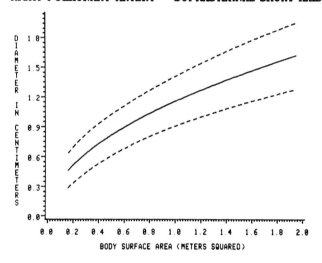

MAIN PULMONARY ARTERY – PARASTERNAL SHORT AXIS

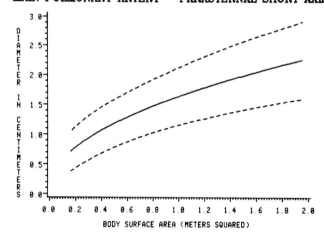

FIG 4–14.
Relations between measurements of the right and main pulmonary arteries in different echocardiographic views and the body surface area in 110 normal children. Where possible, the measurements for these graphs were made in diastole and in an axial direction. The *dashed lines* are the tolerance limits, weighted for body surface area, for prediction of normal values for 80% of the future population with 50% confidence. (From Snider AR, Enderlein MA, Teitel DF, et al: *Am J Cardiol* 1984; 53:221. Used by permission.)

axis views.[73, 74] In more recent studies, however, the apical four-chamber and two-chamber views have been used for several reasons.[72, 75] The apical four-chamber and two-chamber views are orthogonal views around the left ventricular long axis and, as such, satisfy the requirements for volume analysis of an ellipse. These two views also provide imaging of a larger area of the ventricle. In children, the apical long-axis view is preferable to the apical two-chamber view because it contains three anatomic reference points (the apex, the mitral valve, and the aortic valve) with which to standardize the position of the imaging plane.[72] Methods that require multiple short-axis images are no longer in

widespread use because of the difficulty and time requirements of obtaining a number of high-quality short-axis views. In obtaining the apex views, the transducer should be applied posteriorly over the apex impulse. The examiner should then attempt to maximize the size of the left ventricle in the apex views. When the size of the left ventricle is maximized in some patients, the apex will be seen curving out of the plane. In these cases, the error caused by exclusion of the apex is smaller than the error caused by foreshortening the basal portion of the ventricular cavity.

The various geometric models that have been used to

calculate left ventricular volumes are illustrated in Figure 4–16. In the most accurate and widely used method, algorithm I in Figure 4–16 is applied to paired orthogonal apical views. This algorithm is known as the modified Simpson's rule or the method of discs because it treats the ventricle as a stack of discs or slices. In this formula, the left ventricular volume is obtained by summation of the volumes of 20 equal cylinders whose areas are determined from diameters a_i and b_i and whose lengths are $1/20$ of the long-axis length (L) of the left ventricle. One advantage of this model is that it is independent of ventricular geometry. In method II in Figure 4–16, areas A_1, A_2, and A_3 are planimetered areas of three parasternal short-axis views and L is the long-axis length of the left ventricle usually measured from the apical long-axis view. The left ventricular volume is then calculated according to Simpson's rule as the sum of the volumes of a cylinder, a truncated cone, and another cone. Method III in Figure 4–16 is an expansion of method

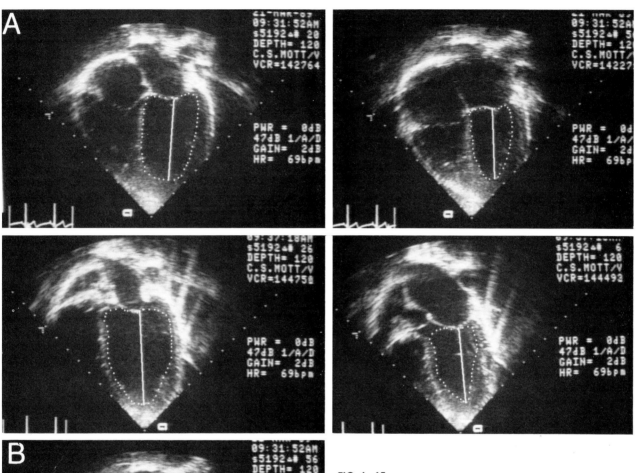

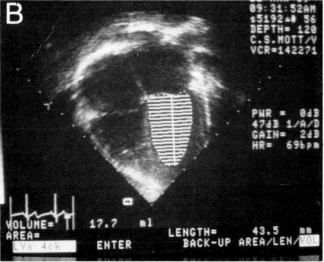

FIG 4–15.
A, illustration of the method used to measure left ventricular volume from the two-dimensional echocardiogram using paired orthogonal views. Using the apical four-chamber *(top)* and long-axis *(bottom)* views, the left ventricular endocardial surfaces are traced at end-diastole *(left)* and end-systole *(right)*. The tracings are made along the interface between the tissue and blood pool and cut across the base of the papillary muscles. The *solid line* indicates the major-axis length of the left ventricle. **B,** from the tracings made in **A,** the computer divides the ventricle along its major axis into 20 equal cylinders. The left ventricular volume is obtained by summation of the volumes of the 20 equal cylinders. In the case shown in **A** and **B,** the ejection fraction determined from biplane Simpson's rule method was 61%.

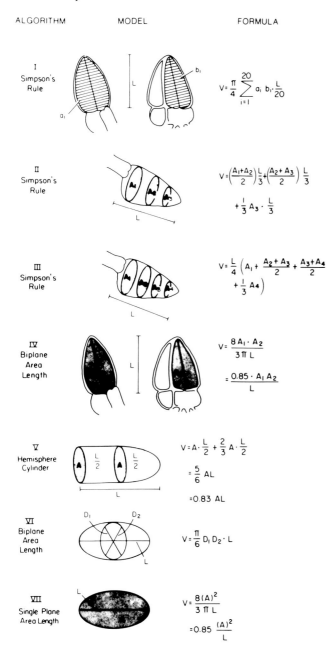

ALGORITHM   MODEL   FORMULA

I
Simpson's Rule

$V = \dfrac{\pi}{4} \displaystyle\sum_{i=1}^{20} a_i \, b_i \cdot \dfrac{L}{20}$

II
Simpson's Rule

$V = \left(\dfrac{A_1 + A_2}{2}\right)\dfrac{L}{3} + \left(\dfrac{A_2 + A_3}{2}\right)\dfrac{L}{3}$
$\quad + \dfrac{1}{3} A_3 \cdot \dfrac{L}{3}$

III
Simpson's Rule

$V = \dfrac{L}{4}\left(A_1 + \dfrac{A_2 + A_3}{2} + \dfrac{A_3 + A_4}{2}\right.$
$\quad \left. + \dfrac{1}{3} A_4\right)$

IV
Biplane Area Length

$V = \dfrac{8 A_1 \cdot A_2}{3\pi L}$
$\quad = \dfrac{0.85 \cdot A_1 A_2}{L}$

V
Hemisphere Cylinder

$V = A \cdot \dfrac{L}{2} + \dfrac{2}{3} A \cdot \dfrac{L}{2}$
$\quad = \dfrac{5}{6} AL$
$\quad = 0.83\,AL$

VI
Biplane Area Length

$V = \dfrac{\pi}{6} D_1 D_2 \cdot L$

VII
Single Plane Area Length

$V = \dfrac{8(A)^2}{3\pi L}$
$\quad = 0.85 \dfrac{(A)^2}{L}$

FIG 4–16.
Illustration of the various biplane and single-plane methods used to calculate chamber volume. A detailed description of each model and the algorithm for that model are contained in the text of this chapter. (From Silverman NH, Snider AR: *Two-dimensional Echocardiography in Congenital Heart Disease.* Norwalk, Appleton-Century-Crofts, 1982, pp 250–251. Used by permission.)

II. One problem with these two methods is the assumption that the short-axis slices are equidistant. Because of the lack of anatomic landmarks in the left ventricle, it is unlikely that three or four equidistant short-axis views could be obtained during a clinical echocardiogram. In method IV of Figure 4–16 (the biplane area-length method), the left ventricular volume is calculated as the volume of an ellipse with long-axis length L and orthogonal areas A_1 and A_2. For this calculation, orthogonal apical views are used. In the hemisphere cylinder or bullet formula (method V, Fig 4–16), the left ventricular volume is calculated as the sums of the volumes of a hemisphere and a cylinder. In this model, the area A is obtained by planimetry of the parasternal short-axis view at the level of the papillary muscles or mitral valve, and the length L is measured from an apical two-chamber view. In method VI of Figure 4–16, the left ventricular volume is calculated as the volume of an ellipse. The length L is obtained from an apical two-chamber view, and the diameters D_1 and D_2 are obtained from a parasternal short-axis view. In the single plane area-length method (method VII in Fig 4–16), the longest length and the planimetered area of a single apical view is used to calculate left ventricular volume. This method is acceptable when only one apical view is available for analysis.

Excellent correlations have been found between echocardiographic and angiographic estimates of left ventricular volumes and ejection fraction.[71–74] In most studies, echocardiographic volumes have been smaller than angiographic volumes, probably because of angiographic contrast filling of trabecular interspaces. In a study of left ventricular volume determination in 20 children with congenital heart disease,[72] multiple two-dimensional echocardiographic methods correlated well with angiographic methods for estimation of end-diastolic volume (correlation coefficients of 0.96 to 0.97). End-systolic volumes calculated from two-dimensional echocardiography also correlated closely with those measured at angiography (correlation coefficients 0.88 to 0.92); however, correlations were not as close as those observed for end-diastolic volumes, and there was a consistent overestimation of end-systolic volumes by the echocardiographic techniques. The discrepancy in the end-systolic volumes could not be explained on the basis of inaccurate area tracings because the endocardium is more easily seen at end-systole than at end-diastole. It is likely that the error in end-systolic volumes was caused by an inability to select a frame that occurred precisely at end-systole. With rapid heart rates, a frame rate of 30/sec does not allow sufficient sampling to provide a true end-systolic frame. In this study, stroke volume derived from two-dimensional echocardiography closely approximated that measured at angiography (correlation coefficient 0.92 to 0.95); however, correlations for ejection fraction were much lower (correlation coefficients 0.68 to 0.82). In estimating stroke volume and ejection fraction, the echocardiographic techniques underestimated the angiographic measurements. The variability between echocardiographic and angiographic measurements of stroke volume and ejection fraction may have been caused by changes in the patient's physiologic state at the times of the two examinations (heart rates were significantly different).

All of these echocardiographic studies show that two-dimensional echocardiography can determine left ventricular volumes and ejection fraction with an acceptable degree of accuracy. In general, more precise measurements are obtained using paired orthogonal apical views and a modified Simpson's rule, which is independent of ventricular geometry. Single-plane methods should be used with caution, as these methods may not provide accurate results if ventricular asynergy is present.

Left Atrial Volumes

Left atrial areas can be traced from several different echocardiographic views, and volumes can be derived using single plane and biplane methods. In one study,[76, 77] the left atrium was imaged in parasternal long-axis, apical four-chamber, and apical two-chamber views. In each view, the volumes were determined from a single-plane area-length method; for the paired apical views, volumes were determined from a biplane Simpson's rule method. Left atrial volumes measured by two-dimensional echocardiography correlated well with those measured at angiography (correlation coefficients 0.78 to 0.86).

When measuring left atrial volumes with two-dimensional echocardiography, care must be taken to image clearly the superior and posterior extents of the left atrial cavity. In tracing the left atrial area, the pulmonary veins and left atrial appendage are excluded by drawing the line through their junction with the atrium. The mitral valve leaflets must be opposed during the measurement; the tracing is drawn along the atrial surface of the mitral leaflets. The long-axis length is drawn from the center of the closed mitral valve leaflets to the posterosuperior left atrial wall.

Normal values are available for left atrial volumes measured by two-dimensional echocardiography in adult subjects.[78] Specific normal values for each echocardiographic view and algorithm must be used, and adjustments must be made for sex or body-surface area.

Right Ventricular Volumes and Ejection Fraction

Right ventricular volume analysis by two-dimensional echocardiography is a much more controversial technique than left ventricular volume analysis. The irregular geometric shape of the right ventricle does not easily satisfy the requirements of most of the standard volume equations. Nevertheless, several approaches have been suggested for measuring right ventricular volumes and ejection fraction.

Watanabe and colleagues[79] assessed right ventricular volume by applying Simpson's rule to two orthogonal apical views. To obtain the apical view that was perpendicular to the standard apical four-chamber view, these investigators examined patients lying prone on a specially constructed table. Echocardiographic estimates of ventricular volume were only about one-half of angiographic values, probably because the entire right ventricular outflow tract was excluded in the calculation.

Starling and associates[80] measured right ventricular volume from a subcostal four-chamber view and a subcostal sagittal view of the right ventricular outflow tract. In the pyramidal volume formula (volume = area × height ÷ 3) that was used, area was obtained from the four-cham-

ber view and height was measured from the right ventricular outflow view. Echocardiographic estimates of right ventricular volume correlated with radionuclide angiography counts (correlation coefficients 0.76 and 0.82 for end-diastole and end-systole). Ejection fractions measured by the two techniques also correlated (correlation coefficient 0.80).

Silverman and Hudson[81] used a summation approach to calculate right ventricular volume. Volumes of the right ventricle were determined by a single-plane area-length method from both the parasternal short-axis and apical four-chamber views. The single-plane volumes grossly underestimated the volume of the right ventricle measured by angiography; therefore, the single-plane volumes were added together to obtain a total right ventricular volume. Using this technique, right ventricular volumes and ejection fraction estimated by echocardiography correlated well with those measured by angiography (correlation coefficients = 0.81 for end-diastolic volume, 0.85 for end-systolic volume, and 0.82 for ejection fraction).

Levine and associates[82] calculated right ventricular volumes from two-dimensional echocardiography using the prolate ellipsoid model (volume = 2/3 × area × length). The apical four-chamber view and the parasternal long-axis view of the right ventricular outflow tract were used. Volumes calculated using the area from the apical four-chamber view combined with the length from the right ventricular outflow tract view and volumes calculated using the area from the right ventricular outflow view combined with the length from the four-chamber view correlated very well with measured cast volumes (correlation coefficients 0.94 and 0.91 respectively). This echocardiographic technique is particularly useful because it involves the simple product of only two measurements—a cross-sectional area and an intersecting length.

Right Atrial Volumes

Right atrial volumes can be calculated from the two-dimensional echocardiogram using the same techniques described previously for left atrial volume. Normal values are available for right atrial volumes measured from the apical four-chamber view in adult subjects.[78] Right atrial volume varies with sex and body-surface area.

Measurement of Left Ventricular Mass

M-mode echocardiographic techniques for estimating left ventricular mass have been widely used; however, these techniques cannot be used in the presence of asymmetric ventricular hypertrophy and are relatively insensitive for detecting serial changes in an individual patient. Therefore, two-dimensional echocardiographic techniques for calculating left ventricular mass have been developed. The two methods suitable for clinical use are a short-axis area-length method[83, 84] and a truncated ellipsoid model.[85]

In either method, a parasternal short-axis view at the level of the papillary muscles is obtained. From an end-diastolic frame, the total area (A_1) enclosed by the epicardium, the cavity area (A_2), and the myocardial area ($A_m = A_1 - A_2$) are measured. The papillary muscles are considered to be part of the cavity area. From the area values, the cavity minor radius (b) and mean wall thickness (t) can be calculated:

$$b = \sqrt{\frac{A^2}{\pi}}$$

$$t = \sqrt{\frac{A_1}{\pi}} - \sqrt{\frac{A_2}{\pi}}$$

The left ventricular long-axis length (L) is measured from apical four- or two-chamber views. For the short-axis area-length technique, the following formula is used[83, 84]:

$$\text{Left ventricular mass} = 1.055 \times 5/6\ A_m L$$

where

	1.055	= specific gravity of myocardium
	A_m	= myocardial area from short axis
	L	= apical long-axis length

For the truncated ellipsoid model,[85] the long-axis length is divided into two segments. The segment between the apex and the cavity minor radius is called the semi-major axis (a), and the segment between the cavity minor radius (b) and the mitral valve is called the truncated semi-major axis (d). The following formulae are then used to calculate mass (x is the myocardial area from short axis):

$$V = \pi \left\{ (b+t)^2 \int_0^{d+a+t} \left[1 - \frac{(x-d)^2}{(a+t)^2} \right] dx \right.$$

$$- b^2 \int_0^{d+a} \left[1 - \frac{(x-d)^2}{a^2} \right] dx \right\}$$

$$= \pi \left\{ (b+t)^2 \left[\frac{2}{3}(a+t) + d - \frac{d^3}{3(a+t)^2} \right] \right.$$

$$- b^2 \left[\frac{2}{3}a + d - \frac{d^3}{3a^2} \right] \right\}$$

$$\text{MASS} = 1.05\ V$$

Left ventricular mass calculated from both of these techniques has correlated well with that measured postmortem (correlation coefficients of 0.93 to 0.98).[83–85]

QUANTITATIVE DOPPLER ECHOCARDIOGRAPHY

The introduction of Doppler echocardiography has had the greatest impact on the ability to quantitate the hemodynamic severity of cardiac disease noninvasively. With M-mode and two-dimensional echocardiography, quantitation of the severity of a cardiac defect is limited to observing secondary hemodynamic consequences of the defect (i.e., chamber dilatation, wall thickening). With Doppler echocardiography, information about blood flow (i.e., ve-

locity and direction) is used to calculate directly the severity of the cardiac defect. Like M-mode echocardiography, Doppler echocardiography has excellent temporal resolution because of its fast sampling rates (thousands of cycles/sec) and provides a useful technique for accurate timing of intracardiac flow.

Measurement of Pressure Gradients

Theoretical Considerations

When fluid flows in a rigid tube, the volumetric flow is equal to the velocity of the fluid times the cross-sectional area of the tube. Figure 4–17 shows fluid flowing in a tube with a constricted area (A_2). If there is no loss of fluid from the tube, the volumetric flow at area 1 must be the same as the volumetric flow at area 2, or $V_1 A_1 = V_2 A_2$. Therefore, when a constant volume of fluid passes through a restricted area, a higher velocity must be generated. This acceleration of fluid to a higher velocity is called convective acceleration and is achieved by a drop in pressure across the area of obstruction. The Bernoulli equation shows the relationship between the pressure drop and the velocity:

$$P_1 - P_2 = \tfrac{1}{2}\rho(V_2^2 - V_1^2) + \rho \int_1^2 \frac{d\vec{V}}{dt}\vec{ds} + R(\vec{V})$$

where

	P_1	= pressure proximal to the obstruction
	P_2	= pressure distal to the obstruction
	V_1	= velocity proximal to the obstruction
	V_2	= velocity in the jet distal to the obstruction
	ρ	= mass density of blood
	$\vec{dV}$	= change in velocity that occurs over the time period dt
	$\vec{ds}$	= distance over which the decrease in pressure occurs
	R	= viscous resistance in the vessel
	V	= velocity of blood flow

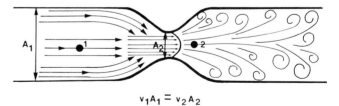

$$v_1 A_1 = v_2 A_2$$

A = vessel cross–sectional area
v = velocity

FIG 4–17.
Diagrammatic representation of fluid flowing in a rigid tube with a constricted area (A_2). If there is no loss of fluid from the tube, the volumetric flow at the normal area (A_1) must be the same as the volumetric flow at A_2. Therefore, $V_1 A_1 = V_2 A_2$, where A = vessel cross-sectional area and v = the velocity of flow in the tube. (From Snider AR: Doppler echocardiography: Basic principles and clinical applications, in Buda AJ, Delp E (ed): *Digital Cardiac Imaging.* Boston, Martinus Nijhoff Publishers, 1985, p 192. Used by permission.)

The first term in the equation represents the component of the pressure drop associated with convective acceleration. The middle term represents the pressure drop generated by flow acceleration (velocity changes with time) or the pressure drop associated with overcoming inertial forces. The third term is the pressure drop associated with overcoming viscous friction along the flow path. Since the velocity proximal to the jet is much smaller than the velocity in the jet, V_1^2 is negligible for practical purposes. Also, because the velocity profile in the inlet of an obstructive orifice is flat, viscous friction in the center of the lumen can be neglected. In clinical applications, the pressure drop required to overcome inertial forces is negligible. For blood, $1/2 \rho$ is approximately 4. From these assumptions, a simplified Bernoulli equation can be derived to calculate the pressure drop across the obstruction:

$$P_1 - P_2 = 4V_2^2$$

For V_2 in m/sec, the pressure drop is in mm Hg.[86–88]

The simplified Bernoulli equation can be used to estimate the pressure gradient across a stenotic valve, a regurgitant valve, or a septal defect. To obtain an accurate assessment of the pressure gradient, meticulous attention must be given to the techniques used to record the peak velocity of the jet. When using the Bernoulli equation to calculate the pressure drop across an obstructive orifice, a Doppler recording of the peak velocity in the jet core (where flow is laminar) is used. In practice, the echocardiographer angles the ultrasound beam until the highest-pitched (the most clear and tonelike) audio signal is found. When the highest-pitched signals are detected on the audio output of the Doppler system or the highest velocities are recorded on the graphic display of the Doppler, the ultrasound beam can be assumed to be nearly parallel to the direction of jet flow and no correction for cosine θ is made (see Chapter 1). Wall filter settings in the range of 400 to 800 Hz will eliminate the high amplitude, low frequency wall noises, making it easier to evaluate the audio signal from the jet. As soon as the pure tonal qualities of the jet are heard, minor adjustments in the position of the Doppler beam are made until a clear peak velocity can be seen on the graphic display of the Doppler waveform. Figure 4–18 is a continuous-wave Doppler recording of the ascending aorta from the apical four-chamber view. The peak velocity of the ascending aortic jet is 4.0 m/sec. From the Bernoulli equation, the predicted pressure drop is 4 times 4^2 or 64 mm Hg. Alternatively, if the examiner cannot align the Doppler beam parallel to the jet flow, a correction for the intercept angle can be made by dividing the recorded velocity by cosine θ. As discussed in Chapter 1, angle correction can lead to significant errors in estimating the velocity and therefore this approach is not recommended.

To obtain the most accurate prediction of the peak gradient, the peak velocity of the jet should be recorded from several different echocardiographic windows. The highest value obtained for the peak velocity is then used in the Bernoulli equation to predict the peak gradient.

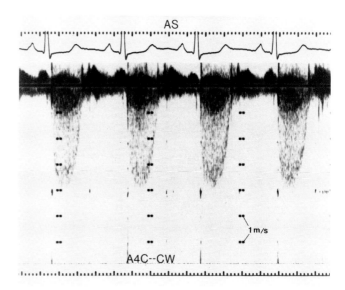

FIG 4–18.
Continuous-wave Doppler recording of the ascending aorta from the cardiac apex of a 16-year-old girl with a bicuspid aortic valve. The peak velocity of the aortic jet is 4 m/sec. This predicts a pressure gradient across the aortic valve of 4×4^2 or 64 mm Hg. Note the lower velocity signals that arise from the blood flow in the left ventricle superimposed on the high-velocity aortic jet. AS = aortic stenosis.

Studies in children have shown that the peak velocity of the jet can be recorded with equal accuracy using either continuous-wave or high pulse repetition frequency Doppler techniques.[89]

The pressure gradient calculated from the Bernoulli equation is the peak instantaneous pressure gradient and not the peak-to-peak pressure gradient measured at cardiac catheterization (Fig 4–19). The peak-to-peak pressure gradient is an artificial measurement that does not occur in the circulation in real time. Instead, many instantaneous differences in pressure occur at each point in time throughout the cardiac cycle. It is the largest of these instantaneous pressure differences—the peak instantaneous pressure gradient or the peak pressure gradient—that is estimated by the Bernoulli equation. The peak instantaneous pressure gradient is larger than the peak-to-peak pressure gradient.[90] The difference between the two is most marked in patients with mild to moderate obstruction in whom the arterial pressure increases more during systole. The difference is less apparent in patients with severe obstructions. For example, in severe aortic stenosis with a very narrowed pulse pressure, the pressure difference is more evenly maintained throughout systole.[86]

In addition to the peak instantaneous pressure gradient, the mean pressure gradient can be calculated from the Doppler recording of the jet. The mean pressure gradient is the average of all the instantaneous pressure gradients throughout the period of flow. The mean pressure gradient is usually calculated by tracing the outermost border of the jet with a digitizing system and a computer. The analysis system measures the peak velocity and calculates the instantaneous gradient every 3 to 5 msec. The computer averages these instantaneous gradients to obtain the mean gradient. The mean gradient is *not* calculated by substituting the mean velocity in the simplified Bernoulli equation.

Clinical studies using the Bernoulli equation have shown excellent correlation between the pressure gradient predicted by Doppler ultrasound and the pressure gradient measured at cardiac catheterization in patients with mitral stenosis,[87, 88, 91] aortic stenosis,[91-97] pulmonary stenosis,[98-100] pulmonary artery bands,[101] and prosthetic valves.[102, 103] In most studies, the correlation coefficients are high, and the standard error of the estimate approximates 5 to 10 mm Hg. In general, the Doppler jets are easier to record in children because better penetration is possible.[89] From several studies on adult patients with aortic stenosis, the correlation was poorer in subjects over 50 years old.[92] In these patients, it is likely that calcification of the aortic valve leads to greater variations in jet direction and greater jet diversion. Also, some studies of adults have shown poor correlation with catheterization gradients in

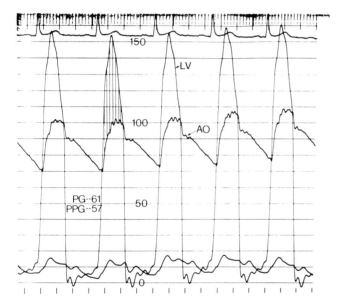

FIG 4–19.
Simultaneous pressure recordings from the left ventricle (LV) and ascending aorta (AO) at the time of cardiac catheterization from a patient with aortic valve stenosis. The peak-to-peak pressure gradient (PPG) is 57 mm HG. The peak instantaneous gradient (PG) is the largest of all the instantaneous differences in pressure that occurred at each point in time throughout the cardiac cycle. In this case, the PG was 61 mm Hg. The pressure gradient predicted by the simplified Bernoulli equation is the peak instantaneous pressure gradient and not the peak-to-peak pressure gradient. (From Snider AR: Doppler echocardiography in congenital heart disease, in Berger M (ed): *Doppler Echocardiography in Heart Disease.* New York, Marcel Dekker Inc, 1987, p 226. Used by permission.)

patients whose peak velocity exceeded 3.5 m/sec.[92] This is probably related to difficulties in detecting the low-amplitude peak velocity signal in adult patients and does not appear to be a limiting factor in pediatric patients.[89]

Limitations of the Simplified Bernoulli Equation

Two general types of inaccuracies can occur when the simplified Bernoulli equation is used to predict the pressure gradient. These include errors that occur because of the assumptions used in deriving the simplified Bernoulli equation and technical errors that occur when the peak velocity of the jet is measured. One assumption made in using the simplified Bernoulli equation is that the velocity proximal to the obstruction is small relative to the jet velocity, so that V_1^2 can be ignored in the equation. In the example of a stenotic semilunar valve, the velocity in the outflow tract of the ventricle is usually 0.7 to 1 m/sec; the overestimation in peak pressure drop that occurs by neglecting this velocity is 2 to 4 mm Hg. Therefore, in clinical practice, a proximal velocity of less than 1 m/sec can usually be ignored with minimal error. With a proximal velocity of greater than 1 m/sec, the error becomes greater and this velocity should not be omitted from the Bernoulli equation. Instead, the pressure gradient should be calculated from an expanded Bernoulli equation:

$$P_1 - P_2 = 4(V_2^2 - V_1^2)$$

In the clinical setting, elevated proximal velocities can be encountered in several situations including:

1. Across a valve that is both stenotic and regurgitant.
2. When both an intracardiac shunt plus valve stenosis are present (i.e., an atrial septal defect with pulmonary valve stenosis).
3. When multiple levels of obstruction in series are present (i.e., a bicuspid aortic valve with coarctation of the aorta).[104]
4. When valve gradients are assessed during exercise.

Figure 4–20 is a continuous-wave Doppler recording of the descending aorta obtained from the suprasternal notch of a patient with both aortic stenosis and coarctation of the aorta. The darker velocities are signals that arise from blood flow in the descending aorta proximal to the coarctation. In this patient the proximal velocity is elevated because of the downstream persistence of jet flow across a stenotic, bicuspid aortic valve. The higher velocity, low amplitude signals arise from the jet flow distal to the coarctation. As can be seen in this example, failure to take the elevated proximal velocity into account leads to an overestimation of the coarctation gradient. If the gray-scale of the continuous-wave Doppler recording is of sufficient quality, the proximal velocity can be measured directly from the continuous-wave Doppler recording of the jet flow, as it was in this case. Otherwise, the proximal velocity must be measured separately with pulsed Doppler techniques.

Another assumption made in simplifying the Ber-

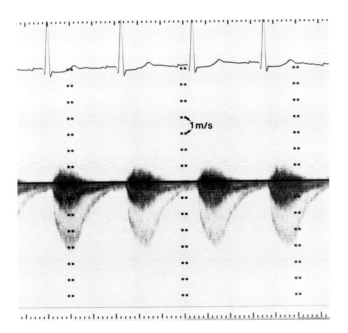

FIG 4–20.
Continuous-wave Doppler recording from the suprasternal notch of an infant with severe coarctation of the aorta. The higher amplitude, lower velocity signals from the descending aorta proximal to the coarctation can be seen superimposed on the lower amplitude, higher velocity signals from the jet flow in the descending aorta distal to the coarctation. The peak velocity of the descending aortic jet is 4 m/sec. The peak velocity of flow in the descending aorta proximal to the coarctation is elevated to approximately 1.8 m/sec. Failure to take into account the elevated proximal velocities would lead to an overestimation of the coarctation gradient in this patient.

noulli equation is that the pressure drop caused by viscous friction is negligible. Viscous resistance, caused by friction between neighboring fluid elements, depends not only on the local velocity but also on the entire velocity profile. The velocity profile in a stenotic valve inlet is flat, and viscous friction in the center of the lumen can be neglected. Following this assumption, Holen and associates[105] have shown that the pressure drop caused by viscous friction can be ignored for orifices 8 mm in diameter (area = 0.5 cm²). With orifice diameters of 3.5 mm (area ≤0.1 cm²) or less, use of the simplified Bernoulli equation underestimated the pressure drop. The underestimation was greater for lower velocities (<3 m/sec), and accuracy was acceptable for velocities greater than 3 m/sec. For a 1.5 mm orifice, the estimated pressure drop was about one-half the actual pressure drop. These observations have been confirmed by Vasko and colleagues,[106] who used a plastic flow model. The Doppler-predicted pressure drop for circular orifices of 8 to 10 mm diameter was very close to the pressure drop measured by mercury manometers. In actuality, the ratio of the inflow tract diameter and the orifice diameter is probably the limiting factor. In clinical practice, ignoring

the pressure drop caused by viscous resistance usually results in acceptable accuracy because orifice diameters of 3.5 mm or less are seldom encountered.

Finally, during rapid increases in velocity (i.e., during valve opening and closure), inertia causes a delay in the velocity curve compared with the pressure. In general, the pressure drop associated with flow acceleration is negligible. However, for high-velocity jets that extend for some distance past the obstruction (i.e., in severe tunnel subaortic stenosis), ignoring the pressure drop associated with flow acceleration can result in a significant underestimation of the true pressure drop.[86]

The second major type of error that occurs when the Bernoulli equation is used to predict the transvalvular pressure gradient are technical errors in detecting the maximum velocity of the jet. These include errors in alignment of the Doppler beam and jet blood flow, errors in detecting the low-amplitude peak velocity signal, and changes in peak velocity caused by alterations in the patient's physiologic state. As stated above, the audio and spectral outputs are used to align the Doppler ultrasound beam parallel with the jet flow and thus detect the peak velocity of the jet. To obtain the best alignment between the Doppler beam and the jet flow, several different echocardiographic windows should be tried. In the clinical setting, technical errors in performing the Doppler ultrasound examination usually result in an underestimation of the actual pressure drop. Although it is uncommon, overestimation of the pressure gradient can occur when angle correction is used to calculate the peak velocity in the jet. Errors in measuring the intercept angle from the two-dimensional echocardiographic image were discussed in Chapter 1.

Another type of technical error that can occur is related to the amplitude of the peak velocity. Because only a small number of scatterers or red blood cells are actually moving at the peak velocity of the jet, the amplitude or power of the returning signal is low, and difficulties can arise in discerning the faint peak-velocity signal on the graphic display. This is more often a problem in adult patients who are obese or who have chronic lung disease. In these patients the Doppler signal is very attenuated and sampling sites are often quite distant from the transducer. The amplitude of the peak velocity can be increased by using an echocardiographic window as close to the sampling site as possible (to decrease attenuation) or by using a transducer with higher emitted power (low carrier frequency).

The third type of technical error that can occur in using the Doppler ultrasound technique to predict the measured pressure gradient is caused by variations in the patient's physiologic state. A thorough and careful Doppler examination is time-consuming and, in children with congenital heart disease, usually follows a lengthy M-mode and two-dimensional echocardiographic examination. Young children often find it very difficult to lie still for such a long period of time and will often become fretful or agitated just as the Doppler examination begins. Because the hemodynamic assessment of the severity of the defect is usually the most important part of the echocardiographic examination, we do not hesitate to sedate children to obtain the most accurate Doppler examination. If the heart rate and cardiac output during the Doppler examination are different from those during cardiac catheterization, discrepancies will occur between the Doppler and the catheterization estimates of the severity of the defect. Stevenson and associates[107] have shown that in unsedated children, Doppler estimates of the pressure gradient averaged 41.5% (range 3% to 275%) greater than pressure gradients measured in the same children sedated at cardiac catheterization. Because it is the sedated catheterization gradients that are currently used to make decisions on interventional therapy, the Doppler measurements should be obtained when the patient is in the same physiologic state. Oral sedatives such as chloral hydrate (50 to 100 mg/kg, not to exceed 1 gm) can be used safely, and their effects wear off quickly.

Prediction of Intracardiac Pressures

Doppler echocardiography allows estimation of right ventricular, pulmonary artery, left ventricular, and left atrial pressures. Because estimation of pulmonary artery pressure is most useful and the least prone to error, it will be considered first.

Right Heart Pressures

Because pulmonary artery and right ventricular systolic pressures are nearly equal in the absence of disease that involves the right ventricular outflow tract, the pulmonary valve, or the supravalvular region, pulmonary artery systolic pressure is commonly estimated by techniques that measure right ventricular systolic pressure. In the method most commonly used, the tricuspid regurgitation jet is used to calculate the right ventricular-right atrial pressure gradient. Pulmonary artery systolic pressure can also be calculated directly by noting the timing of the peak pulmonary artery pressure.

Pulmonary artery systolic pressure from the tricuspid regurgitation jet.—Doppler echocardiographic evidence of tricuspid regurgitation is common in patients with pulmonary hypertension, as well as in normal patients who have no physical evidence of tricuspid valve disease.[108] The tricuspid regurgitation jet (Fig 4–21) can be recorded by placing the transducer at the cardiac apex and obtaining a four-chamber view. The ultrasound beam is directed through the tricuspid valve and aligned parallel to the high-velocity jet between the right ventricle and the right atrium. Careful adjustment of the location of the transducer and the ultrasound beam is essential to assure a small Doppler angle and accurate quantification of actual velocity. Pansystolic velocities from the right ventricle into the right atrium are directed away from the transducer and are thus shown below the baseline on the spectral recording. The peak systolic right ventricular-right atrial pressure gradient is calculated using the Bernoulli equation and the peak velocity of the tricuspid regurgitation jet[109]:

$$RVSP - RA = 4(V)^2$$

and

$$RVSP = 4(V)^2 + RA$$

where   RVSP   = right ventricular systolic pressure
RA   = right atrial systolic pressure
V   = peak velocity of the tricuspid regurgitation jet

Several techniques are used to estimate right atrial pressure. If a central venous line is present, right atrial pressure can be measured directly. Physical examination allows determination of the height of the jugular venous pulse, although even in experienced hands this method can be inexact. Data from the physical examination, echocardiogram, and chest x-ray can be combined to determine if right atrial pressure is normal or abnormal. An arbitrary 10 mm Hg is added to the gradient if the above-mentioned parameters are normal. For example, at the time of the Doppler study, the patient shown in Figure 4–21 had a right atrial pressure of 36 mm Hg measured by a central venous line. The peak velocity of the tricuspid regurgitation jet is 2.5 m/sec, which predicts a systolic tricuspid valve pressure gradient of $4(2.5)^2$ or 25 mm Hg. The patient had no evidence of obstruction near the pulmonary valve; therefore, the pulmonary artery systolic pressure (which equalled the right ventricular systolic pressure) was estimated to be 25 + 36 = 61 mm Hg. Using this technique, there has been excellent correlation between Doppler and invasive measurements of right ventricular and pulmonary artery systolic pressures.[109]

Berger and colleagues simplified this approach by regressing the tricuspid valve gradient derived by Doppler against the pulmonary artery systolic pressure measured at catheterization.[109] This regression equation allows direct calculation of pulmonary artery systolic pressure without determination of right atrial pressure:

$$PA = 4V^2 \times 1.23 \text{ mm Hg}$$

where   PA   = pulmonary artery systolic pressure
V   = peak velocity of the tricuspid regurgitation jet

Pulmonary artery systolic pressure from the ventricular septal defect jet.—In patients with a ventricular septal defect, right ventricular systolic pressure can be estimated using a Doppler recording of the peak velocity across the septum (Fig 4–22). Peak systolic pressure gradient between the right and left ventricle is calculated using the Bernoulli equation:

$$LVSP - RVSP = 4(VSD)^2$$

where   LVSP   = left ventricular systolic pressure
RVSP   = right ventricular systolic pressure
VSD   = peak velocity of the ventricular septal defect jet

If there is no evidence of left ventricular outflow obstruction, then the systolic blood pressure is nearly equal to the left ventricular systolic pressure and:

$$RVSP = SBP - 4(VSD)^2$$

where   SBP   = systolic blood pressure

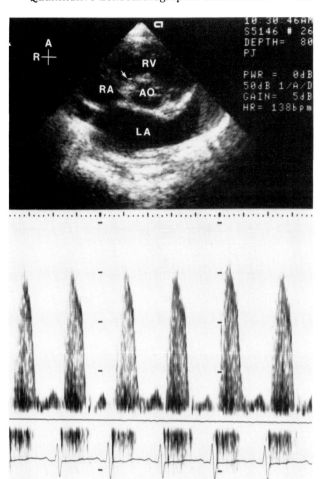

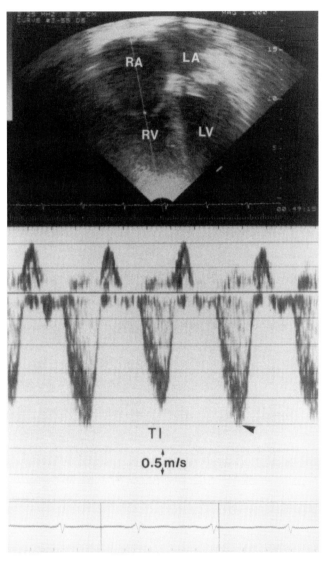

FIG 4–21.
High pulse repetition frequency Doppler recording *(bottom)* from the apical four-chamber view *(top)* of a patient with multivalvular disease. The sample volume is positioned in the right atrium (RA) proximal to the tricuspid valve. The Doppler spectral tracing shows signals below the baseline in systole that indicate flow from the right ventricle (RV) to the RA in systole, or tricuspid insufficiency (TI). The peak velocity of the TI jet *(arrow)* is 2.5 m/sec. This predicts a pressure gradient of 4×2.5^2 or 25 mm Hg between the RA and RV in systole. RA pressure was measured by a central venous line to be 36 mm Hg. Peak RV systolic pressure is therefore 36 + 25, or 61 mm Hg. *LA* = left atrium; *LV* = left ventricle. (From Snider AR: *Echocardiography* 1987; 4:306. Used by permission.)

FIG 4–22.
Continuous-wave Doppler recording *(bottom)* from the parasternal short-axis view *(top)* of an infant with a membranous ventricular septal defect. The top frame shows the position of the continuous-wave Doppler beam at the time of the recording. The *arrow* points to the transmit focal zone of the continuous-wave Doppler. The peak velocity of the jet flow across the ventricular septal defect is 3.2 m/sec. This predicts a pressure gradient from the left ventricle to the right ventricle (RV) of 41 mm Hg. *A* = anterior; *AO* = aorta; *LA* = left atrium; and *R* = right atrium.

If right ventricular outflow obstruction is also absent, right ventricular systolic pressure is close to pulmonary artery systolic pressure. Thus, this approach allows detection of pulmonary hypertension in patients with ventricular septal defect and the absence of left or right ventricular outflow tract obstruction. Using this approach, several investigators have reported excellent correlations between Doppler and catheterization-determined right ventricular systolic pressure (correlation coefficients = 0.93 to 0.95).[86, 110, 111]

Multiple ultrasound windows are used to assure the smallest Doppler angle. The left parasternal and subcostal windows provide the highest Doppler frequency shifts. In general, the jet through perimembranous ventricular septal defects is directed anteriorly and to the right; therefore, the transducer is placed at the mid left sternal border and aimed posteriorly, leftward, and inferiorly.[110] Muscular ventricular septal defects are usually more easily interrogated from a subcostal or apical window. If unusual orientation of the jet is suspected, direct visualization of the jet with two-dimensional color-flow imaging can be helpful in aligning the ultrasound beam parallel to the jet.

The ventricular septal defect approach to estimating pulmonary artery systolic pressure has two potential technical problems. First, cuff blood pressure is used to estimate central aortic pressure. With this assumption, the nonsimultaneous measurement of the blood pressure and the Doppler recording and the increased systolic pressure frequently noted in the peripheral arteries are potential sources of error. Second, Doppler ultrasound predicts the peak instantaneous pressure gradient between the left and right ventricles during systole. At catheterization, the peak-to-peak pressure gradient between the two ventricles is measured. It is possible to have no peak-to-peak gradient at catheterization and a significant peak instantaneous gradient by Doppler. Because of differences in timing of the left and right ventricular pressures, velocities of up to 2.5 m/sec (and instantaneous gradients of up to 25 mm Hg) have been reported in patients with systemic right ventricular systolic pressure at cardiac catheterization.[110]

Diastolic pulmonary artery pressure from the pulmonary regurgitation jet.—Pulmonary regurgitation can be recorded on the Doppler examination in about 70% of normal children, in a large percentage of patients with congenital heart disease, and in nearly all patients with pulmonary hypertension.[108] Quantification of diastolic velocities in patients with pulmonary regurgitation is helpful in calculating pulmonary artery end-diastolic pressure. It should be remembered that the severity of pulmonary regurgitation, pulmonary hypertension, and right ventricular function all affect the end-diastolic pressure gradient across the pulmonary valve. In the presence of mild pulmonary regurgitation, normal right ventricular end-diastolic pressure, and low pulmonary artery diastolic pressure, pulmonic regurgitation Doppler velocities return to the baseline at end-diastole[86] (Fig 4–23). The low end-diastolic velocity indicates a low end-diastolic pulmonary artery-right ventricular pressure gradient. Unfortunately, low end-diastolic velocities can also be detected in patients with severe pulmonary regurgitation and elevation of right ventricular end-diastolic pressure. In patients with elevated pulmonary artery systolic and diastolic pressures and pulmonary regurgitation that is less than severe, the velocity of the pulmonary regurgitation jet is high at the end of diastole (Fig 4–24).

Masuyama and co-workers[112] showed that the end-diastolic pulmonary artery pressure can be calculated accurately using the pulmonary regurgitation jet. From the Bernoulli equation and the peak velocity of the pulmonary

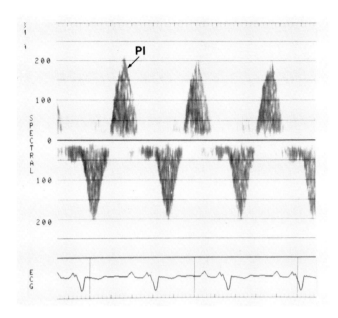

FIG 4–23.
Continuous-wave Doppler tracing from a patient with pulmonary insufficiency (PI) following repair of tetralogy of Fallot. In this patient, there was mild PI, normal right ventricular end-diastolic pressure, and low pulmonary artery diastolic pressure. Thus, the Doppler velocity of the PI jet returned to the baseline at end-diastole, indicating a low end-diastolic pulmonary artery-right ventricular pressure gradient.

regurgitation jet at end-diastole, the diastolic pressure gradient between the pulmonary artery and right ventricle can be calculated as:

$$PADP - RVED = 4(V)^2$$

where   PADP   = pulmonary artery diastolic pressure
             RVED   = right ventricular end-diastolic pressure
             V   = peak velocity of pulmonary regurgitation jet at end-diastole

If right atrial diastolic pressure is known and assumed to be equal to right ventricular end-diastolic pressure, then:

$$PADP = 4(V)^2 + RA$$

where   RA   = right atrial diastolic pressure

Using this technique, good correlations have been found between Doppler and catheterization measurements of the pulmonary artery-right ventricular end-diastolic pressure gradient (correlation coefficient = 0.94, standard error of estimate = 3 mm Hg). If right atrial or right ventricular end-diastolic pressures are unknown, pulmonary artery end-diastolic pressure can be calculated using a regression equation:

$$4(V)^2 = 0.61\ PADP - 2.0$$

Detection of pulmonary hypertension using Doppler time intervals.—In patients who have no tricuspid regurgitation or ventricular septal defect, time intervals derived from the pulmonary artery Doppler tracing can be helpful in detecting pulmonary hypertension.

Measurement of the right ventricular isovolumic relaxation time provides a technique for assessing the pulmonary artery pressure. This time interval between the pulmonary valve closure and tricuspid valve opening was first investigated in 1967 by Burstin[113] using a phonocardiogram and a right ventricular apexcardiogram. These investigators constructed a nomogram relating the isovolumic relaxation time at a given heart rate to the systolic pulmonary artery pressure. Using this nomogram, good correlation with invasive measurements was found in a large group of children with congenital heart disease. Subsequently, Hatle and co-workers[114] measured right ventricular isovolumic relaxation time from the Doppler spectral tracing and a phonocardiogram and used Burstin's nomogram to predict systolic pulmonary artery pressure. Excellent correlation was found between Doppler and catheterization measurements of pulmonary artery pressure. Using the Doppler instrument, pulmonary and tricuspid flows with valve movement are recorded along with a simultaneous phonocardiogram. Tricuspid valve opening can be timed from the tricuspid Doppler tracing, and pulmonary valve closure can be timed from the phonocardiogram. The timing of the pulmonary valve closure on the pulmonary Doppler tracing can be helpful in locating the pulmonary valve closure on the phonocardiogram. The right

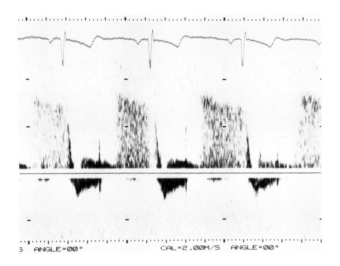

FIG 4–24.
Continuous-wave Doppler tracing from the left parasternal region of a patient with pulmonary vascular obstructive disease and pulmonary insufficiency. The signals that arise from the pulmonary insufficiency jet are displayed above the baseline in diastole. The velocity of the pulmonary regurgitation signals remains high at the end of diastole (approximately 3 m/sec). This indicates a significant gradient between the pulmonary artery and right ventricle at end-diastole because of elevated pulmonary artery diastolic pressure.

ventricular isovolumic relaxation time is quite short when pulmonary artery pressure is normal and lengthens as pressure increases, provided the relaxation rate of the right ventricle is normal. The interval is also lengthened with a slow heart rate, which is taken into account in Burstin's nomogram. When using Doppler ultrasound to record the valve movements, the tracing should be made with the sample volume in the valve orifice so that the opening movement of the valve from the beginning of diastole is recorded. The estimation of pulmonary artery pressure from the relaxation time is based on the assumption that the right atrial pressure is normal.[114] With an elevated right atrial pressure (i.e., pericardial constriction, severe tricuspid insufficiency, congestive heart failure), the tricuspid valve will open earlier and the pulmonary artery pressure will be underestimated. In addition, in infants with heart rates of 140 beats/min or more, difficulty may arise in measuring the short isovolumic relaxation period.[86] If, however, the interval is longer than 10 msec at high heart rates, then pulmonary artery hypertension is probably present.

The morphology of the pulmonary artery Doppler recording can provide important information about the pulmonary artery pressure. In pulmonary hypertension, peak velocity is unchanged; however, the acceleration rate (upslope) is increased and the acceleration time (time from beginning of flow to the peak velocity) is shortened. Also, the decrease in systolic velocity occurs earlier, so that less flow or reverse flow is seen in late systole.[115, 116] This early decrease in systolic flow often creates the appearance of notching on the pulmonary artery Doppler tracing. The severity of the pulmonary artery Doppler flow abnormalities can be assessed by measuring the acceleration time and the ratio of the acceleration time to the right ventricular ejection time (Fig 4–25). Kitabatake and associates[115] noted that acceleration time (the time from onset to peak pulmonary velocity) is shortened in patients with pulmonary hypertension. In this study, patients with mean pulmonary artery pressure <20 mm Hg had acceleration times of 137 ± 24 msec. Patients with mean pulmonary artery pressure >20 mm Hg had acceleration times of 97 ± 20 msec. The ratio of acceleration time to right ventricular ejection time correlated well with the log of the mean pulmonary artery pressure (AT/ET = .45 ± .05 in normal patients and .30 ± .06 in patients with pulmonary hypertension). Hatle and Angelsen[86] found a ratio of acceleration time to ejection time of 0.36 or more in normal patients (mean = 0.41 ± 0.03) and in nearly all patients with increased pulmonary artery pressure and normal pulmonary vascular resistance. In patients with increased pulmonary artery pressure and resistance, the ratio was lower (0.30 ± 0.05). In addition, these investigators measured the percentage of flow in each one-third of systole on the pulmonary artery Doppler tracing. In patients with elevated pulmonary vascular resistance, the percentage of flow in the last one-third of systole was smaller than in normal patients or in patients with elevated pressures and normal resistance. The usefulness of the ratio of acceleration time to ejection time has been confirmed by other studies.[117–119]

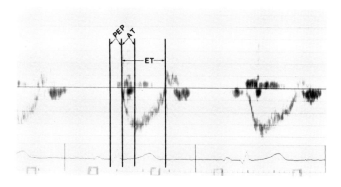

FIG 4–25.
Doppler recording from the left parasternal region of the main pulmonary artery, demonstrating the technique used to measure pulmonary artery systolic time intervals. The pre-ejection period (PEP) is measured from the beginning of the QRS complex on the electrocardiogram to the onset of flow on the Doppler tracing. The acceleration time (AT) is measured from the onset of flow to the peak velocity of flow on the Doppler tracing. The ejection time (ET) is measured from the beginning of flow to the end of flow on the pulmonary artery Doppler tracing.

From the pulmonary artery Doppler recording and the electrocardiogram, the right ventricular pre-ejection period (RVPEP), the right ventricular ejection time (ET), and the ratio of the two (RVPEP/ET) can be measured. This ratio is usually elevated when pulmonary vascular resistance is elevated. Hatle and Angelsen[86] reported that no patient had elevated pulmonary resistance if both ratios were normal (RVPEP/ET <0.34 and RVAT/ET >0.36). Isobe and coworkers[120] recently noted that the ratio of right ventricular pre-ejection period divided by acceleration time was the best predictor of pulmonary hypertension. Ratios of greater than 1.1 were found in 93% of patients with pulmonary hypertension, whereas 97% of normal patients had ratios of less than 1.1. Since factors other than pulmonary artery pressure can alter the Doppler time intervals (age, heart rate, sample volume position, right ventricular preload and function), pulmonary artery pressure based on these measurements should be interpreted with caution.[121, 122]

Left Heart Pressures

In the presence of aortic valve disease, left ventricular systolic and diastolic pressures can be calculated by using systolic stenotic and diastolic regurgitant jets, the Bernoulli equation, and sphygmomanometer blood pressures.

Left ventricular systolic pressure.—In normal patients, left ventricular systolic pressure is estimated easily by measuring systolic blood pressure. In patients with aortic stenosis, left ventricular peak systolic pressure can be calculated from Doppler measurement of the peak gradient across the aortic valve in systole and the simultaneous measurement of arm systolic blood pressure. Using the Bernoulli equation, the aortic valve pressure gradient is determined as[86, 91, 92]:

$$LVSP - AOS = 4(V)^2$$

where   LVSP = left ventricular systolic pressure
AOS = aortic systolic pressure
V = peak velocity of aortic stenosis jet

If arm systolic blood pressure is used to approximate aortic systolic pressure, then:

$$LVSP = 4(V)^2 + SBP$$

where   SBP = systolic blood pressure

When this technique is used, four possible sources of error can be encountered. First, the pressure gradient can be underestimated if the Doppler recording is obtained from a site other than the high-velocity jet in the valve orifice or if the Doppler angle exceeds 25°. Second, cuff systolic pressure overestimates central aortic pressure, and use of cuff blood pressure, rather than central aortic pressure, would overestimate left ventricular systolic pressure. Third, the sphygmomanometer can lead to over- or underestimation of true brachial artery pressure by 5 to 10 mm Hg. Fourth, it is difficult to measure the cuff blood pressure and the transvalvular pressure gradient simultaneously; nonsimultaneous measurements have the potential to cause over- or underestimation of the true left ventricular systolic pressure.

Left ventricular diastolic pressure.—Left ventricular end-diastolic pressure can be estimated in the presence of aortic regurgitation. As shown in Figure 4–26, the transducer is placed at the cardiac apex and a five-chamber view is obtained. The Doppler ultrasound beam is oriented parallel to the diastolic high velocity jet from the aorta into the left ventricle. The Doppler tracing shows diastolic velocities that are directed toward the transducer and decrease in a linear way from an early diastolic peak. Because left ventricular end-diastolic pressure is to be calculated, end-diastolic velocities are used to determine the end-diastolic aortic-left ventricular pressure gradient:

$$AOD - LVED = 4(V)^2$$

where   AOD = aortic diastolic pressure
LVED = left ventricular end-diastolic pressure
V = peak velocity of the aortic regurgitation jet at end-diastole

If diastolic blood pressure is used to estimate aortic diastolic pressure, then:

$$LVED = DBP - 4(V)^2$$

where   DBP = cuff diastolic blood pressure

There are several potential errors in the use of this technique. First, the very nature of the calculation tends to magnify the potential error because a relatively small number (the end-diastolic pressure) is derived by subtracting

---

two larger numbers (diastolic pressure gradient from the cuff diastolic blood pressure). Second, in most cases the end-diastolic velocity is moderate to high (2.5 to 5.0 m/sec) and is squared; therefore, small errors in the velocity result in large errors in the squared velocity required to calculate the gradient. Third, cuff diastolic blood pressure

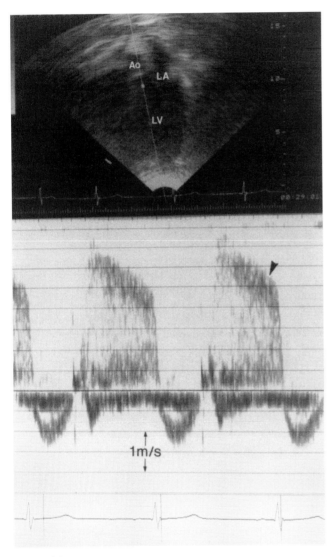

FIG 4-26.
High pulse repetition frequency Doppler recording from the left ventricular (LV) outflow tract of a patient with aortic insufficiency. The two-dimensional image of the apical view *(top)* shows the position of the sample volume just beneath the aortic (AO) valve at the time of the Doppler recording. The Doppler spectral tracing *(bottom)* shows Doppler signals above the baseline in diastole, indicating blood flow toward the transducer from the AO to the LV in diastole (aortic insufficiency). The peak velocity of the aortic insufficiency jet at end-diastole *(arrow)* is 2.7 m/sec. This predicts an AO to LV pressure gradient at end-diastole of 4×2.7^2 or 29 mm Hg. The patient's arm diastolic blood pressure was 45 mm Hg. Left ventricular end-diastolic pressure is therefore 45 − 29 or 16 mm Hg. LA = left atrium. (From Snider AR: *Echocardiography* 1987; 4:311. Used by permission.)

$$LAS = SBP - 4(V)^2$$

where   SBP = cuff systolic blood pressure

The potential errors in this approach are similar to those noted for left ventricular diastolic pressure calculation in the presence of aortic regurgitation. Despite these limitations, the approach can be applied successfully in some patients.[123]

Measurement of Valve Area

Continuity Equation

Doppler ultrasound measurement of the peak velocity of the jet flow through a stenotic valve has been used to determine the transvalvular pressure gradient. For a fixed degree of valve stenosis, however, the transvalvular pressure gradient varies with the volume flow across the valve. Thus, a high pressure gradient can be found in the absence of severe stenosis when transvalvular volume flow is increased, and a low pressure gradient can be found in the presence of severe stenosis when ventricular output is low. In these situations, calculation of the stenotic valve area is a useful method for determining the severity of the stenosis, independent of the volume flow across the valve.

In the initial studies in children, a Doppler echocardiographic method based on measurement of transvalvular gradient at one site and volume flow at another intracardiac site was used.[124] The formula for valve area was:

$$A = \frac{SV}{0.88 \times V_2 \times VET}$$

where   A   = valve area
SV = stroke volume in cc^3
V_2 = peak velocity of the jet in cm/sec
VET = systolic ejection time in seconds

Using this equation, good correlations were found between Doppler-derived valve area and valve area estimated at catheterization, using the Gorlin equation in children with pulmonary or aortic valve stenosis (correlation coefficient = 0.90). The problem with this method, however, is that Doppler measurements must be made from two intracardiac sites, which is technically difficult in many patients.

Subsequent investigators reported the noninvasive estimate of valve area using Doppler ultrasound measurements from one intracardiac site and the continuity equation.[125-130] The continuity equation (see Fig 4–17) states that if there is no loss of fluid from a system, the volumetric flow at area 1 must be the same as the volumetric flow at area 2. Because the volumetric flow is the mean velocity times the cross-sectional area of flow, then:

$$A_1V_1 = A_2V_2$$

where A_1 and A_2 = cross-sectional areas at positions 1 and 2
V_1 and V_2 = mean velocities at positions 1 and 2

The continuity equation is a basic principle of flow from which the Gorlin equation is partially derived.

In clinical applications, A_2 is the effective area of the stenotic valve and V_2 is the jet-flow velocity through the stenotic valve. A_1 and V_1 are the cross-sectional area and flow velocity proximal to the stenotic orifice. The most common application of this equation has been the noninvasive calculation of aortic valve area. In this circumstance, A_2 is the area of the stenotic aortic valve, V_2 is the mean velocity through the stenotic aortic valve, A_1 is the cross-sectional area of the left ventricular outflow tract, and V_1 is the mean velocity of flow in the left ventricular outflow tract. Stenotic aortic valve area is calculated as:

$$CSA_{AV} = \frac{CSA_{LVOT} \times V_{LVOT}}{V_{AV}}$$

where CSA_{AV} = cross-sectional area of aortic valve
CSA_{LVOT} = cross-sectional area of left ventricular outflow tract
V_{LVOT} = mean velocity of left ventricular outflow tract
V_{AV} = mean velocity across aortic valve

Because mean velocity equals the velocity time integral divided by the flow duration and the flow duration is nearly equal at both sites, this equation can be further simplified:

$$CSA_{AV} = \frac{CSA_{LVOT} \times VTI_{LVOT}}{VTI_{AV}}$$

where   VTI = velocity time integral

In addition, examination of the velocity curves at both sites shows that each curve resembles the contour of half an ellipse, both sharing a common axis (the left ventricular ejection time) but having a different peak velocity. For a half-ellipse configuration:

$$VTI = LVET \times PkV \times \pi/2$$

where   LVET = left ventricular ejection time
PkV = peak velocity

Combining these two equations provides an even simpler form of the continuity equation[127, 131]:

$$CSA_{AV} = \frac{CSA_{LVOT} \times PkV_{LVOT}}{PkV_{AV}}$$

Doppler estimates of aortic valve area derived from the continuity equation (and either velocity time integrals or peak velocities) have correlated well with valve area measured at cardiac catheterization using the Gorlin equation.[125-131] Theoretically, any intracardiac site or combination of sites that have the same volume flow could be used in the continuity equation. For example, the stenotic mitral valve area could be calculated using the velocity time integral of the mitral stenosis jet, the velocity time integral of the left ventricular outflow tract Doppler, and the cross-sectional area of the left ventricular outflow tract, if the stroke volume is the same at both sites.[132] For calculation of the aortic valve area, the left ventricular outflow tract site has been the most widely used for several reasons:

1. In most patients, the left ventricular outflow tract can be measured with greater ease and accuracy than any other area in the heart.
2. The left ventricular outflow tract is nearly circular, hence its cross-sectional area can be calculated from one diameter measurement.
3. The cross-sectional area of the left ventricular outflow tract is constant throughout systole. Sites such as the mitral and tricuspid valve have constantly changing cross-sectional areas throughout diastole.

In spite of these advantages, inaccurate measurement of the left ventricular outflow tract diameter is the greatest source of error when the continuity equation in used. For example, an accurate measurement of the left ventricular outflow tract diameter is particularly difficult to obtain when there is a calcified aortic valve or basal septal hypertrophy.[125] Left ventricular outflow tract diameter is best measured from the parasternal long-axis view because in this view measurement of the outflow tract diameter is in the direction of axial resolution of the equipment. The diameter is measured just at the base of the aortic valve cusps in early systole, from inner edge to inner edge. Another potential source of error in the Doppler technique is in measurement of the left ventricular outflow tract mean velocity. The left ventricular outflow tract velocity is recorded with pulsed Doppler echocardiography from an apical four-chamber view, with the transducer tilted anteriorly to visualize the aortic valve. The sample volume is moved from the inferior portion of the outflow tract toward the aortic valve until the velocities begin to increase steeply. The tracing obtained prior to the steeply increasing velocities is used to calculate the velocity time integral or peak velocity of the left ventricular outflow tract.[125]

For several reasons, Doppler calculation of valve area using the continuity equation is more practical than Doppler calculations based on the Gorlin equation. With the continuity equation, there is no need to calculate heart rate or systolic ejection period. In addition, the continuity equation has the major advantage of being unaffected by the presence of valve insufficiency, even when it is severe.[133] The Gorlin method, however, underestimates valve area in the presence of valve insufficiency.

Calculation of Mitral Valve Area From Pressure Half-Time

The velocity across the mitral valve is increased with obstruction or with increased flow across the valve. However, the rate of decline in the velocity from the early peak velocity is altered by obstruction rather than flow. As the stenosis becomes more severe, the diastolic gradient between the left atrium and the left ventricle is maintained

for a longer period of time and, thus results in a slower decline in the gradient throughout diastole. The rate of decline in the pressure gradient can be expressed in terms of the pressure half-time, which is the time needed for the initial peak diastolic gradient to decline by 50%.[86] Because of the quadratic relationship between pressure and velocity, the velocity at which the initial peak pressure drop is halved is obtained by dividing the initial peak velocity by the square root of 2 (or 1.4). The time between the initial peak velocity and the velocity whose value is peak velocity divided by 1.4 is the pressure half-time (Fig 4–28). Pressure half-time is less than 60 msec in normal patients, 100 to 400 msec in patients with mitral stenosis, and associated with a valve area of less than 1.0 cm² when greater than 220 msec. Hatle and Angelsen[86] showed that a good estimate of mitral valve area can be obtained by dividing 220 (an empirically derived constant) by the pressure half-time:

$$\text{Mitral valve area (cm}^2) = \frac{220}{\text{pressure half-time (msec)}}$$

Using a mathematical analysis of the Doppler waveform of the mitral stenosis jet, Yang and Goldberg[134] simplified the pressure half-time method for calculation of the mitral valve area. In their method, a line is drawn from the peak E velocity, through any point on the downslope from the peak E velocity, and extrapolated to the baseline. The time from peak E to the point at which this line crosses the baseline (called AC time) is measured. Mitral valve area is then calculated as:

$$\text{MVA} = 750/\text{AC}$$

This technique requires drawing one line with a straight edge and reading AC off the horizontal scale of the Doppler tracing.

Several studies have shown good correlation between mitral valve area determined by the pressure half-time method and mitral valve area determined by two-dimensional echocardiography or cardiac catheterization (the Gorlin formula).[135–137] However, the pressure half-time is not only inversely proportional to the effective valve area but also directly proportional to the left atrial and left ventricular compliance and the square root of the initial transmitral pressure gradient.[138] It is likely that the accuracy of the pressure half-time method of estimating mitral valve area is caused by the tendency of chamber compliance and initial pressure gradient to change in opposite directions, thus offsetting their effects on the pressure half-time. Immediately after valvotomy, however, the magnitude and directions of these changes is such that the pressure half-time method does not provide accurate assessment of mitral valve area.[139] Another problem with the pressure half-time method is that the empiric constant of 220 was derived from adult patients with relatively slow heart rates. This constant does not apply to young children with fast heart rates. If the measured pressure half-time is less than 60 msec, the mitral valve area measured by the pressure half-time method is essentially meaningless.

Quantitation of Volumetric Flow

Collection and Measurement of the Data

Both systemic and pulmonary blood flows can be calculated from the two-dimensional and Doppler echocardiograms using the following equations for volumetric flow[140-147]:

$$SV = \frac{V \times CSA \times RR}{1000 \; cc/L}$$

where   SV   = stroke volume (cc/beat)
           V   = mean velocity (cm/sec)
        CSA   = cross-sectional area of flow (cm²)
        RR   = R-to-R interval (s/beat)

Because the cardiac output equals the stroke volume times the heart rate and the heart rate equals 60/R-R interval, the volumetric flow or cardiac output is:

$$\text{Volumetric flow (L/min)} = \frac{V \times CSA \times 60 \; s/min}{1,000 \; cc/L}$$

Usually, the pulmonary artery mean velocity and diameter are used to calculate pulmonary blood flow, and the mean velocity and diameter of the ascending aorta are used to calculate systemic blood flow; however, other sites can be used, depending on whether an intracardiac shunt is present and, if so, where it is located. If an intracardiac left-to-right shunt is present, its magnitude can be calculated directly as pulmonary blood flow minus systemic blood flow; it can be assessed indirectly by calculating the ratio of the pulmonary and systemic blood flows or the Qp/Qs.

The calculation of volumetric flow requires measurement of the temporal mean flow velocity and the vessel cross-sectional area. In measuring the mean velocity, a fundamental assumption is that flow is laminar and organized and that the velocity profile is uniform across the vessel or valve inlet.[86] Under these circumstances, a single sampling of the flow velocity in the center of the vessel is recorded. Care is taken to align the Doppler beam parallel with flow in the vessel so that the maximal velocities are recorded and so that no correction for intercept angle needs to be made. The mean velocity is then calculated as the integrated area under the Doppler curve or the velocity time integral divided by the flow period of the traced beats. Figure 4–29 is an example of the technique used to calculate aortic mean velocity. From the apical four-chamber view, the transducer is tilted anteriorly to visualize the aortic valve and ascending aorta. The sample volume is positioned just above the aortic valve leaflets with the Doppler beam as closely parallel as possible to the flow. Using a computer program, the Doppler velocity curve is integrated by tracing the densest area of the Doppler curve or the modal velocity over several consecutive cardiac cycles.[148]

If a computer program is not available for integrating the area under the Doppler curve, it can be calculated manually. When a straight line is drawn from the peak velocity to the baseline, the Doppler spectral tracing can be divided into two right-angle triangles. The area of a right-angle triangle is one-half the base times the height, both of which can be measured directly from the Doppler tracings. The area of the forward and reverse triangles are then added to obtain the total area under the Doppler spectral tracing.

For systemic blood flow, aortic velocity can be recorded from many windows including suprasternal, apical, and subcostal approaches. We prefer the apical view because it is easy to obtain in most patients and because it is possible to position the sample volume parallel with flow across the annulus and close to the valve leaflets. In

FIG 4–28.

Illustration of the method used to calculate the pressure half-time of the mitral valve Doppler recording in an adolescent female with rheumatic mitral stenosis. The freeze-frame image *(right)* is an apical four-chamber view showing the position of the sample volume in the left ventricle (LV) just distal to the mitral valve at the time of the Doppler spectral recording. The mitral valve Doppler recording is shown on the left. The peak velocity of the mitral valve Doppler in early diastole is 1.77 m/sec. The initial pressure drop is halved where the peak velocity falls to 1.77/1.4 or 1.26 m/sec. The pressure half-time is the time between the peak velocity and the time when the velocity falls to 1.26 m/sec. In this example, the pressure half-time is 230 msec. The mitral valve area is 220 divided by the pressure half-time or 0.96 cm².

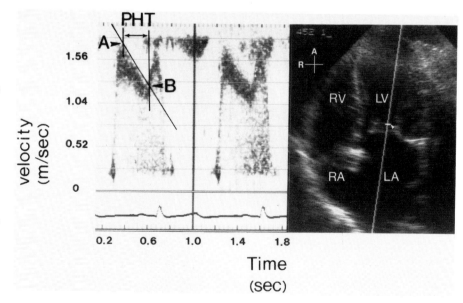

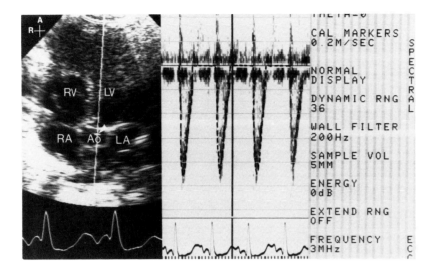

FIG 4–29.
Example of the methods used to calculate the cardiac output or systemic blood flow. The freeze-frame image *(left)* shows the position of the sample volume *(arrow)* in the ascending aorta (AO) at the time of the Doppler spectral recording. The Doppler recording *(right)* shows normal forward flow in the AO away from the transducer and below the baseline. The *dashed lines* indicate the area of the Doppler curve that was traced to determine the mean velocity. The volumetric blood flow is equal to the mean velocity times the vessel cross-sectional area. In this example, the mean velocity of the traced beats was 19.2 cm/sec. The aortic cross-sectional area was .64 cm². The systemic blood flow is equal to 19.2 cm/sec × 0.64 cm² × 60 sec/min × 1,000 cc/L^{-1} which is equal to 0.737 L/min. The patient's body surface area was 0.20 m²; therefore, the cardiac index was equal to 0.737 ÷ 0.20 = 3.65 L/min/m².

the suprasternal view, it is often not possible to sample aortic flow just at the valve leaflets at an acceptable angle; frequently, flow must be sampled in the ascending aorta several centimeters above the valve. If aortic mean velocity is measured in the ascending aorta, the vessel cross-sectional area should be measured at the same location. It is difficult to measure the aortic diameter accurately at this location because of difficulties in imaging the anterior aortic wall from the suprasternal notch and because the aortic diameter is measured in the direction of the lateral resolution of the equipment. The pulmonary artery mean velocity is calculated from the pulmonary artery Doppler tracing in a similar manner. Usually, acceptable pulmonary artery Doppler tracings can be obtained from the parasternal short-axis view or from the subcostal view of the right ventricular outflow tract.[149] Frequently, with a large shunt or a shunt whose location is close to the pulmonary artery (i.e., a ventricular septal defect), the Doppler tracing shows spectral broadening or signs of disturbed flow. In these cases, a uniform velocity profile in the main pulmonary artery cannot be assumed and another site should be chosen to calculate pulmonary blood flow (e.g., the mitral valve for a patient with a ventricular septal defect). Also, the main pulmonary artery Doppler tracing cannot be used to calculate pulmonary blood flow if any pulmonary stenosis accompanies the shunt because in this instance as well, the velocity profile is not uniform across the vessel lumen.

If the atrioventricular valves are used to calculate pulmonary or systemic blood flow, the velocity signals are usually recorded from the apical four-chamber view and the Doppler curve is traced throughout diastole.[150]

The vessel cross-sectional area is usually calculated by measuring the vessel diameter from the two-dimensional echocardiogram and assuming that the vessel is circular, so that cross-sectional area equals $\pi (d^2)/4$. There are many different techniques for measuring vessel diameters. In our laboratory, we measure the aorta and pulmonary artery from inner edge to inner edge in early systole at the level of the valve annulus.[151] We use the inner-edge measurements because this technique gives the closest approximation of the actual flow diameter. It is known that systolic expansion accounts for a 5% to 10% change in aortic cross-sectional area and a 2% to 18% change in pulmonary artery cross-sectional area throughout systole. The increase in cross-sectional area occurs early in systole simultaneously with the upstroke of the pressure curve, so that the majority of the flow in the aorta or pulmonary artery occurs when the vessel is at or near its peak systolic dimension. The vessel diameter is measured at the valve annulus because it is the smallest area, or the flow-limiting point, in the vessel where maximal flow velocity should theoretically occur.

For the aortic diameter, the parasternal long-axis view is preferable because in this view the diameter is measured in the direction of the axial resolution of the equipment (Fig 4–30). For the pulmonary artery flow diameter, the parasternal long-axis view of the right ventricle is preferred because in this view it is easier to visualize the origin of the pulmonary valve leaflets and the left lateral wall of the main pulmonary artery away from the lung. Measurements of the pulmonary flow diameter are made in the same manner as for the aorta (see Fig 4–30).

There are many other methods for measuring aortic

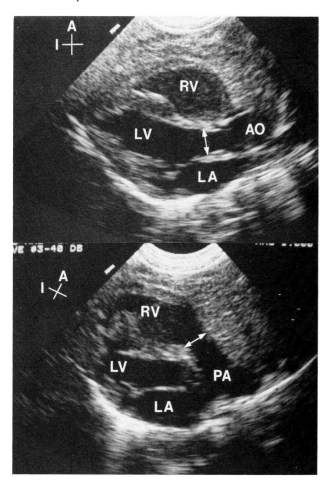

FIG 4–30.
Methods used to measure vessel diameter for calculation of volumetric flow. In the *top frame,* the aortic (AO) diameter is measured from a parasternal long-axis view in the direction of axial resolution of the equipment. The diameter is measured from inner edge to inner edge at the base of the aortic valve leaflets *(arrow).* In the *bottom frame,* the pulmonary artery (PA) diameter is measured from a parasternal long-axis view of the right ventricular (RV) outflow tract. This diameter is also measured from inner edge to inner edge at the base of the pulmonary valve leaflets. *A* = anterior; *I* = inferior; *LA* = left atrium; and *LV* = left ventricle.

sition the plane exactly at the origin of the valve leaflets. If the plane is superior to the origin of the valve leaflets, the diameter of the aorta will be larger because the plane is actually through the sinuses of Valsalva. Figure 4–32 shows measurements of the aorta from the suprasternal long-axis view. In this patient, aortic diameters ranged from 1.79 to 1.88 in the suprasternal view. It is difficult to obtain reliable aortic flow diameters from the suprasternal notch position for several reasons: (1) it is difficult to clearly resolve the anterior aortic wall separate from the sternum; (2) the measurement is made in the direction of the lateral

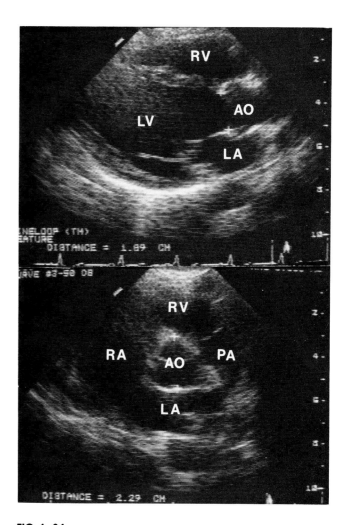

FIG 4–31.
Aortic diameters from the same patient measured in different views. In the *top frame,* the aorta (AO) is measured in the parasternal long-axis view in the direction of axial resolution of the equipment and has a diameter of 1.89 cm. From this diameter, the calculated cross-sectional area is 2.8 cm². In the *bottom frame,* the aorta is also measured in the direction of the axial resolution, this time from a parasternal short-axis view. The diameter measured 2.29 cm, which is a cross-sectional area of 4.1 cm². Note that a small difference in diameter when squared produces a large difference in vessel cross-sectional area. *LA* = left atrium; *LV* = left ventricle; *PA* = pulmonary artery; *RA* = right atrium; and *RV* = right ventricle.

and pulmonary flow diameters. Figure 4–31 shows aortic diameters measured from different views in the same patient. In the top frame, the aorta is measured in the parasternal long-axis view in the direction of axial resolution of the equipment and has a diameter of 1.89 cm. From this diameter, the calculated cross-sectional area is 2.8 cm². In the bottom frame, the aorta is also measured in the direction of the axial resolution, this time from the parasternal short-axis view. The diameter measures 2.29 cm, which is a cross-sectional area of 4.1 cm². Note that a small difference in diameter when squared produces a large difference in vessel cross-sectional area.

In the parasternal short-axis view, it is difficult to po-

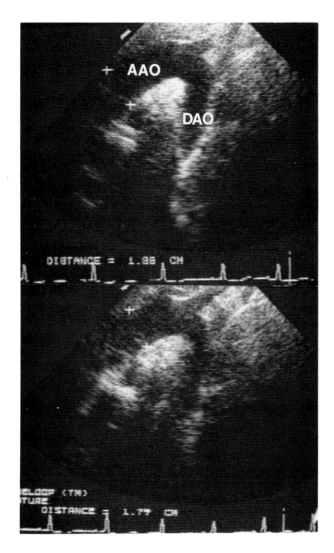

FIG 4–32.
Measurements of the aorta from the suprasternal long-axis view in the same patient. Aortic diameters ranged from 1.79 to 1.88 in the suprasternal long-axis view, depending on the level at which the measurement was made. *AAO* = ascending aorta; *DAO* = descending aorta.

parasternal long- and short-axis views. In this example, the diameters measured from the two views were nearly equal (1.96 and 1.99 cm). If widely discrepant values for the pulmonary diameter are obtained from different views in the same patient, the echocardiographer must use judgment and select the view that provides the clearest image of both walls of the pulmonary artery.

For the pulmonary artery, accurate measurement of the vessel diameter is much more difficult. First, it is usually not possible to image the pulmonary artery in a view that will allow measurement of the diameter in the direction of the axial resolution. Second, it may be difficult to visualize the left lateral border of the main pulmonary artery because of the adjacent lung tissue. Placing the patient in a steep left lateral decubitus position will optimize visualization of the left border of the pulmonary artery. Third, Stewart and colleagues[152] have shown that with increasing volumetric flow, pulmonary artery diameter increases to a far greater extent than aortic diameter. With increasing volume flow from 0.5 to 1.0 L/min, aortic mean velocity increased linearly and aortic diameter increased very slightly. No further changes were observed with increasing flow rates from 2 to 5 L/min. With increasing pulmonary blood flow, there was a consistent increase in pulmonary artery diameter throughout the entire range of flows. Pulmonary artery mean velocity increased as well, but the percent increase in pulmonary artery mean velocity

resolution of the equipment, which increases the measurement errors; and (3) the caliber of the ascending aorta can change dramatically between the valve and the arch vessels, making it difficult to decide exactly at what point to measure the aortic diameter. The aorta can also be measured from an M-mode echocardiogram (Fig 4–33). In this patient (the same as in Figures 4–31 and 4–32), the M-mode aortic diameter was 1.99 cm measured from inner edge to inner edge in early systole. If M-mode diameters of the aorta are used, care should be taken to position the M-mode cursor exactly perpendicular to the aortic root and through the maximum diameter of the aorta at the origin of the valve leaflets.[151]

Figure 4–34 shows examples of measurements of the pulmonary artery diameter from the same patient in both

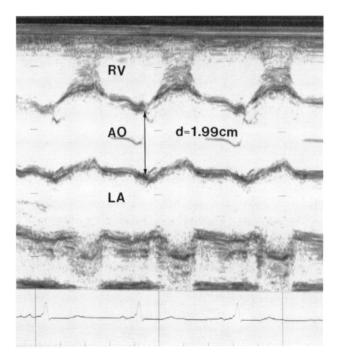

FIG 4–33.
Measurement of the aorta (AO) from the same patient as in Figure 4–32, this time using the M-mode echocardiogram. The AO diameter is measured from inner edge to inner edge at the beginning of systole. From the M-mode echocardiogram, the AO diameter was 1.99 cm. *LA* = left atrium; *RV* = right ventricle.

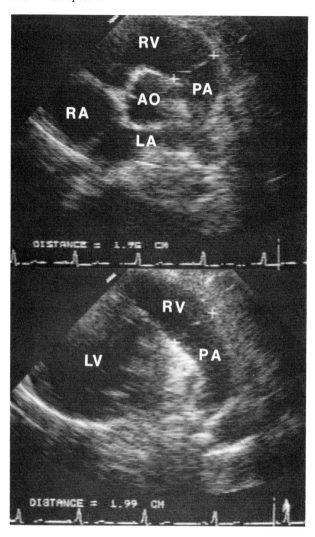

FIG 4–34.
Measurement of the pulmonary artery (PA) diameter in the same patient from the parasternal short-axis view *(top)* and the parasternal long-axis view of the right ventricular (RV) outflow tract *(bottom)*. From the parasternal short-axis view, the diameter measured 1.96 cm. From the parasternal long-axis view, the diameter measured 1.99 cm. The PA diameter is measured from inner edge to inner edge at the base of the valve leaflets. *AO* = aorta; *LA* = left atrium; *LV* = left ventricle; and *RA* = right atrium.

was less than the percent increase in aortic mean velocity for the same change in volumetric flow. Thus, at different volume flows there is far greater variability in pulmonary artery diameter than in aortic diameter. Pulmonary artery diameter, then, can never be assumed to be constant in a given patient when assessing serial changes in pulmonary blood flow.

If the mitral and tricuspid valves are used to calculate systemic or pulmonary blood flow, several different methodologies have been described for calculating cross-sectional area. These methods include the mitral valve orifice

method of Fisher, assumption of a circular orifice, and assumption of an elliptical orifice.[150, 153]

Clinical Applications

In general, in patients with left-to-right shunts, Doppler-derived values for pulmonary and systemic blood flows and Qp/Qs have correlated well with the same values determined at cardiac catheterization using the Fick technique.[140, 154, 155] For systemic blood flow, correlation coefficients in several clinical studies have ranged from 0.78 to 0.91; standard errors of the estimate have ranged from 0.60 to 0.81 L/min. For pulmonary blood flow, correlation coefficients have ranged from 0.72 to 0.88, and standard errors from 1.11 to 2.4 L/min. For Qp/Qs, correlation coefficients have been 0.85 in three different studies, with standard errors of around 0.48.

In children with atrial septal defects, systemic blood flow can be calculated from the aortic or mitral valve sites, assuming no mitral or aortic insufficiency is present. Pulmonary blood flow can be calculated from the main pulmonary artery or tricuspid valve sites, assuming there is no pulmonary stenosis or tricuspid insufficiency. In the case of a ventricular septal defect, systemic blood flow can be calculated from aortic or tricuspid valve sites. Pulmonary blood flow can be calculated from the main pulmonary artery if there is no pulmonary stenosis and if there is minimal spectral broadening of the pulmonary artery Doppler recording. Pulmonary blood flow can be calculated from the mitral valve site if the atrial septum is intact and if there is no mitral insufficiency. For the patent ductus arteriosus, systemic blood flow can be calculated from the tricuspid valve or the right ventricular outflow tract proximal to the patent ductus arteriosus. Use of the left ventricular outflow or ascending aorta sites will overestimate systemic blood flow because of the distal communication between the aorta and pulmonary artery. Pulmonary blood flow can be calculated from the mitral valve or aortic valve sites. Use of the pulmonary valve site will underestimate pulmonary blood flow because of the distal communication.

Limitations of the Technique

There are several possible sources of error when Doppler ultrasound is used to calculate the volumetric flow. First, errors can occur in the measurement of the mean velocity from the Doppler spectral tracing. Gardin and colleagues[151] have shown that in general there is good reproducibility in measurement of the mean velocity. For the aortic mean velocity, intraobserver variability in their study was 3.2% ± 2.9%, interobserver variability was 5.4% ± 3.4%, and the day-to-day variability was 3.8% ± 3.1%. Potential sources of error in measuring the Doppler mean velocity include errors in determining the intercept angle and the lack of a uniform velocity profile across the vessel lumen.

Inaccurate determination of vessel cross-sectional area is the largest source of error in the Doppler technique.

Errors can occur in determination of vessel cross-sectional area because (1) the instrument's gain settings may be too high or too low to optimize visualization of the vessel walls; (2) the vessel cross-sectional area (especially the main pulmonary artery) changes throughout the cardiac cycle and these changes depend on factors such as pressure, flow, and elasticity in the vessel; and (3) it may be necessary to measure the vessel in the direction of the lateral resolution of the equipment.

Errors in the calculation of flow can occur because additional defects are present. For example, an additional undetected shunt such as a patent ductus arteriosus located downstream from the pulmonary artery sampling site will lead to an underestimation of the total pulmonary flow and Qp/Qs ratio. Semilunar valve regurgitation results in an overestimation of flow caused by failure to measure the regurgitant volume.

Finally, discrepancies can occur between the Doppler and catheterization measurements of flow because of errors in the use of the Fick technique as the gold standard. Variability in measurement of blood flow by the Fick technique occurs because this technique requires that the patient be in a steady state for several minutes, which does not often occur, and because the Fick technique is influenced by the patient's ventilatory rate, room temperature, barometric pressure, and the patient's respiratory exchange ratio.

Quantitation of Valvular Regurgitation

Mapping Techniques

Quantitation of valvular regurgitation continues to be a major clinical problem. Many methods for estimating the severity of the valvular insufficiency have been proposed; however, none allows precise quantitation of the regurgitant volume. The most widely used method for assessing the severity of the regurgitation is mapping the dimensions of the regurgitant jet with pulsed or color-flow Doppler echocardiography. With the pulsed Doppler technique, the sample volume is moved across the cardiac chamber that receives the regurgitant jet in both axial and lateral directions to detect the borders of the jet.[156–158] Describing a jet in this manner can be tedious and difficult, especially if the jet is very eccentric and clings to a cardiac wall or valve leaflet. Color-flow Doppler technology provides a spatial display of regurgitant jet velocities determined at multiple sampling sites and superimposed on the two-dimensional echocardiographic image. The autocorrelation technique used in color Doppler systems allows display of only the mean velocities of the jet and thus may be less sensitive than pulsed Doppler techniques (see Chapter 1). It should be remembered that both of these techniques measure only the velocity vector that is parallel to the sound beam and underestimate velocities not parallel to the sound beam. It should also be remembered that pulsed and color-flow Doppler mapping techniques performed in only one echocardiographic view do not provide a complete picture of a three-dimensional regurgitant jet. Nevertheless, current clinical color Doppler assessment of mitral regurgitation

is based on measurement from a single still frame of the regurgitant jet area or the ratio of jet area to the cross-sectional area of the left atrium.[159, 160] In one color Doppler study, the spatial distribution of the mitral regurgitation jet was measured from a still frame of the parasternal long-axis view in midsystole.[159] Doppler measurements of the maximum extension of the jet into the left atrium from the valve orifice and the total cross-sectional area of the jet were compared to the results of angiography. In this study, the following criteria provided good correlations between the two techniques when used in adult patients:

- 1+ (mild) = jet length < 1.5 cm and area <1.5 cm².
- 2+ (moderate) = jet length ≥ 1.5 and < 3.0 cm and area ≥1.5 and <3.0 cm².
- 3+ (moderate-to-severe) = jet length ≥ 3.0 and < 4.5 and area ≥ 3.0 and < 4.5 cm².
- 4+ (severe) = jet length ≥ 4.5 and area ≥ 4.5 cm².

Helmcke and colleagues[160] measured the area of the mitral regurgitation jet in three echocardiographic planes (parasternal long- and short-axis and apical four-chamber views). Using the plane that showed the largest area of the jet, they calculated the ratio of maximum regurgitant jet area to the area of the left atrium in that plane. The ratio was under 20% in patients with angiographic grade 1+ mitral regurgitation, between 20% and 40% with 2+ regurgitation, and more than 40% with severe regurgitation. Other parameters such as maximal linear and transverse jet dimensions correlated less well with angiography.

Aortic insufficiency has also been graded according to the length, area, and width of the jet as imaged by color-flow Doppler. Perry and colleagues[161] found that the maximal length and area of the aortic insufficiency jet was poorly predictive of the angiographic grade. These investigators found that the width of the jet at its origin, relative to the width of the left ventricular outflow tract (from parasternal long- or short-axis views), was the best predictor of the angiographic grading of the insufficiency. This ratio measured 19% in most patients with 1+ insufficiency, 30% with 2+, 56% with 3+, and 80% with 4+ insufficiency. The ratio measured in this study is in actuality a measurement of the diameter of the regurgitant orifice.

Mitral and tricuspid regurgitation occur into atria that are static, symmetric chambers; hence, assessment of these lesions is less complex than assessment of aortic insufficiency. In aortic insufficiency, the regurgitant jet flows into the left ventricular outflow tract, which is a more dynamic structure bounded by a mobile mitral valve leaflet and the ventricular septum. In addition, velocities from the aortic insufficiency jet may be difficult to separate from simultaneous mitral inflow velocities.[162] Furthermore, mapping techniques in general are based on the assumption that the spatial distribution of the regurgitant jet reflects the regurgitant volume. The spatial distribution of a regurgitant jet on a color-flow Doppler mean-velocity map depends on many factors. First, the jet area reflects not only the blood flow in the regurgitant jet but also the blood flow that is entrained and displaced in its path.[162] Second, in vivo and in vitro studies have shown that the maximum length, width, and area of the jet are influenced by the pressure gradient across the regurgitant orifice, the heart rate, the cardiac output, and the orifice area.[161, 163] Third, the spatial display of jet flow on a color Doppler system is particularly affected by instrument settings[164] such as the overall color gains, wall filter settings, transducer frequency, pulse repetition frequency, threshold settings for flow detection, and variance algorithm. Thus, reproducible spatial displays of the jet area are difficult to obtain from machine to machine and even for a given machine. Fourth, measurements of the jet made from a single two-dimensional view may not represent the three-dimensional aspects of jet flow. The direction and expansion of a regurgitant jet may vary significantly between planes, and the shape and direction of the jet may vary throughout the cardiac and respiratory cycle. Doppler mapping techniques, therefore, are valid only for a specific set of physiologic and technical variables. Assessments derived from the mapping technique may not be comparable from machine to machine, from patient to patient, or in the same patient over time. Nevertheless, in many centers Doppler color-flow mapping techniques continue to be used because they provide a good correlation with the "not-so-gold" standard—angiographic grading.[162] When using these semiquantitative techniques, it is necessary to keep in mind the technical and hemodynamic factors that influence the spatial display of jets.

Measurement of Regurgitant Fraction

Regurgitant fraction can be calculated from the Doppler examination when there is regurgitation of a single valve and the absence of a shunt.[165–167] In patients with isolated mitral or aortic regurgitation, volume flows are calculated at the mitral and aortic valves using Doppler ultrasound techniques (see the description of volumetric flow calculation in this chapter). Regurgitant fraction is calculated as the difference in the two flows, divided by the flow through the regurgitant valve. Using this technique, good correlations have been obtained with regurgitant fraction measured at cardiac catheterization.[165] In an alternative method, a combination of two-dimensional and pulsed Doppler techniques has been used to calculate regurgitant fraction in patients with isolated mitral regurgitation.[166] Diastolic and systolic volumes of the left ventricle are calculated from the two-dimensional echocardiogram and used to derive left ventricular stroke volume. The forward stroke volume is obtained from the aortic valve site using pulsed Doppler echocardiography. The regurgitant fraction is calculated as left ventricular stroke volume minus forward stroke volume divided by left ventricular stroke volume.

Quantitation of Semilunar Valve Regurgitation from Diastolic Runoff

With semilunar valve regurgitation, reverse laminar flow signals can be recorded in the great artery downstream

from the regurgitant valve (Fig 4–35). Several studies have shown that the area (or velocity time integral) of the retrograde diastolic flow signals increases with increasing severity of the valvular regurgitation.[168–170] For aortic insufficiency, the ratio of the velocity time integral of the reverse flow to that of the forward flow has correlated well with angiographic grading of the amount of insufficiency. Using an ascending aorta Doppler recording, Quinones and colleagues[168] showed that this ratio (expressed as a percentage) was 8.9 ± 2.9 for $1+$ insufficiency, 23.6 ± 4.2 for $2+$, 35.7 ± 5.0 for $3+$, and 50.2 ± 6.5 for $4+$ insufficiency. Boughner[169] used the descending thoracic aorta flow velocity signals to calculate the ratio of the reverse to the forward flow areas and found a good correlation between the ratio and regurgitant fraction measured at catheterization. Takenaka and colleagues[170] showed that holodiastolic retrograde flow was present on the Doppler examination of the abdominal aorta in all patients with angiographic grade $3+$ or $4+$ aortic insufficiency.

Quantitation of Aortic Insufficiency With Continuous-Wave Doppler

The high-velocity aortic insufficiency jet can be displayed unambiguously using continuous-wave Doppler techniques. From the continuous-wave Doppler tracing, indexes of the rate and timing of deceleration of regurgitant blood flow velocities can be measured. These indexes, which reflect the rate of decline in the diastolic pressure

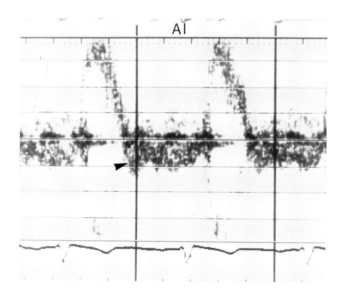

FIG 4–35.
Pulsed Doppler recording of the ascending aorta from the suprasternal notch of a patient with severe aortic insufficiency (AI). Normal forward flow signals are seen in systole above the baseline, indicating flow from the left ventricle to the aorta in systole toward the transducer. In diastole, flow signals are seen below the baseline (arrow), indicating retrograde flow of blood from the ascending aorta to the left ventricle in diastole. This amount of retrograde diastolic flow is usually associated with significant AI.

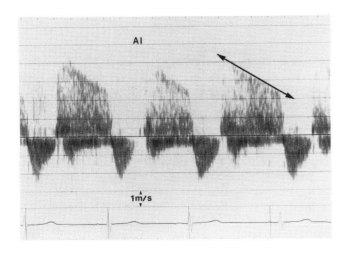

FIG 4–36.
Continuous-wave Doppler tracing from the cardiac apex of a patient with aortic insufficiency (AI). The flow signals above the baseline in diastole arise from the AI jet, which is directed toward the transducer from the aorta to the left ventricle. The deceleration rate of the AI jet is measured as the slope of a line drawn between the peak velocity and the shoulder of the tracing at end-diastole.

difference between the aorta and left ventricle, bear some correlation to the severity of the regurgitation. Some commonly measured indexes are the deceleration rate (measured as the slope of a line drawn between the peak velocity and the shoulder at end-diastole, as shown in Figure 4–36), the half-time index (the interval between the peak velocity and one-half the peak velocity), and the pressure half-time (time required for the initial peak transvalvular pressure gradient to be halved, as described previously for the mitral valve pressure half-time).[171–175] The pressure half-time (also referred to as the velocity half-time) can be calculated from a simplified equation[172]:

$$VHT = (0.29)(\frac{F}{S})$$

where VHT = velocity half-time
F = peak Doppler shift
S = slope of a line between two cursors, one placed at the early diastolic peak of the velocity profile, the second placed visually to define the linear rate of diastolic velocity decay

This simplified approach has two major benefits that the standard methods for calculation of pressure half-time do not have. First, the entire velocity profile can be used to determine the rate of decay, thus increasing the accuracy; second, this half-time approach is independent of the intercept angle between the Doppler beam and the jet (Doppler shifts implicitly containing the intercept angle are found in the numerator (F) and denominator (S) of the equation).[172]

Values for these indexes, shown in Table 4–7, have correlated well with angiographic grading of the insufficiency and with regurgitant fraction measured at cardiac catheterization. In general, a deceleration slope of > 2 m/sec² distinguishes patients with mild aortic insufficiency from those with moderate and severe insufficiency[171]; and, a slope of >3 m/sec² is found only in patients with 3 + to 4 + insufficiency at angiography.[175] Also, a pressure half-time of > 400 msec indicates mild insufficiency, while a pressure half-time of <400 msec indicates 3 + to 4 + insufficiency and regurgitant fraction >40%.[172]

The magnitude of the regurgitation is not the only factor that affects the time course of the diastolic transvalvular pressure drop in patients with aortic insufficiency. This pressure drop also depends on ventricular loading conditions, ventricular compliance, and associated lesions.[174, 175] For example, a patient with mild aortic insufficiency and a noncompliant left ventricle may have a rapid deceleration rate. In addition, the values given in Table 4–7 were derived from adult patients with relatively slow heart rates. We have observed that these numbers lose their predictive value in infants with fast heart rates; therefore, it is likely that heart rate also affects the time course of the pressure gradient decay. When these indexes are used to assess the severity of aortic insufficiency, care must be taken to consider other factors that might be affecting the indexes.

Assessment of Ventricular Function

Ventricular Systolic Function

Doppler echocardiography evaluates intracardiac blood flow and provides an estimate of ventricular performance that is independent of ventricular geometry. Cardiac output is one ejection-phase index of function that can be calculated from the Doppler examination. Doppler-derived values for cardiac output have correlated closely with those measured invasively. Stroke volume or cardiac output can be measured for the left ventricle by using the aortic mean velocity and cross-sectional area and for the right ventricle by using the pulmonary artery mean velocity and cross-sectional area (see the section on volumetric flow in this chapter).

Catheterization and animal studies have shown that peak aortic acceleration is a good index of global left ventricular performance.[176, 177] Doppler echocardiography pro-

TABLE 4–7.
Deceleration Slopes From Continuous-Wave Doppler Recordings of Aortic Insufficiency*

Source	Mild AI	Moderate AI	Severe AI
Labovitz et al.[171]	1.6 ± 0.5	2.7 ± 0.5	4.7 ± 1.5
Masuyama et al.[173]	1.5 ± 0.5	2.2 ± 0.4	4.0 ± 1.0
Beyer et al.[174]	1.8 ± 0.7	2.5 ± 1.3	5.7 ± 2.1

*Data are given as mean ± SD; slopes are in m/sec². AI = aortic insufficiency.

vides a noninvasive technique for the measurement of aortic peak velocity, acceleration rates and times, and deceleration rates and times. Pulsed Doppler tracings from the ascending aorta have been used to distinguish normal patients from patients with impaired systolic function (dilated cardiomyopathy patients).[178] With no overlap of data, peak aortic flow velocity distinguished normal subjects (mean 92 cm/sec, range 72 to 120 cm/sec) from cardiomyopathy patients (mean 47 cm/sec, range 35 to 62). The aortic velocity time integral also distinguished between the two patient groups, with no overlap (normal patients = mean 15.7 cm and range 12.6 to 22.5 cm; cardiomyopathy = mean 6.7 cm and range 3.5 to 9.1 cm). The aortic acceleration time, measured from the onset of flow to the time of the peak aortic velocity, was significantly shorter in the cardiomyopathy patients (mean 73 msec, range 55 to 98 msec) compared with normal patients (mean 98 msec, range 83 to 118 msec); however, between the groups there was considerable overlap in data. Mean aortic acceleration, calculated as peak aortic velocity divided by acceleration time, was also significantly reduced in cardiomyopathy patients (mean 659 cm/sec^2, range 389 to 921 cm/sec^2; normal patients = mean 955 cm/sec^2, range 735 to 1,318 cm/sec^2); again, there was overlap in data points for the two groups. Deceleration time (from aortic peak velocity to end of systole) and mean deceleration rate (peak aortic velocity divided by deceleration time) were lower in cardiomyopathy patients but were less useful indexes for discriminating the two patient groups.

Sabbah and colleagues[179] have measured peak aortic velocity and peak acceleration rate in the ascending aorta using a continuous-wave Doppler transducer applied to the suprasternal notch. Measurements were obtained in patients at the time of cardiac catheterization. The peak acceleration rate is the largest of all the instantaneous values for the slope of the aortic velocity curve measured during the acceleration time (the time between the onset of flow and the aortic peak velocity). This value is different from the mean acceleration rate, which is the peak aortic velocity divided by the acceleration time. In patients with angiographic ejection fraction of >60%, peak aortic acceleration was 19 ± 5 m/sec^2. In patients with ejection fraction of 41% to 60%, peak acceleration was significantly lower (12 ± 2 m/sec^2, p < .001). In patients with ejection fraction <40%, peak acceleration was lower (8 ± 2 m/sec^2) than in patients with ejection fraction of > 60% (p < .001). An excellent correlation was found between peak aortic acceleration and ejection fraction (r = .90).

The effects of varying preload, heart rate, and inotropic state on the Doppler indexes of left ventricular performance have been studied in open-chest dogs.[180] Within a given animal, Doppler measurements of peak aortic velocity correlated closely with maximum aortic flow (r = 0.96) and maximum aortic acceleration (r = 0.95), both measured with an electromagnetic flow probe around the ascending aorta. Peak aortic velocity also correlated with maximum left ventricular dP/dt (r = 0.92). Doppler values for mean aortic acceleration also correlated with invasive

indexes; however, there was greater interobserver variability with this Doppler parameter. The Doppler measurements of peak aortic velocity and mean aortic acceleration provided a method to assess changes in left ventricular performance under conditions of varying preload, heart rate, and inotropic state.

Aortic velocity and acceleration have been used to assess left ventricular function in patients with acute myocardial infarction.[181, 182] When measured within 18 hours of a patient's admission for an acute myocardial infarction, the Doppler indexes correlated closely with the patient's clinical status using the Forrester classification[183] and with subsequent survival. The Doppler indexes have also been compared to the results of exercise stress testing performed three to four weeks after acute myocardial infarction. Aortic peak velocity and acceleration and the aortic velocity time integral were lower at peak exercise in patients with positive exercise stress tests ($\geq$1 mm of ST segment depression in any lead) than in those with negative stress tests.

An indirect assessment of left and right ventricular systolic performance can also be obtained by examining the shape of the Doppler velocity curves of the mitral or tricuspid insufficiency jets.[86] If the rate of rise of the systolic pressure in the ventricle is impaired, the increase in the velocity of the insufficiency jet is slower. In this case, the time from the onset of the insufficiency flow to the peak velocity of the insufficiency jet is prolonged (Fig 4–37). To make this type of assessment, a clear recording of the entire Doppler envelope throughout systole is required.

Ventricular Diastolic Function

Several different indexes of left ventricular diastolic function have been derived from the mitral valve inflow Doppler.[184–190] For this technique, a range-gated pulsed Doppler examination of the left ventricular inflow tract is performed (Fig 4–38). From the apical four-chamber view, the Doppler cursor line and sample volume are placed in the mitral valve orifice at an angle as nearly parallel as possible to the flow. The sample volume position is adjusted to record the maximum velocity through the mitral valve. This point is usually found distal to the annulus near the tips of the mitral valve leaflets. As will be discussed below, the position of the sample volume is critical if standardized results are to be obtained. An adequate mitral valve Doppler examination consists of clear identification of the opening and closure points of the mitral valve and the peak velocities at rapid ventricular filling, the peak E velocity, and during atrial contraction, the peak A velocity.

From the mitral valve Doppler tracing, several types of indexes of left ventricular diastolic filling can be calculated. First, diastolic time intervals reflecting the time course of relaxation can be calculated. The isovolumic relaxation time can be measured from the aortic closing component of the second heart sound to the onset of the diastolic flow velocity and usually requires a phonocardiogram to be recorded simultaneously with the mitral valve Doppler tracing. In some patients, it is possible to record aortic

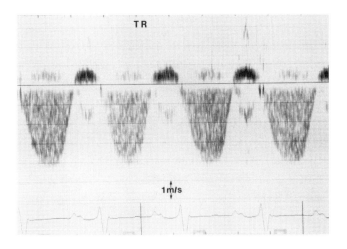

FIG 4–37.

Continuous-wave Doppler tracing from the cardiac apex of an infant with hypoplastic left heart syndrome, status post Norwood I procedure. This infant had markedly depressed right ventricular systolic function. From the cardiac apex, a tricuspid regurgitation (TR) jet was recorded (flow signals in systole below the baseline). In this case, the time from the onset of the regurgitant flow to the peak velocity of the regurgitant jet is prolonged. The rate of increase in velocity of the regurgitant jet is slower because the rate of rise of systolic pressure in the ventricle is impaired.

valve closure and mitral valve opening simultaneously using a continuous-wave Doppler transducer positioned at the cardiac apex, and, from this tracing, to measure isovolumic relaxation time (Fig 4–39). The isovolumic relaxation time is 71 ± 14 msec in normal adults and is prolonged in some patients with impaired left ventricular relaxation.[191] The time from the onset of diastolic flow to the peak E velocity (the acceleration time) can be measured and is 100 ± 10 msec in normal adults.[192] The deceleration time can be measured from the peak E velocity to the time

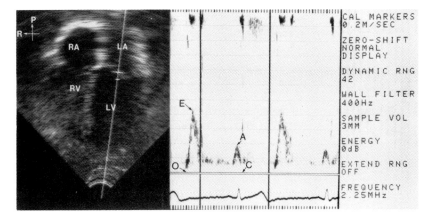

FIG 4–38.

Range-gated pulsed Doppler recording from the left ventricular (LV) inflow tract, demonstrating the technique used to obtain a mitral valve Doppler tracing for analysis of LV diastolic filling. The Doppler cursor line is placed through the mitral valve funnel at an angle as nearly parallel to the flow as possible. The sample volume position is placed near the tips of the mitral valve leaflets. The freeze-frame image, *left,* shows the position of the sample volume at the time of the Doppler spectral recording. The Doppler spectral recording, *right,* shows a typical pattern of left ventricular diastolic filling. Peak velocities of forward flow occur during rapid ventricular filling *(peak E)* and during atrial contraction *(peak A).* The O point represents the onset of flow through the mitral valve Doppler; the C point represents closure of the mitral valve leaflets. *LA* = left atrium; *P* = posterior; *R* = right; *RA* = right atrium; and *RV* = right ventricle.

when the Doppler curve returns from peak E velocity to the baseline. This time period is 193 ± 23 msec in normal subjects.[191] The duration of the early diastolic flow period can be measured from the onset of diastolic flow to the time when the Doppler curve returns from peak E velocity to the baseline. This time period is 214 ± 26 msec in normal subjects and has been reported to be prolonged in patients with left ventricular outflow obstruction.[186, 188] The time from the onset of diastolic flow to the point where the peak E velocity falls to the value of peak E/1.4 has been measured and corresponds well with M-mode measurements of the rapid filling period (normal patients = 130 ± 20 msec).[185] Finally, the acceleration and deceleration half-times of early diastolic rapid inflow have been used to describe the time course of relaxation.[187] These time periods are measured as the intervals between the peak E velocity and 50% of the peak E velocity on the ascending limb (acceleration half-time) and the descending limb (deceleration half-time) of early diastolic inflow.

Acceleration and deceleration half-times of the transmitral inflow velocity have been reported to be prolonged in patients with myocardial infarction (acceleration half-time >73 msec, deceleration half-time >100 msec) compared to normal subjects (acceleration half-time = 62 ± 18 msec, deceleration half-time = 73 ± 24 msec).[187]

A second type of diastolic parameter that has been measured from the mitral valve Doppler tracings are indexes of velocity and acceleration. The peak velocity during rapid filling, or the peak E velocity, can be measured and is 0.60 to 0.68 m/sec in normal subjects. The peak velocity during atrial contraction, or the peak A velocity, is 0.38 to 0.48 m/sec in normal subjects.[192–195] The ratio of the peak E to peak A velocities (E/A ratio) and the ratio of the peak A to peak E velocities (A/E ratio) have been used to describe the pattern of left ventricular diastolic filling. Values for the E/A ratio in normal subjects have ranged from 1.7 ± 0.4 to 2.5 ± 0.9.[186, 192, 196] Normal values for the

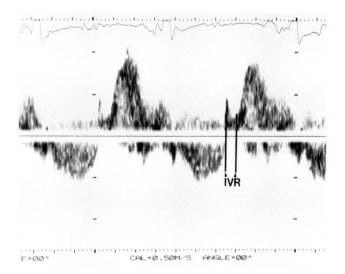

E=00°   CAL=0.50M/S   ANGLE=00°

FIG 4–39.
Technique for measuring isovolumic relaxation time (IVR) from the continuous-wave Doppler. The Doppler transducer is positioned at the cardiac apex and aimed so that it records left ventricular outflow tract velocities in systole below the baseline and left ventricular inflow velocities in diastole above the baseline. The time interval from the aortic valve closure signal and the onset of forward flow in diastole is the IVR.

A/E ratio have ranged from 0.44 ±0.2 to 0.66 ±0.2.[187, 193, 195] The deceleration of early diastolic flow can be measured as the slope of a straight line drawn from the peak E velocity to the point where peak E decreases by half on the descending limb of the early diastolic inflow. In normal subjects, values for the deceleration slope have ranged from 355 ±67 cm/sec² to 399 ±110 cm/sec².[193, 195]

Abnormalities of the mitral valve peak velocities, velocity ratios, and deceleration rates have been reported in a number of disease states. Kitabatake and co-workers[193] found that the peak E velocity and deceleration were significantly reduced in patients with hypertension, hypertrophic cardiomyopathy, and myocardial infarction. In this study, peak A velocity was significantly increased in patients with hypertension and myocardial infarction but not in patients with hypertrophic cardiomyopathy. They concluded that early diastolic filling was impaired in all three disease states and was accompanied by a compensatory increase in filling during atrial contraction in patients with hypertension and myocardial infarction. In patients with hypertrophic cardiomyopathy, the compensatory mechanism appeared to be a prolongation of rapid filling rather than an increased filling during atrial contraction. Spirito and colleagues[186, 188] reported similar abnormalities in a group of patients with left ventricular outflow obstruction. In this patient group, the deceleration and E/A velocity ratio were significantly reduced, compared with normal adults. Takenaka and colleagues reported different Doppler patterns of left ventricular diastolic filling in different

subgroups of patients with hypertrophic cardiomyopathy.[195] In patients with hypertrophic cardiomyopathy and systolic anterior motion of the mitral valve, no significant differences were observed in peak E velocity, peak A velocity, A/E velocity ratio, and deceleration, compared with normal subjects. Patients with hypertrophic cardiomyopathy and no systolic anterior motion of the mitral valve, however, had decreased peak E velocity, increased A/E velocity ratio, and reduced deceleration of early diastolic flow compared to normal subjects. Mitral regurgitation was detected in all patients with systolic anterior motion of the mitral valve and in only 33% of patients without systolic anterior motion of the mitral valve. The authors postulated that increased left ventricular early diastolic filling caused by mitral regurgitation or a less extensive myopathic process reported previously to occur in patients with systolic anterior motion accounted for the differences in left ventricular diastolic filling observed in subgroups of patients with hypertrophic cardiomyopathy. In a similar study, Takenaka and co-workers compared mitral valve Doppler recordings from patients with dilated cardiomyopathy with and without mitral regurgitation to recordings of normal subjects.[197] Compared to normal subjects, cardiomyopathy patients without mitral regurgitation had a reduced peak E velocity and an increased A/E velocity ratio. Cardiomyopathy patients with mitral regurgitation had normal peak E and peak A velocities and normal A/E velocity ratio but a shortened deceleration half-time. These findings suggest that in patients with dilated cardiomyopathy mitral regurgitation can mask filling abnormalities on the mitral valve Doppler examination.

A third type of parameter that can be measured from the mitral valve Doppler examination are indexes of peak and mean left ventricular filling rates. Doppler peak filling rates are calculated as peak E velocity times the mitral annulus cross-sectional area (calculated as $\pi d^2/4$ where d = the annulus diameter measured from the two-dimensional echocardiogram).[184] Normalized peak filling rate is calculated as peak filling rate divided by left ventricular end-diastolic volume (measured from the two-dimensional echocardiogram). In a study by Rokey and colleagues, no differences were found between Doppler and angiographic estimates of peak filling rate (296 vs. 283 ml/sec) and normalized peak filling rate (1.9 vs. 2.0 sec⁻¹). In general, patients with reduced angiographic peak filling rates often had peak E velocity less than 0.45 m/sec, and E/A velocity ratio of less than 1.0.[184]

Additional filling rates have been calculated from the mitral valve Doppler examination by Pearson and colleagues.[196] These investigators calculated (1) peak atrial filling rate as the product of peak A velocity and mitral annular cross-sectional area (normal patients = 225 ± 72 ml/sec), (2) mean filling rate as the product of mean diastolic velocity and mitral annular cross-sectional area, and (3) the rapid filling index as the quotient of peak early diastolic filling rate divided by mean filling rate (normal patients = 2.3 ± 0.3).

Recent studies have shown that peak filling rate can be normalized to mitral stroke volume using the following derived equation:[198]

$$PFR\ (SV/sec) = \frac{peak\ E\ (cm/sec)}{MV\ VTI\ (cm)}$$

where PFR (SV/sec) = peak filling rate normalized to stroke volume

MV VTI = velocity time integral of mitral valve Doppler

This index correlates well with radionuclide peak filling rate normalized for stroke volume (correlation coefficient = 0.91). This index also accounts for cardiac output without the need to calculate left ventricular end-diastolic volume. Values for the index are independent of sample volume position. Normal values for the peak filling rate normalized to mitral stroke volume are 6.0 ± 1.2 SV/sec for patients 18 to 45 years old and 3.9 ± 1.0 SV/sec for patients 57 to 89 years old.

A fourth type of diastolic parameter that has been used to describe the patterns of left ventricular filling are the Doppler area fractions or filling fractions.[185] The Doppler area fractions describe the percentage of the mitral valve Doppler envelope present in the various phases of diastole.

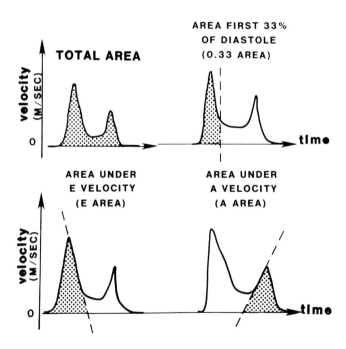

FIG 4–40.
Diagram of the technique used to measure various areas under the mitral valve Doppler tracing. The 0.33 area is measured as the area of the Doppler tracing at the completion of one-third of the total diastolic time. The *E and A areas* are measured as triangular areas under the Doppler tracing obtained by extrapolating a straight line down from the peak E and the peak A velocities to the baseline.

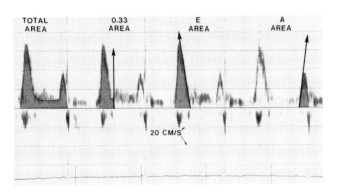

FIG 4–41.
Actual mitral valve Doppler tracing demonstrating the methods used in our laboratory to measure the 0.33 area, the E area, and the A area.

Because the mitral valve cross-sectional area changes throughout diastole, calculation of the absolute volumetric flow in the different portions of diastole would be extremely difficult. Because the volumetric flow is the product of the velocity time integral (the integrated area under the Doppler curve) and the mitral valve cross-sectional area, approximate values for the fraction of filling of the left ventricle in the different phases of diastole can be obtained by measuring several areas under the Doppler curve and dividing these areas by the total area under the Doppler curve. Using this methodology, the area or filling fractions in the first 33% (.33 area fraction), during early diastolic inflow (E area fraction), and during atrial contraction (A area fraction) can be calculated (Fig 4–40). In the studies from our laboratory, the E area and A area were measured as the triangular portion under the Doppler curve formed by extrapolating a straight line down from the peak E and peak A velocities to the baseline (Fig 4–41).[185, 192, 199, 200] Other methods have been used to define the filling fractions during early and late diastolic inflow. These include dividing the Doppler curve with a straight line in the middle of the slow filling period into early and late filling fractions[189] or drawing the triangular E area and defining all the remaining area under the Doppler curve as filling caused by atrial contraction (Fig 4–42). Table 4–8 shows values for the Doppler area fractions obtained in our laboratory in normal children. It is interesting that our value for the percentage of the total Doppler area that occurs under the peak E velocity (0.62 ± 0.07) is identical to Hanrath's value for the percentage of the total change in left ventricular diastolic dimension that occurs in rapid filling on the digitized M-mode echocardiogram (0.62 ± 0.10).[64] Similarly, our value for the fraction of the total Doppler curve that occurs under the peak A velocity (0.20 ± 0.07) is very close to Hanrath's value for the percentage of total change in left ventricular dimension that occurs during atrial contraction (0.16 ± 0.10).

Mitral valve Doppler area fractions have been used to detect abnormalities in left ventricular filling in a variety

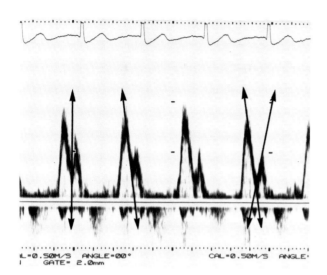

FIG 4–42.
Mitral valve Doppler tracing demonstrating the methods that have been used to calculate the filling during early and late diastole. In the first beat, the mitral valve Doppler tracing is divided in half in the middle of the slow filling period. Areas are measured in the first half and the second half of diastole. In the second beat, the *triangular E area* is measured and all the remaining area of the Doppler curve is defined as filling caused by atrial contraction. The fourth beat illustrates the method used in our laboratory.

of disease states.[185, 189, 192, 196, 199–205] We studied left ventricular diastolic filling in a group of children with systemic hypertension and found that, compared with age-matched normal children, they had a decreased percentage of the total Doppler area occurring in the first one-third of diastole and an increased percentage of the total Doppler area occurring under the A wave (Fig 4–43).[185] Also, the peak A velocity was higher in the children with systemic hypertension. Diastolic filling abnormalities were detectable by mitral valve Doppler ultrasound techniques when the M-mode indexes of diastolic function were still normal and before the development of systolic function abnormalities or left ventricular hypertrophy on the M-mode echocardiogram.

In addition, using mitral valve Doppler techniques, we have evaluated left ventricular diastolic filling in a group of children with hypertrophic cardiomyopathy and no mitral regurgitation.[199] These children had a decreased peak E velocity and a decreased percentage of the total Doppler area occurring in the first one-third of diastole. In these children, there was no compensatory increase in the percentage of the total Doppler area occurring during atrial contraction (Fig 4–44).

Figures 4–45, 4–46, and 4–47 summarize our results of measuring mitral valve Doppler indexes pre– and post–balloon angioplasty in children with either aortic stenosis or coarctation of the aorta.[200] As shown in the figures, children with left ventricular outflow tract obstruction had a decreased 0.33 area fraction and an increased A area frac-

TABLE 4–8.
Doppler Areas and Area Fractions in Normal Children (N = 24)

Doppler Areas	Normal Values*
0.33 area (m)	0.076 ± 0.020
0.33 area/total area	0.58 ± 0.082
E area (m)	0.086 ± 0.018
E area/total area	0.62 ± 0.07
A area (m)	0.036 ± 0.010
A area/total area	0.20 ± 0.07
E area/A area	2.5 ± 0.69

*Values are given as mean ± SD.

tion compared to age-matched normal children. There were no changes in the mitral valve Doppler indexes immediately after successful relief of the left ventricular outflow gradient, suggesting that afterload mismatch was not the cause of the Doppler abnormalities.

As the mitral valve Doppler indexes came into more frequent use, different investigators reported different transmitral flow patterns in groups of patients with the same disease. It became clear that factors other than left ventricular relaxation properties alone had a major influence on transmitral flow velocity patterns. Recent studies in human subjects[191] and in the animal laboratory[206] have helped elucidate many of the factors that determine transmitral flow.

Courtois and colleagues[206] made simultaneous recordings of the left atrial pressure, left ventricular pressure, and

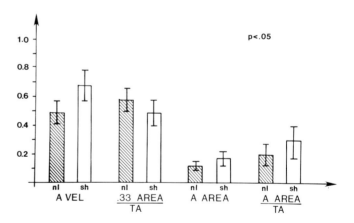

FIG 4–43.
Diagrammatic representation of the diastolic filling abnormalities found in a group of children with systemic hypertension (SH) when compared to a group of normal children (NL). The SH patients had an elevated peak A velocity. In addition, in the SH children, a decreased percentage of the total Doppler area occurred in the first one-third of diastole and an increased percentage of the total Doppler area occurred during atrial contraction. Thus, these children had a shift in diastolic filling toward late diastole. (From Snider AR, Gidding SS, Rocchini AP, et al: Doppler evaluation of left ventricular diastolic filling in children with systemic hypertension. *Am J Cardiol* 1985; 56:924. Used by permission.)

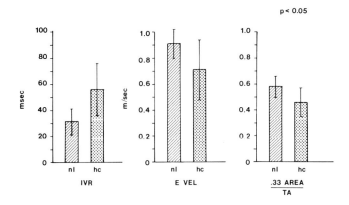

FIG 4–44.
Left ventricular diastolic filling abnormalities found in a group of children with hypertrophic cardiomyopathy (HC) and no mitral regurgitation, compared to normal (NL) age-matched children. The HC patients had a prolonged isovolumic relaxation time (IVR) and a decreased peak E velocity. In addition, in the HC patients, a decreased percentage of the total Doppler area occurred in the first one-third of diastole.

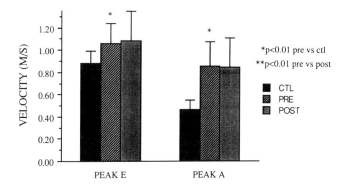

FIG 4–45.
Mitral valve Doppler indexes measured pre– and post–balloon angioplasty in children with either aortic senosis or coarctation of the aorta. The Doppler indexes were compared with those of a control (CTL) group of age-matched normal children. Preangioplasty, children with left ventricular outflow obstruction had an increase in peak E and peak A velocities compared to normal age-matched children. Postangioplasty, there were no changes in the mitral valve Doppler indexes. (From Meliones JN, Snider AR, Serwer GA, et al: *Am J Cardiol* 1989; 63:234. Used by permission.)

mitral valve Doppler tracing in open-chest dogs. Figure 4–48, from their study, shows that when left ventricular pressure decreases to a value equal to left atrial pressure (the first crossover point shown as X_1), the mitral valve opens and the onset of flow occurs on the mitral valve Doppler trace. Both pressures decrease rapidly after mitral valve opening, with a short duration of transvalvular pressure difference. The peak E velocity occurs at the second crossover point X_2, which corresponds closely in time with the left ventricular minimum pressure. Deceleration from the

peak E velocity begins with the onset of the increase in left ventricular diastolic pressure (the rapid filling wave) and ends at the third crossover point X_3. In mid-diastole, the two pressures appear to be equal, increasing slowly together; then left atrial pressure increases with atrial contraction, producing flow across the mitral valve at the A wave of the Doppler trace.

Appleton and colleagues[191] analyzed mitral valve Doppler recordings and catheterization data in patients with coronary artery disease, congestive cardiomyopathy, and

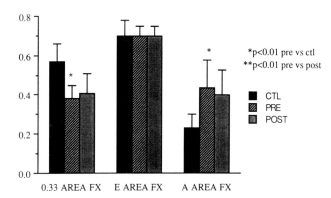

FIG 4–46.
Doppler area fractions in a group of children with either aortic stenosis or coarctation of the aorta measured pre- and post-balloon angioplasty. Preangioplasty, children with left ventricular outflow tract obstruction had a decrease in the 0.33 area fraction and an increase in the A area fraction compared to normal age-matched children (CTL). Postangioplasty, these Doppler abnormalities did not change in spite of successful relief of the left ventricular outflow tract gradient. (From Meliones JN, Snider AR, Serwer GA, et al: *Am J Cardiol* 1989; 63:234. Used by permission.)

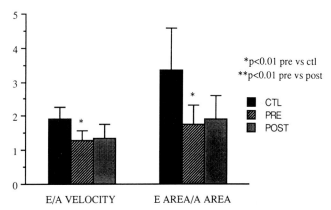

FIG 4–47.
Doppler indexes measured pre- and post-balloon angioplasty in children with either aortic stenosis or coarctation of the aorta. Preangioplasty, the children with left ventricular outflow tract obstruction had a decrease in the E/A velocity and area ratios compared to control (CTL) children. Postangioplasty, these abnormal ratios did not change. (From Meliones JN, Snider AR, Serwer GA, et al: *Am J Cardiol* 1989; 63:235. Used by permission.)

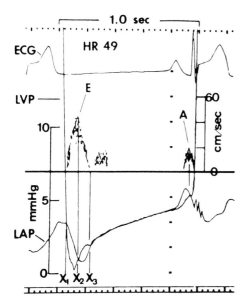

FIG 4–48.
Simultaneous recordings of the left atrial pressure (LAP), left ventricular pressure (LVP), and mitral valve Doppler tracing from an open-chest dog. The timing of events in this figure is explained in detail in the chapter text. A = peak velocity at atrial contraction; E = peak velocity during rapid ventricular filling; and ECG = electrocardiogram. (From Courtois M, Kovacs SJ Jr, Ludbrook PA: *Circulation* 1988; 78:667. Used by permission.)

restrictive myocardial disease. These investigators found two distinct patterns of transmitral flow that related not to the disease itself but to the patient's hemodynamic state. Pattern I, shown in Figure 4–49, was observed when there was impaired left ventricular relaxation (as suggested by a prolonged time constant, T, of isovolumic relaxation) in the presence of normal left atrial pressure. In patients with this pattern (Fig 4–50), a slower rate of left ventricular isovolumic pressure fall results in a later mitral valve opening, a longer isovolumic relaxation time, a reduced early diastolic transmitral pressure gradient, and a resultant decrease in peak E velocity. With less filling in early diastole, the percentage of left ventricular filling with atrial contraction would likely be increased as a compensatory mechanism. The prolonged fall in left ventricular pressure causes a prolonged mitral deceleration time.

Pattern II (see Fig 4–49) had a more normal appearance but tended to occur in more symptomatic patients. This pattern occurred in patients with increased filling pressures, an abnormally increased left ventricular rapid filling wave, and prolonged time constant T. In these patients (Fig 4–51), an elevated left atrial pressure produced a normal or shortened isovolumic relaxation time and normal or increased peak E velocity and, thus, masked the expected Doppler relaxation abnormalities. The abnormal left ventricular filling wave (the type seen in restrictive disease) and the abrupt increase in left ventricular diastolic pressure led to premature cessation of mitral flow and a short

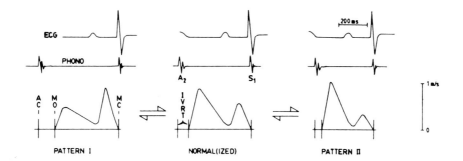

FIG 4–49.
Patterns of left ventricular diastolic filling observed in patients with coronary artery disease, congestive cardiomyopathy, and restrictive myocardial disease. In these groups of patients, there were two distinct patterns of transmitral flow that related not to the disease itself, but to the patient's hemodynamic state. *Pattern I* was observed when there was impaired left ventricular relaxation (as suggested by a prolonged time constant, T, of isovolumic relaxation) in the presence of normal left atrial pressure. Patients with this pattern had a slower rate of left ventricular isovolumic pressure fall, later mitral valve opening, a longer isovolumic relaxation time, a reduced early diastolic transmitral gradient, and a resultant decrease in peak E velocity. *Pattern II* had a more normal appearance but tended to occur in more symptomatic patients—those with increased filling pressure, an abnormally increased left ventricular rapid filling wave, and a prolonged time constant T. These patients had a normal or shortened isovolumic relaxation time and a normal or increased peak E velocity. The abnormal left ventricular filling wave and abrupt increase in left ventricular diastolic pressure led to premature cessation of mitral flow and a short deceleration time. Some patients with reduced left ventricular relaxation had a moderate increase in left atrial pressure, which masked relaxation abnormalities by normalizing the early diastolic transmitral pressure gradient. These patients had a mitral valve Doppler pattern intermediate between Pattern I and Pattern II. *AC* = aortic valve closure; *MO* = mitral valve opening; *MC* = mitral valve closure; and *IVR* = isovolumic relaxation. (From Appleton CP, Hatle LK, Popp RL: *J Am Coll Cardiol* 1988; 12:135. Used by permission.)

deceleration time. Most patients with pattern II had left atrial enlargement and decreased peak A velocity. The decreased peak A velocity may be caused by systolic atrial dysfunction or an elevated left ventricular pressure at the time of atrial contraction.

Some patients with reduced left ventricular relaxation had a moderate increase in left atrial pressure, which masked relaxation abnormalities by normalizing the early diastolic transmitral pressure gradient (see Fig 4–49 and 4–51).

What can be expected clinically, then, is a spectrum of mitral flow velocity patterns (Fig 4–52). In patients with normal left atrial pressure, the reduced left ventricular relaxation rate is the predominant factor responsible for prolonged isovolumic relaxation time, decreased peak E velocity, prolonged deceleration time, and increased peak A velocity. As left atrial pressure increases, early diastolic transmitral pressure gradient and mitral flow velocity pattern return to normal, despite the presence of reduced left ventricular relaxation. In patients with increased left atrial pressure and marked reduction in left ventricular compliance, the effects of diminished compliance overwhelm the effects of reduced relaxation, resulting in shortened isovolumic relaxation time, increased peak E velocity, short-

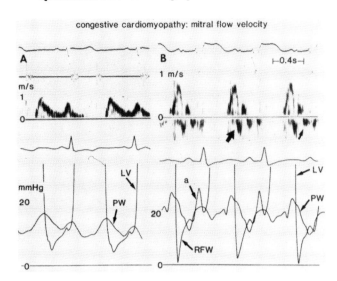

FIG 4–51.
Mitral flow velocity recordings and left ventricular (LV) and pulmonary wedge (PW) pressures in two patients with congestive cardiomyopathy. The pulmonary wedge pressure has been shifted for the estimated time delay. In *patient A,* the left ventricular isovolumic relaxation time, mitral flow velocities, and pressures are within normal limits. In *patient B,* the isovolumic relaxation time and mitral deceleration time are markedly shortened. The early, abrupt cessation of forward flow velocity is followed by mid-diastolic flow reversal (diastolic mitral regurgitation, *large arrow*) which corresponds in time to the peak of the marked left ventricular rapid filling wave (RFW) and an apparent left ventricular-left atrial pressure reversal. With atrial contraction, a short period of forward flow with a low velocity is re-established and is accompanied by a marked further increase in left ventricular pressure (A). A second flow reversal is also seen after atrial contraction *(small arrow).* (From Appleton CP, Hatle LK, Popp RL: *J Am Coll Cardiol* 1988; 12:432. Used by permission.)

ened deceleration time, and decreased peak A velocity.

The major determinant of the peak early mitral flow velocity is the instantaneous left atrial to left ventricular pressure difference in early diastole.[207] Many factors affect this instantaneous pressure gradient, and much investigative work is needed to determine which of these factors influence the patterns of transmitral flow velocity in any individual patient. The factors include: (1) the left atrial pressure at the time of mitral opening; (2) the rate of relaxation of the left ventricle; (3) the wall and chamber compliance of the left atrium and left ventricle; (4) the end-systolic left ventricular volume; (5) the passive viscoelastic properties of the myocardium; and (6) the presence of valvular obstruction. Valvular obstruction might be an alteration in the valve orifice so subtle that only a physiologic gradient is present, perhaps caused by alteration in the mitral valve chordal apparatus as a result of left ventricular hypertrophy or dilatation.

When using the Doppler indexes of diastolic function in the clinical setting, it is necessary to keep in mind other factors that affect these indexes. For example, the Doppler time intervals and peak velocities vary with cardiac cycle

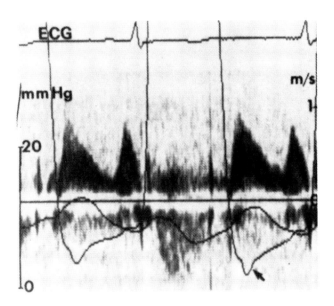

FIG 4–50.
Example of a patient with Pattern I transmitral Doppler abnormality. This figure shows the mitral valve Doppler tracing recorded simultaneously with the left ventricular and pulmonary wedge pressures. The slow rate of fall in left ventricular isovolumic pressure results in a later mitral valve opening and a prolonged isovolumic relaxation time. Also, there is a reduced early diastolic transmitral pressure gradient and resulting decrease in peak E velocity. With less filling in early diastole, the percentage of left ventricular filling with atrial contraction is increased. The prolonged fall in left ventricular pressure also causes a prolonged mitral deceleration time. (From Appleton CP, Hatle LK, Popp RL: *J Am Coll Cardiol* 1988; 12:436. Used by permission.)

Normal LA Pressure →	Increased LA Pressure →	Increased LA pressure
Reduced LV Relax	Reduced LV Relaxation	Reduced LV Compliance
Normal LV Pressure		Reduced LV Relaxation
↑ IVR	nl IVR	↓ IVR
↓ Peak E	nl Peak E	↗ Peak E
↑ DT	nl DT	↓ DT
↑ Peak A	nl Peak A	↓ Peak A

FIG 4–52.
The spectrum of mitral valve diastolic flow patterns that can be found clinically. In patients with normal left atrial (LA) pressure, the reduced left ventricular (LV) relaxation rate is the predominant factor responsible for prolonged isovolumic relaxation time (IVR), decreased peak E velocity, prolonged deceleration time (DT), and increased peak A velocity. As left atrial pressure increases, early diastolic transmitral pressure gradient and mitral flow velocity pattern return toward normal, despite the presence of reduced LV relaxation. In patients with increased LA pressure and marked reduction in LV compliance, the effects of diminished compliance overwhelm the effects of reduced relaxation, resulting in the shortened IVR, increased peak E velocity, shortened DT, and decreased peak A velocity.

lengths.[208] Peak velocities also vary with patient age and ventricular loading conditions.[194, 209–215] The peak E and peak A velocity tend to decrease and increase respectively with aging; the A/E velocity ratio shows a significant increase with aging. Also, the peak A velocity and the A/E velocity ratio tend to be increased in the fetus in utero and in the first few days after birth.[216] The position of the sample volume can alter the Doppler tracing. Doppler tracings obtained from the left atrium just proximal to the mitral valve have a peak E velocity 25% lower and a peak A velocity 22% lower than tracings obtained at the tips of the mitral valve leaflets. The A/E ratio is the same at both sites.[217] The mitral valve Doppler indexes vary with the phases of respiration. In normal adults, peak E velocity decreases on inspiration by 9%; peak A velocity remains unchanged.[218] In normal children, peak E velocity decreases by 8% and peak A velocity is unchanged. Thus, E/A velocity and area ratios decrease by 14% and 12%.[219]

Currently, little information is available on the use of Doppler echocardiography to assess right ventricular diastolic function. Using the tricuspid valve inflow Doppler, peak velocities during early and late diastolic filling, peak filling rates, and filling fractions of the right ventricle can be calculated. In the future, it can be expected that these measurements will be used to analyze right ventricular diastolic filling in a variety of disease states.

In summary, Doppler echocardiography provides a noninvasive technique for the evaluation of ventricular performance that is independent of ventricular geometry. This application of the Doppler technique is still in its infancy. Much investigative work is needed to correlate the invasive and noninvasive measurements of ventricular function and to determine the effect of factors such as heart rate, loading conditions, and cardiac drugs on the Doppler

indexes of function. In the future, it is likely that Doppler color-flow mapping techniques will provide additional information on ventricular emptying and filling patterns that will be important in the noninvasive assessment of cardiac function.

REFERENCES

1. Epstein ML, Goldberg SJ, Allen HD, et al: Great vessel, cardiac chamber and wall growth patterns in normal children. *Circulation* 1975; 51:1124–1129.
2. Gutgesell HP, Paquet M, Duff DF, et al: Evaluation of left ventricular size and function by echocardiography. Results in normal children. *Circulation* 1977; 56:457–462.
3. Henry WL, Ware J, Gardin JM, et al: Echocardiographic measurements in normal subjects. Growth-related changes that occur between infancy and early adulthood. *Circulation* 1978; 57:278–285.
4. Roge CLL, Silverman NH, Hart PA, et al: Cardiac structure growth pattern determined by echocardiography. *Circulation* 1978; 57:285–290.
5. Henry WL, Gardin JM, Ware JH: Echocardiographic measurements in normal subjects from infancy to old age. *Circulation* 1980; 62:1054–1061.
6. Panidis IP, Ross J, Ren J-F, et al: Comparison of independent and derived M-mode echocardiographic measurements. *Am J Cardiol* 1984; 54:694–696.
7. Sahn DJ, DeMaria A, Kisslo J, et al: Recommendations regarding quantitation in M-mode echocardiography: Results of a survey of echocardiographic measurements. *Circulation* 1978; 58:1072–1083.
8. Devereux RB, Reichek N: Echocardiographic determination of left ventricular mass in man. *Circulation* 1977; 55:613–618.
9. Devereux RB, Casale PN, Kligfield P, et al: Performance of primary and derived M-mode echocardiographic measurements for detection of left ventricular hypertrophy in necropsied subjects and in patients with systemic hypertension, mitral regurgitation, and dilated cardiomyopathy. *Am J Cardiol* 1986; 57:1388–1393.
10. Devereux RB, Alonso DR, Lutas EM, et al: Echocardiographic assessment of left ventricular hypertrophy: Comparison to necropsy findings. *Am J Cardiol* 1986; 57:450–458.
11. Daniels SR, Meyer RA, Liang Y, et al: Echocardiographically determined left ventricular mass index in normal children, adolescents, and young adults. *J Am Coll Cardiol* 1988; 12:703–708.
12. Feigenbaum H: *Echocardiography*, ed 4. Philadelphia, Lea and Febiger, 1986.
13. Hirschfeld S, Meyer R, Schwartz DC, et al: Measurement of right and left ventricular systolic time intervals by echocardiography. *Circulation* 1975; 51:304–309.
14. Weissler AM, Harris LC, White GD: Left-ventricular ejection time index in man. *J Appl Physiol* 1963; 18:919–923.
15. Riggs T, Hirschfeld S, Borkat G, et al: Assessment of the pulmonary vascular bed by echocardiographic right ventricular systolic time intervals. *Circulation* 1978; 57:939–947.

16. Hirschfeld S, Meyer R, Schwartz DC, et al: The echocardiographic assessment of pulmonary artery pressure and pulmonary vascular resistance. *Circulation* 1975; 52:642–650.
17. Golde D, Burstin L: Systolic phases of the cardiac cycle in children. *Circulation* 1970; 42:1029–1036.
18. Weissler AM, Harris WS, Schoenfeld CD: Systolic time intervals in heart failure in man. *Circulation* 1968; 37:149–159.
19. Spitaels S, Arbogast R, Fuoron JC, et al: The influence of heart rate and age on the systolic and diastolic time intervals in children. *Circulation* 1974; 49:1107–1115.
20. Weissler AM, Harris WS, Schoenfeld CD: Bedside techniques for the evaluation of left ventricular function in man. *Am J Cardiol* 1969; 23:277–284.
21. Spooner EW, Perry BL, Stern AM, et al: Estimation of pulmonary/systemic resistance ratios from echocardiographic systolic time intervals in young patients with congenital or acquired heart disease. *Am J Cardiol* 1978; 42:810–816.
22. Kerber RE, Martins JB, Barnes R, et al: Effects of acute hemodynamic alterations on pulmonic valve motion. Experimental and clinical echocardiographic studies. *Circulation* 1979; 60:1074–1081.
23. Rees AH, Rao PS, Ribby JJ, et al: Echocardiographic shunt in isolated ventricular septal defects. *Eur J Cardiol* 1978; 7:25.
24. Baylen B, Meyer RA, Korfhagen J, et al: Left ventricular performance in the critically ill premature infant with patent ductus arteriosus and pulmonary disease. *Circulation* 1977; 55:182–188.
25. McDonald IG: Echocardiographic assessment of left ventricular function in aortic valve disease. *Circulation* 1976; 53:860–864.
26. Ghafour AS, Gutgesell HP: Echocardiographic evaluation of left ventricular function in children with congestive cardiomyopathy. *Am J Cardiol* 1979; 44:1332–1338.
27. Sahn DJ, Deely WJ, Hagen AD, et al: Echocardiographic assessment of left ventricular performance in normal newborns. *Circulation* 1974; 49:232–236.
28. Sahn DJ, Vaucher Y, Williams DE, et al: Echocardiographic detection of large left to right shunts and cardiomyopathies in infants and children. *Am J Cardiol* 1976; 38:73–79.
29. Colan SD, Borow KM, Newmann A: Left ventricular end-systolic wall stress-velocity of fiber shortening relation: A load independent index of myocardial contractility. *J Am Coll Cardiol* 1984; 4:715–724.
30. Gibson DG, Brown DJ: Measurement of instantaneous left ventricular dimension and filling rate in man using echocardiography. *Br Heart J* 1973; 35:1141–1149.
31. Gibson DG, Brown DJ: Assessment of left ventricular systolic function in man from simultaneous echocardiographic and pressure measurements. *Br Heart J* 1976; 38:8–17.
32. Kugler JD, Gutgesell HP, Nihill MR: Instantaneous rates of left ventricular wall motion in infants and children. Computer-assisted determination from single-cycle echocardiograms. *Pediatr Cardiol* 1979; 1:15–21.
33. Upton MT, Gibson DG: The study of left ventricular function from digitized echocardiograms. *Prog Cardiovasc Dis* 1978; 20:359–384.
34. St. John Sutton MS, Hagler DJ, Tajik AJ, et al: Cardiac function in the normal newborn. Additional information by computer analysis of the M-mode echocardiogram. *Circulation* 1978; 57:1198–1204.
35. Friedman MJ, Sahn DJ: Computer-assisted analysis of M-mode echocardiogram: Is it a "gold mine"? *Pediatr Cardiol* 1979; 1:47–50.
36. Hofstetter R, Mayr A, Von Bernuth G: Computer analysis of cardiac contractility variables obtained by M-mode echocardiography in normal newborns. *Br Heart J* 1982; 48:525–528.
37. Traill TA, Gibson DG, Brown DJ: Study of left ventricular wall thickness and dimension changes using echocardiography. *Br Heart J* 1978; 40:162–169.
38. Shapiro E, Marier DL, St. John Sutton MG, et al: Regional non-uniformity of wall dynamics in normal left ventricle. *Br Heart J* 1981; 45:264–270.
39. Massie BM, Schiller NB, Ratshin RA, et al: Mitral-septal separation: A new echocardiographic index of left ventricular function. *Am J Cardiol* 1977; 39:1008–1016.
40. Ginzton LE, Kulick D: Mitral valve E-point septal separation as an indicator of ejection fraction in patients with reversed septal motion. *Chest* 1985; 88:429–431.
41. Ahmadpour H, Shah AA, Allen JW, et al: Mitral E point septal separation: A reliable index of left ventricular performance in coronary artery disease. *Am Heart J* 1983; 106:21–28.
42. Engle SJ, DiSessa TG, Perloff JK, et al: Mitral valve E point to ventricular septal separation in infants and children. *Am J Cardiol* 1983; 52:1084–1087.
43. Reichek N, Wilson J, St. John Sutton M, et al: Noninvasive determination of left ventricular end-systolic stress: Validation of the method and initial application. *Circulation* 1982; 65:99–108.
44. Grossman W, Jones D, McLaurin LP: Wall stress and patterns of hypertrophy in the human left ventricle. *J Clin Invest* 1975; 56:56–64.
45. Gault JH, Ross J Jr, Braunwald E: Contractile state of the left ventricle in man: Instantaneous tension-velocity-length relations in patients with and without disease of the left ventricular myocardium. *Circ Res* 1968; 22:451–459.
46. Quinones MA, Mokotoff DM, Nouri S, et al: Noninvasive quantification of left ventricular wall stress: Validation of method and application to assessment of chronic pressure overload. *Am J Cardiol* 1980; 45:782–790.
47. DePace NL, Ren J-F, Iskandrian AS, et al: Correlation of echocardiographic wall stress and left ventricular pressure and function in aortic stenosis. *Circulation* 1983; 67:854–859.
48. Sandler H, Dodge HT: Left ventricular tension and stress in man. *Circ Res* 1963; 13:71–104.
49. Graham TP Jr, Franklin RCG, Wyse RKH, et al: Left ventricular wall stress and contractile function in childhood: Normal values and comparison of Fontan repair versus palliation only in patients with tricuspid atresia. *Circulation* 1986; 74(suppl 1):61–69.

50. Carabello BA, Green LH, Grossman W, et al: Hemo-dynamic determinants of prognosis of aortic valve replacement in critical aortic stenosis and advanced congestive heart failure. *Circulation* 1980; 62:42–48.

51. Borow KM, Neumann A, Lang R: Milrinone v. dobu-tamine: Contribution of afterload reduction and aug-mented inotropic state to improved left ventricular performance. *Circulation* 1986; 73(suppl 3):153–161.

52. Weber KT, Janicki JS: Myocardial oxygen consump-tion: The role of wall force and shortening. *Am J Physiol* 1977; 233:H421–H427.

53. Suga H, Sugawa K: Instantaneous pressure-volume relationship and their ratio in the excised, supported canine left ventricle. *Circ Res* 1974; 35:117–126.

54. Weber KT, Janicki JS, Hefner LL: Left ventricular force-length relations of isovolumic and ejecting contractions. *Am J Physiol* 1976; 231:337–343.

55. Marsh JD, Green LH, Wynne J, et al: Left ventricular end-systolic pressure dimension and stress-length relations in normal human subjects. *Am J Cardiol* 1979; 44:1311–1317.

56. Borow KM, Green LH, Grossman W, et al: Left ven-tricular end-systolic stress-shortening and stress-length relations in humans: Normal values and sen-sitivity to inotropic state. *Am J Cardiol* 1982; 50:1301–1308.

57. Colan SD, Borow KM, Neumann A: Use of the cali-brated carotid pulse tracing for calculation of left ventricular pressure and wall stress throughout ejec-tion. *Am Heart J* 1985; 109:1306–1310.

58. Colan SD, Borow KM, MacPherson D, et al: Use of the indirect axillary pulse tracing for noninvasive determination of ejection time, upstroke time, and left ventricular wall stress throughout ejection in in-fants and young children. *Am J Cardiol* 1984; 53:1154–1158.

59. Borow KM, Neumann A, Wynne J: Sensitivity of end-systolic pressure-dimension and pressure-vol-ume relations to the inotropic state in humans. *Cir-culation* 1982; 62:988–997.

60. Hanrath P, Mathey DG, Kremer P, et al: Effect of ver-apamil on left ventricular relaxation time and re-gional left ventricular filling in hypertrophic cardiomyopathy. *Am J Cardiol* 1980; 45:1258–1264.

61. Bahler RC, Vrobel TR, Martin P: The relation of heart rate and shortening fraction to echocardi-ographic indexes of left ventricular relaxation in normal subjects. *J Am Coll Cardiol* 1983; 2:926–933.

62. Fifer MA, Borow KM, Colan SD, et al: Early diastolic left ventricular function in children and adults with aortic stenosis. *J Am Coll Cardiol* 1985; 5:1147–1154.

63. St. John Sutton MG, Tajik AJ, Gibson DG, et al: Echo-cardiographic assessment of left ventricular filling and septal and posterior wall dynamics in idiopathic hypertrophic subaortic stenosis. *Circulation* 1978; 50:512–520.

64. Hanrath P, Mathey DG, Siegert R, et al: Left ventric-ular relaxation and filling pattern in different forms of left ventricular hypertrophy: An echocardi-ographic study. *Am J Cardiol* 1980; 45:15–23.

65. Schnittger I, Gordon EP, Fitzgerald PJ, et al: Stan-dardized intracardiac measurements of two-dimen-sional echocardiography. *J Am Coll Cardiol* 1983; 2:934–938.

66. Snider AR, Enderlein MA, Teitel DF, et al: Two-di-mensional echocardiographic determination of aortic and pulmonary artery sizes from infancy to adult-hood in normal subjects. *Am J Cardiol* 1984; 53:218–224.

67. Gutgesell HP, Bricker JT, Colvin EV, et al: Atrioven-tricular valve anular diameter: Two-dimensional echocardiographic-autopsy correlation. *Am J Cardiol* 1984; 533:1652–1655.

68. Bommer W, Weinert L, Neumann A, et al: Determi-nation of right atrial and right ventricular size by two-dimensional echocardiography. *Circulation* 1979; 60:91–100.

69. Triulzi M, Gillam LD, Gentile F, et al: Normal adult cross-sectional echocardiographic values: Linear di-mensions and chamber areas. *Echocardiography* 1984; 1:403–409.

70. King DH, Smith EO, Huhta JC, et al: Mitral and tri-cuspid valve annular diameter in normal children determined by two-dimensional echocardiography. *Am J Cardiol* 1985; 55:787–789.

71. Folland ED, Parisi AF, Moynihan PF, et al: Assess-ment of left ventricular ejection fraction and vol-umes by real-time, two-dimensional echocardi-ography. A comparison of cineangiographic and radionuclide techniques. *Circulation* 1979; 60:760–766.

72. Silverman NH, Ports TA, Snider AR, et al: Determi-nation of left ventricular volume in children: Echo-cardiographic and angiographic comparisons. *Circulation* 1980; 62:548–557.

73. Mercier JC, DiSessa TG, Jarmakani JM, et al: Two-dimensional echocardiographic assessment of left ventricular volumes and ejection fraction in chil-dren. *Circulation* 1982; 65:962–969.

74. Schiller NB, Acquatella H, Ports TA, et al: Left ven-tricular volume from paired biplane two-dimen-sional echocardiography. *Circulation* 1979; 60:547–555.

75. Wahr DW, Wang YS, Schiller NB: Left ventricular volumes determined by two-dimensional echocar-diography in a normal adult population. *J Am Coll Cardiol* 1983; 1:863–868.

76. Schabelman SE, Schiller NB, Anschultz RA, et al: Comparison of four two-dimensional echocardi-ographic views for measuring left atrial size. *Am J Cardiol* 1978; 41:391–396.

77. Schabelman S, Schiller NB, Silverman NH, et al: Left atrial volume estimation by two-dimensional echocardiography. *Cathet Cardiovasc Diagn* 1981; 7:165–178.

78. Wang Y, Gutman JM, Heilbron D, et al: Atrial vol-ume in a normal adult population by two-dimen-sional echocardiography. *Chest* 1984; 86:595–601.

79. Watanabe T, Katsume H, Matsukubo H, et al: Esti-mation of right ventricular volume with two-di-mensional echocardiography. *Am J Cardiol* 1982; 49:1946–1953.

80. Starling MR, Crawford MH, Sorensen SG, et al: A new two-dimensional echocardiographic technique for evaluating right ventricular size and perform-

ance in patients with obstructive lung disease. *Circulation* 1982; 66:612–620.

81. Silverman NH, Hudson S: Evaluation of right ventricular volume and ejection fraction in children by two-dimensional echocardiography. *Pediatr Cardiol* 1983; 4:197–203.

82. Levine RA, Gibson TC, Aretz T, et al: Echocardiographic measurements of right ventricular volume. *Circulation* 1984; 69:497–505.

83. Wyatt HL, Heng MK, Meerbaum S, et al: Cross-sectional echocardiography: Analysis of mathematical models for quantifying mass of the left ventricle in dogs. *Circulation* 1979; 60:1104–1113.

84. Reichek N, Helak J, Plappert T, et al: Anatomic validation of left ventricular mass estimates from clinical two-dimensional echocardiography: Initial results. *Circulation* 1983; 67:348–352.

85. Schiller NB, Skioldebrand CG, Schiller EJ, et al: Canine left ventricular mass estimation by two-dimensional echocardiography. *Circulation* 1983; 68:210–216.

86. Hatle L, Angelsen B: *Doppler Ultrasound in Cardiology*, ed 2. Philadelphia, Lea & Febiger, 1985.

87. Holen J, Aaslid R, Landmark K, et al: Determination of pressure gradient in mitral stenosis with a non-invasive ultrasound Doppler technique. *Acta Med Scand* 1976; 199:455–460.

88. Hatle L, Brubakk A, Tromsdal A, et al: Noninvasive assessment of pressure drop in mitral stenosis by Doppler ultrasound. *Br Heart J* 1978; 40:131–140.

89. Snider AR, Stevenson JG, French JW, et al: Comparison of high pulse repetition frequency and continuous-wave Doppler for velocity measurement and gradient prediction in children with valvular and congenital heart disease. *J Am Coll Cardiol* 1986; 7:873–879.

90. Currie PJ, Hagler DJ, Seward JB, et al: Instantaneous pressure gradient: A simultaneous Doppler and dual catheter correlative study. *J Am Coll Cardiol* 1986; 7:800–806.

91. Stamm RB, Martin RP: Quantification of pressure gradients across stenotic valves by Doppler ultrasound. *J Am Coll Cardiol* 1983; 2:707–718.

92. Hatle L, Angelsen BA, Tromsdal A: Noninvasive assessment of aortic stenosis by Doppler ultrasound. *Br Heart J* 1980; 43:284–292.

93. Young JB, Quinones MA, Waggoner AD, et al: Diagnosis and quantification of aortic stenosis with pulsed Doppler echocardiography. *Am J Cardiol* 1980; 45:487–494.

94. Berger M, Berdoff RL, Gallerstein PE, et al: Evaluation of aortic stenosis by continuous wave Doppler ultrasound. *J Am Coll Cardiol* 1984; 3:150–156.

95. Lima CO, Sahn DJ, Valdes-Cruz LM, et al: Prediction of the severity of left ventricular outflow tract obstruction by quantitative two-dimensional echocardiographic Doppler studies. *Circulation* 1983; 68:348–354.

96. Yeaker M, Yock PG, Popp RL: Comparison of Doppler-derived pressure gradient to that determined at cardiac catheterization in adults with aortic valve stenosis: Implications for management. *Am J Cardiol* 1986; 57:644–648.

97. Smith MD, Dawson PL, Elion JL, et al: Correlation of continuous wave Doppler velocities with cardiac catheterization gradients: An experimental model of aortic stenosis. *J Am Coll Cardiol* 1985; 6:1306–1314.

98. Lima CO, Sahn DJ, Valdes-Cruz LM, et al: Noninvasive prediction of transvalvular pressure gradient in patients with pulmonary stenosis by quantitative two-dimensional echocardiographic Doppler studies. *Circulation* 1983; 67:866–871.

99. Johnson GL, Kwan OL, Handshoe S, et al: Accuracy of combined two-dimensional echocardiography and continuous-wave Doppler recordings in the estimation of pressure gradient in right ventricular outlet obstruction. *J Am Coll Cardiol* 1984; 3:1013–1018.

100. Frantz EG, Silverman NH: Doppler ultrasound evaluation of valvar pulmonary stenosis from multiple transducer positions in children requiring pulmonary valvuloplasty. *Am J Cardiol* 1988; 61:844–849.

101. Fyfe DA, Currie PJ, Seward JB, et al: Continuous-wave Doppler determination of the pressure gradient across pulmonary artery bands: Hemodynamic correlation in 20 patients. *Mayo Clin Proc* 1984; 59:744–750.

102. Holen J, Hoie J, Semb B: Obstructive characteristics of Bjork-Shiley, Hancock, and Lillehei-Kastor prosthetic mitral valves in the immediate postoperative period. *Acta Med Scand* 1978; 204:5–11.

103. Holen J, Simonsen S, Froysaker T: An ultrasound Doppler technique for the noninvasive determination of the pressure gradient in the Bjork-Shiley mitral valve. *Circulation* 1979; 59:436–442.

104. Marx GR, Allen HD: Accuracy and pitfalls of Doppler evaluation of the pressure gradient in aortic coarctation. *J Am Coll Cardiol* 1986; 7:1379–1385.

105. Holen J, Aaslid R, Landmark K, et al: Determination of effective orifice area in mitral stenosis from noninvasive ultrasound Doppler data and mitral flow rate. *Acta Med Scand* 1977; 201:83–88.

106. Vasko SD, Goldberg SJ, Requarth JA, et al: Factors affecting accuracy of in vitro valvar pressure gradient estimates by Doppler ultrasound. *Am J Cardiol* 1984; 54:893–896.

107. Stevenson JG, Kawabori I, French JW: Critical importance of sedation when measuring pressure gradients by Doppler (abstract). *Circulation* 1984; 70(suppl 2):363.

108. Yock PG, Naasz C, Schnittger I, et al: Doppler tricuspid and pulmonic regurgitation in normals: Is it real? *Circulation* 1984; 70(suppl 2):40.

109. Berger M, Haimowitz A, Van Tosh A, et al: Quantitative assessment of pulmonary hypertension in patient with tricuspid regurgitation using continuous wave Doppler ultrasound. *J Am Coll Cardiol* 1985; 6:359–365.

110. Murphy DJ Jr, Ludomirsky A, Huhta JC: Continuous-wave Doppler in children with ventricular septal defect: Noninvasive estimation of interventricular pressure gradient. *Am J Cardiol* 1986; 57:428–432.

111. Silbert DR, Brunson AC, Schiff R, et al: Determination of right ventricular pressure in the presence of

a ventricular septal defect using continuous wave Doppler ultrasound. *J Am Coll Cardiol* 1986; 8:379–384.

112. Masuyama T, Kodama K, Kitabatake A, et al: Continuous-wave Doppler echocardiographic detection of pulmonary regurgitation and its application to noninvasive estimation of pulmonary artery pressure. *Circulation* 1986; 74:484–492.

113. Burstin L: Determination of pressure in the pulmonary artery by external graphic recordings. *Br Heart J* 1967; 29:396–404.

114. Hatle L, Angelsen BAJ, Tromsdal A: Non-invasive estimation of pulmonary artery systolic pressure with Doppler ultrasound. *Br Heart J* 1981; 45:157–165.

115. Kitabatake A, Inoue M, Asao M, et al: Noninvasive evaluation of pulmonary hypertension by a pulsed Doppler technique. *Circulation* 1983; 68:302–309.

116. Dabestani A, Mahan G, Gardin JM, et al: Evaluation of pulmonary artery pressure and resistance by pulsed Doppler echocardiography. *Am J Cardiol* 1987; 59:662–668.

117. Kosturakis D, Goldberg SJ, Allen HD, et al: Doppler echocardiographic prediction of pulmonary arterial hypertension in congenital heart disease. *Am J Cardiol* 1984; 53:1110–1115.

118. Martin-Duran R, Larman M, Trugeda A, et al: Comparison of Doppler-determined elevated pulmonary arterial pressure with pressure measured at cardiac catheterization. *Am J Cardiol* 1986; 57:859–863.

119. Matsuda M, Sekiguchi T, Sugishita Y, et al: Reliability of non-invasive estimates of pulmonary hypertension by pulsed Doppler echocardiography. *Br Heart J* 1986; 56:158–164.

120. Isobe M, Yazaki Y, Takaku F, et al: Prediction of pulmonary arterial pressure in adults by pulsed Doppler echocardiography. *Am J Cardiol* 1986; 57:316–321.

121. Serwer GA, Cougle AG, Eckerd JM, et al: Factors affecting use of the Doppler-determined time from flow onset to maximal pulmonary artery velocity for measurement of pulmonary artery pressure in children. *Am J Cardiol* 1986; 58:352–356.

122. Panidis IP, Ross J, Mintz GS: Effect of sampling site on assessment of pulmonary artery blood flow by Doppler echocardiography. *Am J Cardiol* 1986; 58:1145–1147.

123. Nishimura RA, Tajik A: Determination of left-sided pressure gradients by utilizing Doppler aortic and mitral regurgitant signals: Validation by simultaneous dual catheter and Doppler studies. *J Am Coll Cardiol* 1988; 11:317–321.

124. Kosturakis D, Allen HD, Goldberg SJ, et al: Noninvasive quantification of stenotic semilunar valve areas by Doppler echocardiography. *J Am Coll Cardiol* 1984; 3:1256–1262.

125. Skjaerpe T, Hegrenaes L, Hatle L: Non-invasive estimation of valve area in patients with aortic stenosis by Doppler ultrasound and two-dimensional echocardiography. *Circulation* 1985; 72:810–818.

126. Otto CM, Pearlman AS, Comess KA, et al: Determination of the stenotic aortic valve area in adults using Doppler echocardiography. *J Am Coll Cardiol* 1986; 7:509–517.

127. Zoghbi WA, Farmer KL, Soto JG, et al: Accurate noninvasive quantification of stenotic aortic valve area by Doppler echocardiography. *Circulation* 1986; 73:452–459.

128. Richards KL, Cannon SR, Miller JF, et al: Calculation of aortic valve area by Doppler echocardiography: A direct application of the continuity equation. *Circulation* 1986; 73:964–969.

129. Teirstein P, Yeager M, Yock PG, et al: Doppler echocardiographic measurement of aortic valve area in aortic stenosis: A noninvasive application of the Gorlin formula. *J Am Coll Cardiol* 1986; 8:1059–1065.

130. Oh JK, Taliercio CP, Holmes DR Jr, et al: Prediction of the severity of aortic stenosis by Doppler aortic valve area determination: Prospective Doppler-catheterization correlation in 100 patients. *J Am Coll Cardiol* 1988; 11:1227–1234.

131. Otto CM, Pearlman AS, Gardner CL, et al: Simplification of the Doppler continuity equation for calculating stenotic aortic valve area. *J Am Soc Echo* 1988; 1:155–157.

132. Nakatani S, Masuyama T, Kodama K, et al: Value and limitations of Doppler echocardiography in the quantification of stenotic mitral valve area: Comparison of the pressure half-time and the continuity equation methods. *Circulation* 1988; 77:78–85.

133. Grayburn PA, Smith MD, Harrison MR, et al: Pivotal role of aortic valve area calculation by the continuity equation for Doppler assessment of aortic stenosis in patients with combined aortic stenosis and regurgitation. *Am J Cardiol* 1988; 61:376–381.

134. Yang SS, Goldberg H: Simplified Doppler estimation of mitral valve area. *Am J Cardiol* 1985; 56:488–489.

135. Smith MD, Handshoe R, Handshoe S, et al: Comparative accuracy of two-dimensional echocardiography and Doppler pressure half-time methods in assessing severity of mitral stenosis in patients with and without prior commissurotomy. *Circulation* 1986; 73:100–107.

136. Grayburn PA, Smith MD, Gurley JC, et al: Effect of aortic regurgitation on the assessment of mitral valve orifice area by Doppler pressure half-time in mitral stenosis. *Am J Cardiol* 1987; 60:322–326.

137. Gonzalez MA, Child JS, Krivokapich J: Comparison of two-dimensional and Doppler echocardiography and intracardiac hemodynamics for quantification of mitral stenosis. *Am J Cardiol* 1987; 60:327–332.

138. Thomas JD, Weyman AE: Doppler mitral pressure half-time: A clinical tool in search of theoretical justification. *J Am Coll Cardiol* 1987; 10:923–929.

139. Thomas JD, Wilkins GT, Choong CYP, et al: Inaccuracy of mitral pressure half-time immediately after percutaneous mitral valvotomy. *Circulation* 1988; 78:980–993.

140. Goldberg SJ, Sahn DJ, Allen HD, et al: Evaluation of pulmonary and systemic blood flow by 2-dimensional Doppler echocardiography using fast Fourier transform spectral analysis. *Am J Cardiol* 1982; 50:1394–1400.

141. Colocousis JS, Huntsman LL, Curreri PW: Estimation of stroke volume changes by ultrasonic Doppler. *Circulation* 1977; 56:914–924.

142. Huntsman LL, Stewart DK, Barnes SR, et al: Noninvasive Doppler determination of cardiac output in man. Clinical validation. *Circulation* 1983; 67:593–602.

143. Alverson DC, Eldridge M, Dillon T, et al: Noninvasive pulsed Doppler determination of cardiac output in neonates and children. *J Pediatr* 1982; 101:46–50.

144. Nishimura RA, Callahan MJ, Schaff HV, et al: Noninvasive measurement of cardiac output by continuous wave Doppler echocardiography: Initial experience and review of the literature. *Mayo Clin Proc* 1984; 59:484–489.

145. Valdes-Cruz LM, Horowitz S, Mesel E, et al: A pulsed Doppler echocardiographic method for calculation of pulmonary and systemic flow: Accuracy in a canine model with ventricular septal defect. *Circulation* 1983; 68:597–602.

146. Valdes-Cruz LM, Horowitz S, Mesel E, et al: A pulsed Doppler echocardiographic method for calculating pulmonary and systemic blood flow in atrial level shunt: Validation studies in animals and initial human experience. *Circulation* 1984; 69:80–86.

147. Meijboom EJ, Valdes-Cruz LM, Horowitz S, et al: A two-dimensional Doppler echocardiographic method for calculation of pulmonary and systemic blood flow in a canine model with a variable-sized left-to-right extracardiac shunt. *Circulation* 1983; 68:437–445.

148. Lewis JF, Kuo LC, Nelson JG, et al: Pulsed Doppler echocardiographic determination of stroke volume and cardiac output: Clinical validation of two new methods using the apical window. *Circulation* 1984; 70:425–431.

149. Lighty GW Jr, Gargiulo A, Kronzon I, et al: Comparison of multiple views for the evaluation of pulmonary arterial blood flow by Doppler echocardiography. *Circulation* 1986; 74:1002–1006.

150. Loeber CP, Goldberg SJ, Allen HD: Doppler echocardiographic comparison of flows distal to the four cardiac valves. *J Am Coll Cardiol* 1984; 4:268–272.

151. Gardin JM, Tobis JM, Dabestani A, et al: Superiority of two-dimensional measurement of aortic vessel diameter in Doppler echocardiographic estimates of left ventricular stroke volume. *J Am Coll Cardiol* 1985; 6:66–74.

152. Stewart WJ, Jiang L, Mich R, et al: Variable effects of changes in flow rate through the aortic, pulmonary, and mitral valves on valve area and flow velocity: Impact on quantitative Doppler flow calculations. *J Am Coll Cardiol* 1985; 6:653–662.

153. Fisher DC, Sahn DJ, Friedman MJ, et al: The mitral valve orifice method for noninvasive two-dimensional echo Doppler determinations of cardiac output. *Circulation* 1983; 67:872–877.

154. Sanders SP, Yeager S, Williams RG: Measurements of systemic and pulmonary blood flow and QP/QS ratio using Doppler and two-dimensional echocardiography. *Am J Cardiol* 1983; 51:952–956.

155. Barron JV, Sahn DJ, Valdes-Cruz LM, et al: Clinical utility of two-dimensional Doppler echocardiographic techniques for estimating pulmonary to systemic blood flow ratios in children with left to right shunting atrial septal defect, ventricular septal defect, or patent ductus arteriosus. *J Am Coll Cardiol* 1984; 3:169–178.

156. Abbasi AS, Allen MW, DeChistofaro D, et al: Detection and estimation of the degree of mitral regurgitation by range-gated pulsed Doppler echocardiography. *Circulation* 1980; 61:143–147.

157. Miyatake K, Kinoshita N, Nagata S, et al: Intracardiac flow pattern in mitral regurgitation studied with combined use of the ultrasonic pulsed Doppler technique and cross-sectional echocardiography. *Am J Cardiol* 1980; 45:155–162.

158. Ciobanu M, Abbasi AS, Allen M, et al: Pulsed Doppler echocardiography in the diagnosis and estimation of severity of aortic insufficiency. *Am J Cardiol* 1982; 49:339–343.

159. Miyatake K, Izumi S, Okamoto M, et al: Semiquantitative grading of severity of mitral regurgitation by real-time two-dimensional Doppler flow imaging technique. *J Am Coll Cardiol* 1986; 7:82–88.

160. Helmcke F, Nanda NC, Hsiung MC, et al: Color Doppler assessment of mitral regurgitation with orthogonal planes. *Circulation* 1987; 75:175–183.

161. Perry GJ, Helmcke F, Nanda NC, et al: Evaluation of aortic insufficiency by Doppler color flow mapping. *J Am Coll Cardiol* 1987; 9:952–959.

162. Bolger AF, Eigler NL, Maurer G: Quantifying valvular regurgitation. Limitations and inherent assumptions of Doppler techniques. *Circulation* 1988; 78:1316–1318.

163. Switzer DF, Yoganathan AP, Nanda NC, et al: Calibration of color Doppler flow mapping during extreme hemodynamic conditions in vitro: A foundation for a reliable quantitative grading system for aortic incompetence. *Circulation* 1987; 75:837–846.

164. Sahn DJ: Instrumentation and physical factors related to visualization of stenotic and regurgitant jets by Doppler color flow mapping. *J Am Coll Cardiol* 1988; 12:1354–1365.

165. Rokey R, Sterling LL, Zoghbi WA, et al: Determination of regurgitant fraction by pulsed Doppler two-dimensional echocardiography. *J Am Coll Cardiol* 1986; 7:1273–1278.

166. Blumlein S, Bouchard A, Schiller NB, et al: Quantitation of mitral regurgitation by Doppler echocardiography. *Circulation* 1986; 74:306–314.

167. Goldberg SJ, Allen HD: Quantitative assessment by Doppler echocardiography of pulmonary or aortic regurgitation. *Am J Cardiol* 1985; 56:131–135.

168. Quinones MA, Young JB, Waggoner AD, et al: Assessment of pulsed Doppler echocardiography in detection and quantification of aortic and mitral regurgitation. *Br Heart J* 1980; 44:612–620.

169. Boughner DR: Assessment of aortic insufficiency by transcutaneous Doppler ultrasound. *Circulation* 1975; 52:874–879.

170. Takenaka K, Dabestani A, Gardin JM, et al: A simple Doppler echocardiographic method for estimating severity of aortic regurgitation. *Am J Cardiol* 1986; 57:1340–1343.

171. Labovitz AJ, Ferrara RP, Kern MJ, et al: Quantitative evaluation of aortic insufficiency by continu-

ous wave Doppler echocardiography. *J Am Coll Cardiol* 1986; 8:1341–1347.

172. Teague SM, Heinsimer JA, Anderson JL, et al: Quantification of aortic regurgitation utilizing continuous wave Doppler ultrasound. *J Am Coll Cardiol* 1986; 8:592–599.

173. Masuyama T, Kodama K, Kitabatake A, et al: Noninvasive evaluation of aortic regurgitation by continuous-wave Doppler echocardiography. *Circulation* 1986; 73:460–466.

174. Beyer RW, Ramirez M, Josephson MA, et al: Correlation of continuous-wave Doppler assessment of chronic aortic regurgitation with hemodynamics and angiography. *Am J Cardiol* 1987; 60:852–856.

175. Grayburn PA, Handshoe R, Smith MD, et al: Quantitative assessment of the hemodynamic consequences of aortic regurgitation by means of continuous wave Doppler recordings. *J Am Coll Cardiol* 1987; 10:135–141.

176. Noble MIM, Trenchard D, Guz A: Left ventricular ejection in conscious dogs, 1. Measurement and significance of the maximum acceleration of blood from the left ventricle. *Circ Res* 1966; 19:139–143.

177. Stein PD, Sabbah HN: Ventricular performance measured during ejection. Studies in patients of the rate of change of ventricular power. *Am Heart J* 1976; 91:599–606.

178. Gardin JM, Iseri LT, Elkayam U, et al: Evaluation of dilated cardiomyopathy by pulsed Doppler echocardiography. *Am Heart J* 1983; 106:1057–1065.

179. Sabbah HN, Khaja F, Brymer JF, et al: Noninvasive evaluation of left ventricular performance based on peak aortic blood acceleration measured with a continuous-wave Doppler velocity meter. *Circulation* 1986; 74:323–329.

180. Wallmeyer K, Wann LS, Sagar KB, et al: The influence of preload and heart rate on Doppler echocardiographic indexes of left ventricular performance: Comparison with invasive indexes in an experimental preparation. *Circulation* 1986; 74:181–186.

181. Mehta N, Bennett DE: Impaired left ventricular function in acute myocardial infarction assessed by Doppler measurement of ascending aortic blood velocity and maximum acceleration. *Am J Cardiol* 1986; 57:1052–1058.

182. Mehta N, Bennett D, Mannering D, et al: Usefulness of noninvasive Doppler measurement of ascending aortic blood velocity and acceleration in detecting impairment of the left ventricular functional response to exercise three weeks after acute myocardial infarction. *Am J Cardiol* 1986; 58:879–884.

183. Forrester JS, Diamond GA, Swan HJC: Correlative classification of clinical and hemodynamic function after acute myocardial infarction. *Am J Cardiol* 1977; 39:137–142.

184. Rokey R, Kuo LC, Zoghbi WA, et al: Determination of parameters of left ventricular diastolic filling with pulsed Doppler echocardiography: Comparison with cineangiography. *Circulation* 1985; 71:543–550.

185. Snider AR, Gidding SS, Rocchini AP, et al: Doppler evaluation of left ventricular diastolic filling in children with systemic hypertension. *Am J Cardiol* 1985; 56:921–926.

186. Spirito P, Maron BJ, Bonow RO: Noninvasive assessment of left ventricular diastolic function: Comparative analysis of Doppler echocardiographic and radionuclide angiographic techniques. *J Am Coll Cardiol* 1986; 7:518–526.

187. Fuji J, Yazaki Y, Sawada H, et al: Noninvasive assessment of left and right ventricular filling in myocardial infarction with a two-dimensional Doppler echocardiographic method. *J Am Coll Cardiol* 1985; 5:1155–1160.

188. Spirito P, Maron BJ, Bellotti P, et al: Noninvasive assessment of left ventricular diastolic function: Comparative analysis of pulsed Doppler ultrasound and digitized M-mode echocardiography. *Am J Cardiol* 1986; 58:837–843.

189. Friedman BJ, Drinkovic N, Miles H, et al: Assessment of left ventricular diastolic function: Comparison of Doppler echocardiography and gated blood pool scintigraphy. *J Am Coll Cardiol* 1986; 8:1348–1354.

190. Pearson AC, Goodgold H, Labovitz AJ: Comparison of pulsed Doppler echocardiography and radionuclide angiography in the assessment of left ventricular filling. *Am J Cardiol* 1988; 61:446–454.

191. Appleton CP, Hatle LK, Popp RL: Relation of transmitral flow velocity patterns to left ventricular diastolic function: New insights from a combined hemodynamic and Doppler echocardiographic study. *J Am Coll Cardiol* 1988; 12:426–440.

192. Wind BE, Snider AR, Buda AG, et al: Pulsed Doppler assessment of left ventricular diastolic filling in patients with coronary artery disease before and immediately after coronary angioplasty. *Am J Cardiol* 1987; 59:1041–1046.

193. Kitabatake A, Inoue M, Asao M, et al: Transmitral blood flow reflecting diastolic behavior of the left ventricle in health and disease: A study by pulsed Doppler technique. *Jpn Circ J* 1982; 46:92–102.

194. Miyatake K, Okamoto M, Kinoshita N, et al: Augmentation of atrial contribution to left ventricular inflow with aging as assessed by intracardiac Doppler flowmetry. *Am J Cardiol* 1984; 53:586–589.

195. Takenaka K, Dabestani A, Gardin J, et al: Left ventricular filling in hypertrophic cardiomyopathy: A pulsed Doppler echocardiographic study. *J Am Coll Cardiol* 1986; 7:1263–1271.

196. Pearson AC, Schiff M, Mrosek D, et al: Left ventricular diastolic function in weight lifters. *Am J Cardiol* 1986; 58:1254–1259.

197. Takenaka AK, Dabestani A, Gardin JM, et al: Pulsed Doppler echocardiographic study of left ventricular filling in dilated cardiomyopathy. *Am J Cardiol* 1986; 58:143–147.

198. Bowman LK, Forrester AL, Jaffe CC, et al: Peak filling rate normalized to mitral stroke volume: A new Doppler echocardiographic filling index validated by radionuclide angiographic technique. *J Am Coll Cardiol* 1988; 12:937–943.

199. Gidding SS, Snider AR, Rocchini AP, et al: Left ventricular diastolic filling in children with hypertrophic cardiomyopathy: Assessment with pulsed Doppler echocardiography. *J Am Coll Cardiol* 1986; 8:310–316.

200. Meliones JN, Snider AR, Serwer GA, et al: Pulsed

Doppler assessment of left ventricular diastolic filling in children with left ventricular outflow obstruction before and after balloon angioplasty. *Am J Cardiol* 1989; 63:231–236.

201. Finkelhor RS, Hanak LJ, Bahler RC: Left ventricular filling in endurance-trained subjects. *J Am Coll Cardiol* 1986; 8:289–293.

202. Masuyama T, Kodama K, Nakatani S, et al: Effects of changes in coronary stenosis of left ventricular diastolic filling assessed with pulsed Doppler echocardiography. *J Am Coll Cardiol* 1988; 11:744–751.

203. Phillips RA, Coplan NL, Krakoff LR, et al: Doppler echocardiographic analysis of left ventricular filling in treated hypertensive patients. *J Am Coll Cardiol* 1987; 9:317–322.

204. Maron BJ, Spirito P, Green KJ, et al: Noninvasive assessment of left ventricular diastolic function by pulsed Doppler echocardiography in patients with hypertrophic cardiomyopathy. *J Am Coll Cardiol* 1987; 10:733–742.

205. Appleton RS, Graham TP, Cotton RB, et al: Altered early left ventricular diastolic cardiac function in the premature infant. *Am J Cardiol* 1987; 59:1391–1394.

206. Courtois M, Kovacs SJ Jr, Ludbrook PA: Transmitral pressure-flow velocity relation: Importance of regional pressure gradients in the left ventricle during diastole. *Circulation* 1988; 78:661–671.

207. Ishida Y, Meisner JS, Tsujioka K, et al: Left ventricular filling dynamics: Influence of left ventricular relaxation and left atrial pressure. *Circulation* 1986; 74:187–196.

208. Danielson R, Nordrehaug JE, Vik-mo H: Importance of adjusting left ventricular diastolic peak filling rate for heart rate. *Am J Cardiol* 1988; 61:489–491.

209. Sartori MP, Quinones MA, Kuo LC: Relation of Doppler-derived left ventricular filling parameters to age and radius/thickness ratio in normal and pathologic states. *Am J Cardiol* 1987; 59:1179–1182.

210. Bryg RJ, Williams GA, Labovitz AJ: Effect of aging on left ventricular diastolic filling in normal subjects. *Am J Cardiol* 1987; 59:971–974.

211. Kuo LC, Quinones MA, Rokey R, et al: Quantification of atrial contribution to left ventricular filling by pulsed Doppler echocardiography and the effect of age in normal and diseased hearts. *Am J Cardiol* 1987; 59:1174–1178.

212. Choong CY, Abascal VM, Thomas JD, et al: Combined influence of ventricular loading and relaxation on the transmitral flow velocity profile in dogs measured by Doppler echocardiography. *Circulation* 1988; 78:672–683.

213. Takenaka K, Dabestani A, Waffarn F, et al: Effect of left ventricular size on early diastolic left ventricular filling in neonates and in adults. *Am J Cardiol* 1987; 59:138–141.

214. Choong CY, Herrman HC, Weyman AE, et al: Preload dependence of Doppler-derived indexes of left ventricular diastolic function in humans. *J Am Coll Cardiol* 1987; 10:800–808.

215. Shaikh MA, Levine SJ: Effect of mitral regurgitation on diastolic filling with left ventricular hypertrophy. *Am J Cardiol* 1988; 61:590–594.

216. Reed KL, Sahn DJ, Scagnelli S, et al: Doppler echocardiographic studies of diastolic function in the human fetal heart: Changes during gestation. *J Am Coll Cardiol* 1986; 8:391–395.

217. Gardin JM, Dabestani A, Takenaka K, et al: Effect of imaging view and sample volume location on evaluation of mitral flow velocity by pulsed Doppler echocardiography. *Am J Cardiol* 1986; 57:1335–1339.

218. Dabestani A, Takenaka K, Allen B, et al: Effects of spontaneous respiration on diastolic left ventricular filling assessed by pulsed Doppler echocardiography. *Am J Cardiol* 1988; 61:1356–1358.

219. Riggs TW, Snider AR: Respiratory influence on right and left ventricular diastolic function in normal children. *Am J Cardiol* 1989; 63:858–861.

Defects in Cardiac Septation

Defects in septation of the atria, ventricles, or conotruncus are the single largest group of congenital cardiac anomalies encountered. The echocardiographer must be able to diagnose these defects accurately and assess their effects upon the patient. While septation defects are often present in association with complex cardiac anomalies, this chapter will review conditions in which the septation defect is the primary cardiac abnormality. The anatomy of cardiac septation as well as the echocardiographic views required to image these defects will be discussed, along with the role of ancillary techniques such as Doppler flow studies and contrast studies.

ATRIAL SEPTATION

Anatomy

Regions of the Atrial Septum

The atrial septum is generally divided into three regions based upon the embryologic derivation of the area. The most superior region, referred to as the sinus venosus region, extends from the superior portion of the atrial septum to the region of the fossa ovalis. It is bounded by the posterior wall of the atria (running along a line that joins the superior to the inferior vena cava), the right atrial appendage, and the limbus of the fossa ovalis. The sinus venosus region lies in close proximity to the right-sided pulmonary veins and the entrance of the superior vena cava into the right atrium. Thus, defects in this region of the septum are superior and posterior, with minimal or no septal tissue separating the defect from the posterior atrial wall. The entrances of the superior vena cava and the right pulmonary veins lie adjacent to this area and may be closely related to the sinus venosus defect.

Lying inferior and anterior to the sinus venosus region is the fossa ovalis, which forms the central portion of the atrial septum. This is a very thin portion of the atrial septum which, in a high percentage of people, is probe patent

because the flap valve of the foramen ovale has failed to seal to the limbus. This region is often referred to as the secundum portion of the atrial septum and is bounded by the limbus—the elevated margins that form the rim of the fossa ovalis. The limbus consists of two major muscle bundles. The superior limbic band arises from the posterior right atrial wall, courses along the superior border of the fossa ovalis, and inserts into the central fibrous body. The inferior limbic band arises near the inferior vena caval orifice, runs along the inferior border of the fossa ovalis, and inserts into the central fibrous body. The medial end of the eustachian valve is inserted into the inferior edge of the inferior limbic band. Defects in the secundum region are the most common form of abnormalities of the atrial septum. These defects are found in the region inferior to the sinus venosus septum, superior to the atrioventricular septum, and bounded by the limbic bands. Tissue margins separate these defects from the atrial walls and the atrioventricular valves. However, the tissue rim may be small, especially along the posterior margin.

Finally, lying inferior to the fossa ovalis is the atrioventricular portion of the atrial septum (the primum portion of the atrial septum), bounded by the atrioventricular valves, the posterior atrial wall, and the fossa ovalis. This region is formed in conjunction with the atrioventricular valves and the inlet portion of the ventricular septum; defects in this region of the atrial septum are associated with defects of the atrioventricular valves and/or inlet ventricular septum. This type of atrial septal defect will be discussed in conjunction with the atrioventricular septal defects.

Echocardiographic Views

Views for imaging the atrial septum must be chosen to maximize echo reflectivity from the thin septum. The atrial septum should be visualized from multiple aspects in order to assess the size, shape, and location of the defect

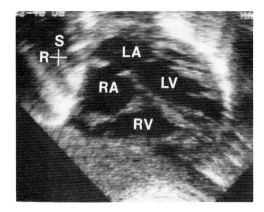

FIG 5–1.
Subcostal four-chamber view from a child with a large secundum atrial septal defect located in the midportion of the atrial septum. The edges of the defect act as specular reflectors of ultrasound and thus are very bright. *LA* = left atrium; *LV* = left ventricle; *R* = right; *RA* = right atrium; *RV* = right ventricle; and *S* = superior.

as well as its relationship to adjacent structures. Particular care must be taken to assess the relationship of the defect to the superior vena cava, the pulmonary veins, and the coronary sinus. Additional views of the ventricles are used to determine the presence of secondary findings associated with the hemodynamic consequences of an atrial septal defect.

Differentiation of Defects From Artifactual Drop-out

Because the atrial septum is a relatively thin structure, especially in the region of the fossa ovalis, care must be taken to distinguish true defects from loss of targets. Views that image the atrial septum aligned parallel with the ultrasound beam must be avoided. In addition, the edges of true defects are often more echogenic, producing the so-called T artifact.[1] The T artifact gives the edges of the defect a broadened appearance, forming the visual image of a T. The T artifact is thought to be caused by the edges of the defect acting as specular reflectors, scattering the reflected sound energy, and thus broadening the apparent edge of the defect. The presence of such an artifact clearly marks the defect borders, distinguishing it from artifactual echo dropout. Some defects, however, may not produce a T artifact and thus may be difficult to distinguish from artifactual echo dropout. In these situations, the defect must be imaged in multiple views and secondary indicators such as right atrial and ventricular dilatation must be evaluated. Doppler and contrast studies, as discussed later, may be helpful.

Subcostal Four-Chamber View

The subcostal four-chamber view permits imaging of the atrial septum along its anterior-posterior axis from the region of the superior vena cava to the region of the atrioventricular valves; this is the preferred view for imaging the atrial septum (Fig 5–1).[2] In this view, the septum runs almost perpendicular to the ultrasound beam, permitting

measurement of the defect size along its long axis. Because the septum is thin (particularly in its midportion), placing the septum perpendicular to the sound beam helps distinguish a true defect from artifactual dropout. This view permits easy separation of superior sinus venosus defects from secundum defects, and allows evaluation of the relation of the superior vena cava to the defect. The size of the right atrium can also be evaluated. Right atrial size is an important secondary indicator of the size of the atrial septal defect.

This view also permits evaluation of the entrance of the pulmonary veins into the heart. Because there is a high incidence of abnormal insertion of the pulmonary veins into the heart, particularly in the presence of a sinus venosus defect, evaluation of pulmonary venous drainage is very important (Fig 5–2).[3] Even if one right pulmonary vein is seen entering the left atrium, the proximal superior vena cava must be closely evaluated to detect the abnormal entrance of other pulmonary veins.

Sweeping the scan plane posteriorly, the posterior-inferior portion of the atrial septum can be evaluated. Defects in this area of the septum are rare[4] but can be located near the orifice of the coronary sinus. The coronary sinus can be traced leftward and does not open into the left atrium, whereas low atrial septal defects communicate with the left atrium. Unlike primum atrial septal defects, these defects are separated from the atrioventricular valves by a rim of tissue. Finally, such defects may be associated with the absence of the left atrial-coronary sinus septum and drainage of the coronary sinus into the left atrium.

Aneurysms of the atrial septum comprised of tissue attached to the edges of the atrial septal defect also are well seen in this view (Fig 5–3). These structures are quite

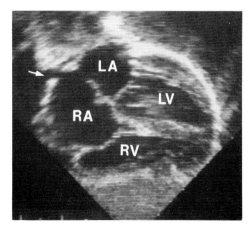

FIG 5–2.
Subcostal four-chamber view from a patient with a large sinus venosus atrial septal defect and anomalous drainage of the right upper pulmonary vein *(arrow)*. The sinus venosus atrial septal defect is located in the most superior and posterior portion of the atrial septum. This type of defect is often associated with anomalous drainage of the right pulmonary veins. *LA* = left atrium; *LV* = left ventricle; *RA* = right atrium; and *RV* = right ventricle.

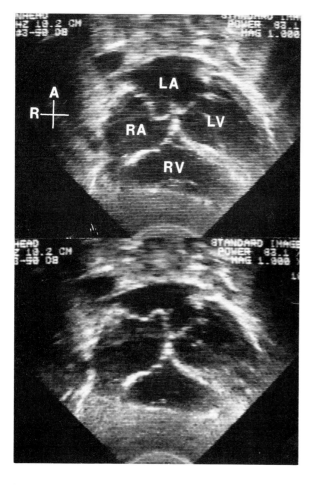

FIG 5–3.
Subcostal four-chamber view from a patient with an atrial septal
aneurysm. In the *top frame,* the atrial septal aneurysm bulges prominently into the right atrium (RA). In the *bottom frame,* the atrial
septal aneurysm bulges into the left atrium (LA). This phasic motion
of the atrial septal aneurysm reflects phasic differences in pressure
between the two atria. A = anterior; LV = left ventricle; R = right; and
RV = right ventricle.

thin walled and billow into the right atrium.[5,6] Their position and prominence varies throughout the cardiac and
respiratory cycle as the pressure difference between the
atria changes (Figs 5–4 and 5–5). Atrial septal aneurysms
are usually patent but may be intact with no resultant
shunting. Doppler and contrast studies are useful for detecting aneurysm patency. Atrial septal aneurysms must
be distinguished from other right atrial masses that are
more clinically significant. Large aneurysms may extend
to, and in some instances through, the tricuspid valve.
      Other structures within the atria that may be imaged
include the eustachian valve associated with the entrance
of the inferior vena cava into the right atrium. The eustachian valve can be visualized up to its insertion into the
primum atrial septum. The eustachian valve may be quite
prominent and must not be confused with the atrial septum. Abnormal persistence of this structure may result in

obstruction to flow into the right ventricle, as will be discussed in a subsequent chapter. Also present may be a
Chiari's network, which consists of a spider-web-like structure that extends from the orifice of the superior vena cava
to the orifice of the inferior vena cava. This structure is
thin and delicate, and while it is usually not mistaken for
the atrial septum, it must be differentiated from other right
atrial pathology.[7] Finally, the coronary sinus ostia may be
very large, especially if there is a persistent left superior
vena cava. Care must be exercised to distinguish this from
a posterior-inferior atrial septal defect.

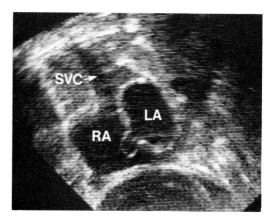

FIG 5–4.
Subcostal sagittal view from a patient with a prominent aneurysm
in the region of the foramen ovale. In this view, the aneurysm bows
into the right atrium (RA). LA = left atrium; SVC = superior vena cava.

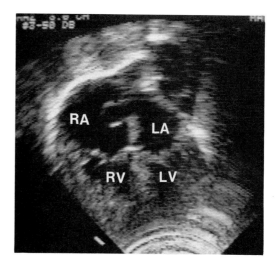

FIG 5–5.
Apical four-chamber view from a patient with an atrial septal aneu-
rysm. The atrial septal aneurysm is seen bowing into the right atrium
(RA). Atrial septal aneurysms are often seen during spontaneous
closure or diminution in size of atrial septal defects. LA = left atrium;
LV = left ventricle; and RV = right ventricle.

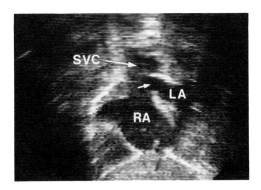

FIG 5–6.
Subcostal sagittal view from a patient with a large sinus venosus atrial septal defect *(arrow)*. This defect is located in the superior and posterior portion of the atrial septum just beneath the superior vena cava (SVC). Note the right atrial appendage anteriorly. *LA* = left atrium; *RA* = right atrium.

Subcostal Sagittal View

Turning the transducer 90° from the subcostal four-chamber view permits imaging of the atrial septum along its superior-inferior axis in a plane orthogonal to the previous view. This view is analogous to the lateral angiogram, with the left atrium posterior to the right atrium. Sweeping the transducer from right to left in this axis allows evaluation of the largest dimension of the atrial septal defect. This dimension can be compared to the dimension measured in the subcostal four-chamber view. Equal dimensions imply a circular defect, while unequal dimensions imply an ellipsoid-shaped defect. The combined use of these two subcostal views also permits evaluation of the amount of tissue rim surrounding the defect, which is important surgically (Figs 5–4 and 5–6). In addition, some defects will be seen in this projection that will not be appreciated in the coronal view. Sweeping the scan plane further rightward, it is possible to see the right upper pulmonary vein coursing superiorly to enter the left atrium (Fig 5–7).

Parasternal Short-Axis View

In the parasternal short-axis view at the base of the heart, the atrial septum is seen posterior to the aortic root running in an anterior-posterior orientation. While defects in the septum are not well seen in this view because the beam orientation is parallel to the septum, the sizes of both atria can be appreciated. In the presence of an atrial septal defect, the right atrium is considerably larger than the left atrium.[8]

In the parasternal short-axis view at the level of the ventricles, the hemodynamic evidence of right ventricular volume overload can be detected. With a sizeable left-to-right atrial shunt, the right ventricle becomes enlarged and circular-shaped in diastole (Fig 5–8). In diastole, the left ventricle may be crescent-shaped. With a significant increase in right ventricular preload, ventricular septal mo-

tion becomes paradoxical, moving anteriorly rather than posteriorly in systole.

Parasternal Long-Axis View

While the atrial septum is not seen at all in this view, secondary signs of right ventricular volume overload are seen. The right ventricle is enlarged and hyperdynamic. The increased shortening fraction of the right ventricle creates a vigorous to-and-fro motion of the outflow tract in the long-axis view. In addition, abnormal septal motion can be seen on the M-mode record. The normal posterior systolic septal motion is replaced by an anterior systolic motion known as paradoxical septal motion.[9,10] The cause

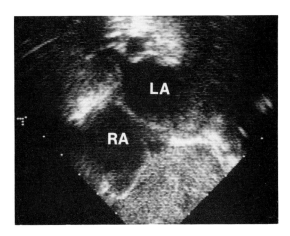

FIG 5–7.
Subcostal sagittal view with the plane of sound tilted far toward the patient's right to image the right upper pulmonary vein as it enters the left atrium (LA). *RA* = right atrium.

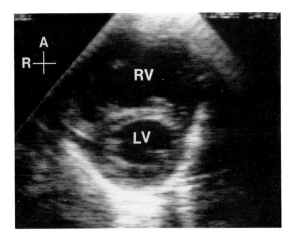

FIG 5–8.
Parasternal short-axis view of the left ventricle (LV) from a patient with a large secundum atrial septal defect. Note the marked dilatation of the right ventricle (RV). *A* = anterior; *R* = right.

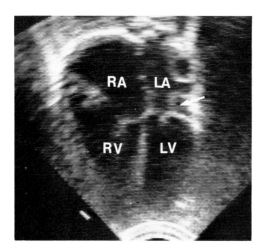

FIG 5–9.
Apical four-chamber view from a patient with a secundum atrial septal defect and a large coronary sinus *(arrow)*, caused by persistent left superior vena cava draining to the coronary sinus. Note the marked dilatation of the right atrium (RA) and right ventricle (RV). *LA* = left atrium; *LV* = left ventricle.

of this abnormal motion is believed to be the leftward and anterior rotation of the right ventricle about the left ventricle when right ventricular volume overload is present. Weyman and colleagues showed that the *diastolic* position of the interventricular septum and the relation of the right and left ventricles is markedly altered, with some flattening of the septum and left ventricle.[10] Nevertheless, the systolic shape and position of the septum are normal. Thus, the manner of motion of the septum from diastole to systole is altered. These findings have been confirmed in children by Agata and coworkers.[11]

Apical Four-Chamber View

In the apical four-chamber view, atrial septal defects are difficult to diagnose with certainty because in this view the atrial septum is aligned parallel with the ultrasound beam. Thus, artifactual echo dropout is frequently seen in the region of the thin fossa ovalis. Visualization of the atrial septum can be optimized by sliding the transducer medially from the cardiac apex toward the sternal border. This transducer position provides a low parasternal four-chamber view for imaging the atrial septum at an angle nearly perpendicular to the sound beam. In patients in whom the subcostal views are difficult to obtain (i.e., in obese patients or patients with subxyphoid chest tubes), the low parasternal four-chamber view provides an alternative method for imaging the atrial septum in the direction of the axial resolution of the equipment.

The apical four-chamber view is particularly useful for assessing right atrial and right ventricular dilatation. In this view, the degree of right heart enlargement is easily assessed by comparing the right- and left-sided cardiac chambers (Fig 5–9).

Contrast Studies

Peripheral venous contrast studies have been used to detect interatrial communications.[12–14] Positive results (i.e., the presence of contrast echoes in the left atrium) and negative results (i.e., a negative washout of contrast echoes from blood shunted across the defect) have been used as diagnostic evidence of an atrial septal defect. Studies of the instantaneous pressure gradient between the left and right atria have shown that right-to-left shunting occurs even when the predominate shunt is in a left-to-right direction.[15] However, this right-to-left shunt is transient, occurring during ventricular systole, and is easily missed. With even a mild decrease in right ventricular compliance, a net right-to-left shunt occurs with visualization of contrast echoes in the left heart. This is less common in children because ventricular compliance tends to remain normal. In cooperative children, the performance of a Valsalva maneuver will transiently elevate right atrial pressure and create a right-to-left shunt.

Initially, contrast studies were used as a diagnostic aid when the atrial defect was difficult to image. With technologic improvements, defect imaging has improved considerably and contrast studies are often not required to document the presence of a defect. In certain situations, such as the presence of an atrial septal aneurysm, contrast studies are helpful in determining septal patency. Also, contrast echocardiography is important in determining a patient's susceptibility to paradoxical emboli.

The contrast technique requires the rapid injection of saline into a peripheral vein. Most injections have been performed using an upper extremity vessel. Because the flow patterns are different from the superior vena cava and the inferior vena cava, injections into upper extremity and lower extremity vessels may produce different results.[15] Thus, all injections should be made into upper extremity vessels to permit comparisons with published data. Also, agitation of the saline before injection increases the echogenicity of the saline.

For detection of an interatrial shunt with contrast echocardiography, the apical and subcostal four-chamber views are preferred. These views permit imaging of all four cardiac chambers simultaneously, thus allowing diagnosis of the level of the right-to-left shunt. A positive study is one in which contrast echoes are clearly seen in the left atrium. Diagnosis of an atrial defect based on observation of a negative washout of contrast echoes from the right atrium is fraught with inaccuracy because the inflow of contrast-free blood from the inferior vena cava and the coronary sinus can create a negative washout.

Doppler Studies

In children with atrial septal defects, Doppler echocardiography has been especially useful for detecting the left-to-right shunting of blood across the defect. Doppler examination of the right atrium can be performed from the left or right parasternal location, the cardiac apex, or the subcostal position; however, the subcostal and right parasternal positions provide the best windows for alignment of the Doppler beam parallel with shunt flow. In patients with an isolated atrial septal defect, right atrial Doppler examination shows disturbed flow above the baseline (toward the transducer), beginning in midsystole and extending into early diastole (Figs 5–10 and 5–11). This flow generally reaches its maximum velocity in late systole. A second short period of left-to-right shunt appears as disturbed flow above the baseline at the time of atrial contraction. In addition, almost all patients with a simple atrial septal defect exhibit a short period of disturbed flow below the baseline (away from the transducer) in early systole.[16, 17] These variations in the direction of shunt flow correspond to the differences in pressures that exist between the left and right atria throughout the cardiac cycle.[15] The greatest pressure difference and the largest amount of left-to-right shunting occurs in the last half of systole, when left atrial pressure exceeds right atrial pressure (especially at the end of systole, corresponding to the peak of the left atrial V wave). Another period of left-to-right shunting occurs with atrial contraction, and a small right-to-left shunt occurs in early systole, when right atrial pressure exceeds left atrial pressure because of the unequal activation times of the two atria. In most cases, the peak velocity of the left-to-right shunt in late systole is 1 to 1.5 m/sec, indicating a maximum pressure difference between the atria of roughly 5 mm Hg. A very high velocity jet can occasionally be recorded across the atrial septum and usually indicates a restrictive atrial communication with a large pressure difference between the atria (i.e., a stretched-open, patent foramen ovale).[18]

In addition, atrial septal defects cause an increase in flow velocity (because of the increased volume of flow) across the tricuspid and pulmonary valves. Flow velocities across the mitral and aortic valves are often slightly decreased. Several investigators have found a close correlation between the ratios of the right- and left-sided flow velocities (i.e., pulmonary artery/aorta and tricuspid/mitral) and the ratio of pulmonary to systemic flow measured at cardiac catheterization.[16] The pulmonary and systemic blood flows can be calculated with Doppler echocardiography using the techniques outlined in Chapter 4.

Shunting across the atrial septal defect varies with respiration. With inspiration, the pressure difference between the two atria at late systole decreases and the left-to-right flow velocities decrease. On the other hand, the flow reversal in early systole is more apparent during inspiration, when less left-to-right shunting occurs.

Doppler echocardiography is an extremely sensitive technique for detecting flow across an atrial septal defect. The Doppler examination is especially useful for confirming the presence of an atrial septal defect when one cannot be imaged with certainty on the two-dimensional echocardiogram and for excluding an atrial septal defect when an area of echocardiographic dropout is seen in the atrial

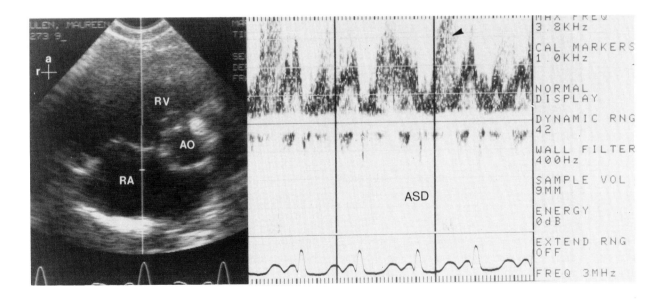

FIG 5–10.
Pulsed Doppler recording from the parasternal short-axis view of a small child with an atrial septal defect. The freeze-frame image *(left)* shows the position of the sample volume in the right atrium (RA) at the time of the Doppler spectral recording. The Doppler tracing *(right)* shows disturbed flow above the baseline (toward the transducer), beginning at mid-systole and extending into early diastole. This flow reaches its maximum velocity in late systole *(arrow).*

A second short period of left-to-right shunting appears as disturbed flow above the baseline at the time of atrial contraction. *A* = anterior; *AO* = aorta; *R* = right; and *RV* = right ventricle. (From Snider AR: Doppler echocardiography in congenital heart disease, in Berger M (ed): *Doppler Echocardiography in Heart Disease*, New York, Marcel, Dekker, 1987, p 271. Used by permission.)

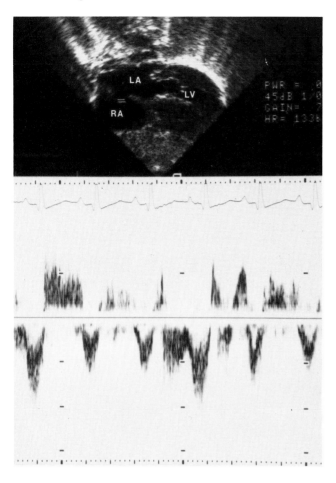

FIG 5–11.
Pulsed Doppler tracing from a patient with bidirectional atrial shunting. The freeze-frame image of the subcostal four-chamber view *(top)* shows the position of the sample volume adjacent to the atrial septal defect at the time of the recording. The Doppler flow signals below the baseline indicate flow at atrial contraction extending into early systole from the right atrium (RA) to the left atrium (LA) away from the transducer. Throughout most of systole and extending into diastole, the Doppler flow signals above the baseline indicate flow toward the transducer from the LA to the RA. *LV =* left ventricle.

septum on the two-dimensional echocardiogram. In a recent study, Doppler echocardiography showed the characteristic patterns of atrial septal shunting in 30 of 31 patients with catheterization-proven atrial septal defect. Doppler patterns suggesting an atrial left to right shunt were not found in 15 normal patients.[17, 18]

Doppler color-flow mapping techniques can be used to detect shunting across an atrial septal defect (Plates 9 and 10). This technique is particularly useful for confirming the presence of an atrial septal defect in those patients in whom direct imaging of the atrial septum is technically inadequate and in distinguishing a true atrial septal defect from artifactual echocardiographic dropout in the thin region of the fossa ovalis. On the Doppler color-flow mapping

examination from the subcostal four-chamber view, flow across the atrial septum appears as an area of red flow (flow toward the transducer), with some evidence of disturbed flow on the variance map.

VENTRICULAR SEPTATION

Anatomy

Regions of the Ventricular Septum

Morphologically, the ventricular septum is composed of two parts: the membranous septum and the muscular septum. The membranous septum is relatively small, bounded superiorly by the aortic valve at the junction of the right and noncoronary cusps and inferiorly by the muscular septum. This is a relatively small structure even in the adult heart, where it may measure only 5 mm in diameter. Viewed from the right ventricle, the membranous septum is divided into two sections by the septal leaflet of the tricuspid valve. These sections are the pars atrioventricularis, which lies above the tricuspid valve, and the pars interventricularis, which lies beneath the septal leaflet of the tricuspid valve. Viewed from the left ventricle, the membranous septum lies in the superior portion of the left ventricular outflow tract just beneath the aortic valve. In addition, the membranous septum is a very thin structure and like the central portion of the atrial septum, may not be well imaged in all planes, giving the false impression of a defect being present in some views.

Radiating out from the membranous septum like the spokes of a wheel is the muscular septum, which typically is divided into three regions. The first is the inlet portion, which lies inferior to the membranous septum and between the two atrioventricular valves. This is the superior, posterior one-third of the muscular septum. The inferior borders of the inlet septum are bounded by the chordal attachments of the atrioventricular valves.

The second portion of the muscular septum is the trabecular septum, which extends from the membranous septum to the cardiac apex. It is the largest portion of the ventricular septum and does not lie entirely in the same plane. Multiple defects may be present in this portion of the septum.

Finally, the superior and anterior portion is the infundibular or outlet septum, which lies superior to the trabecular septum and inferior to the great vessels. From the right ventricular aspect, the infundibular septum lies above an imaginary line drawn from the membranous septum through the papillary muscle of the conus to the anterior infundibular wall. Thus, portions of the outlet septum lie above and below the crista supraventricularis. From the left ventricular side, the outlet septum lies under the right coronary cusp of the aortic valve.

Ventricular septal defects can occur in any of the four portions of the ventricular septum that have different embryologic derivations (membranous, inlet, trabecular, outlet) but usually occur along the fusion lines between the different portions of the septum. With two-dimensional

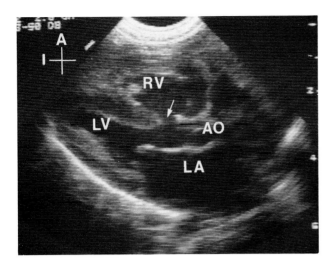

FIG 5–12.
Parasternal long-axis view from a patient with a membranous ventricular septal defect *(arrow)*. The membranous ventricular septal defect is located superiorly just beneath the aortic (AO) valve. *A* = anterior; *I* = inferior; *LA* = left atrium; *LV* = left ventricle; and *RV* = right ventricle.

echocardiography, defects are classified as being entirely within a portion of the septum (i.e., trabecular defects) or on a fusion line between two or more portions of the ventricular septum (i.e., perimembranous outlet, perimembranous inlet defects). Defects need to be assessed according to their location and size. It must also be determined if they are completely rimmed by muscular tissue or partially bordered by valve annulus and if there is any malalignment of the septal components bordering on the defect. Thus, anatomically, the echocardiographic examination should address the following questions:

1. What segments of the septum are involved?
2. What is the size of the defect?
3. What are the borders of the defect?
4. Is septal component malalignment present or absent?
5. What is the relation of the cardiac valves to the defect?
6. What is the relation of the atrioventricular valve chordal attachments to the defect?
7. How many defects are present?

Echocardiographic Views

Parasternal Long-Axis View

This echocardiographic plane images the ventricular septum along its long axis, traversing predominantly the infundibular septum and the trabecular septum.[19] The septum, however, does not lie in a single plane, and thus only specific portions of these segments are imaged. With slight rightward rotation of the scan plane off the major axis of the left ventricle, the membranous septum is imaged (Fig

5–12). The distinction between the infundibular septum and the membranous septum becomes somewhat blurred in this view; imaging in other views is often necessary to distinguish between defects of the infundibular septum and the membranous septum. When malalignment of the septum and the aorta is present, the defect must be in the infundibular septum (Fig 5–13). Finally, leftward rotation of the scan plane results in imaging the right ventricular outflow tract and the superior portion of the infundibular septum above the crista supraventricularis and just beneath the pulmonary valve (Fig 5–14). In summary, this is the best view for imaging defects in all portions of the infundibular septum and in many segments of the trabecular septum. Although the membranous septum can also be seen, other views may be superior for imaging it.

Small ventricular septal defects, particularly in the muscular septum, can be difficult to image. The presence of the T-artifact described for atrial septal defects[1] greatly enhances the ability to distinguish a true defect from artifactual target dropout (Fig 5–15). Color Doppler mapping is also helpful, as will be discussed later.

Parasternal Short-Axis View

The parasternal short-axis view, with the scan plane passing just inferior to the aortic valve, images the tricuspid valve, the membranous septum, the infundibular septum, and the pulmonary valve. This is the best view to image the membranous septum and to assess fully the extent of the defect in this portion of the septum (Fig 5–16). This view also allows assessment of the extension of the membranous defect into the adjacent infundibular septum and permits evaluation of the extent of malposition of the aortic root in entities such as tetralogy of Fallot. With this view, defects in the infundibular septum can be further classified as being below the crista supraventricularis (to the right of midline closer to the tricuspid valve) or above the crista (to the left of midline adjacent to the pulmonary valve as shown in Figure 5–14, bottom).

As the plane of sound is tilted inferiorly toward the cardiac apex, a short-axis view through the two atrioventricular valves can be obtained. This view allows visualization of the inlet septum (posteriorly and between the atrioventricular valves) as well as an anterior, superior portion of the trabecular septum (Fig 5–17,A and B).

Next, the scan plane can be tilted inferiorly to the level of the papillary muscles, which permits evaluation of the more inferior segments of the trabecular septum. Because the septum is imaged perpendicular to the scan plane, the resolution is maximized for imaging relatively small muscular defects (Fig 5–17,C). In addition, the presence of the T-artifact is helpful in defining the edges of the muscular defects. Many small defects do not cut straight across the septum, but follow a tortuous route through the septum. They are initially suspected when breaks are noted in the left-sided septal endocardial echo. Not all such breaks are true defects, although any break must be closely inspected to determine if it is a small ventricular septal defect.

Apical Four-Chamber View

The apical four-chamber view, with the scan plane passing through the tricuspid and mitral valves, images the inlet portion of the heart and is the best view for imaging the inlet septum. This view shows the extension of the defect toward the atrioventricular valves and the amount of tissue, if any, that remains between the valves and the defect (Fig 5–18). Even though the septum is parallel to the plane of sound, the imaging of large defects is preserved. Defects in the trabecular septum (the inferior two-thirds of the septum) can be detected in this view as well (Fig 5–18,B). Scanning ventrally from the inlet region allows imaging of the outlet portion of the heart and the infundibular septum. This view should be performed to confirm the diagnosis of an outlet defect that may have been suspected from the previous views. This view will also provide information about the alignment of the muscular and infundibular septa. Finally and most important, the chordal attachments of the atrioventricular valves can be fully assessed. This is critical when there is malalignment of the atrial and the inlet ventricular septa, as the atrioventricular valves may straddle the septum and make repair very difficult (Fig 5–19).[20] Careful assessment of the point of chordal attachment is critical to distinguish between a straddling valve, where some chordal attachments cross through the defect and insert into the opposite ven-

tricle, and an overriding valve, where the valve leaflet may float through the defect during diastole while the chordal attachments remain within the appropriate ventricle.

Subcostal Four-Chamber View

The subcostal four-chamber view provides information similar to the apical four-chamber view. However, the scan plane can be swept from the most dorsal aspects up to the outlet regions, permitting a thorough evaluation of the inlet and outlet regions (Figs 5–20 and 5–21). This view is particularly useful in assessing defects closely associated with the tricuspid valve and assessing the integrity of the portion of the trabecular septum closely associated with the inlet region of the heart.

Subcostal Sagittal View

Rotation of the scan plane from the subcostal four-chamber view provides the examiner with a subcostal sagittal view similar to the lateral angiogram. This view permits evaluation of the inferior trabecular septum, with the septum aligned perpendicular to the scan lines. It also provides an orthogonal view to the subcostal four-chamber plane and thus permits evaluation of the size of the defect in two different dimensions (Fig 5–22). It is particularly useful for assessing trabecular septal defects and defects closely related to the pulmonary valve.

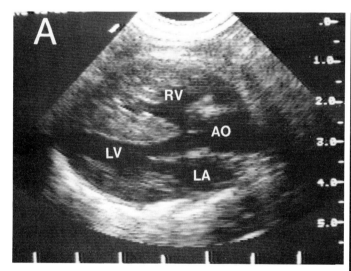
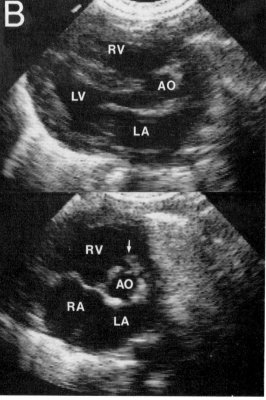

FIG 5–13.
A, parasternal long-axis view from a patient with pulmonary atresia and a ventricular septal defect. This ventricular septal defect is located in the outlet septum and associated with marked aortic (AO) override or septal-AO discontinuity. *LA* = left atrium; *LV* = left ventricle; and *RV* = right ventricle. **B,** parasternal long-axis view *(top)* from a patient with a small ventricular septal defect in the outlet septum and a minor amount of aortic (AO) override. Parasternal short-axis view *(bottom)* from the same patient. In this view mild malalignment between the infundibular septum *(arrow)* and the remainder of the membranous and outlet septum is seen. This defect is located within the crista supraventricularis. *LA* = left atrium; *LV* = left ventricle; and *RV* = right ventricle.

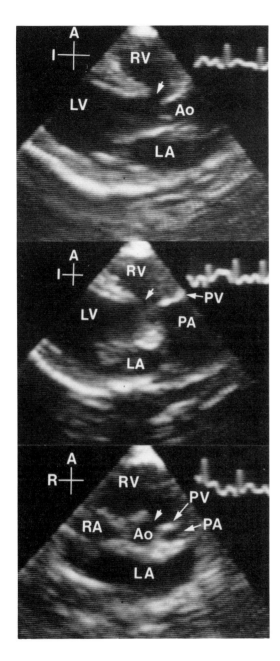

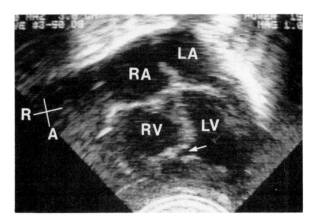

FIG 5–15.
Apical four-chamber view from a patient with a small ventricular septal defect *(arrow)* located in the apical portion of the trabecular septum. This figure shows that the edges of a ventricular septal defect are very bright and form a T artifact; this helps distinguish a real defect from artificial echo dropout. *A* = anterior; *LA* = left atrium; *LV* = left ventricle; *R* = right; *RA* = right atrium; and *RV* = right ventricle.

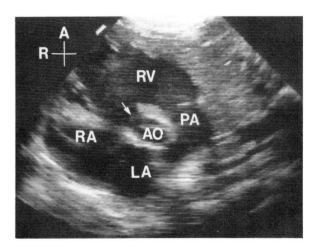

FIG 5–16.
Parasternal short-axis view at the base of the heart from a patient with a perimembranous outlet ventricular septal defect *(arrow)*. The defect extends from the region of the septal leaflet of the tricuspid valve and is located just beneath the aortic (AO) valve. *A* = anterior; *LA* = left atrium; *PA* = pulmonary artery; *R* = right; *RA* = right atrium; and *RV* = right ventricle.

FIG 5–14.
Parasternal views from a patient with an outlet defect located above the crista supraventricularis (supracristal ventricular septal defect). In the parasternal long-axis view *(top)*, the defect *(arrow)* is located just beneath the aortic (Ao) root. From this view alone, it is not possible to tell if the defect is above or below the crista supraventricularis. In the *middle frame*, the plane of sound has been tilted toward the patient's left to obtain a parasternal long-axis view of the right ventricular (RV) outflow tract. In this view, the defect *(arrow)* can be seen extending to the septum just beneath the pulmonary valve (PV). This indicates that the defect is located above the crista supraventricularis. In the parasternal short-axis view *(bottom)*, the ventricular septal defect *(arrow)* is located far to the left between the Ao and PV. *A* = anterior; *I* = inferior; *LA* = left atrium; *LV* = left ventricle; *PA* = pulmonary artery; and *RA* = right atrium.

Sensitivity and Specificity of Two-Dimensional Echocardiography

Two-dimensional echocardiography has been reported to be 100% sensitive in the detection of outlet and inlet ventricular septal defects. In infants less than 1 year of age, the sensitivity for detecting membranous ventricular septal defects has ranged from 74% to 87%.[21–23] Trabecular ventricular septal defects are the most difficult to

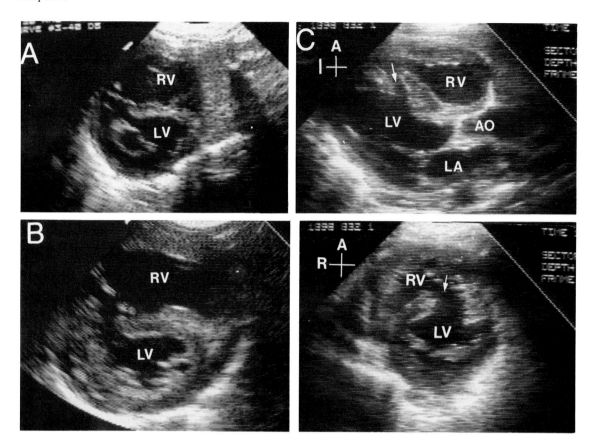

FIG 5–17.
A, parasternal short-axis view at the level of the atrioventricular valves in a patient with a large inlet ventricular septal defect, situated posteriorly between the leaflets of the two atrioventricular valves. **B,** parasternal short-axis view at the level of the left ventricular (LV) papillary muscles in a patient with a large inlet ventricular septal defect extending into the trabecular septum. This defect is located posteriorly and extends inferiorly. **C,** parasternal long-axis *(top)* and short-axis *(bottom)* views from a patient with a sizeable muscular ventricular septal defect *(arrows)*. This defect is located in the inferior or apical portion of the ventricular septum. Unlike the defect shown in Figure 5–17B, this defect is located anteriorly and is not related to the atrioventricular valves. *A* = anterior; *AO* = aorta; *I* = inferior; *LA* = left atrium; *LV* = left ventricle; *R* = right; and *RV* = right ventricle.

detect with two-dimensional echocardiography, and sensitivity has been reported to be as low as 30% in some prospective studies. Several factors make direct visualization of these muscular ventricular septal defects very difficult. First, they can occur anywhere in the wide area of the septum that is the trabecular septum. Second, these defects are often serpiginous, so that the right septal surface of the defect may not be visualized simultaneously with the left septal surface of the defect. Third, these defects may change size and virtually obliterate in systole. Finally, they may be hidden on the right septal surface by septo-parietal muscle bundles within the right ventricle. With the introduction of pulsed, continuous-wave, and color-flow Doppler techniques, the sensitivity in detecting ventricular septal defects has improved considerably.

Indirect Evidence of a Ventricular Septal Defect

In patients with a moderate-sized or large ventricular septal defect and normal pulmonary vascular resistance, the increased pulmonary blood flow and increased pulmonary venous return cause dilatation of the left atrium and left ventricle. Enlargement of the left heart can be detected in the parasternal and apical long-axis views and in the apical and subcostal four-chamber views. In the four-chamber views, the atrial septum bulges prominently, with its convexity toward the right. Because of the increased left ventricular preload, the left ventricular stroke volume is increased. Exaggerated septal and left ventricular posterior wall motion can be seen in several views. These signs of left ventricular volume overload are not specific for ventricular septal defects but can be seen in other defects causing left ventricular volume overload (i.e., in patent ductus arteriosus or mitral insufficiency).

Recent studies have shown a poor correlation between left atrial size and shunt magnitude, especially in older children. This may relate to several factors, including a decrease in compliance or distensibility of the left atrium with advancing age, or persistent left atrial enlargement

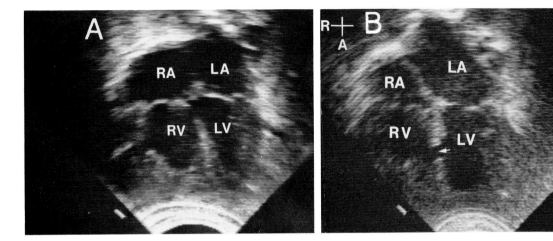

FIG 5–18.
A, apical four-chamber view from a patient with a large inlet ventricular septal defect. This defect is located superiorly and posteriorly between the atrioventricular valves. Note that the atrioventricular valves are at separate heights, which distinguishes this patient from one with an atrioventricular septal defect. **B,** apical four-chamber view from a patient with a midmuscular *(arrow)* ventricular septal defect. This defect is also located posteriorly but, unlike the defect shown in Figure 5–18A, is located in the middle one-third of the ventricular septum. Thus, the defect is located entirely within the trabecular septum. *A* = anterior; *LA* = left atrium; *LV* = left ventricle; *R* = right; *RA* = right atrium; and *RV* = right ventricle.

following spontaneous closure of a previously large ventricular septal defect. In an infant or young child in whom the left atrium is extremely compliant and spontaneous closure of the ventricular septal defect has not begun, left atrial size is a better indicator of the shunt volume.

In patients with small ventricular septal defects, the left atrium and left ventricle are usually of normal size. If the defect is not visualized in these patients, the two-dimensional echocardiogram may appear entirely normal.

In patients with an isolated ventricular septal defect and normal pulmonary vascular resistance, the right ventricular anterior wall and left ventricular posterior wall are of normal thickness. If a thickened left ventricular posterior wall is present, additional defects such as coarctation of the aorta or aortic valve stenosis should be sought. In patients with an isolated ventricular septal defect and elevated pulmonary vascular resistance, the right ventricular anterior wall thickness is increased and the left atrium and left ventricle are often of normal size.

Contrast Studies

Echocardiographic contrast studies are a mechanism for evaluating the hemodynamic effects of ventricular septal defects. Before Doppler techniques were developed for assessing right ventricular systolic pressure, contrast studies provided a means of assessing the degree of right ventricular hypertension. This method was based upon the discovery of a transient right-to-left shunt through the ventricular septal defect that occurred in diastole with moderate elevation of right ventricular pressure, even though there was no net right-to-left shunt.[24] With a nonrestrictive defect and equalization of the right and left ventricular

pressures, a small but definite right-to-left shunt was present, even though the predominant shunt was left-to-right. This was easily seen using both M-mode and two-dimensional techniques. Such studies are useful for assessing the presence of right-to-left shunting and the ventricular flow patterns. However, their usefulness for assessing the degree

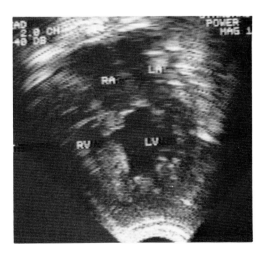

FIG 5–19.
Apical four-chamber view from a patient with a large inlet ventricular septal defect and malalignment between the atrial and ventricular septa. As a result, the tricuspid valve overrides the ventricular septal defect. In this patient, all of the tricuspid valve chordal attachments were into the right ventricle (RV); therefore, the tricuspid valve did not straddle the defect. *LA* = left atrium; *LV* = left ventricle; and *RA* = right atrium.

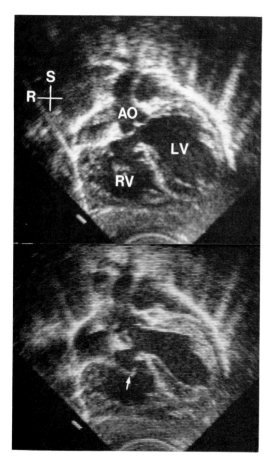

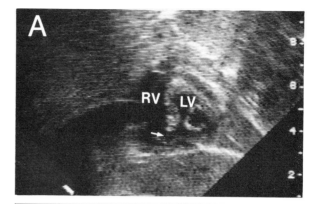

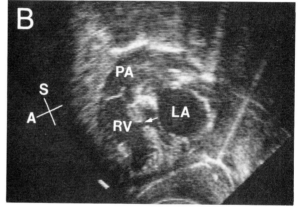

FIG 5–20.
Subcostal four-chamber views through the left ventricular (LV) out-flow tract of a patient with a large outlet ventricular septal defect and aortic (AO) override. In the *top frame,* taken in diastole, the aortic valve is seen to override the ventricular septum. In the *bottom frame,* taken during systole, a chordal attachment *(arrow)* of the tricuspid valve to the crest of the ventricular septum is seen. *R* = right; *RV* = right ventricle; and *S* = superior.

FIG 5–22.
A, subcostal sagittal view from a patient with a large inlet ventricular septal defect *(arrow)*. The inlet ventricular septal defect is located posteriorly and superiorly in the ventricular septum. **B,** subcostal sagittal view from a patient with a membranous ventricular septal defect *(arrow)*. This defect is located high in the ventricular septum just beneath the aortic valve and is separated from the pulmonary valve by the outlet septum above. *A* = anterior; *LA* = left atrium; *PA* = pulmonary artery; *RV* = right ventricle; and *S* = superior.

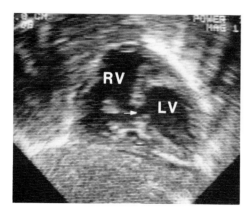

FIG 5–21.
Subcostal coronal view of the right ventricular (RV) outflow tract from a patient with an apical muscular ventricular septal defect *(arrow)*. *LV* = left ventricle.

of right ventricular hypertension has largely been supplanted by Doppler techniques.

Doppler Evaluation
Doppler evaluation of ventricular septal defects is useful in many ways. For small defects that are difficult to image, particularly those in the trabecular septum, the finding of a high velocity systolic jet from the left to the right ventricle is diagnostic of such a small defect.[25] The use of color Doppler to localize small defects is now preferable to single-gated Doppler studies because this technique is more rapid and multiple defects are readily apparent.

In children with ventricular septal defects and left ventricular pressure higher than right ventricular pressure, a systolic jet can be recorded in the right ventricle on the Doppler examination.[16, 25–27] The right ventricle can be scanned with either continuous-wave or pulsed Doppler ultrasound; scanning can be performed from several locations, including left parasternal, apical, and subcostal positions. From a left parasternal position, the jet from the ventricular septal defect is oriented toward the transducer and usually extends throughout systole (Fig 5–23). In most instances, the systolic velocities are high because left ventricular systolic pressure is much higher than right ventricular systolic pressure; however, with very large defects and systemic right ventricular pressure, systolic velocities may be low (less than 2.5 m/sec) or not recorded at all.[28] Although left-to-right shunting occurs throughout systole in most small or moderate-sized ventricular septal defects, in some small muscular ventricular septal defects the systolic jet occupies only a short portion of early systole, presumably because the muscular defect closes in midsystole with ventricular contraction. In most small or moderate-

sized ventricular septal defects, left-to-right shunting also extends into diastole because left ventricular diastolic pressure exceeds right ventricular diastolic pressure.[16] In these cases, a low-velocity diastolic flow is seen on the Doppler examination, which peaks in early diastole and with atrial contraction (Fig 5–24). This diastolic shunt flow will disappear if there are associated lesions (i.e., severe tricuspid or pulmonary insufficiency) that cause an elevated right ventricular diastolic pressure. In patients with large left-to-right ventricular shunts, Doppler examination of the pulmonary artery shows an increased velocity (because of increased flow) and spectral broadening (because of the persistence of disturbed flow downstream from the defect).

Doppler color-flow mapping has had major application in the rapid detection of septal defects (Plates 11 to 15). With this technique, blood flow can be seen crossing defects that are too small to be visualized directly on the two-dimensional echocardiogram. In a recent study, the abilities of color Doppler and angiography to detect multiple muscular ventricular septal defects were compared. The color Doppler technique correctly identified 72% of all patients proven by angiography to have multiple muscular defects. No false-positive diagnoses were made with the color Doppler technique.[29]

In patients with ventricular septal defects and no right or left ventricular outflow obstruction, the pressure difference between the left and right ventricles can be calculated from the peak velocity of the systolic jet.[16] For this calculation, a simplified Bernoulli equation is used (Fig 5–25):

$$\text{Pressure gradient} = 4 \times (\text{peak velocity})^2$$

If the arm blood pressure is obtained at the time of the Doppler examination, the right ventricular systolic pressure can be calculated as:

$$\text{RV systolic pressure} = \text{systolic arm blood pressure} - 4 \times (\text{peak velocity})^2$$

Using this equation, good correlations have been found between Doppler and cardiac catheterization measurements of right ventricular systolic pressure.[28, 30] If an adequate recording of the peak velocity of the jet through the ventricular septal defect cannot be obtained, the right ventricular systolic pressure can be estimated from the peak velocity of the tricuspid insufficiency jet using the following equation:

$$\text{RV systolic pressure} = 4 \times (\text{peak velocity})^2 + \text{right atrial pressure}$$

Most children, and especially those with right ventricular hypertension, have at least a small tricuspid insufficiency jet that can be used to estimate right ventricular systolic pressure. Right atrial pressure can be estimated from the amount of jugular venous distension, can be assumed to

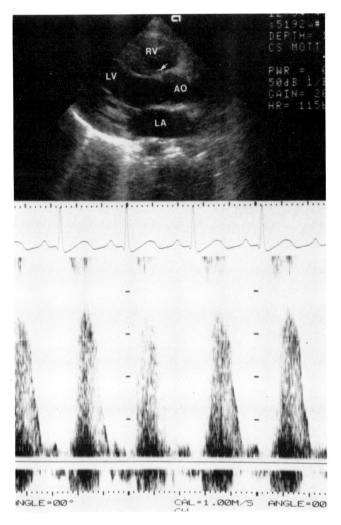

FIG 5–23.
Doppler recording *(bottom)* from the parasternal long-axis view *(top)* of a patient with a tiny membranous ventricular septal defect. Flow through the ventricular septal defect from the left ventricle (LV) to the right ventricle (RV) is toward the transducer and therefore displayed above the baseline in systole. The peak velocity of the systolic jet is 3.5 m/sec, which predicts a 49 mm Hg pressure gradient across the defect. AO = aorta; LA = left atrium.

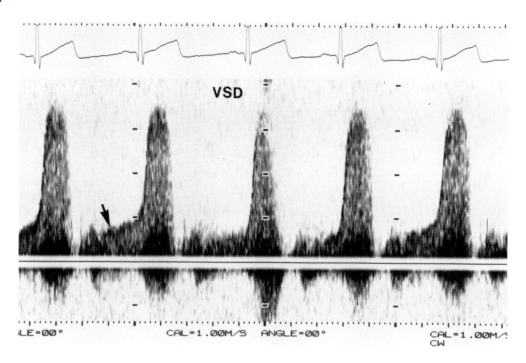

FIG 5–24.
Continuous-wave Doppler recording from the low parasternal region of a patient with a muscular ventricular septal defect. In systole, a high-velocity jet is seen above the baseline, indicating a large pressure gradient in systole between the left ventricle and right ventricle. In addition, flow signals are seen above the baseline *(arrow)* throughout diastole, indicating continued flow across the ventricular septal defect during diastole because of a diastolic pressure gradient between the left ventricle and right ventricle. This type of tracing is often seen in very restrictive ventricular septal defects in which a pressure gradient exists in systole and diastole between the ventricles.

be normal (8 to 10 mm Hg), or can be measured if a central venous line is in place.

As discussed in Chapter 4, the Doppler technique is also useful for quantitation of the pulmonary and systemic blood flows in children with ventricular septal defects.

Associated Lesions

In addition to evaluating the ventricular septal defect, the examiner must closely evaluate the heart for associated defects. The most common such lesion is the ventricular septal aneurysm,[31] which is comprised of thin tissue arising from the margins of the defect. The defect itself may be large; yet, because of obstruction of flow by the aneurysm tissue, the degree of left-to-right shunting may be small. In some cases, the formation of an aneurysm may be a prelude to spontaneous closure.[32] The aneurysm is highly mobile, protruding into the right ventricle during systole and realigning with the ventricular septum in diastole. Because the walls of the aneurysm are thin, multiple views are often needed to accurately identify it. The parasternal long- and short-axis views and the apical four-chamber view tend to be most useful (Figs 5–26 to 5–28). Care must be taken to distinguish the aneurysm from redundant atrioventricular valve tissue, particularly the tricuspid valve. Such redundant tissue is most often seen in atrioventricular septal defects and is less common in isolated ventricular septal defects.[33]

Doppler examination of the aneurysm, particularly color-flow mapping, is mandatory to assess the patency of this structure. Most ventricular septal aneurysms are associated with less than systemic right ventricular pressure.[31] Nevertheless, because large left-to-right shunts may be present, careful assessment of pulmonary artery pressure is essential. Ventricular septal aneurysms often develop by incorporation of tissue from the septal leaflet of the tricuspid valve in the aneurysm. Involvement of the tricuspid septal leaflet may result in tricuspid regurgitation or left ventricular-to-right atrial shunting through the ventricular septal defect. Both of these associated defects can be detected by Doppler techniques.

Regurgitation of the atrioventricular valves is also common in children with ventricular septal defects. When left ventricular dilatation is present, mitral valve regurgitation is common and usually does not represent an intrinsic defect of the valve itself. Likewise, enlargement of the left atrium may result in stretching of the foramen ovale with a resultant left-to-right atrial shunt detectable by Doppler exam in the absence of a true atrial septal defect. This distinction can usually be made by careful examination of the atrial septum, as described previously.

Aortic regurgitation, a not infrequently associated lesion,[34, 35] usually occurs in older children and is more common in infundibular septal defects that permit prolapse of an aortic valve cusp. However, aortic regurgitation can also

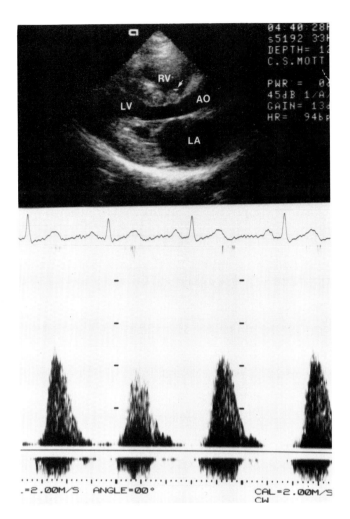

FIG 5–25.
Continuous-wave Doppler recording *(bottom)* from the parasternal long-axis view *(top)* of a patient with a small membranous ventricular septal defect. The *arrow* in the *top frame* indicates the position of the continuous-wave cursor line and transmit focus at the time of the Doppler recording. In the *bottom frame,* the Doppler tracing shows a high-velocity systolic flow directed toward the transducer and above the baseline. The peak velocity of this flow is 4.6 m/sec. The pressure gradient from the left ventricle (LV) to the right ventricle (RV) predicted by the simplified Bernoulli equation is 4×4.6^2 or 85 mm Hg. *AO* = aorta; *LA* = left atrium.

and trabecular septa. The concept of septal malalignment is important because of the serious consequences this malalignment has upon cardiac structure and function. Atrioventricular malalignment has been briefly reviewed above,

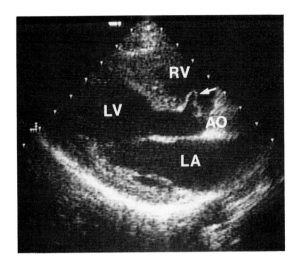

FIG 5–26.
Parasternal long-axis view from a patient with a membranous ventricular septal defect in the process of closing spontaneously by formation of a ventricular septal aneurysm *(arrow)*. The ventricular septal aneurysm is seen protruding into the right ventricle (RV). *AO* = aorta; *LA* = left atrium; and *LV* = left ventricle.

be associated with defects of the membranous septum as well. Careful Doppler examination of the left ventricular outflow tract is required, as well as careful imaging of the defect, to determine if a prolapsed aortic cusp is present.

Defects of Septal Malalignment

Malalignment may occur between the inlet ventricular septum and the atrial septum or between the infundibular

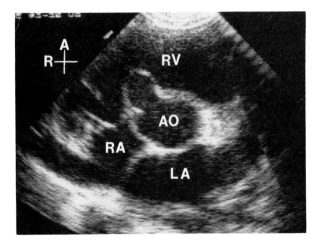

FIG 5–27.
Parasternal short-axis view from a patient with a membranous ventricular septal defect and a large ventricular septal aneurysm. The ventricular septal aneurysm is seen bulging into the right ventricle (RV). The aneurysm is located just adjacent to the septal leaflet of the tricuspid valve. The base of the aneurysm reflects the size of the original defect. *A* = anterior; *AO* = aorta; *LA* = left atrium; *R* = right; and *RA* = right atrium.

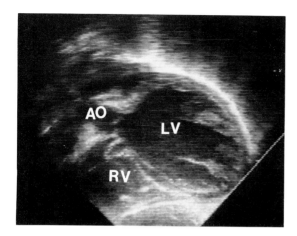

FIG 5–28.
Subcostal coronal view of the left ventricular (LV) outflow tract from a patient with a ventricular septal aneurysm. The ventricular septal aneurysm is seen just beneath the aortic (AO) valve and protruding into the right ventricle (RV).

in the discussion of straddling atrioventricular valves; because it usually occurs in the context of complex segmental abnormalities, it will be more fully discussed later. Malalignment of different segments of the ventricular septum will be discussed in this section.

When a coarctation and a ventricular septal defect coexist, the morphology of the ventricular septal defect may be altered in such a way that blood is diverted away from the aortic valve and subaortic obstruction is created.[36] Morphologic studies have shown the outlet septum to be deviated posteriorly and leftward, extending into the left ventricular outflow tract. The defect itself may also show extension into the membranous septum and/or the trabecular septum. The aortic annulus may be narrowed, and anomalies of the mitral valve may be present. While this type of defect does not occur in all patients with a concomitant coarctation, its incidence is high enough to warrant close examination when a coarctation is present.

Echocardiographically, this posterior deviation of the outlet septum is best seen in the parasternal long-axis view (Fig 5–29). The outlet septum extends posteriorly from the aortic annulus clearly malaligned with the trabecular septum.[37] Care must be taken to inspect this area closely. Doppler studies may show no gradient present when the ventricular septal defect is open, only to show a large gradient after closure. The surgical approach must be to resect this outlet septum when closing the defect if it has the potential for significant obstruction postoperatively.

In some infundibular ventricular septal defects, the infundibular septum is displaced anteriorly, creating aortic override without right ventricular outflow tract narrowing. These defects are generally quite large and are associated with systemic pulmonary artery pressure. Because of their natural history, they have been referred to as Eisenmenger ventricular septal defects (as opposed to Eisenmenger syndrome, which is the development of irreversible pulmo-

nary vascular changes associated with any type of intracardiac shunt).

Tetralogy of Fallot

Anterior and rightward deviation of the infundibular septum produces tetralogy of Fallot, with dextroposition and enlargement of the aorta and narrowing of the entire right ventricular outflow tract.[38, 39] The septal defect may be solely infundibular or it may extend into the membranous septum, which is the most common situation; in some cases it may extend into the inlet septum. The defect is usually situated anterior and superior to the tricuspid valve and beneath the right and noncoronary aortic cusps. The aortic root is enlarged, and the right ventricular outflow tract, the pulmonary annulus, and pulmonary arteries are small. The degree of aortic override is a function of the magnitude of malalignment and abnormal rotation of the infundibular and trabecular septa. Because its length is normal,[39] the outflow tract is not truly underdeveloped. Yet it is narrowed, producing the obstruction characteristic of tetralogy of Fallot.

The major views used to assess this lesion are the parasternal long-axis and short-axis views and the apical and subcostal four-chamber views.[40–42] The pulmonary arteries are assessed from the suprasternal notch views, as will be discussed below. Although the parasternal long-axis view allows estimation of the degree of septal override, it is not by itself diagnostic of tetralogy of Fallot (Fig 5–30). In this view, an isolated ventricular septal defect without right ventricular outflow tract obstruction, pulmonary atresia with a ventricular septal defect, and truncus arteriosus all may have the same general appearance. In this view, the examiner must assess the degree of aortic override, the presence or absence of aortic-mitral continuity, the size of the right ventricle, and the size of the aortic

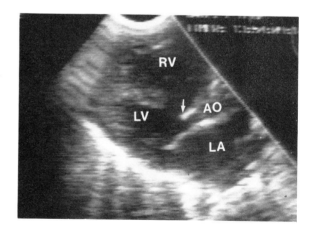

FIG 5–29.
Parasternal long-axis view from a patient with a large outlet ventricular septal defect and posterior deviation of the infundibular septum into the left ventricular (LV) outflow tract (arrow). This deviation causes marked subaortic stenosis. AO = aorta; LA = left atrium; and RV = right ventricle.

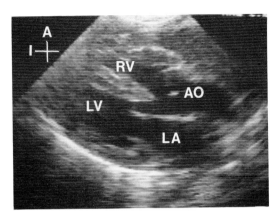

FIG 5–30.
Parasternal long-axis view from an infant with tetralogy of Fallot. A large outlet ventricular septal defect is present. There is discontinuity between the septum and the anterior wall of the aorta (AO). *A* = anterior; *I* = inferior; *LA* = left atrium; *LV* = left ventricle; and *RV* = right ventricle.

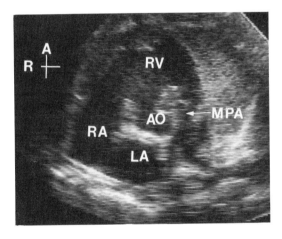

FIG 5–31.
Parasternal short-axis view from a patient with tetralogy of Fallot. There is uniform hypoplasia of the entire right ventricular (RV) outflow tract. The pulmonary valve annulus and the main pulmonary artery (MPA) are very small, as are the pulmonary artery branches. A large perimembranous outlet ventricular septal defect is present. *A* = anterior; *AO* = aorta; *LA* = left atrium; *R* = right; and *RA* = right atrium.

root. Finally, a careful search for defects of the trabecular septum must be made.

The parasternal short-axis view allows assessment of the degree of extension of the septal defect into other areas of the ventricular septum and the degree of narrowing of the right ventricular outflow tract (Fig 5–31). In the most usual form, the ventricular septal defect extends to the right, toward the tricuspid valve, and involves the membranous septum. In rare instances, the outlet defect extends to the left, above the crista supraventricularis and just be-

low the pulmonary valve. In the parasternal short-axis view in tetralogy of Fallot, the entire right ventricular outflow tract is narrowed (Fig 5–32), although a patent pulmonary valve with antegrade flow is seen by Doppler examination of the main pulmonary artery. The pulmonary valve is located anterior, superior, and leftward of the aortic valve. In pulmonary atresia with a ventricular septal defect, no pulmonary valve echo can be found in the parasternal short-axis view, and there is no Doppler evidence of antegrade blood flow in the main pulmonary artery. Usually, an imperforate membrane occupies the position where a pulmonary valve would normally be found; however, the right ventricular outflow tract sometimes ends blindly, with no evidence of a main pulmonary artery segment. Measurement of the pulmonary valve annulus diameter, which may be useful for planning the appropriate surgical approach, can be made in the parasternal short-axis view.

A small percentage of patients with tetralogy of Fallot have absence of the pulmonary valve leaflets, an unguarded pulmonary valve annulus, and severe pulmonary regurgitation. In the parasternal short-axis view in these patients, linear bright echoes are often seen in the location normally occupied by the valve leaflets, even though there is no echocardiographic evidence of valve leaflet motion (Fig 5–33). The bright echoes usually arise from the fibrous annulus or from a rim of tissue around the annulus. The main and branch pulmonary arteries (especially the right pulmonary artery) are massively dilated because of the severe pulmonary regurgitation. In addition, the right ventricle is dilated and has exaggerated contractility. Doppler echocardiography shows evidence of severe pulmonary regurgitation.

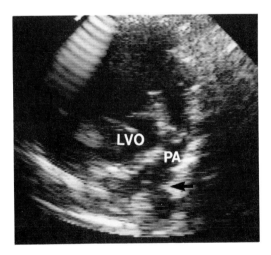

FIG 5–32.
Parasternal short-axis view from a patient with tetralogy of Fallot. The entire right ventricular (RV) outflow tract is underdeveloped. The pulmonary valve annulus is small and the pulmonary valve leaflets are thickened. There is narrowing at the pulmonary artery bifurcation *(arrow)*. *LVO* = left ventricular outflow tract; *PA* = pulmonary artery.

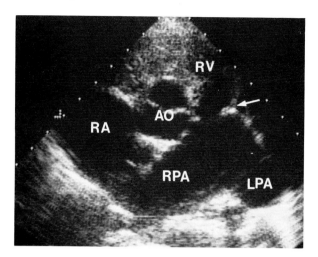

FIG 5–33.
Parasternal short-axis view from a patient with tetralogy of Fallot and an absent pulmonary valve. In the area of the pulmonary valve annulus *(arrow)*, no evidence of leaflet tissue is seen. The right ventricle (RV) is massively dilated because of severe pulmonary regurgitation. In addition, the right pulmonary artery (RPA) is also dilated because of the combination of pulmonary stenosis and pulmonary regurgitation. *AO* = aorta; *RA* = right atrium.

Another small percentage of patients with tetralogy of Fallot have anomalous origin of the left anterior descending coronary artery from the right main coronary artery. After its origin from the right coronary artery, the left anterior descending coronary artery crosses the right ventricular outflow tract anteriorly to reach the ventricular septum. In most infants, the bifurcation of the left main coronary artery can easily be visualized in the parasternal short-axis view. Failure to image a bifurcation of the left main coronary artery into two distinct, clearly seen branches is a warning of the possible diagnosis of anomalous origin of the left anterior descending coronary artery. If the diagnosis is suspected, the anomalous artery can often be visualized coursing anterior to the right ventricular outflow tract in the parasternal short-axis view.

The apical four-chamber view is used to assess the degree of infundibular—trabecular septal malalignment, with the resultant rightward deviation of the aorta. This is also a useful view from which to assess the left ventricular outflow tract (Fig 5–34). Obstruction either from a discrete membrane or fibromuscular ridge may coexist and may be difficult to assess from the pressure gradient measurement alone. Doppler interrogation of flow from this position is useful in assessing both atrioventricular and aortic valve insufficiency.

The subcostal views in both the coronal and sagittal projections are extremely useful for assessing the right ventricular outflow tract (Figs 5–35 and 5–36). In the coronal projection, the scan plane is angled anteriorly, bringing the right ventricular outflow tract into view. The degree of infundibular hypoplasia and the degree of muscular hypertrophy are assessed. Particular attention must be paid

to the crista supraventricularis and the presence or absence of additional muscle bands that may coexist more inferior within the ventricle. The sagittal view also provides an excellent assessment of the right ventricular outflow tract in a view orthogonal to the coronal view. Together, these two views provide the anatomic detail needed to plan a surgical approach.

Of paramount importance is careful assessment of the size of the branch pulmonary arteries as far distally as possible. This is particularly important if a surgical systemic-to-pulmonary artery shunt has been placed. The best views for pulmonary artery evaluation are the suprasternal

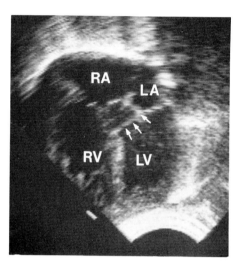

FIG 5–34.
Apical four-chamber view from a patient with tetralogy of Fallot. This view was taken in systole, with the atrioventricular valves in the closed position and with the transducer tilted slightly anteriorly to visualize a mitral valve chord *(arrow)* crossing the ventricular septal defect to insert into a papillary muscle in the right ventricle (RV). *LA* = left atrium; *LV* = left ventricle; and *RA* = right atrium.

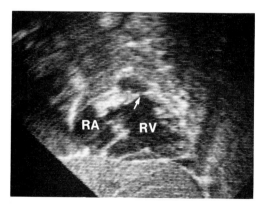

FIG 5–35.
Subcostal coronal view of the right ventricle (RV) from a patient with tetralogy of Fallot and severe infundibular pulmonary stenosis. A prominent muscle bundle *(arrow)* is seen crossing the RV outflow tract in the area of the crista supraventricularis. *RA* = right atrium.

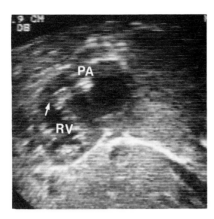

FIG 5–36.
Subcostal sagittal view of the right ventricle (RV) from a patient with tetralogy of Fallot and marked muscular infundibular stenosis *(arrow)*. *PA* = pulmonary artery.

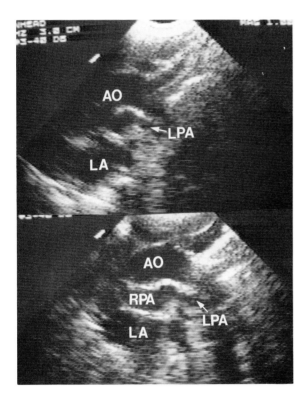

FIG 5–37.
Suprasternal views from a patient with tetralogy of Fallot and uniform narrowing of the left pulmonary artery (LPA). In the suprasternal long-axis view *(top)*, the LPA becomes very narrow at its origin from the main pulmonary artery. In the suprasternal short-axis view *(bottom)*, the confluence of the right pulmonary artery (RPA) and LPA is seen. In this view, the discrepancy in the sizes of the branch pulmonary arteries is quite evident. *AO* = aorta; *LA* = left atrium.

long- and short-axis views (Figs 5–37 and 5–38). The suprasternal short-axis view is obtained to image the pulmonary artery bifurcation, which is seen to the left of the aorta. The right pulmonary artery, seen coursing under the aorta, can be followed usually to the origin of the upper lobe branch. The diameter of the right pulmonary artery should be measured as it passes behind the ascending aorta. If the transducer is moved inferiorly and tilted superiorly, a long segment of the left pulmonary artery can frequently be seen. This view is particularly useful for determining if the right and left pulmonary arteries are anatomically continuous.

The suprasternal long-axis view is used to assess the left pulmonary artery as it arches posteriorly and leftward. Its diameter can be measured at this point. This measurement and the size of the right pulmonary artery are then compared with the diameter of the descending aorta, measured from a transverse view of the abdomen at the level of the diaphragm. These measurements can then be compared to published data to allow assessment of the adequacy of the pulmonary artery size for total repair.[43] In general, the ratio of the sum of the pulmonary artery diameters to the descending aortic diameter should exceed 1.5. Finally, the aortic arch is imaged with the arch anatomy visualized. By noting the position of the tracheal air column, the position of the arch relative to the trachea can be determined. This allows diagnosis of a right aortic arch, as will be discussed in a subsequent chapter.

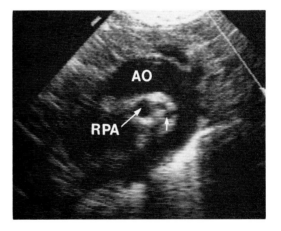

FIG 5–38.
Suprasternal long-axis view from a newborn infant with severe tetralogy of Fallot and a patent ductus arteriosus *(arrow)*. The patent ductus arteriosus is long, tortuous, and oriented in a reverse fashion. There is no evidence of narrowing of the aortic (AO) isthmus. These findings suggest altered fetal flow pathways caused by severe right ventricular outflow tract obstruction in utero. *RPA* = right pulmonary artery.

ANOMALIES OF THE ATRIOVENTRICULAR REGION

Anatomy

Atrioventricular septal defects occur because of failure of partitioning of the embryonic atrioventricular canal. This results in a confluent defect that involves the ostium primum, the atrioventricular canal, and the interventricular foramen. Atrioventricular septal defects have a common atrioventricular valve that contains superior (anterior) and inferior (posterior) bridging leaflets, as well as left lateral, right lateral, and right accessory leaflets.[44, 45] The common atrioventricular valve can have an undivided common orifice or can be divided into right- and left-sided orifices by a tongue of tissue that connects the superior and inferior bridging leaflets. The common atrioventricular valve can be displaced downward into the ventricle and anchored to the crest of the muscular septum, thus allowing left-to-right shunting to occur only above the valve at atrial level (the so-called partial form), or it can float freely in the septal defect, allowing shunting to occur above and below the valve at atrial and ventricular levels (the so-called complete form). In addition, depending on the position of the valve leaflets, intermediate forms of atrioventricular septal defects (incomplete forms) can occur.

Two-dimensional echocardiography has been particularly useful for defining the morphology and attachments of the atrioventricular valve leaflets, for determining the level of the left-to-right shunt, and for estimating the sizes of the right and left ventricles.[46] Some two-dimensional echocardiographic findings common to all variants of atrioventricular septal defect include (1) deficiency of the inlet portion of the ventricular septum; (2) displacement of the atrioventricular valve inferiorly; (3) lack of two separate fibrous valve rings at different distances from the cardiac apex; and (4) attachment of the left half of the common atrioventricular valve to the ventricular septum, with resulting orientation of the valve into the left ventricular outflow tract. From a surgical perspective, the important anatomic questions that need to be addressed are:

1. What is the extent of the atrial communication?
2. What is the extent of the ventricular communication and the nature of the tissue that separates the atrioventricular valves from the trabecular septum?
3. What is the anatomy of the atrioventricular valves and their chordal attachments?
4. What is the distribution of the atrioventricular valve tissue between the two ventricles?
5. What is the degree of atrioventricular valve insufficiency?
6. What is the degree of ventriculoatrial septal malalignment and what are the resultant sizes of the ventricular inflow tracts?
7. Are other associated lesions present?

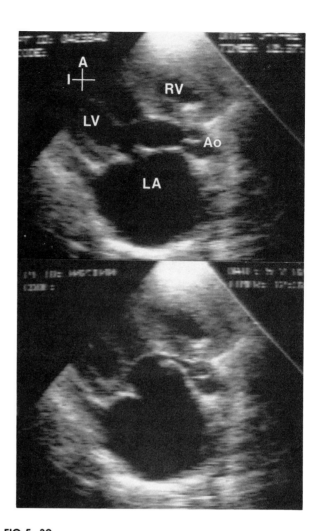

FIG 5–39.
Parasternal long-axis views in systole *(top)* and diastole *(bottom)* from a patient with an atrioventricular septal defect. Note the orientation of the left half of the common atrioventricular valve into the left ventricular (LV) outflow tract. This creates the appearance of a gooseneck deformity of the LV outflow tract. A = anterior; AO = aorta; I = inferior; LA = left atrium; and RV = right ventricle.

Echocardiographic Views

Parasternal Long Axis View

The parasternal long-axis view provides little information for evaluating the ventricular septal defect, as the inlet septum is not seen in this view. However, the inferior and anterior displacement of the left atrioventricular valve is seen with the leaflet tips pointing up toward the septum rather than toward the ventricular apex (Fig 5–39).[46] This orientation of the left atrioventricular valve often gives the examiner the first clue that an atrioventricular septal defect is present. In addition, the left ventricular outflow tract needs to be carefully evaluated for the presence of chordal attachments of the atrioventricular valve apparatus crossing the outflow tract (Fig 5–40). Discrete membranous sub-aortic obstruction may also be present.[47, 48]

This view is also useful for evaluating associated defects of the outlet septum and the trabecular septum. The concomitant occurrence of atrioventricular septal defect and tetralogy of Fallot is well described,[49] and associated trabecular or muscular defects are common. The left ventricular, right ventricular, and left atrial size should also be noted.

Parasternal Short-Axis View

The parasternal short-axis view at the level of the papillary muscles is useful for determining the number and location of the papillary muscles of the left ventricle,[50] the presence of a cleft in the anterior mitral valve leaflet,[46] and the presence of associated trabecular defects. The left ventricular papillary muscles are displaced in atrioventricular septal defects, with the anterolateral papillary muscle rotated anteriorly, moving from about 5-o'clock to 3-o'clock if the left ventricular cross-section is seen as a clock face. While this is of little clinical significance, the absence of one papillary muscle often creates a situation that necessitates valve replacement (Fig 5–41). Such abnormalities have been reported in as many as 20% of patients with atrioventricular septal defects.[50] Also, if chordal attachments are not equally divided between the papillary muscles, this is apparent and raises the possibility of an unrepairable atrioventricular valve (Fig 5–42).

Scanning slightly superiorly, the anterior valve leaflet is seen. Clefts are easily recognized by the diastolic separation of this leaflet into two segments with their tips pointing toward the ventricular septum (Fig 5–43).[46] The cleft is most easily seen when there are two separate atrioventricular valve orifices. In this situation, the cleft in the anterior mitral leaflet actually represents a space between

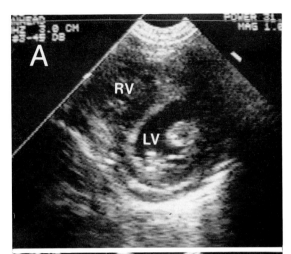

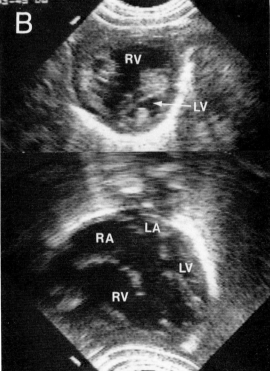

FIG 5–41.

A, parasternal short-axis view at the level of the papillary muscles in a patient with atrioventricular septal defect. The papillary muscles are rotated counterclockwise from their position in the normal left ventricle (LV). This rotation is commonly found in patients with atrioventricular septal defect. The anterolateral papillary muscle is considerably larger than the posteromedial papillary muscle. **B,** parasternal short-axis *(top)* and apical four-chamber *(bottom)* views from a patient with an atrioventricular septal defect and a small left ventricle (LV). This patient had a single papillary muscle in the LV. In addition, only a small portion of the common atrioventricular valve orifice was committed to the LV. *LA* = left atrium; *RA* = right atrium; and *RV* = right ventricle.

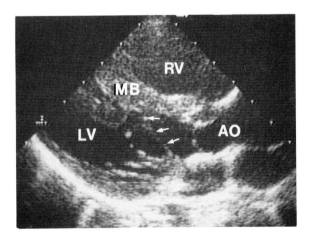

FIG 5–40.

Parasternal long-axis view from a patient with an atrioventricular septal defect. Chordae from the left half of the common atrioventricular valve *(arrows)* cross the defect and insert into a prominent muscle bundle (MB) that lies along the right side of the ventricular septum. *AO* = aorta; *LV* = left ventricle; and *RV* = right ventricle.

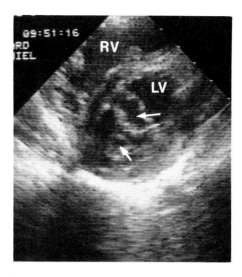

FIG 5–42.
Parasternal short-axis view from a patient with an atrioventricular septal defect and a double-orifice mitral valve. The atrioventricular valve is divided by aberrant tissue connections into a large orifice and a smaller accessory orifice (arrows). Double-orifice mitral valve with unequal orifice sizes is common in atrioventricular septal defect. LV = left ventricle; RV = right ventricle.

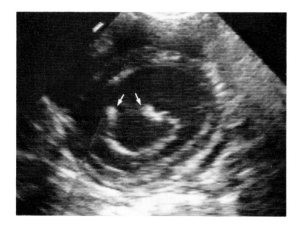

FIG 5–43.
Parasternal short-axis view of the left atrioventricular valve of a patient with atrioventricular septal defect. A cleft, seen in the anterior mitral valve leaflet (arrows), really represents the space between the left halves of the superior and inferior bridging leaflets.

the left halves of the anterior and posterior bridging leaflets. In reality, clefts or spaces can exist between any of the five leaflets of the common atrioventricular valve; regurgitation can occur through any of these clefts. Color-flow mapping techniques permit direct visualization of the origin of insufficiency jets in patients with atrioventricular septal defect. In color-flow Doppler, most patients can be seen to have valve insufficiency jets that originate from several clefts or spaces between the valve leaflets.

Continued superior angulation to image the area just inferior to the aortic valve permits evaluation of any extension of the septal defect into the membranous septum. Frequently, redundant atrioventricular valve tissue can be seen protruding into the right ventricle in systole near the right atrioventricular valve. This tissue closely resembles a ventricular septal aneurysm and has been called a tricuspid pouch (Fig 5–44). Defects are not confined to the inlet or membranous septum and may extend through the membranous septum into the infundibular septum, especially if concomitant defects such as tetralogy of Fallot are present.

Apical Four-Chamber View
Because the apical four-chamber view permits detailed examination of the inlet portion of the heart, it is very important in describing atrioventricular septal defects.[51] The examination should begin with imaging of the atrioventricular valve tissue, the inlet ventricular septum, and the atrial septum (Fig 5–45). This permits assessment of the degree of atrial communication, the degree of ventricular communication, and the distribution of the atrioventricular valve tissue between the two ventricles. Although an inferior or primum atrial septal defect is usually present, this is not always the case (Figs 5–46 and 5–47).[51, 52] For example, the bridging tongue of tissue that divides the common atrioventricular valve into two separate orifices can be fused to the inferior rim of the atrial septum, thus obliterating the atrial communication and allowing shunting only at the ventricular level.

Considered next are the ventricles and their relative sizes, which may be assessed qualitatively from inspection of the relative ventricular sizes or quantitatively from the ratio of right ventricular to left ventricular end-diastolic

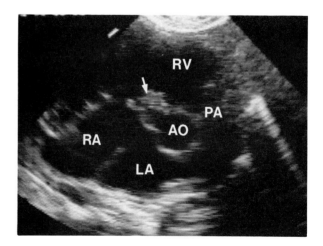

FIG 5–44.
Parasternal short-axis view from a patient with an atrioventricular septal defect and a tricuspid pouch (arrow). The tricuspid pouch really represents accessory atrioventricular valve tissue in the region of the atrioventricular septal defect. AO = aorta; LA = left atrium; PA = pulmonary artery; RA = right atrium; and RV = right ventricle.

atrioventricular valve into two orifices adheres to the crest of the muscular septum. Also, the ventricular communication may be partially or completely closed by either matted chordal attachments to the septal crest or by atrioventricular valve tissue that usually arises from the right half of the anterior bridging leaflet (Fig 5–51).[54] Such pouches need to be identified, for they often require surgical resection at the time of repair, leaving a ventricular communication that will then need to be closed.

Finally, close examination of the atrioventricular valve

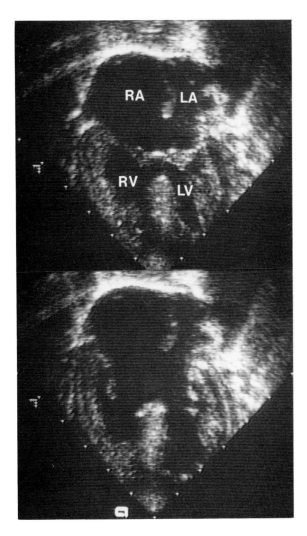

FIG 5–45.
Apical four-chamber views in systole *(above)* and diastole *(below)* from a patient with an atrioventricular septal defect. When the atrioventricular valve opens in diastole, a large deficiency in the inlet ventricular septum can be seen. In systole, the valve is attached to the crest of the ventricular septum by chordae. Because the atrioventricular valve is not tethered to the crest of the ventricular septum, shunting can occur at both atrial and ventricular levels. Note that there is a common atrioventricular valve, instead of two separate atrioventricular valves situated at separate heights in the ventricles. The common atrioventricular valve is displaced inferiorly into the heart because of the deficiency in the inlet ventricular septum. *LA* = left atrium; *LV* = left ventricle; *RA* = right atrium; and *RV* = right ventricle.

dimensions.[53] In this view, assessment of the chordal attachments is just as important as determination of the ventricular sizes (Fig 5–48). Unequal division of the atrioventricular valve tissue between the two ventricles is surgically important, often making repair impossible (Figs 5–49 and 5–50). Next, the degree of inlet septal deficiency is examined. Large ventricular communications may be present, or no ventricular communication may be present if the bridging tongue of tissue that divides the common

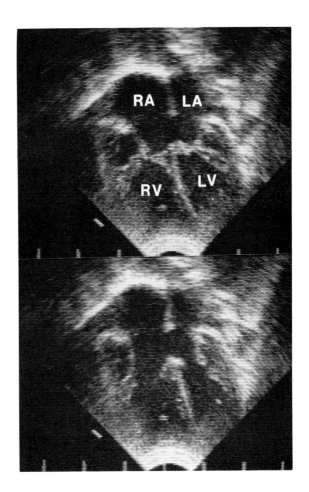

FIG 5–46.
Apical four-chamber views in systole *(above)* and diastole *(below)* from a patient with an atrioventricular septal defect. In this patient, the common atrioventricular valve had a bridging tongue of tissue that connected the superior and inferior bridging leaflets. This tongue of tissue divided the common atrioventricular valve into two separate orifices. In addition, the atrioventricular valve was tethered to the crest of the ventricular septum along the length of the bridging tongue of tissue. Therefore, shunting could occur only at atrial level. The common atrioventricular valve is displaced inferiorly in the heart and anchored to the crest of the ventricular septum. When the valve is closed in systole, there is no ventricular septal defect. This type of atrioventricular septal defect is commonly called a primum atrial septal defect. *LA* = left atrium; *LV* = left ventricle; *RA* = right atrium; and *RV* = right ventricle.

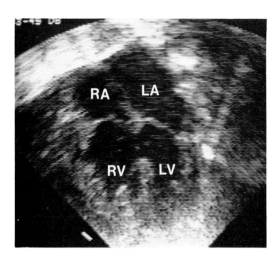

FIG 5–47.
Apical four-chamber view from a patient with an atrioventricular septal defect. This patient, like the one in Figure 5–46, had a common atrioventricular valve with two separate orifices. In this patient, however, the common atrioventricular valve was attached along the bridging tongue of tissue to the undersurface of the atrial septum. Thus, in systole, shunting could occur only at ventricular level. There is no atrial septal defect. This defect is commonly called a ventricular septal defect of the atrioventricular canal type. Both the right half and left half of the common atrioventricular valve prolapse in systole. *LA* = left atrium; *LV* = left ventricle; *RA* = right atrium; and *RV* = right ventricle.

tissue itself is performed. The apical four-chamber view is useful for assessing chordal attachments; the number of valve orifices, however, cannot be determined from this view and are better evaluated with subcostal views.

Chordal attachments of the valve leaflets are well visualized in the apical four-chamber view. The degree of chordal attachment to the crest of the septum is seen. Chordae that cross from one side of the atrioventricular valve to insert in the contralateral ventricle create a difficult surgical problem. This situation can be imaged by carefully tracking the major chordae individually, from the valve leaflet to their point of attachment in the ventricle.

The relationship of the remaining atrial septum to the remaining ventricular septum must also be assessed. With severe malalignment caused by leftward deviation of the atrial septum, the right atrium now has access to both atrioventricular orifices, producing a double-outlet right atrium.[55] In this entity, the only outlet of the left atrium is usually through the atrial septal defect. This lesion has been encountered most frequently in the presence of an atrioventricular septal defect, although this is not a requirement. The embryologic primum atrial septum may deviate leftward and fuse with the left lateral endocardial cushion. A number of venous anomalies are associated with this lesion, particularly drainage of the left superior vena cava to the left atrium and anomalous return of the pulmonary veins.

Subcostal Four-Chamber and Short-Axis Views

The subcostal views provide detailed imaging of the atrial septum to evaluate the extent of the atrial communication, detailed imaging of the atrioventricular valve anatomy and the relationship of the valve tissue to the inlet portion of the heart, and detailed imaging of the ventricular septum. The subcostal four-chamber view, used first, provides a close look at the atrial septum (Fig 5–52). Also, the presence or absence of an associated secundum defect is evaluated. If the atrial septum were totally absent, as in common atrium, it would be easily evident in this view. From the subcostal four-chamber view, the plane of sound

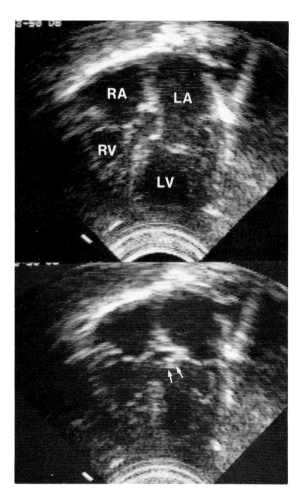

FIG 5–48.
Apical four-chamber views in diastole *(above)* and systole *(below)* from a patient with an atrioventricular septal defect identical to that shown in Figure 5–47. When the common atrioventricular valve opens in diastole *(above)* it can be seen tethered to the lower rim of the atrial septum. Shunting can occur only at ventricular level. When the common atrioventricular valve is closed in systole *(below)*, a prominent chord *(arrow)* can be seen crossing from the left half of the atrioventricular valve through the ventricular septal defect. This chord is inserted into the right ventricle (RV). *LA* = left atrium; *LV* = left ventricle; and *RA* = right atrium.

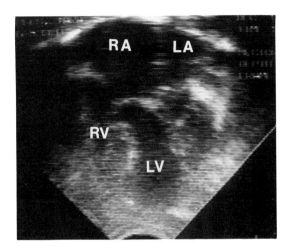

FIG 5–49.
Apical four-chamber view from a patient with an unbalanced form of atrioventricular septal defect. There is marked malalignment between the atrial and ventricular septa. In this case, the malalignment is such that the right ventricle (RV) is small and underdeveloped. *LA* = left atrium; *LV* = left ventricle; and *RA* = right atrium.

is tilted anteriorly toward the left ventricular outflow tract. In this position, the characteristic gooseneck deformity or elongation of the left ventricular outflow tract is seen (Fig 5–53). The gooseneck deformity is created by the inferior and anterior displacement of the atrioventricular valve.

By rotating the transducer midway between the subcostal coronal and the sagittal view, the atrioventricular valve is seen well en face (Fig 5–54). The number of orifices is easily seen, as is the degree of commitment of the atrioventricular valve tissue to each ventricle. The valve area committed to each ventricle can be measured and indicates if the valve tissue is evenly committed to both ventricles or if it favors one over the other. These data, used in conjunction with measurement of ventricular sizes, allow accurate estimation of the degree of ventricular hypoplasia. The presence of a double orifice mitral valve can also be appreciated in this view. In double-orifice mitral valve, the left half of the common atrioventricular valve usually opens in diastole into one large and one small accessory orifice. Evaluation of the number of valve orifices and the commitment of the valve tissue to each ventricle is best accomplished if the subcostal sagittal images are reviewed in slow motion or frame by frame. This can be accomplished using the slow motion review mode of the videotape player or the memory loop function present on most instruments.

Rotating farther into the subcostal sagittal plane permits evaluation of the relation of the atrioventricular valve to the septum in a view orthogonal to that provided by the subcostal and apical four-chamber views. In particular, the presence of redundant right-sided valve tissue, which may extend through the ventricular septal defect, is seen as a billowing of the tissue into the right ventricle during sys-

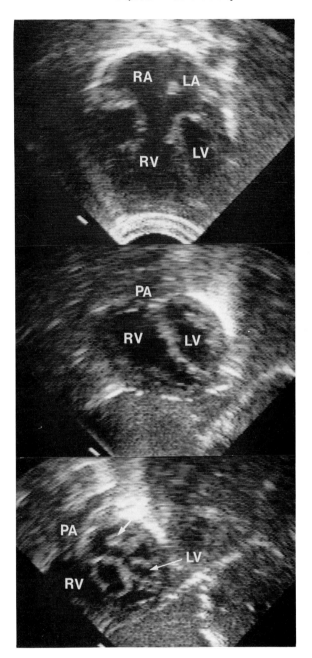

FIG 5–50.
Echocardiographic views from an infant with an unbalanced atrioventricular septal defect and a small left ventricle (LV). In the apical four-chamber view *(top)*, the left half of the atrioventricular valve is small and the left atrium (LA) and LV are small. In this patient, shunting occurred only at atrial level. In the subcostal short-axis view at the level of the papillary muscles *(middle)*, the discrepancy in size between the LV and the right ventricle (RV) is apparent. In the subcostal short-axis view through the atrioventricular valve *(bottom)*, the portion of the common atrioventricular valve committed to the RV is of good size. The portion of the atrioventricular valve committed to the LV is considerably smaller and consists of a large inferior orifice and a small superior accessory orifice *(arrows)*. *RA* = right atrium; *PA* = pulmonary artery.

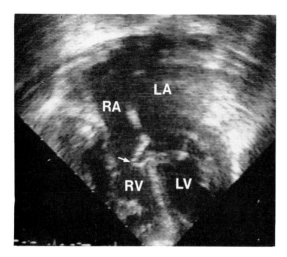

FIG 5–51.
Apical four-chamber view from a patient with an atrioventricular septal defect. Accessory atrioventricular valve tissue *(arrow),* also known as a tricuspid pouch, occludes the ventricular septal defect. *LA* = left atrium; *LV* = left ventricle; *RA* = right atrium; and *RV* = right ventricle.

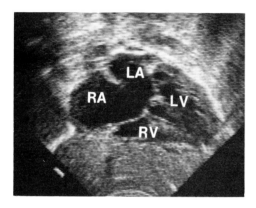

FIG 5–52.
Subcostal four-chamber view from a patient with an atrioventricular septal defect. The common atrioventricular valve is displaced inferiorly into the heart, and a large primum atrial septal defect is present. *LA* = left atrium; *LV* = left ventricle; *RA* = right atrium; and *RV* = right ventricle.

tole. The sagittal plane provides another view for assessing chordal attachments of the atrioventricular valve and for detecting other defects such as subaortic membranous obstruction or an additional muscular defect (Fig 5–55).

Doppler Studies

Pulsed and color-flow Doppler techniques have been especially useful for defining the complex patterns of intracardiac shunting and valve regurgitation that occur in patients with atrioventricular septal defects. Deformities of the common atrioventricular valve are such that insuf-

ficiency jets can be directed anywhere in the left or right atria. Color-flow mapping provides a technique for the rapid visualization of these eccentric jets (Plates 16 and 17).

The jet flow across the atrioventricular septal defect should be evaluated as well. Atrial shunting can occur from the left atrium to the right atrium or obligatory shunting can occur from the left ventricle to the right atrium. Shunting from the left ventricle to the right ventricle can also be detected.

Finally, because subvalvular obstruction of both outflow tracts is common, the right and left ventricular outflow tracts must be carefully evaluated. This obstruction can take the form of either muscular obstruction or, especially on the left side, chordal insertions into the septum crossing the outflow tract. Although many such attachments create no obstruction, only careful Doppler assessment can make this differentiation.

SEPTATION OF THE CONOTRUNCUS AND AORTIC SAC

Anatomy

The final group of cardiac septation anomalies to be discussed are those that involve the conotruncal septum. Defects of this region result in a direct communication between the aorta and pulmonary artery that may or may not be associated with a defect of the ventricular septum. The most common of these anomalies is persistent truncus arteriosus. In this deformity, there is failure of partitioning of the distal conus, truncus arteriosus, and aortic sac. This

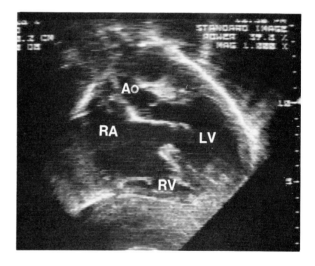

FIG 5–53.
Subcostal coronal view of the left ventricular (LV) outflow tract from a patient with an atrioventricular septal defect. In this view, displacement of the common atrioventricular valve inferiorly and into the LV outflow tract can be seen. This displacement and the attachments of the valve chordae to the ventricular septum create the appearance of a long, narrowed LV outflow tract (gooseneck deformity). *AO* = aorta; *RA* = right atrium; and *RV* = right ventricle.

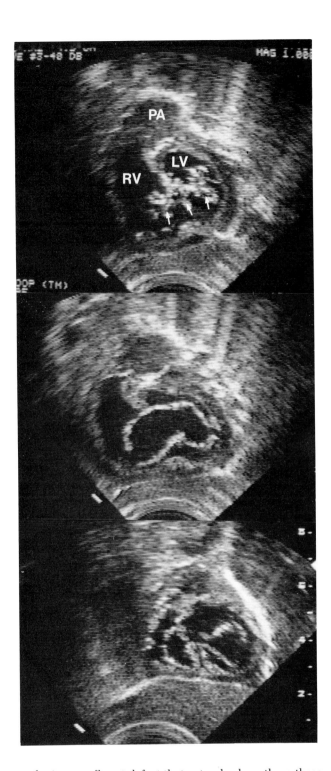

FIG 5–54.
Subcostal short-axis views through the common atrioventricular valve in two patients with atrioventricular septal defect. The *top and middle frames* were obtained from a patient with a common atrioventricular valve and a common atrioventricular valve orifice (the so-called complete form of atrioventricular septal defect). In the *top frame,* the common atrioventricular valve is seen in the closed position in systole. In the *middle frame,* the atrioventricular valve is seen in the open position in diastole. This view shows that there is a common atrioventricular valve orifice, which is equally divided between the right ventricle (RV) and the left ventricle (LV). The proportion of the valve orifice committed to each ventricle can be roughly determined by drawing a straight line from the infundibular septum above to the crest of the muscular septum below. If this is done, then nearly equal areas of the valve orifice are committed to each ventricle. The *bottom frame* was obtained from a patient with a primum atrial septal defect. In this patient, the common atrioventricular valve is divided into two separate orifices. This division occurs because of a bridging tongue of tissue that connects the superior and inferior bridging leaflets. It is important to note that all patients with atrioventricular septal defect have only a single common atrioventricular valve. This valve may be divided into two separate and equally sized orifices; however, there are not two separate atrioventricular valves at separate heights in the heart. *PA* = pulmonary artery.

results in a confluent defect that extends along these three cardiac segments. The confluent defect consists of an outlet ventricular septal defect, a single semilunar valve, and a common arterial trunk that overrides the ventricular septal defect. The ventricular septal defect is bounded inferiorly and anteriorly by the trabecular septum and the two limbs of the trabecula septomarginalis. Superiorly, the defect is bounded by the truncal valve. Posteriorly, the defect is bounded by the posterior limb of the trabecula septomarginalis, the ventriculoinfundibular fold, and the membranous septum. This usually results in separation of the tricuspid valve from the defect. If the defect extends into the membranous septum, however, it may extend to the tricuspid annulus.[56, 57]

The truncal valve usually originates from both ventricles equally but may be situated over one ventricle more than the other. When this occurs, the ventricular sizes must be carefully assessed, as one ventricle may be hypoplastic.

Also, if the valve is shifted more toward the right ventricle, closure of the defect may result in left ventricular outflow tract obstruction, particularly if there is also posterior deviation of the trabecular septum. The truncal valve itself is large and may consist of from one to six leaflets. The valve may be normal, stenotic, and/or regurgitant.

Not only does the truncal septum fail to partition the truncal valve into two separate semilunar valves, but also the septum aortopulmonale fails to form completely and to separate the aortic sac into an ascending aorta and main pulmonary artery. If the majority of the septum aortopulmonale is present, a main pulmonary artery segment is present at the left lateral aspect of the truncus arteriosus (type I). If the septum aortopulmonale is completely absent, the two pulmonary arteries arise by separate, side-by-side

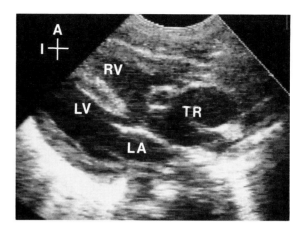

FIG 5–56.
Parasternal long-axis view from an infant with truncus arteriosus. The truncal vessel (TR) can be seen overriding the ventricular septum. A large outlet ventricular septal defect is present. A pulmonary artery can be seen arising from the posterior aspect of the TR. *A* = anterior; *I* = inferior; *LA* = left atrium; *LV* = left ventricle; and *RV* = right ventricle.

orifices from the posterior aspect of the truncus arteriosus (type II). In type III truncus arteriosus, only one true pulmonary artery is present, arising from the ascending aorta. The other lung is supplied by an arterial branch off the aortic arch or descending aorta.

Although the origin(s) of the pulmonary arteries are usually nonrestrictive, stenosis may be present and the branch pulmonary arteries may be hypoplastic. Finally, other anomalies of the pulmonary arteries may be present. The right pulmonary artery may originate from the truncus, while the left pulmonary artery originates from the ductus arteriosus.

In some situations, the proximal truncal septum is present and the ventricular septum is intact, but the septum aortopulmonale is defective. This results in an aorticopulmonary or A-P window. The size of the communication is variable but usually large. In this anomaly there are two separate semilunar valves and a main pulmonary segment. This defect is located in the anterior and leftward wall of the aorta where the main pulmonary artery crosses over the aorta.

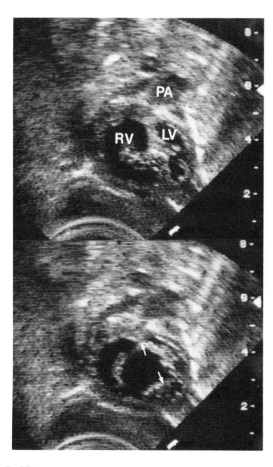

FIG 5–55.
Subcostal short-axis view of the common atrioventricular valve from a patient with an atrioventricular septal defect and a small left ventricle (LV). In the *top frame,* the atrioventricular valve is in the closed position in systole. In the *bottom frame,* the atrioventricular valve is seen in the open position in diastole. There is a common atrioventricular valve orifice. However, if a straight line is drawn from the infundibular septum above *(arrow)* to the rim of the muscular septum below *(arrow),* only a small portion of the total area of the common atrioventricular valve orifice is committed to the LV. *PA* = pulmonary artery; *RV* = right ventricle.

Echocardiographic Views

Parasternal Long-Axis View

In the parasternal long-axis view, the deficiency in the infundibular septum and the aortic override are seen, suggesting the diagnosis.[58] The degree of septal deficiency, the degree of great vessel override, the size of the great vessel, and the left ventricular size all are well evaluated (Figs 5–56 and 5–57). In addition, in some cases of truncus arteriosus, the pulmonary arteries are imaged arising from the posterior aspect of the great vessel, clearly establishing the diagnosis. However, in many instances, the diagnosis of truncus arteriosus cannot be made with certainty in this view because the pulmonary outflow tract is not visual-

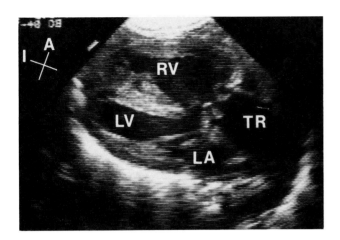

FIG 5–57.
Parasternal long-axis view from a patient with truncus arteriosus and severe truncal valve regurgitation. In this view, the truncal valve leaflets are rolled and nobby. In addition, a regurgitant orifice can be seen in this diastolic frame. *LA* = left atrium; *LV* = left ventricle; *RV* = right ventricle; and *TR* = truncus.

ized. In truncus arteriosus, there is discontinuity between the anterior truncal wall and the ventricular septum; however, the truncal valve is in fibrous continuity with the anterior mitral valve leaflet. Thus, truncus arteriosus, tetralogy of Fallot, and pulmonary atresia/ventricular septal defect can have an identical appearance in the long-axis view.

Parasternal Short-Axis View

The parasternal short-axis view at the level of the truncal valve is the best view for imaging the pulmonary arteries as they arise from the truncal vessel (Fig 5–58).[58] The pulmonary valve is absent and the pulmonary arteries and coronary arteries arise from the truncal vessel. In truncus arteriosus type I, the pulmonary artery branches arise via a short main pulmonary segment from the left lateral aspect of the ascending aorta (Fig 5–58). In truncus arteriosus type II, the two pulmonary artery branches arise from the posterior wall of the ascending aorta via separate (but side-by-side) orifices (Fig 5–59). In truncus arteriosus type III, the pulmonary artery branches arise from the truncal vessel via two widely separated orifices.

The parasternal short-axis view is useful for imaging the ventricular septal defect. In most cases of truncus arteriosus, the defect extends leftward above the crista supraventricularis and most of the membranous septum is intact (Fig 5–60). In addition, this view is useful for evaluating the number and morphology of the truncal valve cusps (Fig 5–61).

Apical Four-Chamber View

The apical four-chamber view permits imaging of the ventricular septal defect and evaluation of truncal valve morphology. Thickened valves may even show a deficiency in diastole or a regurgitant orifice that produces a

leak; leakage, however, must be confirmed by Doppler examination.

Subcostal Views

The subcostal four-chamber view is again useful for evaluating the degree of ventricular septal deficiency and the degree of great vessel malposition. This view is used primarily to evaluate the proximal truncal septum.[59, 60] In truncus arteriosus, the proximal truncal septum is missing, whereas in an aortopulmonary window, the proximal truncal septum is present and the deficiency is in the septum

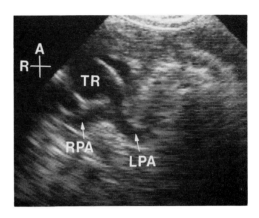

FIG 5–58.
Parasternal short-axis view from an infant with truncus arteriosus. The truncal vessel (TR) can be seen in cross-section. A short main pulmonary artery segment, which bifurcates into a right pulmonary artery (RPA) and a left pulmonary artery (LPA), is seen arising from the left lateral aspect of the TR. This type of truncus arteriosus is known as type I truncus arteriosus. *A* = anterior; *R* = right.

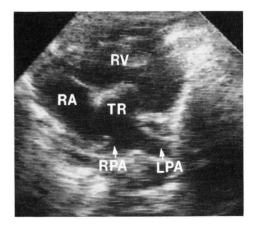

FIG 5–59.
Parasternal short-axis view from an infant with truncus arteriosus. The truncal vessel (TR) is seen in cross-section. The right pulmonary artery (RPA) and the left pulmonary artery (LPA) arise from the posterior aspect of the TR by separate but closely spaced orifices. This is a type II truncus arteriosus. *RA* = right atrium; *RV* = right ventricle.

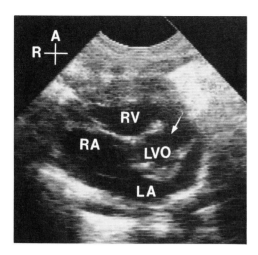

FIG 5–60.
Parasternal short-axis view at the base of the heart from an infant with truncus arteriosus. The ventricular septal defect *(arrow)* is located in the outlet septum above the level of the crista supraventricularis. The defect does not involve the membranous septum. This position of the ventricular septal defect is commonly found in infants with truncus arteriosus. A = anterior; LA = left atrium; LVO = left ventricular outflow tract; R = right; RA = right atrium; and RV = right ventricle.

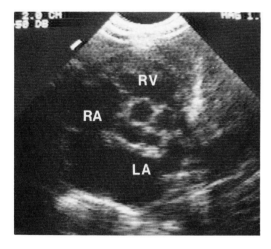

FIG 5–61.
Parasternal short-axis view in a patient with truncus arteriosus. The truncal valve is divided into four cusps (i.e., quadricuspid truncal valve). LA = left atrium; RA = right atrium; and RV = right ventricle.

aortopulmonale. Thus, in aortopulmonary window, there are usually two separate semilunar valves and two separate great arteries; the great arteries, however, communicate through a defect usually in the lateral wall of the ascending aorta (Fig 5–62). The subcostal views are useful for determining how close the defect is to the left main coronary artery.

In truncus arteriosus, the branch pulmonary arteries can often be imaged from the subcostal views. The right

pulmonary artery passes immediately behind the truncal vessel, while the left pulmonary artery dives posteriorly and leftward and thus can be seen to arch over the superior aspect of the left atrium.

Suprasternal Notch Views

The suprasternal notch views are the most useful for imaging the ductus arteriosus, the aortic arch, and the branch pulmonary arteries. Right-sided aortic arch, coarctation, and aortic arch interruption are commonly associated lesions that can be evaluated from these views. In the suprasternal long-axis view, the position of the arch relative to the trachea can be determined by careful scanning from right to left. Next, the aortic arch is imaged by scanning toward the left. The aortic arch must be carefully inspected to rule out an interrupted arch or a coarctation. Finally, a ductus arteriosus must be carefully searched for from the descending aorta to the left pulmonary artery. In

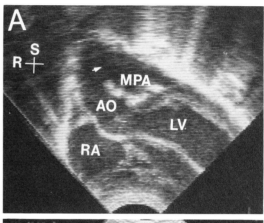

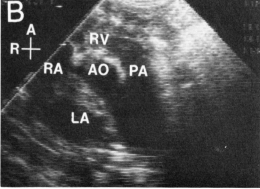

FIG 5–62.
A, subcostal coronal view of the left ventricular (LV) outflow tract from an infant with an aortopulmonary window *(arrow)*. This is a defect in the septum aortopulmonale. The truncal septum forms normally so that separate aortic and pulmonary valves are present. **B,** parasternal short-axis view from the same infant as in Figure 5–62A. The defect in the aortopulmonary septum is well seen in this view. A = anterior; AO = aorta; LA = left atrium; PA = pulmonary artery; R = right; RA = right atrium; and RV = right ventricle.

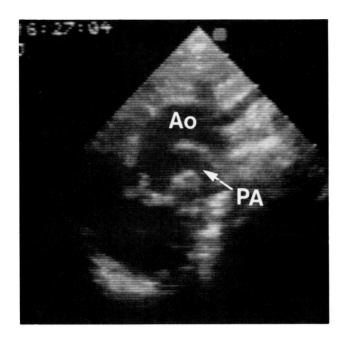

FIG 5–63.
Suprasternal long-axis view from an infant with truncus arteriosus. The truncal vessel gives rise to the aortic arch (AO) and the pulmonary arteries (PA).

the suprasternal views, the branch pulmonary arteries can be traced back to their origin from the truncal vessel (Fig 5–63). These views are useful for detecting branch pulmonary artery stenosis.

Doppler Studies

Doppler interrogation of flow in both pulmonary arteries should be performed from the parasternal and suprasternal views to assess the presence or absence of stenosis at the origin of these vessels. From the apical view, Doppler assessment of the truncal valve can be performed. Stenosis, as well as regurgitation, may be present. In attempting to locate regurgitation, both the left and right sides of the ventricular septum must be scanned, as the jet may lie along either side. Color-flow mapping is quite useful for evaluation of the truncal valve.

REFERENCES

1. Canale JM, Sahn DJ, Allen HD, et al: Factors affecting real-time, cross-sectional echocardiographic imaging of perimembranous ventricular septal defects. *Circulation* 1981; 63:689–697.
2. Shub C, Dimopoulos IN, Seward JB, et al: Sensitivity of two-dimensional echocardiography in the direct visualization of atrial septal defects utilizing a subcostal approach: Experience with 154 patients. *J Am Coll Cardiol* 1983; 4:127–135.
3. Green CE, Gottdiener JS, Goldstein HA: Atrial septal defect. *Semin Radiol* 1985; 20:214–225.
4. Raghib G, Ruttenberg HD, Anderson RC, et al: Termination of left superior vena cava in left atrium, atrial septal defect, and absence of coronary sinus. *Circulation* 1965; 31:906–918.
5. Gondi B, Nanda NC: Two-dimensional echocardiographic features of atrial septal aneurysms. *Circulation* 1981; 63:452–457.
6. Belkin RN, Waugh RA, Kisslo J: Interatrial shunting in atrial septal aneurysm. *Am J Cardiol* 1986; 57:310–312.
7. Weiner JA, Cheitlin MD, Gross BW, et al: Echocardiographic appearance of Chiari's network: Differentiation from right heart pathology. *Circulation* 1981; 63:1104–1109.
8. Ghisla RP, Hannon DW, Meyer RA, et al: Spontaneous closure of isolated secundum atrial septal defects in infants: An echocardiographic study. *Am Heart J* 1985; 109:1327–1333.
9. Meyer RA, Schwartz D, Benzing G, et al: Ventricular septum in right ventricular volume overload. *Am J Cardiol* 1972; 30:349–353.
10. Weyman AE, Wann S, Feigenbaum H, et al: Mechanism of abnormal septal motion in patients with right ventricular volume overload. A cross-sectional echocardiographic study. *Circulation* 1976; 54:179–186.
11. Agata Y, Hiraishi S, Misawa H, et al: Two-dimensional echocardiographic determinants of interventricular septal configurations in right or left ventricular overload. *Am Heart J* 1985; 110:819–825.
12. Fraker TD, Harris PJ, Behar VS, et al: Detection and exclusion of interatrial shunts by two-dimensional echocardiography and peripheral venous injections. *Circulation* 1979; 59:379–384.
13. Valdes-Cruz LM, Pieroni DR, Roland J-MA, et al: Echocardiographic detection of intracavitary right to left shunts following peripheral vein injections. *Circulation* 1976; 54:558–562.
14. Weyman AE, Wann LS, Caldwell RL, et al: Negative contrast echocardiography: A new method for detecting left to right shunts. *Circulation* 1979; 59:498–505.
15. Levin AR, Spach MS, Boineau JP, et al: Atrial pressure-flow dynamics in atrial septal defects (secundum type). *Circulation* 1968; 37:476–488.
16. Hatle L, Angelsen B: *Doppler Ultrasound in Cardiology*, ed 2. Philadelphia, Lea & Febiger, 1985, pp 97–293.
17. Minagoe S, Tei C, Kisanuki A, et al: Noninvasive pulsed Doppler echocardiographic detection of the direction of shunt flow in patients with atrial septal defect: Usefulness of the right parasternal approach. *Circulation* 1985; 71:745–753.
18. Snider AR: Doppler ultrasound in congenital heart disease, in Berger M (ed): *Doppler Ultrasound in Heart Disease*. New York, Marcel Dekker, Inc., 1987, pp 199–311.
19. Hagler DJ, Edwards WD, Seward JB, et al: Standardized nomenclature of the ventricular septum and ventricular septal defects with applications for two-dimensional echocardiography. *Mayo Clin Proc* 1985; 60:741–752.
20. Milo S, Yen S, Macartney FJ, et al: Straddling and overriding atrioventricular valves: Morphology and classification. *Am J Cardiol* 1978; 14:1122–1134.

21. Bierman FZ, Fellows K, Williams RG: Prospective identification of ventricular septal defects in infancy using subxiphoid two-dimensional echocardiography. *Circulation* 1980; 62:807–817.

22. Cheatham JP, Latson LA, Gutgesell HP: Ventricular septal defect in infancy: Detection with two-dimensional echocardiography. *Am J Cardiol* 1981; 47:85–89.

23. Canale JM, Sahn DJ, Allen HD, et al: Factors affecting real-time, cross-sectional echocardiographic imaging of perimembranous ventricular septal defects. *Circulation* 1981; 63:689–697.

24. Serwer GA, Armstrong BE, Anderson PAW, et al: Use of contrast echocardiography for evaluation of right ventricular hemodynamics in the presence of ventricular septal defects. *Circulation* 1978; 58:327–336.

25. Stevenson JG, Kawabori I, Dooley T, et al: Diagnosis of ventricular septal defect by pulsed Doppler echocardiography: Sensitivity, specificity, and limitations. *Circulation* 1978; 58:322–326.

26. Magherini A, Azzolina G, Wiechmann V, et al: Pulsed Doppler echocardiography for diagnosis of ventricular septal defects. *Br Heart J* 1980; 43:143–147.

27. Hatle L, Rokseth R: Noninvasive diagnosis and assessment of ventricular septal defect by Doppler ultrasound. *Acta Med Scand* 1981; 645:47–56.

28. Murphy DJ, Ludomirsky A, Huhta JC: Continuous-wave Doppler in children with ventricular septal defect: Noninvasive estimation of interventricular pressure gradient. *Am J Cardiol* 1986; 57:428–432.

29. Ludomirsky A, Huhta JC, Vick GW III, et al: Color Doppler detection of multiple ventricular septal defects. *Circulation* 1986; 74:1317–1322.

30. Marx GR, Allen HD, Goldberg SJ: Doppler echocardiographic estimation of systolic pulmonary artery pressure in pediatric patients with interventricular communications. *J Am Coll Cardiol* 1985; 6:1132–1137.

31. Snider AR, Silverman NH, Schiller NB, et al: Echocardiographic evaluation of ventricular septal aneurysms. *Circulation* 1979; 59:920–926.

32. Ramaciotti C, Keren A, Silverman NH: Importance of (perimembranous) ventricular septal aneurysm in the natural history of isolated perimembranous ventricular septal defect. *Am J Cardiol* 1986; 57:268–272.

33. Chesler E, Korns ME, Edwards JE: Anomalies of the tricuspid valve, including pouches, resembling aneurysms of the membranous ventricular septum. *Am J Cardiol* 1968; 21:661–668.

34. Criag BG, Smallhorn JF, Burrows P, et al: Cross-sectional echocardiography in the evaluation of aortic valve prolapse associated with ventricular septal defect. *Am Heart J* 1986; 112:800–807.

35. Menahem S, Johns JA, Del Torso S, et al: Evaluation of aortic valve prolapse in ventricular septal defect. *Br Heart J* 1986; 56:242–249.

36. Anderson RH, Lenox CC, Zuberbuhler JR: Morphology of ventricular septal defect associated with coarctation of aorta. *Br Heart J* 1983; 50:176–181.

37. Smallhorn JF, Anderson RH, Macartney FJ: Morphological characteristics of ventricular septal defects associated with coarctation of aorta by cross-sectional echocardiography. *Br Heart J* 1983; 49:485–494.

38. Soto B, Pacifico AD, Ceballos R, et al: Tetralogy of Fallot: An angiographic-pathologic correlative study. *Circulation* 1981; 64:558–566.

39. Becker AE, Connor M, Anderson RH: Tetralogy of Fallot: A morphometric and geometric study. *Am J Cardiol* 1975; 35:402–412.

40. Henry WL, Maron BJ, Griffith JM, et al: Differential diagnosis of anomalies of the great arteries by real-time two-dimensional echocardiography. *Circulation* 1975; 51:283–291.

41. Hagler DJ, Tajik AJ, Seward JB, et al: Wide-angle two-dimensional echocardiographic profiles of conotruncal abnormalities. *Mayo Clin Proc* 1980; 55:73–82.

42. Caldwell RL, Weyman AE, Hurwitz RA, et al: Right ventricular outflow tract assessment by cross-sectional echocardiography in tetralogy of Fallot. *Circulation* 1979; 59:395–402.

43. Blackstone EH, Kirkland JW, Bertranou EG, et al: Preoperative prediction from cineangiograms of postrepair right ventricular pressure in tetralogy of Fallot. *J Thorac Cardiovasc Surg* 1979; 78:542–552.

44. Becker AE, Anderson RH: Atrioventricular septal defects: What's in a name? *J Thorac Cardiovasc Surg* 1982; 83:461–469.

45. Allwork SP: Anatomical-embryological correlates in atrioventricular septal defects. *Br Heart J* 1982; 47:419–429.

46. Hagler DJ, Tajik AJ, Seward JB, et al: Real-time wide-angle sector echocardiography: Atrioventricular canal defects. *Circulation* 1979; 59:140–150.

47. Heydarian M, Griffith BP, Zuberbuhler JR: Partial atrioventricular canal associated with discrete subaortic stenosis. *Am Heart J* 1985; 109:915–917.

48. Spanos PK, Fiddler GI, Mair DD, et al: Repair of AV canal associated with membranous subaortic stenosis. *Mayo Clin Proc* 1977; 52:121–124.

49. Lev M, Agustsson MH, Arcilla R: The pathologic anatomy of common atrioventricular orifice associated with tetralogy of Fallot. *Am J Clin Pathol* 1961; 36:408–416.

50. Chin AJ, Bierman FZ, Sanders SP, et al: Subxyphoid 2-dimensional echocardiographic identification of left ventricular papillary muscle anomalies in complete common atrioventricular canal. *Am J Cardiol* 1983; 51:1695–1699.

51. Silverman NH, Zuberbuhler JR, Anderson RH: Atrioventricular septal defects: Cross-sectional echocardiographic and morphologic comparisons. *Int J Cardiol* 1986; 13:309–331.

52. Virdi IS, Keeton BR, Shore DF: Atrioventricular septal defect with a well developed primum component of the atrial septum. *Int J Cardiol* 1985; 9:243–247.

53. Mehta S, Hirschfeld S, Riggs T, et al: Echocardiographic estimation of ventricular hypoplasia in complete atrioventricular canal. *Circulation* 1979; 59:888–893.

54. Kudo T, Yokoyama M, Imai Y, et al: The tricuspid pouch in endocardial cushion defect. *Am Heart J* 1974; 87:544–549.

55. Westerman GR, Norton JB, Van Devanter SH: Double-outlet right atrium associated with tetralogy of

Fallot and common atrioventricular valve. *J Thorac Cardiovasc Surg* 1986; 91:205–207.

56. Van Praagh R, Van Praagh S: The anatomy of common aorticopulmonary trunk (truncus arteriosus communis) and its embryologic implications. *Am J Cardiol* 1965; 16:406–425.

57. Ceballos R, Soto B, Kirklin JW, et al: Truncus arteriosus. An anatomical-angiographic study. *Br Heart J* 1983; 49:589–599.

58. Rice MJ, Seward JB, Hagler DJ, et al: Definitive diagnosis of truncus arteriosus by two-dimensional echocardiography. *Mayo Clin Proc* 1982; 57:476–481.

59. Smallhorn JF, Anderson RH, Macartney FJ: Two-dimensional echocardiographic assessment of communications between the ascending aorta and pulmonary trunk or individual pulmonary arteries. *Br Heart J* 1982; 47:563–572.

60. Rice MJ, Seward JB, Hagler DJ, et al: Visualization of aortopulmonary window by two-dimensional echocardiography. *Mayo Clin Proc* 1982; 57:482–487.

Abnormalities of Ventriculoarterial Connection

TRANSPOSITION OF THE GREAT ARTERIES

The term transposition describes an abnormal or discordant ventriculoarterial connection in which the aorta arises from the morphologic right ventricle and the pulmonary artery arises from the morphologic left ventricle. The complete echocardiographic evaluation of the child with transposition of the great arteries requires diagnosing not only the ventriculoarterial connections (transposition) but also the atrial situs and atrioventricular connections. The echocardiographic approach to the segmental analysis of the heart is discussed in detail in Chapter 14. In general terms, however, the morphologic right atrium is the chamber that has the eustachian valve of the inferior vena cava and the limbus of the fossa ovalis. The morphologic left atrium has the flap valve of the foramen ovale. The morphologic right ventricle has an atrioventricular valve (the tricuspid valve) that is closer to the cardiac apex and has chordal attachments into the septum. In addition, the right ventricle has septal-parietal free wall muscle bundles, the largest of which is usually the moderator band. The morphologic left ventricle has an atrioventricular valve (the mitral valve) that is farther from the cardiac apex and has chordal attachments into two papillary muscles. The left ventricle has a smooth septal surface devoid of septal-parietal muscle bundles and chordal insertions.

This chapter will review the echocardiographic diagnosis of d- and l-transposition of the great arteries in situs solitus (morphologic right atrium on the patient's right, morphologic left atrium on the left). Transposition complexes in the setting of situs inversus are discussed in Chapter 14. The terms d-transposition or simple transposition of the great arteries will be used to describe a situation where the morphologic right ventricle is located to the right of the morphologic left ventricle (d-bulboventricular loop). The terms l-transposition or l-transposition with

ventricular inversion will be used to describe the situation where the morphologic right ventricle is to the left of the morphologic left ventricle (l-bulboventricular loop).

d-Transposition of the Great Arteries

In the most common form of transposition of the great arteries, the morphologic right atrium on the patient's right is connected to the morphologic right ventricle on the patient's right which, in turn, is connected to the aorta. On the patient's left, the morphologic left atrium is connected to the morphologic left ventricle, which is connected to the pulmonary artery. This defect is called situs solitus, d-loop, d-transposition, or simply d-transposition. In the third term, the d describes the spatial relations of the aortic and pulmonic valves. In more than 80% of cases, the aortic valve is spatially to the right of the pulmonary valve, hence the use of the d. The echocardiographic diagnosis of transposition of the great arteries is based on demonstrating an abnormal connection of the right ventricle to the aorta. The echocardiogram also provides useful information about the spatial relationships of the great arteries. Although the spatial relationships of the great arteries can provide supportive evidence of the diagnosis, they should never be used as the sole diagnostic criterion.

The connections between the ventricles and great arteries can be seen in multiple echocardiographic views; the subcostal views, however, are particularly useful because they provide simultaneous imaging of the entire ventricle, the outflow tract, and the great artery.[1] In the subcostal four-chamber views shown in Figure 6–1, the ventricle on the patient's left has characteristic features of a morphologic left ventricle (smooth septal surface, two papillary muscles) and is connected to a great artery that bifurcates into two branches and is therefore the pulmonary artery. The ventricle on the right has anatomic features of a mor-

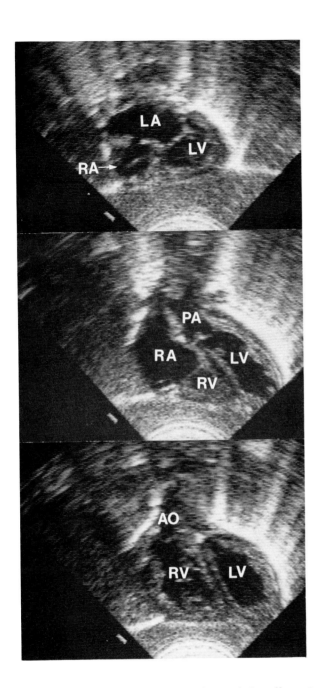

FIG 6–1.
Subcostal four-chamber views from an infant with situs solitus, *d*-loop, and *d*-transposition of the great arteries. From top to bottom, these views were obtained by progressively tilting the transducer from a posterior to a very anterior position. The *top frame* is a very posterior view through the inflow portion of the heart. In this view, the eustachian valve is seen crossing the floor of the right-sided atrium, indicating that this chamber is a morphologic right atrium (RA). The pulmonary veins are seen draining to the left-sided atrium, indicating that this chamber is a morphologic left atrium (LA). Thus, from this view there is situs solitus. The *middle frame* was obtained by tilting the transducer anteriorly to image the midportion of the heart. In this view, the left-sided ventricle is smooth-walled and has features of a morphologic left ventricle (LV). The LV gives rise to a vessel that bifurcates into two branches and is therefore a pulmonary artery (PA). In the *bottom frame*, the plane of sound has been tilted far anteriorly. The right-sided ventricle is triangular and has prominent septal-parietal free wall muscle bundles, indicating that this chamber is a morphologic right ventricle (RV). Thus, there is *d*-bulboventricular looping. The RV gives rise to a long vessel that arches and is therefore the aorta (AO). This substantiates a diagnosis of *d*-transposition of the great arteries.

phologic right ventricle (septoparietal muscle bundles, triangular shape), and gives rise to a vessel that does not bifurcate but, instead, arches out of the plane and is therefore the aorta. These anatomic features are diagnostic of *d*-transposition of the great arteries. The discordant ventriculoarterial connections can also be imaged in the parasternal long-axis views and the subcostal sagittal views (Figs 6–2 and 6–3).

In *d*-transposition of the great arteries (Fig 6–1), the aortic valve is usually superior to the pulmonary valve. The aortic valve is superior because it is supported by a complete muscular infundibulum. The muscular infundibulum of the left ventricle is mostly absorbed so that the pulmonary valve is in fibrous continuity with the mitral valve (Fig 6–2).

Spatial Relations of the Great Arteries

In the normal heart, the right ventricular outflow tract courses from right to left, anterior to the aorta, and reaches the pulmonary valve to the left of the aortic valve. The left ventricular outflow tract courses from left to right and reaches the aortic valve to the right of the pulmonary valve. Thus, in the normal heart, the outflow tracts and great vessels are coiled around one another, and the ventricular septum has a complex spatial curvature. In the normal heart, a cross-sectional view of the aorta will provide a

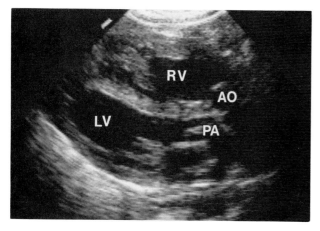

FIG 6–2.
Parasternal long-axis view from an infant with situs solitus, *d*-loop, and *d*-transposition of the great arteries. In this view, the great vessels can be seen in parallel alignment. The posterior great artery bifurcates into two branches and is therefore a pulmonary artery (PA); in addition, it has an acute posterior angulation as it exits the left ventricle (LV). *AO* = aorta; *RV* = right ventricle.

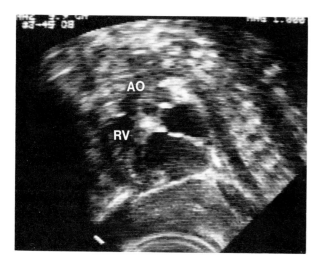

FIG 6–3.
Subcostal sagittal view from an infant with *d*-transposition of the great arteries. In this view, the aortic arch (AO) is seen arising from the anterior right ventricle (RV).

longitudinal view of the pulmonary artery and vice versa (the so-called circle-sausage appearance in the short-axis view).[2] In transposition, the outflow tracts and great arteries are not wrapped around each other; instead, the great arteries exit the heart in a parallel fashion. In addition, the entire muscular septum is much straighter than it is in the normal heart. As a result of these altered spatial relations, in most patients with transposition, the long-axis views are obtained with the plane of sound oriented more vertically than usual; the short-axis views are obtained with the plane of sound oriented more horizontally than usual.

As a result of the parallel arrangements of the great

arteries, longitudinal sections of both vessels can be imaged simultaneously in the parasternal long-axis view (Fig 6–4). In this view, the aortic valve is seen superior and anterior to the pulmonary valve. In the normal heart, the posterior aorta angles anteriorly as it exits the posterior left ventricle. In transposition, the posterior pulmonary artery dives immediately posteriorly toward the lungs as it exits the left ventricle (Figs 6–2 and 6–4).

Because of the parallel arrangement of the great arteries, both vessels will be seen in cross-section in the parasternal short-axis view (Fig 6–5) as double circles.[2–4] In most instances, the semilunar valves will not be seen simultaneously in the short-axis view because they are at separate heights. Thus, a cross-section through the pulmonary valve generally provides an image of the right ventricular outflow tract in cross-section; a cross-section through the aortic valve usually shows the main pulmonary artery and bifurcation.

In the majority of cases of *d*-transposition of the great arteries, the aorta is spatially to the right and anterior (see Fig 6–5); however, other spatial relationships are possible. In a small percentage of cases, the aortic infundibulum and valve may be to the left of the pulmonary valve (Fig 6–6). This spatial relationship is frequently found in patients with *d*-transposition and a large ventricular septal defect and is often referred to as situs solitus, *d*-loop, *l*-transposition. In this nomenclature, the *l* in the third term refers to the spatial position of the aorta (to the left). When the aortic infundibulum is to the left, the curvature of the septum is the same as it is in the normal heart. In another small percentage of patients, the aortic valve may be directly anterior to the pulmonary valve (Fig 6–7).

In the parasternal short-axis view, the bifurcation of the main pulmonary artery into right and left pulmonary

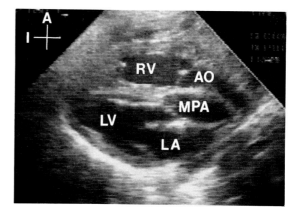

FIG 6–4.
Parasternal long-axis view from an infant with situs solitus, *d*-loop, and *d*-transposition of the great arteries. In this view, the aorta (AO) and main pulmonary artery (MPA) are parallel. The aortic valve is situated slightly superior to the pulmonary valve. These findings are highly suggestive of transposition. *LA* = left atrium; *LV* = left ventricle; and *RV* = right ventricle.

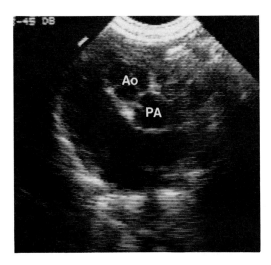

FIG 6–5.
Parasternal short-axis view from an infant with *d*-transposition of the great arteries. Because of the parallel alignment of the great vessels, in the short-axis view the aorta (AO) and the pulmonary artery (PA) are seen in cross-section as double circles. In this patient, the AO was located to the right and anterior of the PA.

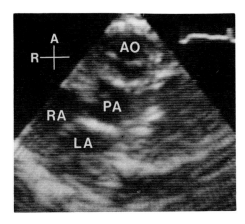

FIG 6–6.
Parasternal short-axis view at the base of the heart from a patient with *d*-transposition of the great arteries and a large ventricular septal defect. In this patient, the aorta (AO) and pulmonary artery (PA) are seen in cross-section as double circles. However, in this patient the AO is to the left and anterior to the PA. *A* = anterior; *LA* = left atrium; *R* = right; and *RA* = right atrium.

Chamber Sizes

In patients with simple transposition, during the first few weeks after birth the pulmonary vascular resistance decreases to a low level. M-mode echocardiographic studies performed at this time show that the right ventricular end-diastolic dimension is much larger than normal, and the left ventricular end-diastolic dimension is less than the fifth percentile of normal.[5] Following re-routing of systemic and venous return with an intra-atrial baffle procedure, the left ventricle is still the low-pressure chamber; therefore, the echocardiographic dimension measurements described above remain unchanged.[6–8] From birth to 20 years of age, patients with simple transposition pre- or

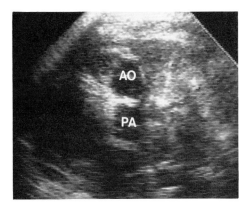

FIG 6–7.
Parasternal short-axis view at the base of the heart from an infant with *d*-transposition of the great arteries. The aorta (AO) and pulmonary artery (PA) are seen in cross-section as double circles. In this case, the AO is directly anterior to the PA.

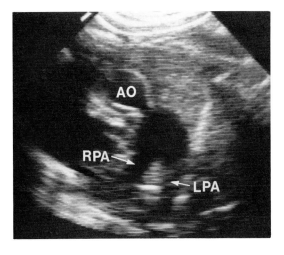

FIG 6–8.
Parasternal short-axis view at the base of the heart, with the plane of sound tilted anteriorly. In this view, the posterior great artery is seen bifurcating into two branches, which proves that the posterior great vessel is a pulmonary artery. *AO* = aorta; *LPA* = left pulmonary artery; and *RPA* = right pulmonary artery.

artery branches can be imaged by tilting the plane of sound superiorly (Fig 6–8). Visualization of a posterior great artery that bifurcates is supportive evidence of transposition of the great arteries. The appearance of double circles in the short-axis views can be created by unusual transducer positions high on the precordium or by unusual cardiac orientation in the chest. Therefore, the visualization of double circles alone, without demonstration of a posterior vessel that bifurcates, is *not* supportive evidence of transposition.

post-intra-atrial baffle procedures have thinner left ventricular posterior wall and septum compared with normal children. From birth to 10 years of age in one large group of children, the left ventricular posterior wall maintained a constant mean diastolic thickness of 2.3 mm.[6] After 10 years of age, the posterior wall thickness increased with increasing body surface area but was always less than normal.[7] Although the septal thickness is less than normal, the ratio of diastolic septal and posterior wall thicknesses is nearly always greater than 1.3, hence the echocardiographic appearance of asymmetric septal hypertrophy.[5] Because of the alterations in cardiac dimensions found on the M-mode echocardiogram in children with transposition, some authors have suggested that the cardiac chamber and wall thicknesses in these children should be compared to normal values derived from children with transposition, rather than to normal values derived from normal children.[7] Other authors have suggested that in children with transposition either pre- or post-baffle procedures measurements of the right ventricle should be compared to measurements of the left ventricle of normal children. Similarly, left ventricular dimensions in transposition should be compared to right ventricular dimensions of normal children.[8]

Because of the high right-ventricular pressure and low left-ventricular pressure, the ventricular septum bulges prominently in systole into the left ventricular outflow tract.[5–8] In about 50% of patients, the motion of the upper portion of the septum is normal, moving posteriorly in systole. In the remaining 50%, septal motion is abnormal, either flat or moving anteriorly in systole.[7] The bulging of the septum into the left ventricular outflow tract can create a dynamic form of subpulmonary stenosis often associated with systolic anterior motion of the mitral valve. It is postulated that the bowing of the septum into the left ventricular outflow tract reduces the cross-sectional area of flow and thus causes a high velocity of flow and a Venturi effect, which leads to anterior motion of the mitral valve. In patients with transposition, the finding of systolic anterior motion of the mitral valve has the opposite implication than the same finding in patients with hypertrophic cardiomyopathy. In transposition, patients with lower left ventricular pressure and smaller left ventricular cavities have a higher incidence of systolic anterior motion of the mitral valve.[5] This finding, then, suggests the absence of significant fixed subpulmonary stenosis.

In patients with simple transposition (pre- or post-baffle procedure), the shortening fraction and mean velocity of circumferential fiber shortening of the left ventricle are higher than normal.[7] The alterations in left ventricular geometry probably account for the observed alterations in indexes of systolic function.

Right ventricular dilatation and hypertrophy can also be seen on the two-dimensional echocardiogram in patients with simple transposition (either pre- or post-baffle procedure). In the apical and subcostal four-chamber views (Fig 6–9), the right atrium and right ventricle are usually considerably larger than the left atrium and left ventricle,

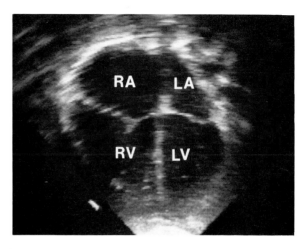

FIG 6–9.
Apical four-chamber view from an infant with situs solitus, *d*-loop, and *d*-transposition of the great arteries. In this view, the marked enlargement of the right atrium (RA) and right ventricle (RV) can be seen. *LA* = left atrium; *LV* = left ventricle.

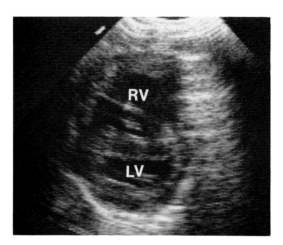

FIG 6–10.
Parasternal short-axis view from an infant with *d*-transposition of the great arteries. In this view, the right ventricle (RV) is circular and dominant, whereas the left ventricle (LV) is crescent-shaped. This suggests that RV pressure is higher than LV pressure.

and the right ventricle is apex-forming. In the short-axis views, the right ventricle is the dominant circular ventricle, and the left ventricle is crescent-shaped (Fig 6–10). The finding of a circular or enlarged left ventricle suggests the presence of left ventricular hypertension, possibly caused by pulmonary stenosis, a left-to-right shunt, or pulmonary hypertension.

Associated Defects

A complete echocardiographic examination of a child with *d*-transposition includes a thorough evaluation of any associated defects. Some of the more frequently occurring defects are reviewed below.

Atrial septal defect/patent ductus arteriosus.—To sur-
vive, infants with *d*-transposition must have mixing of systemic venous and pulmonary venous blood. In a patient
with an intact ventricular septum, mixing usually occurs
through an atrial septal defect, a patent ductus arteriosus,
or both. The echocardiographic examination is ideally
suited for determining the presence and adequacy of these
defects.

In infants with *d*-transposition, the patent ductus arteriosus is easily visualized from the suprasternal long-axis
view (Fig 6 11). Because of the altered spatial relationships of the great vessels, the patent ductus arteriosus is
easier to image in this view in children with *d*-transposi-
tion than it is in children with normal ventriculoarterial
connections. Pulsed and color-flow Doppler echocardiography provide methods for assessing the direction and
magnitude of the ductal shunts (see Chapter 10).

Most patients with transposition have an interatrial
communication in the region of the foramen ovale. Because
the atrial septum is perpendicular to the sound beam in
the subcostal views, these views are particularly useful for
imaging real echocardiographic dropout in the area of the
thin fossa ovalis (Fig 6–12). In infants who need a balloon
atrial septostomy to enlarge the interatrial communication,
the two-dimensional echocardiogram can be used to visualize the catheter during the procedure (Fig 6–13) and to
determine the size of the atrial septal defect after the procedure (Fig 6–14).[9, 10] With this technique, the balloon
catheter is advanced up the inferior vena cava, into the
right atrium, across the atrial septum, and into the left
atrium while it is being imaged from multiple subcostal

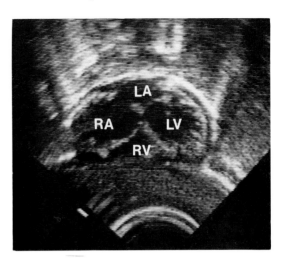

FIG 6–12.
Subcostal four-chamber view from an infant with *d*-transposition
and an interatrial communication. *LA* = left atrium; *LV* = left ventricle;
RA = right atrium; and *RV* = right ventricle.

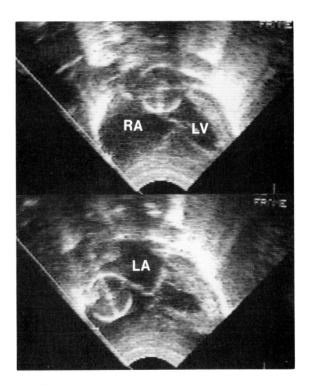

FIG 6–13.
Subcostal four-chamber views obtained from an infant with *d*-trans-
position of the great arteries at the time of atrial septostomy. In the
top frame, the catheter has been positioned in the left atrium (LA)
and the balloon has been inflated. In the *bottom frame*, the balloon
has been pulled back across the atrial septum into the right atrium
(RA). *LV* = left ventricle.

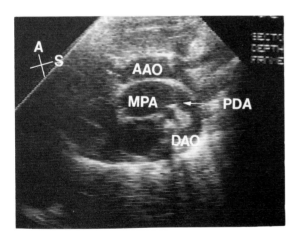

FIG 6–11.
Suprasternal long-axis view from an infant with *d*-transposition of
the great arteries and a patent ductus arteriosus (PDA). Because of
the parallel alignment of the great arteries in infants with *d*-trans-
position, it is common to visualize a long length of the PDA in the
standard suprasternal long-axis view. *A* = anterior; *AAO* = ascending
aorta; *DAO* = descending aorta; *MPA* = main pulmonary artery; and
S = superior.

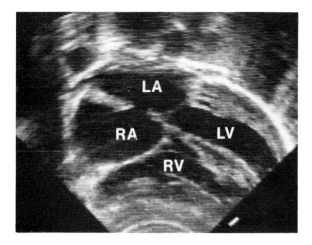

FIG 6–14.
Subcostal four-chamber view from an infant with *d*-transposition of the great arteries who had a previous balloon atrial septostomy. In this infant, the atrial septal defect created by the septostomy is quite small and restrictive. *LA* = left atrium; *LV* = left ventricle; *RA* = right atrium; and *RV* = right ventricle.

views. Before the inflated balloon is pulled back across the atrial septum, its position in the left atrium is verified with two-dimensional echocardiography. Following the balloon septostomy, it is common to image the torn edges of the atrial septum flicking rapidly back and forth across the atrial septal defect. As with the patent ductus arteriosus, pulsed and color-flow Doppler can provide important information about the size and direction of the interatrial shunts.[11]

Ventricular septal defect.—Ventricular septal defects occur in about 33% of patients with *d*-transposition of the great arteries. The majority of these defects are located in the outlet septum and are associated with an overriding pulmonary artery. Another important defect commonly found in *d*-transposition is the perimembranous inlet defect, which extends posteriorly between the mitral and tricuspid valves. Although infundibular malalignment and perimembranous inlet defects are the most common, any type of ventricular septal defect can occur with simple transposition of the great arteries.

In *d*-transposition of the great arteries, anterior displacement of the infundibular septum results in a narrowed right ventricular infundibulum, discontinuity of the infundibular septum and the trabecular septum, and a malaligned outlet ventricular septal defect.[12] This condition has been referred to as *d*-transposition with an outlet ventricular septal defect and an overriding pulmonary artery. The outlet ventricular septal defect can be imaged in several planes; however, the parasternal long-axis view is particularly useful for visualizing the anteriorly displaced infundibular septum and the overriding pulmonary artery (Fig 6–15). Although the pulmonary artery overrides the ventricular septum, more than 50% of the pulmonary artery is committed to the left ventricle, and there is pulmonary-

mitral continuity. These features help distinguish this defect from double-outlet right ventricle with anterior position of the aorta. Hemodynamically, this defect is similar to Taussig-Bing malformation because both have subpulmonary ventricular septal defect. Anatomically, however, these two defects are quite different. In the classic Taussig-Bing form of double-outlet right ventricle, the great arteries are nearly side by side with the aorta rightward and slightly posterior. The pulmonary artery is in its normal position and overrides the ventricular septal defect anteriorly.[12] In *d*-transposition with a ventricular septal defect and overriding pulmonary artery, the aorta is anterior and the pulmonary artery overrides posteriorly (Fig 6–15).

In a patient with a malalignment outlet ventricular septal defect, the uppermost portion of the tricuspid annulus is posterior to the defect. The chordae of the tricuspid valve can attach to the crest of the ventricular septum, to the infundibular septum, or to papillary muscles in the right ventricle. With this type of ventricular septal defect, tricuspid valve abnormalities are frequent, in one series occurring in 65% of patients with a malalignment outlet ventricular septal defect.[13] The types of tricuspid valve anomalies that occur are chordal attachments to the infundibular septum or ventricular septal crest, overriding of the tricuspid annulus, straddling tricuspid valve with chordal attachments into the left ventricle, tricuspid valve tissue protruding through the ventricular septal defect and causing subpulmonary obstruction, and cleft anterior leaflet of the tricuspid valve (Fig 6–16).

The anterior displacement of the infundibular septum causes subaortic narrowing and produces a long, oblique course from the left ventricle to the aorta (Fig 6–17). These anatomic features make intraventricular repair extremely difficult and favor repair with an arterial switch procedure,

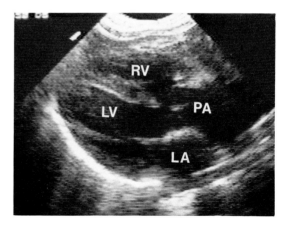

FIG 6–15.
Parasternal long-axis view from an infant with *d*-transposition of the great artery and a large outlet ventricular septal defect. In this patient, the outlet ventricular septal defect was associated with anterior displacement of the conus septum. When this occurs, the pulmonary artery (PA) overrides the ventricular septum. *LA* = left atrium; *LV* = left ventricle; and *RV* = right ventricle.

these cases, muscular subpulmonary obstruction is nearly always present. The posteriorly displaced infundibular septum can be well visualized from parasternal long-axis and subcostal four-chamber views of the left ventricular outflow tract (Fig 6–18). Because of the posterior deviation of the infundibular septum, a direct route from the left ventricle to the aorta is present, and children with this defect are good candidates for repair by way of intraventricular rerouting from the left ventricle to the aorta.[12] With

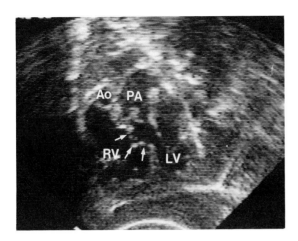

FIG 6–16.
Subcostal sagittal view from an infant with *d*-transposition of the great arteries, a large outlet ventricular septal defect, and an overriding pulmonary artery (PA). Note the discontinuity between the conus septum, situated between the aorta and the PA, and the trabecular septum. A tricuspid valve chord *(arrows)* is seen crossing the area of the outlet ventricular septal defect and inserting into the crest of the trabecular septum. Tricuspid valve abnormalities are frequently found in patients with *d*-transposition, outlet ventricular septal defect, and overriding PA. *AO* = aorta; *LV* = left ventricle; and *RV* = right ventricle.

closure of the ventricular septal defect, and resection of subaortic muscle if necessary (see the section on arterial switch in this chapter).[12] After closure of the ventricular septal defect, the right ventricle always becomes smaller, and right ventricular outflow gradients that were of minor significance preoperatively may become significant. The subaortic narrowing seen in patients with *d*-transposition and a malalignment ventricular septal defect may lead to the development of coarctation and interruption of the aorta. In one review of 129 pathologic specimens with *d*-transposition, 17% had right ventricular outflow obstruction and 7% had associated aortic arch obstruction as well. Anatomic narrowing of the subaortic region was found only in association with a malalignment outlet ventricular septal defect. Aortic arch obstruction was present in 44% of specimens with a malalignment outlet ventricular septal defect and in only 3% of specimens with an intact ventricular septum.[14] Thus, in patients with *d*-transposition and a malalignment outlet ventricular septal defect, a careful search should be made during the echocardiographic examination for evidence of subaortic narrowing or aortic arch obstruction. Subaortic narrowing is best detected from the subcostal four-chamber view of the right ventricle, and aortic coarctation is best visualized from a suprasternal long-axis view.

Other types of outlet ventricular septal defects occur less commonly in children with *d*-transposition. Outlet ventricular septal defects can occur with posterior displacement of the infundibular septum, left ventricular outflow tract narrowing, and posterior malalignment between the infundibular septum and the trabecular septum.[12] In

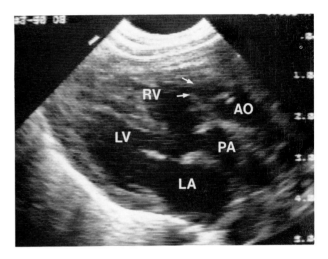

FIG 6–17.
Parasternal long-axis view from an infant with *d*-transposition of the great arteries, a large outlet ventricular septal defect, and an overriding pulmonary artery (PA). In this patient, the anterior displacement of the conus septum has created severe subaortic stenosis *(arrows)*. *AO* = aorta; *LA* = left atrium; *LV* = left ventricle; *PA* = pulmonary artery; and *RV* = right ventricle.

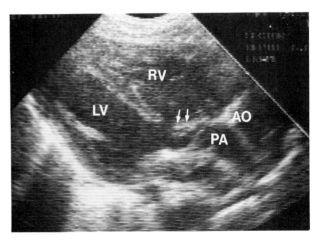

FIG 6–18.
Parasternal long-axis view from an infant with *d*-transposition of the great arteries, an outlet ventricular septal defect, and posterior displacement of the infundibular septum *(arrow)* into the left ventricular (LV) outflow tract. This posterior deviation of the infundibular septum creates subpulmonary stenosis. *AO* = aorta; *LV* = left ventricle; *PA* = pulmonary artery; and *RV* = right ventricle.

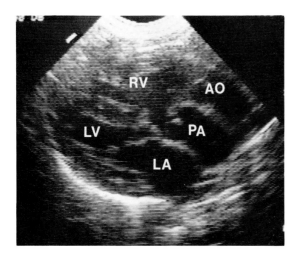

FIG 6–19.
Parasternal long-axis view from an infant with *d*-transposition of the great arteries, a large outlet ventricular septal defect, and a hypoplastic or absent infundibular septum. In these patients, the pulmonary artery (PA) does not override the ventricular septum. When subpulmonary stenosis is present, it is usually not a muscular form of subpulmonary stenosis. In this patient, a discrete subpulmonary membrane can be seen. *AO* = aorta; *LA* = left atrium; *LV* = left ventricle; and *RV* = right ventricle.

this type of defect, the upper portion of the tricuspid annulus and the highest papillary muscle of the tricuspid valve are posterior to the defect. Coarctation of the aorta is not associated with this type of ventricular septal defect.

Another type of outlet ventricular septal defect that occurs infrequently in children with *d*-transposition is a subarterial (subaortic) ventricular septal defect in which the infundibular septum is hypoplastic or absent but not displaced (Fig 6–19).[12] As in other forms of outlet ventricular septal defect, the tricuspid valve and highest papillary muscle are posterior to the defect. Coarctation is not associated with this type of defect. In patients with subarterial ventricular septal defect, the aorta is frequently to the left and anterior (see Fig 6–6).[12] Thus, if the parasternal short-axis view shows a leftward and anterior aorta, the examiner should suspect that a subaortic ventricular septal defect is present.

Perimembranous inlet ventricular septal defects are commonly found in patients with *d*-transposition. In these defects, the infundibular septum is fully developed and normally placed. The roof of this defect extends posteriorly between the mitral and tricuspid valves. Thus, in the apical and subcostal four-chamber views, the mitral and tricuspid valve leaflets are seen touching, with no intervening ventricular septum (Fig 6–20). Because the defect extends posteriorly, the uppermost portion of the tricuspid annulus and the highest papillary muscle and chordae are anterosuperior to the defect.[12] The defect relates, then, primarily to the septal rather than to the anterior leaflet of the tricuspid valve. This type of defect is also associated with tricuspid valve abnormalities of the type described above

for a malalignment outlet defect. In one series, 100% of patients with inlet ventricular septal defect had tricuspid valve abnormalities.[13] Overriding or straddling of the tricuspid valve is most frequently associated with an inlet ventricular septal defect. In its most severe form, tricuspid valve straddle leads to underdevelopment of the right ventricle and aortic arch obstruction. Tricuspid valve override or straddle is easily detectable in the four-chamber views (Figs 6–21 and 6–22). These views also provide a method of judging the relative sizes of the right ventricular and left ventricular inflow tracts.

Other types of ventricular septal defects found in association with *d*-transposition are isolated muscular defects and perimembranous trabecular defects.

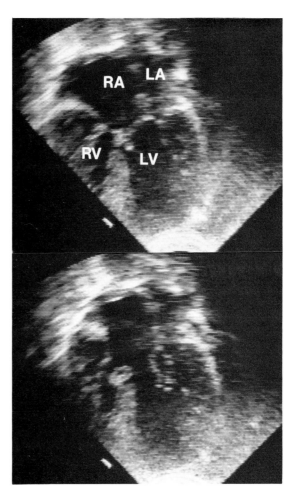

FIG 6–20.
Apical four-chamber views in systole *(above)* and diastole *(below)* from an infant with *d*-transposition of the great arteries, a large inlet ventricular septal defect, and malalignment between the atrial and ventricular septa. As a result, the tricuspid valve overrides the ventricular septum. The tricuspid valve is primarily committed to the right ventricle (RV), which is quite small. Other views in this patient showed that the tricuspid valve also had chordal insertions into the left ventricle (LV). Thus the tricuspid valve both overrode and straddled the ventricular septal defect. *LA* = left atrium; *RA* = right atrium.

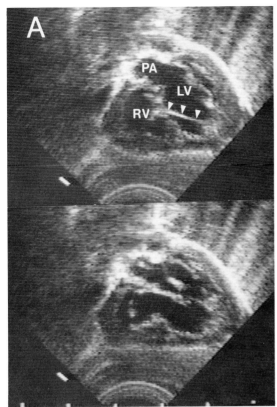

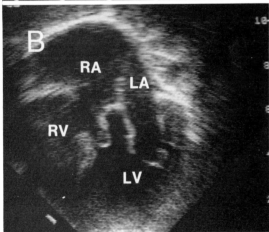

Left ventricular outflow tract obstruction.—Obstruction to the pulmonary outflow occurs in patients with *d*-transposition and an intact ventricular septum and in patients with *d*-transposition and a ventricular septal defect. In children with an intact ventricular septum, dynamic subpulmonary obstruction is common, either pre- or post-intra-atrial baffle procedure. This dynamic obstruction is believed to be caused by a prominent systolic bulging of the ventricular septum into the left ventricular outflow tract.[15] Dynamic subpulmonary obstruction causes systolic anterior motion of the mitral valve, fine frequency fluttering of the pulmonary valve, and midsystolic closure of the pulmonary valve on the M-mode echocardiogram.[5, 8, 15] On the two-dimensional echocardiogram, the left ventricle is thin-walled and crescent-shaped in the short-axis views. Only minimal pressure gradients are detected by pulsed or continuous-wave Doppler techniques.[16]

With significant fixed anatomic obstruction, the left ventricular pressure increases and the left ventricle becomes spherical and thick-walled. The most common forms of fixed pulmonary stenosis that occur in patients with *d*-transposition and an intact ventricular septum are fibrous subpulmonary diaphragm, fibromuscular ridge, and valvular stenosis (usually a bicuspid pulmonary valve). The parasternal long-axis view and the subcostal four-chamber view of the left ventricular outflow tract are particularly useful for imaging fibrous rings and fibromuscular ridges. These views are also useful for detecting the abnormal motion of a domed stenotic pulmonary valve; the parasternal short-axis view, however, is preferable for determining the valve morphology (Fig 6–23).

Figure 6–24 shows the anatomic types of left ventricular outflow tract obstruction that occur in children with *d*-transposition and a ventricular septal defect.[17] Subpulmonary stenosis occurs more commonly in association with a ventricular septal defect, and certain types of subpulmonary stenosis are specific for certain types of ventricular septal defects (Figs 6–25 and 6–26). For example, posterior deviation of the infundibular septum occurs with mala-

FIG 6–21.
A, subcostal coronal views from an infant with *d*-transposition of the great arteries, a large inlet ventricular septal defect, and an overriding and straddling tricuspid valve. In systole *(top)*, the closed tricuspid valve leaflets are seen situated in the middle of the inlet ventricular septal defect. A chordae of the tricuspid valve *(arrows)* is seen inserting into the left ventricle (LV). In diastole *(bottom)*, one tricuspid valve leaflet can be seen inserting into the LV, while the other tricuspid valve leaflet has chordal insertions into the right ventricle (RV). Note the lack of septum intervening between the tricuspid and mitral valve leaflets. **B,** apical four-chamber view from the same patient as in **A.** In this view, the septal leaflet of the tricuspid valve can be seen inserting into the left ventricular (LV) surface of the ventricular septum. Note the malalignment between the atrial and ventricular septa. *LA* = left atrium; *RA* = right atrium; *RV* = right ventricle; and *PA* = pulmonary artery.

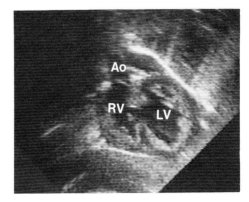

FIG 6–22.
Subcostal coronal view from the same infant as in Figure 6–21. In this patient, the right ventricle (RV) is considerably smaller than the left ventricle (LV). The ventricular septal defect can again be seen. *AO* = aorta.

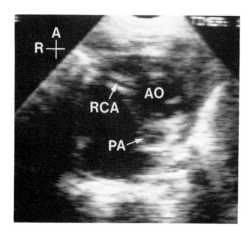

FIG 6–23.
Parasternal short-axis view at the base of the heart from a patient with *d*-transposition of the great arteries, a bicuspid pulmonary valve, and a small pulmonary valve annulus. *A* = anterior; *AO* = aorta; *PA* = pulmonary artery; *R* = right; and *RCA* = right coronary artery.

lignment outlet ventricular septal defect,[12] while accessory tricuspid tissue bowing into the left ventricular outflow tract tends to occur with perimembranous inlet defects.[13] The parasternal long-axis and subcostal views are particularly useful for diagnosing the type of anatomic obstruction. Doppler examination from these views provides measurement of the peak gradient across the obstruction.

Postoperative Evaluation of the Patient With d-Transposition

Arterial switch procedure.—In children with *d*-transposition of the great arteries, anatomic correction with the arterial switch procedure is rapidly gaining widespread acceptance as the operation of choice (Fig 6–27).[18–28] Compared to intra-atrial baffle procedures, the arterial switch procedure offers the advantage of reinstating the left ventricle as the systemic pumping chamber. Long-term complications of intra-atrial baffle procedures, such as arrhythmias, baffle obstructions, and right ventricular failure, are not expected to develop following this type of repair. Two-dimensional and Doppler echocardiography provide important noninvasive techniques for evaluating the child who has had arterial switch repair in infancy. The echocardiographic examination should focus on three major areas: detection of newly created structural abnormalities, detection of residual structural abnormalities, and evaluation of systolic and diastolic function.[29]

The surgical maneuvering required to perform the arterial switch repair can result in newly created structural abnormalities, the most common of which is supravalvular pulmonary stenosis. Structural distortion of the main pulmonary artery above the new pulmonary valve (old aortic valve) is commonly seen by two-dimensional echocardiography. The distortion usually consists of a long segment of narrowing that includes the suture line as well as the large patches over the areas where the coronary arteries

and a surrounding button of the aortic root have been removed (Figs 6–28 and 6–29).[23, 29–31]

The hemodynamic significance of supravalvular pulmonary stenosis is difficult to assess on the basis of imaging information alone. Instead, a Doppler estimate of the peak systolic pressure gradient across the main pulmonary artery should be used. In order to obtain the best alignment between the Doppler ultrasound beam and blood flow, the main pulmonary artery should be interrogated from parasternal, apical, and subcostal approaches. In our experience, significant obstruction above the pulmonary valve is uncommon, occurring in only 9% of patients. Doppler peak gradients indicating mild to moderate supravalvular pulmonary stenosis are found in about 44% of patients.[29] Further follow-up examinations are necessary to determine if

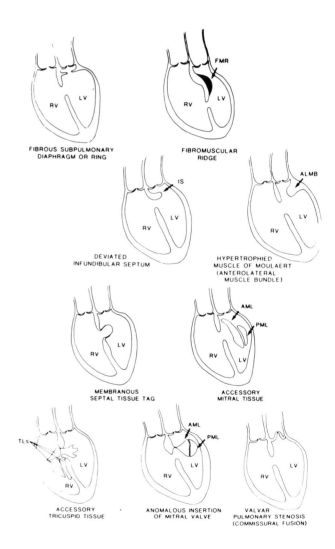

FIG 6–24.
Diagrammatic representation of the types of subpulmonary stenosis that can occur in infants with *d*-transposition of the great arteries. (From Chin AJ, Yeager SB, Sanders SP, et al: *Am J Cardiol* 1985; 55:761. Used by permission.)

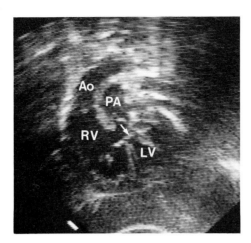

FIG 6–25.
Subcostal sagittal view from an infant with *d*-transposition of the great arteries, a large outlet ventricular septal defect, and a fibrous subpulmonary ring *(arrow)*. *Ao* = aorta; *LV* = left ventricle; *PA* = pulmonary artery; and *RV* = right ventricle.

the mild stenosis detected in these patients will progress to severe obstruction.

Anatomic distortion of the newly created ascending aorta is seen on the two-dimensional echocardiographic examination in all patients after the arterial switch procedure is performed.[29] This distortion occurs where the smaller ascending aorta is sewn to the larger main pulmonary artery above the original pulmonary valve (now the patient's aortic valve). Because of the discrepancy in size between these two structures, the narrowing often appears very severe by two-dimensional imaging, even when Doppler examination shows no evidence of obstruction (Figs 6–30 to 6–32). Thus, the severity of supravalvular aortic stenosis should not be based on imaging information alone, but rather on a careful estimate, using Doppler echocardiography, of the peak gradient across the ascending aorta. Significant supravalvular aortic stenosis is rarely encountered after the arterial switch repair.[29, 31]

Valvular regurgitation can occur as a new finding after the switch procedure or can take on added significance after surgery. For example, what may appear preoperatively to be normal physiologic pulmonary regurgitation in an infant with transposition can persist postoperatively as aortic regurgitation. After the arterial switch, the incidence of aortic insufficiency has ranged from 14% to 40% in various series of patients.[23,29, 31, 32] Despite the discrepancy in incidence, however, in virtually all patients the degree of aortic insufficiency has been trivial to mild.

A small percentage of patients with *d*-transposition of the great arteries have a bicuspid pulmonary valve. After arterial switch repair, these patients have a newly created abnormality—a bicuspid aortic valve. The patients with a bicuspid aortic valve that we have followed have not developed aortic stenosis or regurgitation; however, further follow-up examinations are necessary to determine the fate of the newly created bicuspid aortic valve.[29]

The arterial switch procedure requires the mobilization of small, delicate coronary arteries, thus creating the potential for damage to these vessels, either in the immediate postoperative period or as a late postoperative complication. The two-dimensional echocardiogram is useful for detecting abnormalities in the origin and distribution of the main coronary artery branches preoperatively; to date, however, there are no reports of the use of this technique to detect coronary artery obstruction or kinking postoperatively. It is likely that minor amounts of luminal narrowing will not be detectable by two-dimensional echocardiography because of the limits in resolution.

The coronary arteries can be visualized in 90% of preoperative patients, predominantly with the use of parasternal and apical views. Figure 6–33 shows the coronary artery distribution observed by Pasquini and colleagues in 32 infants with *d*-transposition.[33] The criteria for diagnosing normal coronary artery distribution are (1) imaging separate origins of the right and left coronary arteries from the right and left aortic sinuses in parasternal short- or long-axis views; (2) the absence of a coronary artery between the pulmonary root and the mitral valve in parasternal short-axis, apical four-chamber, or subcostal four-chamber views; and (3) imaging the bifurcation of the left coronary artery in the parasternal short-axis view or the parasternal long-axis view through the right ventricular outflow tract. The criteria for diagnosing the origin of the left circumflex coronary artery from the right coronary artery are (1) visualization of separate origins of the left and right coronary arteries from the left and right aortic sinuses in parasternal views; (2) imaging a coronary artery passing between the pulmonary root and mitral valve in parasternal

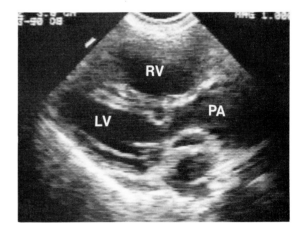

FIG 6–26.
Parasternal long-axis view from an infant with *d*-transposition of the great arteries and a membranous ventricular septal defect. In this patient, a ventricular septal aneurysm is seen bulging in systole into the left ventricular (LV) outflow tract. This type of aneurysm tissue can cause subpulmonary stenosis in infants with *d*-transposition. *PA* = pulmonary artery; *RV* = right ventricle.

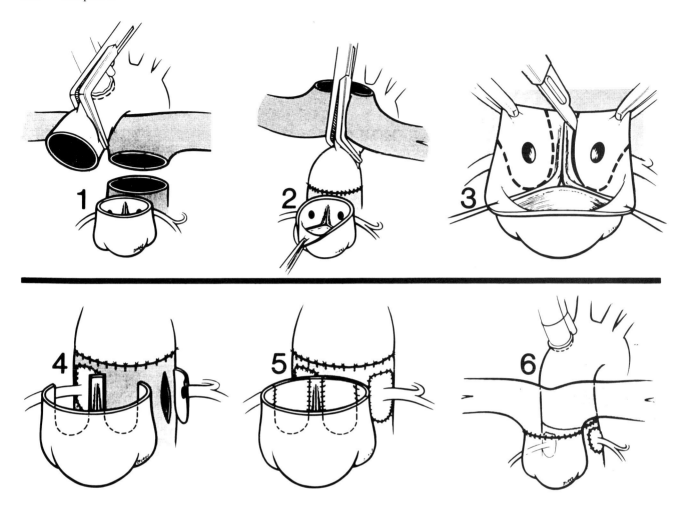

FIG 6–27.
Diagrammatic representation of the arterial switch operation for repair of *d*-transposition of the great arteries. In *step 1*, the anterior aorta and posterior pulmonary artery *(gray stippled area)* have been transected. In *step 2*, the aortic arch is anastomosed to the proximal pulmonary artery and pulmonary valve. In *step 3*, the left and right main coronary arteries and the surrounding button of aortic root tissue are removed. In *step 4*, the coronary arteries and surrounding portion of aortic root are implanted into the original proximal pulmonary artery. In *step 5*, the areas of the aortic root where the coronary arteries were excised are repaired with patches. In *step 6*, the distal main pulmonary artery and branches are anastomosed to the proximal ascending aorta and aortic valve. (From Bove EL, Beekman RH, Snider AR, et al: *Circulation* 1988; 78[suppl 3]:28. Used with permission.)

short-axis or apical and subcostal four-chamber views; and (3) visualization of the left circumflex coronary artery arising from the right coronary artery a few millimeters after its origin and passing posteriorly and leftward in the parasternal short-axis view. The criteria for diagnosis of single right coronary artery include (1) imaging of a single large coronary ostium arising from the right aortic sinus in the parasternal views; (2) identification of the left coronary artery arising from the right and passing leftward behind the pulmonary root in the parasternal short-axis or apical four-chamber view; and (3) imaging of the left coronary artery bifurcation in parasternal views.[33] Visualization of the coronary arteries can be optimized by moving the transducer superiorly and rightward from a standard parasternal short-axis view.

Besides the detection of newly created structural ab-

normalities, the echocardiographic examination is useful for detecting residual structural abnormalities. For example, the Doppler examination is useful for detecting residual shunting across atrial or ventricular septal defect patches or residual coarctation. Although it is fairly common to detect left-to-right shunting across ventricular patches in the first few days postoperatively, residual ventricular septal defects beyond the first postoperative week are uncommon.

The arterial switch procedure has the theoretical advantage of reinstating the left ventricle as the systemic pumping chamber in children with *d*-transposition of the great arteries, thus eliminating the long-term complication of right ventricular failure. However, the arterial switch procedure requires the mobilization of small, delicate, coronary arteries, thus creating the potential for left ventricular ischemia, either in the immediate postoperative period or as a late postoperative complication. In patients evaluated years after the arterial switch repair, M-mode echocardiographic measurements of the left ventricular dimensions, wall thickness, wall stress, and fractional shortening have been normal.[29, 34] Likewise, peak left-ventricular shortening rate measured from the digitized M-mode echocardiogram has been normal after arterial switch repair.[35] M-mode echocardiographic measurements of the left-ventricular end-systolic pressure-dimension and wall stress-shortening relationships—sensitive indexes of contractility—have been normal at varying afterloads in children who have undergone the arterial switch procedure.[34, 36] Two-dimensional echocardiographic evaluation of right and left ventricular wall motion has shown no evidence of regional ischemia.[29, 34] Diastolic indexes of left ventricular function, including normalized peak filling rates and normalized peak wall thinning rates, have also been normal.[34]

In summary, follow-up studies of patients after the arterial switch have shown that distortion of the great arteries is commonly seen by two-dimensional echocardiography, but significant functional abnormalities are uncommon on Doppler examination (9% with significant supravalvular pulmonary stenosis). Right and left ventricular systolic function are well-preserved, although more investigation is needed to assess systolic function during exercise, diastolic function, and the fate of the coronary artery circulation.

Intra-atrial baffle procedures.—In atrial switch procedures, the pulmonary and systemic venous return is rerouted using an intra-atrial baffle. The baffle can be thought of as a conduit that runs between the superior and inferior

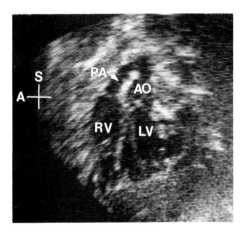

FIG 6–28.
Subcostal coronal view from an infant with *d*-transposition of the great arteries following an arterial switch repair. The pulmonary artery (PA) is narrowed at the point where patches were placed over the areas where the coronary arteries and a surrounding button of aortic root tissue were removed. In this patient, a mild supravalvular pulmonary stenosis gradient was present. *A* = anterior; *AO* = aorta; *LV* = left ventricle; *RV* = right ventricle; and *S* = superior.

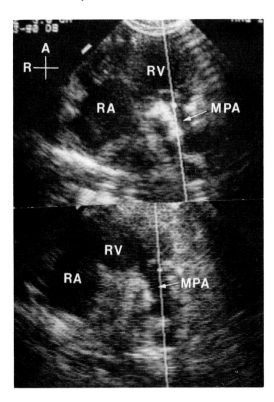

FIG 6–29.
Parasternal short-axis views from a patient with *d*-transposition of the great arteries with an arterial switch repair who developed severe supravalvular pulmonary stenosis. In the *top frame*, a narrowing in the main pulmonary artery (MPA) can be seen. At the time of the Doppler examination, this patient had a 77 mm Hg gradient across the narrowed area. The peak gradient was not obtained at the sample volume position shown in the figure, but obtained distally in the MPA. The *bottom frame* was obtained from the same patient following re-operation for repair of supravalvular pulmonary stenosis. The MPA is considerably wider, and at the time of this study there was no significant gradient remaining. *A* = anterior; *R* = right; *RA* = right atrium; and *RV* = right ventricle. (From Martin MM, Snider AR, Bove EL, et al: *Am J Cardiol* 1989; 63:335.)

venae cavae and the mitral valve.[37] Systemic venous return flows under the conduit to the mitral valve, while pulmonary venous return cascades over the conduit to reach the tricuspid valve. Not all portions of the newly created systemic and pulmonary venous atria can be seen in a single echocardiographic plane. Therefore, visualization of the atria and baffle with multiple echocardiographic views is necessary for complete evaluation of the child who has undergone an atrial switch procedure.

In the parasternal and apical long-axis views, the intra-atrial baffle can be seen stretching obliquely from an anterosuperior to a posteroinferior position (Fig 6–34). Inferior to the baffle, the mid-portion of the systemic venous atrium can be seen communicating with the mitral valve and left ventricle. The superior vena caval and inferior vena caval portions of the systemic venous atrium cannot be seen in this view.[37] Posterior to the baffle, a left-sided portion of the pulmonary venous atrium can be seen. With

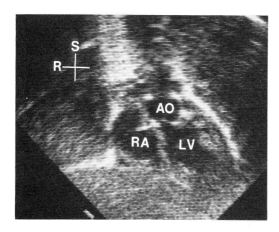

FIG 6–30.
Subcostal coronal view of the left ventricular (LV) outflow tract from a patient with *d*-transposition of the great arteries following arterial switch repair. In this view, there is an apparent narrowing of the ascending aorta (AO) above the sinuses of Valsalva. This apparent narrowing is caused by the discrepancy in size between the original pulmonary valve and the aortic root. In this patient there was no gradient across this area. *R* = right; *RA* = right atrium; and *S* = superior.

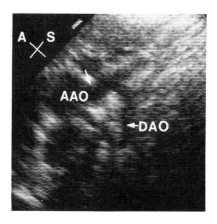

FIG 6–32.
Suprasternal long-axis view from an infant with *d*-transposition of the great arteries following an arterial switch repair. In this view, the area of apparent narrowing *(arrow)* is seen in the ascending aorta (AO). No gradient was present across this area. *A* = anterior; *DAO* = descending aorta; and *S* = superior. (From Martin MM, Snider AR, Bove EL, et al: *Am J Cardiol* 1989; 63:334. Used by permission.)

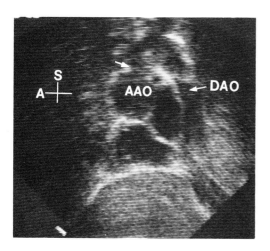

FIG 6–31.
Subcostal sagittal view of a patient with *d*-transposition of the great arteries following an arterial switch repair. A narrowed area *(arrow)* can be seen in the ascending aorta (AAO) above the sinuses of Valsalva. This apparent narrowing is caused by the discrepancy in size between the original pulmonary valve and root and the ascending aorta. There was no pressure gradient by Doppler examination or cardiac catheterization across this area. *A* = anterior; *DAO* = descending aorta; and *S* = superior. (From Martin MM, Snider AR, Bove EL, et al: *Am J Cardiol* 1989; 63:334. Used by permission.)

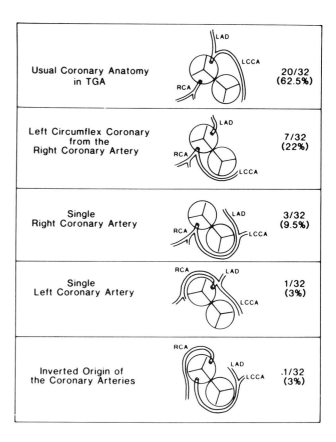

FIG 6–33.
Diagrammatic representation of the coronary artery anatomy found in infants with transposition of the great arteries. From Pasquini L, Sanders SP, Parness IA, et al: Diagnosis of coronary artery anatomy by two-dimensional echocardiography in patients with transposition of the great arteries. *Circulation* 1987; 75:560. Used by permission.)

angulation of the transducer in the long-axis view toward the patient's right hip, the junction of the pulmonary venous atrium and the right ventricle can be imaged. These long-axis views are useful for detecting tricuspid regurgitation or pulmonary venous stenosis with pulsed or color-flow Doppler techniques.

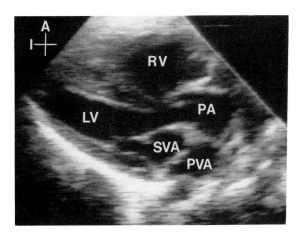

FIG 6–34.
Parasternal long-axis view from a patient with *d*-transposition of the great arteries following an intra-atrial baffle procedure. The baffle can be seen stretching across the atrium and dividing the atrium into a pulmonary venous atrium (PVA) above and a systemic venous atrium (SVA) below. The SVA is continuous with the left ventricle (LV). *A* = anterior; *I* = inferior; *PA* = pulmonary artery; and *RV* = right ventricle.

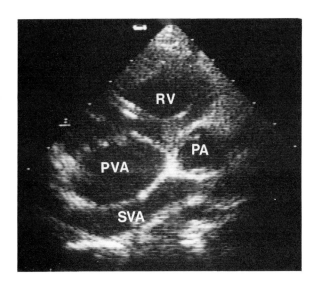

FIG 6–35.
Parasternal short-axis view from an infant with *d*-transposition of the great arteries following an intra-atrial baffle procedure. The baffle can be seen dividing the atrial chamber. In this view, a considerable length of the systemic venous atrium (SVA) stretching between the inferior vena cava and the left ventricle can be seen. In addition, a portion of the pulmonary venous atrium (PVA) can be seen connecting to the right ventricle (RV). *PA* = pulmonary artery.

In the parasternal short-axis view, the baffle courses horizontally from right to left. Above the baffle, the mid-portion of the systemic venous atrium is imaged, while a portion of the pulmonary venous atrium is seen below the baffle (Figs 6–35 and 6–36).

The apical four-chamber view is especially useful for imaging larger portions of both atria. In this view, the plane of sound slices through both walls of the pericardial conduit so that the systemic venous atrium is imaged from its junction with the inferior vena cava to its junction with the mitral valve (Fig 6–37). This view is particularly useful for detecting inferior vena caval obstruction and mitral regurgitation with pulsed and color-flow Doppler. In addition, this view shows a long length of the conduit and

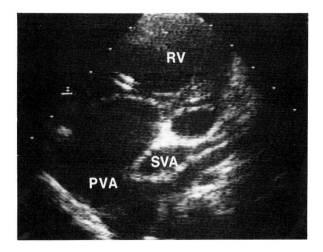

FIG 6–36.
Parasternal short-axis view obtained from the same patient as in Figure 6–35. To obtain this view, the transducer was tilted superiorly to image the entire length of the pulmonary venous atrium (PVA). The pulmonary veins can be seen draining to the pulmonary venous atrium and ultimately to the right ventricle (RV). A portion of the systemic venous atrium (SVA) can also be seen.

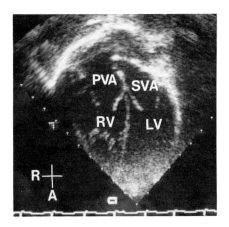

FIG 6–37.
Apical four-chamber view from a patient with *d*-transposition of the great arteries following an intra-atrial baffle procedure. In this view, the plane of sound has been tilted anteriorly to image a considerable portion of the pulmonary venous atrium (PVA). In addition, a section of the systemic venous atrium (SVA) can be seen. *A* = anterior; *LV* = left ventricle; *R* = right; and *RV* = right ventricle.

is useful for detecting baffle leaks with contrast or color-flow Doppler echocardiography. If the plane of sound is tilted anteriorly above the intra-atrial conduit, a large portion of the pulmonary venous atrium (from the pulmonary veins to the tricuspid valve) can be imaged. The sharp angulation of the baffle divides the pulmonary venous atrium into two portions—a portion that communicates with the tricuspid valve and a portion that receives the pulmonary veins. These views are particularly useful for the detection of tricuspid regurgitation or pulmonary venous obstruction with pulsed or color-flow Doppler.

In the subcostal long-axis view in the abdomen, the junction of the inferior vena cava and the systemic venous atrium can be imaged. With rotation of the transducer into a subcostal short-axis view, the junctions of both venae cavae with the systemic venous atrium can be imaged. These views are particularly well suited for the diagnosis of superior or inferior vena caval obstruction using contrast or Doppler echocardiography.

In the suprasternal short-axis view, anterior angulation of the transducer will provide an image in some patients of the superior vena caval junction with the systemic venous atrium. Pulsed and color-flow Doppler examinations can be performed easily from this view to detect superior vena caval obstruction.

Patients who have had a successful intra-atrial baffle procedure have an M-mode echocardiographic profile that resembles that of a preoperative transposition patient. Right ventricular dimension and wall thickness are larger than those of a normal right ventricle and instead resemble the dimensions of a normal left ventricle. Likewise, the left ventricular dimension and wall thickness are smaller than those of a normal left ventricle and resemble the dimensions of a normal right ventricle.[7, 8] Any increase in left ventricular diameter or wall thickness suggests the presence of residual defects such as residual left-to-right shunt, subpulmonary stenosis, or pulmonary hypertension (possibly caused by pulmonary venous obstruction).

Baffle leaks commonly occur after intra-atrial baffle procedures and are usually small. Isolated baffle leaks generally produce bidirectional atrial shunting. With peripheral venous contrast echocardiography, right-to-left baffle leaks can be detected even when the arterial oxygen saturation is normal.[37] After saline injection into a peripheral vein, contrast echoes pass from the systemic venous atrium into the pulmonary venous atrium (Fig 6–38). Baffle left-to-right or right-to-left shunting can also be detected with Doppler color-flow mapping techniques.

Another frequent complication of intra-atrial baffle procedures is superior vena caval obstruction. Peripheral venous contrast echocardiography was the first technique used to detect superior vena caval obstruction (Fig 6–39).[38] With this technique, saline is injected into an upper body vein (arm or scalp vein) while the inferior vena cava (from below the hepatic veins to its junction with the systemic venous atrium) is visualized from the subcostal long-axis view. In patients with no superior vena caval obstruction, contrast echoes are seen filling the systemic venous atrium

from above. No contrast echoes are seen in the lower inferior vena cava. Reflux of contrast echoes can be seen, however, in the upper inferior vena cava and hepatic veins during vigorous atrial contraction. In patients with partial superior vena caval obstruction, contrast echoes arrive first in the systemic venous atrium from the superior vena cava. During subsequent cardiac cycles, contrast echoes are seen in the lower inferior vena cava travelling toward the systemic venous atrium. These contrast echoes reach the lower inferior vena cava through azygous-inferior vena cava collateral veins. In patients with complete superior vena cava obstruction, contrast echoes are seen first in the lower inferior vena cava, flowing toward the heart. No contrast echoes are seen in the systemic venous atrium before contrast echoes appear in the lower inferior vena cava.

Doppler echocardiography is also useful for detecting superior vena caval obstruction.[39, 40] From the suprasternal notch, the Doppler transducer is aimed inferiorly and rightward toward the superior vena cava. Normal superior vena cava flow is directed away from the transducer below the baseline and has a phasic, low-velocity pattern in diastole (see Chapter 3). With partial superior vena caval obstruction, a continuous, disturbed flow pattern is seen below the baseline. Peak velocities of this flow are usually elevated (> 1 m/sec). With complete superior vena caval obstruction, flow velocities in the superior vena cava can be difficult to record. Color-flow Doppler techniques are especially useful for examining superior vena caval flow patterns. Because venous flow is of very low velocity, the color-flow Doppler instrument should be used with minimum wall filter settings and a low velocity scale so that the sensitivity for registering low velocity flow signals will be increased. In many patients, superior vena caval flow can be seen in the suprasternal short-axis view. With no obstruction, areas of blue flow are seen passing from the superior vena cava to the systemic venous atrium. With partial obstruction, the color-flow Doppler variance map may show a mosaic-colored jet just past the area of obstruction. With complete obstruction, areas of red flow may appear in the lower superior vena cava, indicating retrograde flow toward the transducer. The color-flow Doppler examination can also be performed by imaging the superior vena cava from the subcostal short-axis view. The same flow patterns are observed; in this view, however, normal forward flow in the superior vena cava is toward the transducer and is therefore red rather than blue. Also, in the subcostal short-axis view, flow can be seen in the azygous vein on the color Doppler examination. Normal flow in the azygous vein is directed away from the transducer and is therefore blue. An area of red flow in the azygous vein represents partial or complete superior vena caval obstruction.

Inferior vena caval obstruction rarely occurs after intra-atrial baffle procedures. The area of obstruction usually can be visualized directly in the subcostal views of the junction of the inferior vena cava and systemic venous atrium. The inferior vena cava below the obstruction is generally quite dilated. Pulsed Doppler examination shows

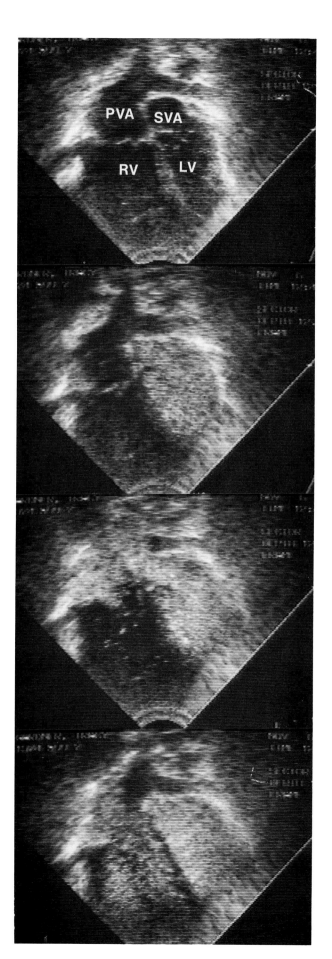

FIG 6–38.
Peripheral venous contrast injection from a patient with *d*-transposition of the great arteries following an intra-atrial baffle procedure. In the *top frame,* the apical four-chamber view is seen before injection of the contrast agent. In the *second frame,* contrast echoes are seen filling the systemic venous atrium (SVA) and the left ventricle (LV). In the *third frame,* contrast echoes have appeared in the pulmonary venous atrium (PVA) because of the presence of a right-to-left baffle leak. In the *bottom frame,* contrast echoes have flowed forward from the PVA to the right ventricle (RV). The pulmonary veins are free of contrast echoes, which proves that the shunt was at atrial level and not at pulmonary level.

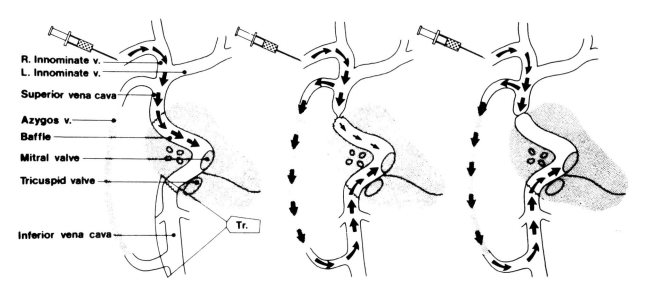

FIG 6–39.
Echocardiographic contrast patterns found in patients after an intra-atrial baffle procedure. A contrast injection is made into an arm or scalp vein while the transducer (TR) is applied in the subcostal long-axis plane to image the junction of the inferior vena cava with the systemic venous atrium. With no superior vena caval obstruction, the contrast echoes (black arrows) fill the systemic venous atrium from above. No contrast echoes are seen in the lower inferior vena cava. In patients with partial superior vena caval obstruction, contrast echoes (middle) fill the systemic venous atrium from above.

Subsequently, contrast echoes appear in the lower inferior vena cava, flowing toward the systemic venous atrium. These contrast echoes arrive in the inferior vena cava by way of azygous-inferior vena cava collateral vessels. In patients with total superior vena caval obstruction, contrast echoes (right) fill the systemic venous atrium entirely from below by way of azygous-inferior vena cava collateral vessels. (From Silverman NH, Snider AR, Colo J, et al: *Circulation* 1981; 64:393. Used by permission.)

a continuous, disturbed flow from the inferior vena cava into the systemic venous atrium. This area of disturbed flow is readily seen on color Doppler examination as a mosaic, high-velocity jet (usually from 1 to 2 m/sec).

Pulmonary venous obstruction is another important complication that can occur following an intra-atrial baffle procedure. Because of the sharp angulation of the baffle, the presence and severity of pulmonary venous obstruction is difficult to determine with two-dimensional echocardiography alone. Pulsed and color-flow Doppler echocardiography are important techniques for detecting the presence and hemodynamic severity of pulmonary venous obstruction.[41, 42] First, the color-flow Doppler examination is performed to seek out areas of disturbed (high-velocity, mosaic) flow across the pulmonary venous ostia or within the body of the pulmonary venous atrium. The color Doppler instrument settings are the same as described above for interrogating the superior vena cava (low wall filters and low velocity scale). Next, the color-flow Doppler map is used to align the pulsed or continuous-wave Doppler beam parallel to the jet flow. Flow in the normal pulmonary vein is of low velocity and biphasic (see Chapter 3). With pulmonary venous obstruction, a high-velocity disturbed flow is present. This flow may be biphasic or continuous. When using the Doppler technique to detect pulmonary venous obstruction, several important factors should be remembered. First, patients with severe pulmonary venous inflow obstruction have abnormally high diastolic flow

velocities, with biphasic or even continuous disturbed flow. Doppler peak diastolic velocity of 2 m/sec or more corresponds to catheterization evidence of severe obstruction (mean gradient ≥16 mm Hg). Second, with large baffle leaks, maximum diastolic flow velocities as high as 1.7 m/sec can be recorded at the junction of the pulmonary vein confluence and the pulmonary venous atrium. Third, on the basis of peak velocity alone, it may not be possible to distinguish mild obstruction from no obstruction. In these patients, color Doppler may be useful for detecting areas of turbulent flow. Finally, severe pulmonary venous narrowing can be present with minimal gradient. For example, stenosis of a single pulmonary vein can result in decreased pulmonary blood flow to the lung segment drained by that stenotic vein. In this case as well, the detection of turbulence may alert the examiner to the diagnosis even when maximum diastolic velocity is normal.

Complete echocardiographic evaluation of a child after an intra-atrial baffle procedure should include assessment of right ventricular function using the techniques outlined in Chapter 4, detection and grading of tricuspid regurgitation, and determination of the severity of left ventricular outflow obstruction.

l-Transposition of the Great Arteries

l-Transposition of the great arteries is a condition in which there is atrioventricular discordance as well as ventriculoarterial discordance. Therefore, in situs solitus, the morphologic right atrium on the patient's right is connected to the morphologic left ventricle on the patient's right which, in turn, is connected to the pulmonary artery. On the left, the morphologic left atrium is connected to the morphologic right ventricle, which is connected to the aorta.[43, 44] This defect is called situs solitus, *l*-loop, *l*-transposition, or simply *l*-transposition. The *l* in the third term describes the spatial relations of the aortic and pulmonic valves. In the majority of cases, the aortic valve is to the left, hence the use of the *l*. Because discordant connections are present at two levels, the circulation is hemodynamically correct (systemic venous blood flows to the pulmonary artery and pulmonary venous blood flows to the aorta); some investigators have called this defect corrected transposition of the great arteries. Because of the confusion in distinguishing this defect from surgically corrected *d*-transposition, we prefer not to use this terminology.

As with *d*-transposition, the echocardiographic diagnosis of *l*-transposition is based on demonstrating abnormal connections between the right ventricle and aorta and also between the atria and the ventricles. The spatial relationships of the great arteries may provide supportive evidence of the diagnosis; however, spatial relationship is never used as the sole diagnostic criterion.

The morphology of the atria, ventricles, and great arteries are determined on the echocardiogram using the criteria outlined under *d*-transposition in this chapter and in Chapter 14. As with *d*-transposition, the connections of the chambers and great vessels can be seen in multiple echocardiographic views; the subcostal views, however, are particularly useful because, by simply tilting the transducer in one view, they provide imaging of all cardiac chambers, great vessels, and connections. In the subcostal four-chamber view shown in Figure 6–40, the atrium on the patient's left receives the four pulmonary veins and is the morphologic left atrium. The ventricle on the patient's left has characteristic features of a morphologic right ventricle (tricuspid valve, prominent septoparietal muscle bundles) and gives rise to a vessel that arches and is therefore the aorta. On the right, the morphologic right atrium is connected to a ventricle that has the anatomic features of a left ventricle (a smooth septal surface, a mitral valve, and two papillary muscles). The morphologic left ventricle on the patient's right is connected to a vessel that bifurcates into two branches and is therefore the pulmonary artery. These anatomic features are diagnostic of *l*-transposition of the great arteries. The discordant atrioventricular and ventriculoarterial connections can also be imaged in the apical four-chamber (Fig 6–41) and subcostal sagittal views.

In *l*-transposition, the aortic valve is usually supported by a complete muscular infundibulum and is therefore located more superiorly than the pulmonary valve (see Fig 6–40). In the majority of cases, the muscular infundibulum of the left ventricle is absorbed so that the pulmonary valve is wedged deeply in the heart between the two atrioventricular valves. Direct valvular continuity exists between the posterior cusp of the pulmonary valve and the anterior leaflet of the mitral valve; however, indirect continuity also exists with the tricuspid valve on the left through the central fibrous body and membranous septum.[43] With a slight tilting of the plane in the parasternal long-axis view, echocardiographic continuity of the pulmonary valve to both right and left atrioventricular valves can be shown.

Spatial Relations

As in *d*-transposition, the ventricular outflow tract and great arteries in *l*-transposition exit the heart in a parallel fashion instead of wrapping around one another. Unlike the normal heart or the heart with *d*-transposition, however, the right ventricle is usually not anterior to the left ventricle in *l*-transposition. Typically, the ventricles are positioned side by side, and the ventricular septum is oriented in a straight line perpendicular to the frontal plane through the thorax. In some cases, the ventricles are arranged in a superior-inferior manner, with the morphologic right ventricle being superior.[45] The unusual spatial relationships of the ventricles, the ventricular septum, and the great arteries lead to several unusual echocardiographic findings of which the examiner should be aware. First, the parasternal long-axis plane is oriented in a much more vertical direction than usual; and, because the ventricles and great arteries are side by side, long-axis views can be obtained through the morphologic left ventricle and pulmonary artery on the right, or through the morphologic right ventricle and aorta on the left. If the transducer is oriented in the usual direction of a normal parasternal long-axis view, it is possible to obtain a long-axis section through the pulmonary valve and left atrioventricular (tricuspid) valve. This unusual view can be obtained because of the indirect fibrous continuity between the pulmonary and tricuspid valves. If a large ventricular septal defect is present, the plane of sound can pass from the pulmonary valve to the left-sided tricuspid valve with no intervening septum and, thus, mimic the appearance of a single ventricle. Even when the parasternal long-axis plane is oriented correctly for *l*-transposition, it is possible to obtain an image that resembles a single ventricle. This occurs because the ventricles are side by side and the plane of sound can pass through an atrioventricular and semilunar valve without passing through any portion of the ventricular septum. The parasternal short-axis view is oriented more horizontally than usual and, in this view, the septum is aligned in a straight anteroposterior direction (Fig 6–42). Second, if the ventricles are positioned in a superior and inferior fashion, it is usually not possible to image both atrioventricular valves simultaneously in the four-chamber views. The plane of sound must be tilted superiorly to image the left-sided, superior tricuspid valve and inferiorly to image the right-sided, inferior mitral valve.

Because of their parallel arrangement, the great arteries are seen in the short-axis views in cross-section as double circles. In the majority of patients with *l*-transposition, the aortic valve is spatially to the left, anterior, and superior to the pulmonary valve; however, as in *d*-transposition, any spatial orientation of the great arteries is possible. Be-

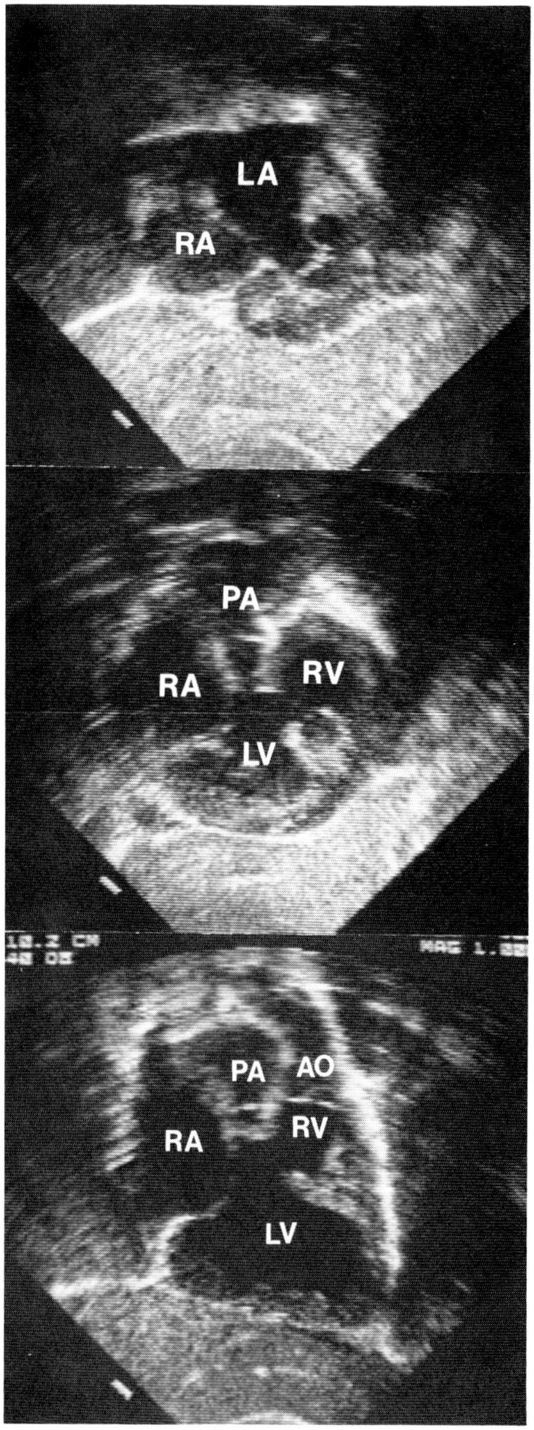

FIG 6–40.
Subcostal coronal views from an infant with situs solitus, *l*-bulbo-
ventricular loop, *l*-transposition of the great arteries, a large ventricular septal defect, and severe subpulmonary stenosis. These views
were obtained by tilting the plane of sound from a posterior to an
anterior position. The *top frame* was obtained by tilting the plane
of sound posteriorly through the inlet of the heart. In this view, the
pulmonary veins can be seen draining to the left-sided atrium,
establishing that this chamber is a morphologic left atrium (LA).
Other views showed that the chamber on the right was a morphologic right atrium (RA). In the *middle frame*, the plane of sound has
been tilted to image the middle portion of the heart. In this plane,
a vessel which bifurcates and is therefore a pulmonary artery (PA)
arises from the right-sided ventricle. This ventricle is smooth-walled
and has features of a morphologic left ventricle (LV). This suggests
that an *l*-bulboventricular loop is present. Note the large ventricular
septal defect and severe subpulmonary narrowing seen in this frame.
In the *bottom frame*, the plane of sound has been tilted far anteriorly. The leftward and superior ventricle is triangular and has
prominent septal-parietal muscle bundles. These features establish
this chamber as a morphologic right ventricle (RV). The aortic (AO)
arch can be seen arising from the RV. The AO is situated at the left
basal aspect of the heart. These findings all demonstrate situs solitus,
l-bulboventricular loop and *l*-transposition of the great arteries.

cause they are at separate heights, the semilunar valves
will not be seen simultaneously in the short-axis view. A
cross-section through the pulmonary valve provides a cross-
section of the right ventricular outflow tract, and a cross-
section through the aortic valve provides an image of the
main pulmonary artery and bifurcation. Imaging of the bifurcation of the posterior great artery into two branches
proves that this vessel is a posterior pulmonary artery and

is strong supportive evidence of ventriculoarterial discordance.

In *l*-transposition, the aortic arch is often situated at
the left upper border of the cardiac silhouette.[46] The ascending aorta passes straight up on the left and then arches,
while the descending aorta passes straight down on the
left behind the ascending aorta. Thus, it is often difficult
to image the entire aortic arch from the standard supra-

sternal notch position. If the transducer is placed in a high left parasternal position (often just under the left clavicle) with the plane of sound vertically aligned, the entire aortic arch can usually be seen (Fig 6–43).

l-Transposition in situs solitus is particularly likely to occur in the presence of dextrocardia.[43] Techniques for

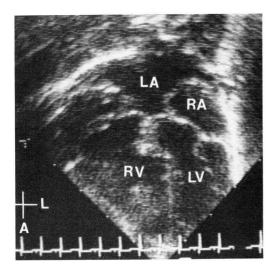

FIG 6–41.
Apical four-chamber view from a patient with situs inversus, *d*-bulbo-ventricular loop, and *d*-transposition of the great arteries. In this view, the pulmonary veins can be seen draining to the right-sided atrium, suggesting that this chamber is a morphologic left atrium (LA). The ventricle on the right has prominent septal parietal muscle bundles and an atrioventricular valve with chordal attachments to the ventricular septum. These findings suggest that the right-sided ventricle is a morphologic right ventricle (RV). Thus, this patient has atrioventricular discordance. *A* = anterior; *L* = left; *LV* = left ventricle; *RA* = right atrium.

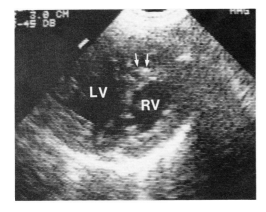

FIG 6–42.
Parasternal short-axis view from a patient with situs solitus, *l*-loop, and *l*-transposition of the great arteries. In this view, the ventricular septum can be seen aligned nearly parallel to the plane of sound. This alignment of the ventricular septum is nearly always found in patients with *l*-bulboventricular loop. Note the moderator band *(arrow)* in the morphologic right ventricle (RV). *LV* = left ventricle.

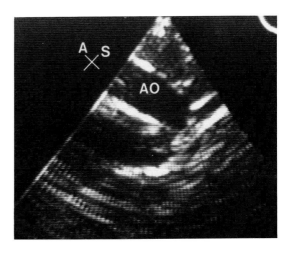

FIG 6–43.
Long-axis view of the aortic (AO) arch from a patient with situs solitus, *l*-loop, and *l*-transposition of the great arteries. Because the AO is positioned at the left basal aspect of the heart, a long-axis view of the arch can be obtained by placing the transducer directly over the ascending AO and under the left clavicle. This results in the orientation of the arch as seen in this frame. *A* = anterior; *S* = superior.

imaging the patient with dextrocardia are discussed in Chapter 14. In this situation, the subcostal views are particularly useful for imaging the rightward orientation of the cardiac apex.

Associated Defects

Tricuspid valve abnormalities.—Abnormalities of the left-sided tricuspid valve occur in about 90% of children with *l*-transposition of the great arteries.[43] The common malformation is an Ebstein-type deformity in which the origin of the valve leaflet is displaced downward so that the basal attachment of the leaflets are from the systemic ventricular wall below the annulus fibrosus. Typically, the anterior leaflet is the least malformed, and the septal and posterior leaflets are the most malformed. Occasionally, the valve leaflets are fused together and are poorly demarcated. The chordae tendinae may be shortened, irregular, and thickened so that they hinder valve motion. The papillary muscles are also frequently deformed. All of these anatomic features result in some loss in the size of the functioning right ventricle (the atrialized portion of the right ventricle is between the annulus and the displaced valve) and a tricuspid valve incapable of closing properly (tricuspid regurgitation).[47] Because both atrioventricular annuli and the basal attachments of the septal and posterior leaflets of the tricuspid valve and the anterior and posterior leaflets of the mitral valve are seen simultaneously, the apical four-chamber view is especially useful for detecting Ebstein deformity of the left-sided tricuspid valve. Pulsed and color Doppler techniques are useful for assessing the presence and severity of tricuspid insufficiency.

In patients with *l*-transposition, deformities of the tricuspid valve other than Ebstein malformation occur and lead to the development of tricuspid regurgitation (physiologic mitral regurgitation). Deformities such as deficient valve leaflet tissue, thickened valve leaflets, dilatation of the annulus fibrosus, abnormal papillary muscles, and shortened chordae tendinae that insert directly into the ventricular wall may all occur and contribute to valvular dysfunction.[47] In a patient with *l*-transposition and a ventricular septal defect (usually perimembranous inlet), chordae can insert through the ventricular septal defect into the morphologic left ventricle (straddling tricuspid valve).

Although it is uncommon, obstruction to right ventricular inflow can occur in patients with *l*-transposition. This obstruction usually takes the form of a stenosing membrane or ring just above the tricuspid valve. On the two-dimensional echocardiogram, the supratricuspid stenosing ring appears as a thin, linear echo just above the left-sided tricuspid valve. Medially, the ring inserts into the left atrial surface just above the crux of the heart and laterally, into the free wall of the left atrium below the appendage.[48] These membranes are seen particularly well in the apical four-chamber view because in this view they are perpendicular to the sound beam. Doppler echocardiography can determine the mean pressure gradient across the obstruction.

Ventricular septal defect.—Ventricular septal defect occurs in about 70% of patients with *l*-transposition[43] and is usually perimembranous in location. However, ventricular septal defects can occur in any portion of the septum (see Fig 6–40). In *l*-transposition, ventricular septal defects are frequently accompanied by other malformations. For example, perimembranous inlet defects may be associated with tricuspid valve straddle, while anterior outlet defects may be associated with mitral valve straddle.

Left ventricular outflow tract obstruction.—Left ventricular outflow tract obstruction occurs in approximately 40% of patients with *l*-transposition. Usually, the stenosis is subvalvular—either a subvalvular diaphragmatic ring or an aneurysm of fibrous tissue that protrudes into the left ventricular outflow tract (see Fig 6–40). This fibrous tissue can originate from the membranous septum, the mitral valve, the tricuspid valve, or the pulmonary valve. The anatomic features of the left ventricular outflow tract are best imaged from apical and subcostal views. With high pulse repetition frequency or continuous-wave Doppler techniques, the peak pressure gradient across the obstruction can be measured. If a nonimaging continuous-wave Doppler transducer is used, care must be taken not to mistake the systolic jets of tricuspid regurgitation or a ventricular septal defect with those of pulmonary stenosis.

Right ventricular outflow tract obstruction.—Right ventricular outflow tract obstruction is rare in patients with *l*-transposition, occurring in only about 10% of patients.[48] Subaortic stenosis can occur in patients with an outlet ventricular septal defect and anterior and leftward displacement of the infundibular septum. Rarely, subaortic

stenosis may occur with an intact ventricular septum and marked hypertrophy of the infundibulum. In these cases, the ascending aorta is usually very hypoplastic. Most patients with *l*-transposition and subaortic stenosis also have aortic coarctation; however, aortic coarctation can occur without subaortic stenosis.[48] The subcostal four-chamber and short-axis views are particularly useful for imaging the right ventricular outflow tract in *l*-transposition. The high left parasternal view described previously is useful for diagnosing coarctation of the aorta.

Double-Outlet Right Ventricle

In double-outlet right ventricle, both great arteries connect primarily to the right ventricle. Thus, in parasternal long- and short-axis views, both great arteries are entirely connected to the right ventricular side of the septum, or the posterior great artery may partially override the septum (Figs 6–44 and 6–45). In cases of double-outlet right ventricle and overriding posterior great artery, more than 50% of the base of the posterior great artery originates in the right ventricle. In its classic form, a muscular infundibulum exists beneath both semilunar valves so that neither is in fibrous continuity with an atrioventricular valve. The thick muscle bundle that separates the subpulmonary and subaortic outflow tracts is known as the outlet (or infundibular) septum or the conus septum[49] and can be visualized easily in the subcostal four-chamber view of the right ventricle. In double-outlet right ventricle, the outlet septum is malaligned relative to the remainder of the septum. The outlet septum is oriented in a sagittal cardiac plane, while the remainder of the septum is usually oriented in

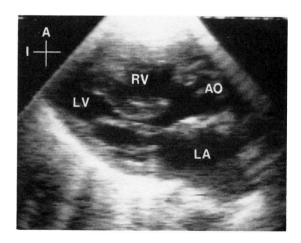

FIG 6–44.
Parasternal long-axis view from an infant with double-outlet right ventricle and side-by-side great arteries. In this view the marked separation (posterior discontinuity) between the anterior mitral valve leaflet and the aortic (AO) valve can be seen. Note that the AO overrides the ventricular septum by more than 50%. *A* = anterior; *I* = inferior; *LA* = left atrium; *LV* = left ventricle; *RV* = right ventricle. (From Snider AR: *Clin Perinatol* 1988; 15:543. Used by permission.)

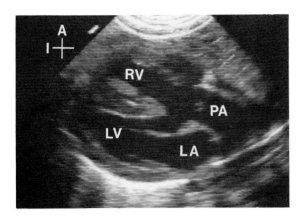

FIG 6–45.
Parasternal long-axis view from an infant with double-outlet right ventricle and *d*-transposition of the great arteries. In this view, the posterior great artery has an immediate posterior sweep suggesting that it is a pulmonary artery (PA). Note the separation between the anterior mitral valve leaflet and the pulmonary valve. The PA overrides the ventricular septum by more than 50%. *A* = anterior; *I* = inferior; *LA* = left atrium; *LV* = left ventricle; *RV* = right ventricle.

a frontal body plane.[49] For this reason, only the outlet septum can be seen in the subcostal four-chamber view of the right ventricle (the remainder of the septum is posterior to and parallel with the imaging plane; Fig 6–46). The remainder of the septum can be seen in long-axis and apical four-chamber views. The muscle bundle that separates a semilunar valve from the atrioventricular valve is called the ventriculoinfundibular fold (also visible in the subcostal views). The muscle bundle along the septal surface of the right ventricle, which in some cases surrounds a ventricular septal defect, is the septal band. Although both great arteries are usually supported by a muscular infundibulum or conus, the conus can be partially or completely absorbed beneath either or both great arteries. In patients with situs solitus, *d*-loop, and double-outlet right ventricle, complete absorption of the conus beneath the posterior or leftward semilunar valve will result in fibrous continuity between that valve and the mitral valve (see Chapter 14 for a discussion of cases in situs inversus or ambiguus). Thus, demonstration of discontinuity between the posterior semilunar valve and the atrioventricular valve on the two-dimensional echocardiogram is supportive, but not diagnostic, evidence of double-outlet right ventricle. On the two-dimensional echocardiogram, the diagnostic feature of double-outlet right ventricle is visualization of two great arteries committed primarily (each more than 50%) to the right ventricle.

Great Vessel Relations

In double-outlet right ventricle, four different spatial relationships of the semilunar valves are possible[50]:

Normal relationship.—The pulmonary arterial trunk is anterior and to the left of the aorta. In the parasternal short-axis view, the great arteries wrap around one another,

creating a circle-sausage appearance. Double-outlet right ventricle and this rare type of great artery relations (approximately 2% of cases) may be difficult to distinguish on the echocardiogram from tetralogy of Fallot.

Side-by-side relationship.—The aorta is to the right of the pulmonary artery and the semilunar valves lie in approximately the same transverse plane. This is the classic and most common type (45%) of great vessel relationship in double-outlet right ventricle.[50] On the parasternal short-axis view, both great vessels are seen in cross-section as double circles lying side by side (Fig 6–47).[51] With cranial angulation of the transducer, the leftward vessel bifurcates, indicating that it is the pulmonary artery. With caudal angulation of the transducer, the ventricular septum

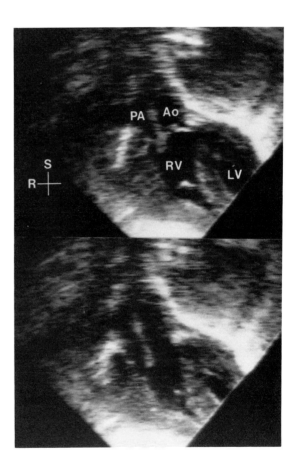

FIG 6–46.
Subcostal coronal views of the right ventricle (RV) from an infant with double-outlet right ventricle and side-by-side great arteries. In the diastolic frame *(top)*, both the pulmonary artery (PA) and the aorta (AO) arise from the RV. Both semilunar valves are located superiorly in the heart and at the same height. In systole *(bottom)*, the parallel alignment of the great vessels is apparent. In this patient, the right-sided vessel bifurcates and is therefore the PA. *LV* = left ventricle; *R* = right; *S* = superior. (From Snider AR: Two-dimensional echocardiography of neonatal cardiac abnormalities, in Maklad NF (ed), *Ultrasound in Perinatology*. New York, Churchill Livingstone, 1986, p 189. Used by permission.)

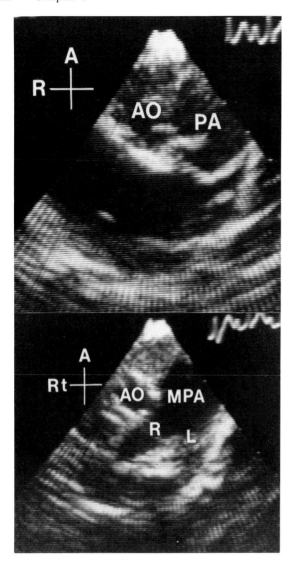

FIG 6–47.
Parasternal short-axis views from an infant with double-outlet right ventricle and side-by-side great arteries. In the *top frame,* the two vessels are seen situated side by side and very anterior in the heart. In the *bottom frame,* the plane of sound has been tilted anteriorly to image the pulmonary artery bifurcation. In this patient, the left-sided vessel bifurcated and was therefore identified as the main pulmonary artery (MPA). *A* = anterior; *AO* = aorta; *L* = left pulmonary artery; *R* = right pulmonary artery; *RT* = right. (From Silverman NH, Snider AR: *Two-Dimensional Echocardiography in Congenital Heart Disease.* Norwalk, Appleton-Century-Crofts, 1982, p 162. Used by permission.)

and left ventricle are seen posterior to the level of both great arteries. Because the great arteries are lying side by side, it is possible to obtain a parasternal long-axis view that passes through the left ventricle and either the pulmonary artery or the aorta by simply tilting the transducer from right to left. With side-by-side great vessels, the two vessels cannot be seen simultaneously in the long-axis view.

Dextromalposition of the great arteries.—The aorta is anterior and to the right of the pulmonary artery (Fig 6–48). Some investigators call this relationship double-outlet right ventricle with *d*-transposition. Here, we reserve the term transposition for cases in which the aorta arises from the right ventricle *and* the pulmonary artery arises from the left ventricle. In the parasternal short-axis view in this case, the great arteries appear in cross-section exactly the same as in *d*-transposition. However, if the plane of sound is angled inferiorly, both great arteries are seen to be anterior to the level of the ventricular septum and left ventricle. In the parasternal long-axis view, both great arteries are seen simultaneously in longitudinal section anterior to the ventricular septum. As in *d*-transposition, when the pulmonary artery is the posterior vessel it has an immediate posterior angulation as it passes toward the lungs.

Levomalposition.—The aorta is anterior and to the left of the pulmonary artery. In the parasternal short-axis views, the vessels appear in cross-section exactly as they do in *l*-transposition.

In the classic form of double-outlet right ventricle, the great arteries are situated at the same height above the ventricular mass because of the persistent muscular conus beneath each vessel (see Figs 6–46 and 6–48). In the parasternal long-axis view, the persistent muscular infundibulum beneath the posterior great artery creates a wide distance between the posterior semilunar valve and the mitral valve (see Fig 6–44). Less commonly, the conus beneath the posterior great artery may be partially or com-

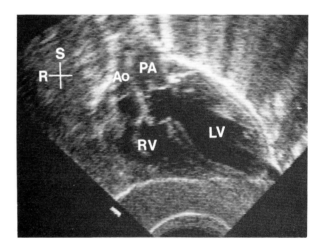

FIG 6–48.
Subcostal coronal view from an infant with double-outlet right ventricle and *d*-malposition of the great arteries. In this view, the malalignment between the conus septum and the trabecular septum is apparent. The pulmonary artery (PA) overrides the ventricular septal defect by more than 50%. The aortic (AO) valve and pulmonary valve are both situated superiorly at the same level above the ventricles. *LV* = left ventricle; *R* = right; *RV* = right ventricle; *S* = superior. (From Snider AR: *Clin Perinatol* 1988; 15:543. Used by permission.)

pletely absorbed. In these cases, it may be extremely difficult to determine if posterior discontinuity is present on the echocardiogram.

Ventricular Septal Defect

Four types of ventricular septal defects occur in patients with double-outlet right ventricle[50]:

Subaortic type.—The ventricular septal defect is more closely related to the aortic valve. If the vessels are located side by side, the subaortic ventricular septal defect is located below the septal limb of the crista supraventricularis. On the subcostal four-chamber views, this defect is located to the right of the conus septum, just beneath the aortic valve. The conus septum separates the defect from the subpulmonary infundibulum. If the vessels are malposed (anterior aorta), the subaortic ventricular septal defect is above the septal limb. In the subcostal view, the defect is located anteriorly beneath the aortic valve and separated from the pulmonary outflow by the conus septum. Subaortic ventricular septal defect occurs in nearly 50% of patients with double outlet right ventricle.[50]

Subpulmonary type.—The ventricular septal defect is more closely related to the pulmonary valve. If the great arteries are side by side, a subpulmonary ventricular septal defect is located above the septal limb of the crista supraventricularis (the original Taussig-Bing form of double-outlet right ventricle). On the subcostal four-chamber views, this defect is located to the left of the conus septum, just beneath the pulmonary valve. The conus septum separates the ventricular septal defect from the subaortic infundibulum. If the great arteries are malposed, the subpulmonary ventricular septal defect lies beneath the septal limb. On the subcostal views, the defect is separated by the conus septum from the aortic outflow.

Doubly committed type.—The ventricular septal defect is subaortic and subpulmonic and therefore is closely related to both semilunar valves. The defect is centered below the semilunar valves and below the crista supraventricularis.

Noncommitted type.—The ventricular septal defect is distant from both semilunar valves (i.e., in the inlet or apical muscular portions of the septum).

In rare cases, especially those with malposition of the great arteries, the ventricular septum can be intact; however, most patients have a large nonrestrictive ventricular septal defect.[50] The most frequent combination of ventricular septal defect and great artery position is side-by-side great arteries with a subaortic defect; this occurs in nearly 50% of patients.[50]

Pulmonary Stenosis

Pulmonary stenosis occurs in nearly half of all patients with double-outlet right ventricle. Pulmonary stenosis can

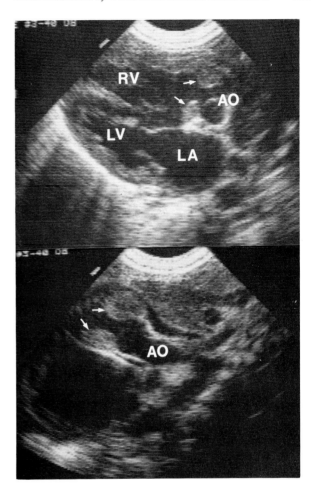

FIG 6–49.
Parasternal long-axis *(top)* and suprasternal long-axis *(bottom)* views from an infant with double-outlet right ventricle, side-by-side great arteries, and severe subaortic stenosis. In the parasternal long-axis view, the aorta (AO) can be seen arising from the right ventricle (RV). There is marked discontinuity between the anterior mitral valve leaflet and the aortic valve caused by the presence of persistent muscular conus. This conus tissue *(arrows)* has contributed to the development of severe muscular subaortic stenosis, which can also be seen in the suprasternal long-axis view of the aortic arch. In the suprasternal long-axis view of the aortic arch, the ascending aorta is tilted superiorly and anteriorly and is not tucked in the heart. This suggests persistent subaortic conus. *LA* = left atrium; *LV* = left ventricle.

be valvular, subvalvular, or both. Subvalvular pulmonary stenosis is usually caused by a hypertrophied conus septum and infundibular muscle bundles. Regardless of the position of the ventricular septal defect, pulmonary stenosis is more frequently encountered in patients with malposition of the great arteries (68%).[50] Doppler echocardiography can be used to assess the hemodynamic severity of the pulmonary stenosis. Parasternal, apical, and subcostal views should be used to find the highest peak velocity of the pulmonary stenosis jet.

Associated Defects

Double-outlet right ventricle can occur as an isolated entity (the so-called simple type) or can be associated with other complex defects (the so-called complex type).[52] In its complex form, double-outlet right ventricle is associated with defects such as total anomalous pulmonary venous return, atrioventricular septal defect, mitral stenosis or atresia, and persistent left superior vena cava. The complex type of double-outlet right ventricle is often associated with situs ambiguus, particularly asplenia.[52]

Patients with either type of double-outlet right ventricle frequently have additional sites of left-to-right shunting, including atrial septal defect (present in 25%), additional ventricular septal defects, and patent ductus arteriosus (9%).[50] Pulsed and color-flow Doppler are useful techniques for detecting additional left-to-right shunts.

Approximately 4% of patients have mitral valve abnormalities including mitral valve straddle, parachute mitral valve, mitral stenosis, and mitral atresia.[50] Two-dimensional echocardiographic and Doppler techniques should be used to detect mitral stenosis or regurgitation. In addition, a small percentage of patients with double-outlet right ventricle have subaortic stenosis and/or aortic coarctation (Fig 6–49). Subaortic stenosis is usually caused by a greatly hypertrophied conus septum and is best detected from parasternal and subcostal views of the right ventricle.[53]

Double-outlet right ventricle is often found in patients with situs solitus, atrioventricular discordance (*l*-loop), and superior-inferior ventricles.[45] In these circumstances, any great vessel relationship is possible, although *l*-malposition is the most common (see Chapter 14).

REFERENCES

1. Bierman FZ, Williams RG: Prospective diagnosis of *d*-transposition of the great arteries in neonates by subxiphoid, two-dimensional echocardiography. *Circulation* 1979; 60:1496–1502.
2. Henry WL, Maron BJ, Griffith JM, et al: Differential diagnosis of anomalies of the great arteries by real-time two-dimensional echocardiography. *Circulation* 1975; 51:283–291.
3. Henry WL, Maron BJ, Griffith JM: Cross-sectional echocardiography in the diagnosis of congenital heart disease. Identification of the relation of the ventricles and great arteries. *Circulation* 1977; 56:267–273.
4. Houston AB, Gregory NL, Coleman EN: Echocardiographic identification of aorta and main pulmonary artery in complete transposition. *Br Heart J* 1978; 40:377–382.
5. Park SC, Neches WH, Zuberbuhler JR, et al: Echocardiographic and hemodynamic correlation in transposition of the great arteries. *Circulation* 1978; 57:291–298.
6. Maroto E, Fouron JC, Douste-Blazy MY, et al: Influence of age on wall thickness, cavity dimensions, and myocardial contractility of the left ventricle in simple transposition of the great arteries. *Circulation* 1983; 67:1311–1317.
7. Carceller AM, Fouron JC, Smallhorn JF, et al: Wall thickness, cavity dimensions, and myocardial contractility of the left ventricle in patients with simple transposition of the great arteries. A multicenter study of patients from 10 to 20 years of age. *Circulation* 1986; 73:622–627.
8. Silverman NH, Payot M, Stanger P, et al: The echocardiographic profile of patients after Mustard's operation. *Circulation* 1978; 58:1083–1093.
9. Bierman FZ, Williams RG: Subxiphoid two-dimensional imaging of the interatrial septum in infants and neonates with congenital heart disease. *Circulation* 1979; 60:80–90.
10. Perry LW, Ruckman RN, Galioto FM Jr, et al: Echocardiographically assisted balloon atrial septostomy. *Pediatrics* 1982; 70:403–408.
11. Satomi G, Nagazawa M, Takao A, et al: Blood flow pattern of the interatrial communication in patients with complete transposition of the great arteries: A pulsed Doppler echocardiographic study. *Circulation* 1986; 73:95–99.
12. Kurosawa H, Van Mierop LHS: Surgical anatomy of the infundibular septum in transposition of the great arteries with ventricular septal defect. *J Thorac Cardiovasc Surg* 1986; 91:123–132.
13. Deal BJ, Chin AJ, Sanders SP, et al: Subxiphoid two-dimensional echocardiographic identification of tricuspid valve abnormalities in transposition of the great arteries with ventricular septal defect. *Am J Cardiol* 1985; 55:1146–1151.
14. Pigott JD, Chin AJ, Weinberg PM, et al: Transposition of the great arteries with aortic arch obstruction. Anatomical review and report of surgical management. *J Thorac Cardiovasc Surg* 1987; 94:82–86.
15. Aziz KU, Paul MH, Muster AJ: Echocardiographic assessment of left ventricular outflow tract in *d*-transposition of the great arteries. *Am J Cardiol* 1978; 41:543–551.
16. Areias JC, Goldberg SJ, Spitaels SEC, et al: An evaluation of range gated pulsed Doppler echocardiography for detecting pulmonary outflow tract obstruction in *d*-transposition of the great vessels. *Am Heart J* 1978; 96:467–474.
17. Chin AJ, Yeager SB, Sanders SP, et al: Accuracy of prospective two-dimensional echocardiographic evaluation of left ventricular outflow tract in complete transposition of the great arteries. *Am J Cardiol* 1985; 55:759–764.
18. Jatene AD, Fontes VF, Souza LCB, et al: Anatomic correction of transposition of the great vessels. *J Thorac Cardiovasc Surg* 1977; 72:364–372.
19. Yacoub MH, Bernhard A, Lange PE, et al: Clinical and hemodynamic results of the two-stage anatomic correction of transposition of the great arteries. *Circulation* 1980; 62(suppl 1):190–196.
20. Hougen TJ, Colan SD, Norwood WI, et al: Hemodynamic results of arterial switch operation for transposition of the great arteries, intact ventricular septum. *Circulation* 1984; 70(suppl 2):26.
21. Lange PE, Sievers HH, Onnasch DGW, et al: Up to 7

years of follow-up after two-stage anatomic correction of simple transposition of the great arteries. *Circulation* 1986; 74(suppl 1):47–52.

22. Brawn WJ, Mee RBB. Early results for anatomic correction of transposition of the great arteries and for double-outlet right ventricle with subpulmonary ventricular septal defect. *J Thorac Cardiovasc Surg* 1988; 95:230–238.
23. Gibbs JL, Qureshi SA, Grieve L, et al: Doppler echocardiography after anatomical correction of transposition of the great arteries. *Br Heart J* 1986; 56:67–72.
24. Sidi D, Planche C, Kachaner J, et al: Anatomic correction of simple transposition of the great arteries in 50 neonates. *Circulation* 1987; 75:429–435.
25. Idriss FS, Ilbawi MN, DeLeon SY, et al: Transposition of the great arteries with intact ventricular septum. Arterial switch in the first month of life. *J Thorac Cardiovasc Surg* 1988; 95:255–262.
26. Ilbawi MN, Idriss FS, DeLeon SY, et al: Preparation of the left ventricle for anatomic correction in patients with simple transposition of the great arteries. Surgical guidelines. *J Thorac Cardiovasc Surg* 1987; 94:87–94.
27. Lecompte Y, Zannini L, Hazan E: Anatomic correction of transposition of the great arteries. *J Thorac Cardiovasc Surg* 1981; 82:629–631.
28. Bove EL, Beekman RH, Snider AR, et al: Arterial repair for transposition of the great arteries and large ventricular septal defect in early infancy. *Circulation* 1988; 78(suppl 3):26–31.
29. Martin MM, Snider AR, Bove EL, et al: Two-dimensional and Doppler echocardiographic evaluation after arterial switch repair in infancy for complete transposition of the great arteries. *Am J Cardiol* 1989; 63:332–336.
30. Paillole C, Sidi D, Kachaner J, et al: Fate of pulmonary artery after anatomic correction of simple transposition of great arteries in newborn infants. *Circulation* 1988; 78:870–876.
31. Wernovsky G, Hougen TJ, Walsh EP, et al: Midterm results after the arterial switch operation for transposition of the great arteries with intact ventricular septum: Clinical, hemodynamic, echocardiographic, and electrophysiologic data. *Circulation* 1988; 77:1333–1344.
32. Martin RP, Ettedqui JA, Qureshi SA, et al: A quantitative evaluation of aortic regurgitation after anatomic correction of transposition of the great arteries. *J Am Coll Cardiol* 1988; 12:1281–1284.
33. Pasquini L, Sanders SP, Parness IA, et al: Diagnosis of coronary artery anatomy by two-dimensional echocardiography in patients with transposition of the great arteries. *Circulation* 1987; 75:557–564.
34. Colan SD, Trowitzsch E, Wernovsky G, et al: Myocardial performance after arterial switch operation for transposition of the great arteries with intact ventricular septum. *Circulation* 1988; 78:132–141.
35. Arensman FW, Radley-Smith R, Grieve L, et al: Computer assisted echocardiographic assessment of left ventricular function before and after anatomic correction of transposition of the great arteries. *Br Heart J* 1986; 55:162–167.
36. Borow KM, Arensman FW, Webb C, et al: Assessment of left ventricular contractile state after ana-

tomic correction of transposition of the great arteries. *Circulation* 1984; 69:106–112.
37. Silverman NH, Snider AR: *Two-Dimensional Echocardiography in Congenital Heart Disease.* Norwalk, Appleton-Century-Crofts, 1982, pp 167–188.
38. Silverman NH, Snider AR, Colo J, et al: Superior vena caval obstruction after Mustard's operation: Detection by two-dimensional contrast echocardiography. *Circulation* 1981; 64:392–396.
39. Wyse RKH, Haworth SG, Taylor JFN, et al: Obstruction of superior vena caval pathway after Mustard's repair. Reliable diagnosis by transcutaneous Doppler ultrasound. *Br Heart J* 1979; 42:162–167.
40. Stevenson JG, Kawabori I, Guntheroth WG, et al: Pulsed Doppler echocardiographic detection of obstruction of systemic venous return after repair of transposition of the great arteries. *Circulation* 1979; 60:1091–1095.
41. Chin AJ, Sanders SP, Williams RG, et al: Two-dimensional echocardiographic assessment of caval and pulmonary venous pathways after the Senning operation. *Am J Cardiol* 1983; 52:118–127.
42. Smallhorn JF, Gow R, Freedom RM, et al: Pulsed Doppler echocardiographic assessment of the pulmonary venous pathway after the Mustard or Senning procedure for transposition of the great arteries. *Circulation* 1986; 73:765–774.
43. Allwork SP, Bentall HH, Becker AE, et al: Congenitally corrected transposition: A morphologic study of 32 cases. *Am J Cardiol* 1976; 38:910–922.
44. Ellis K, Morgan BC, Blumenthal S, et al: Congenitally corrected transposition of the great vessels. *Radiology* 1962; 79:35–49.
45. Carminati M, Valsecchi O, Borghi A, et al: Cross-sectional echocardiographic study of criss-cross hearts and superoinferior ventricles. *Am J Cardiol* 1987; 59:114–118.
46. Lester RG, Anderson RC, Amplatz K, et al: Roentgenologic diagnosis of congenitally corrected transposition of the great vessels. *Am J Roentgen* 1960; 83:985–997.
47. Jaffe RB: Systemic atrioventricular valve regurgitation in corrected transposition of the great vessels. *Am J Cardiol* 1976; 37:395–402.
48. Marino B, Sanders SP, Parness IA, et al: Obstruction of right ventricular inflow and outflow in corrected transposition of the great arteries {S,L,L}: Two-dimensional echocardiographic diagnosis. *J Am Coll Cardiol* 1986; 8:407–411.
49. Stellin G, Zuberbuhler JR, Anderson RH, et al: The surgical anatomy of the Taussig-Bing malformation. *J Thorac Cardiovasc Surg* 1987; 93:560–569.
50. Sridaromont S, Feldt RH, Ritter DG, et al: Double outlet right ventricle: Hemodynamic and anatomic correlations. *Am J Cardiol* 1976; 38:85–94.
51. DiSessa TG, Hagan AD, Pope C, et al: Two-dimensional echocardiographic characteristics of double outlet right ventricle. *Am J Cardiol* 1979; 44:1146–1154.
52. Lev M, Bharati S: Double outlet right ventricle. Association with other cardiovascular anomalies. *Arch Pathol* 1973; 95:117–122.
53. Thanopoulos BD, Dubrow IW, Fisher EA, et al: Double outlet right ventricle with subvalvular aortic stenosis. *Br Heart J* 1979; 41:241–244.

Ventricular Hypoplasia

This chapter discusses conditions that result in underdevelopment of a ventricular cavity as a result of either atresia or severe hypoplasia of one or more segments of the ventricle, usually with some degree of hypoplasia of the remaining segments. Two basic situations may be present. In the first, there may be only one atrioventricular valve, permitting access of only one atrium to a dominant ventricle with only a small second ventricle present. In the second, there may be two atrioventricular valves (or a common atrioventricular valve), allowing both atria direct access to a dominant ventricle with only a rudiment of the second ventricle present that has no direct access to either atria. The first situation is typified by mitral or tricuspid atresia, while the second situation is classified as a double-inlet ventricle. This discussion will focus on hypoplastic right and left ventricle. Double-inlet ventricle and other forms of single ventricle will be discussed in Chapter 14.

Ventricular hypoplasia is a spectrum of defects, ranging from hypoplasia of one or more segments of the affected ventricle to total absence of one or more segments. Classic examples are tricuspid atresia, pulmonary atresia, and hypoplastic left heart syndrome. In the spectrum of ventricular hypoplasia, these are the relatively severe forms, whereas underdevelopment of the apical portion of a ventricle with minimal overall ventricular cavity diminution represents the opposite extreme. In the discussion of right ventricular hypoplasia, inlet and outlet lesions will be considered separately. Left ventricular hypoplasia will be discussed as a single entity because of the similar effects of both inlet and outlet lesions upon the clinical course.

RIGHT VENTRICULAR HYPOPLASIA

Anatomy

The right ventricle consists of three regions: the inlet region, the apical region, and the outlet region. The inlet region consists of the atrioventricular orifice with the valve tissue and tensor apparatus. It is defined by the limits of the chordal attachments of the tricuspid valve and occupies the posterior aspect of the heart. The inlet region leads to the apical region, which is a relatively well demarcated area situated at the apex of the ventricle. The outlet region is superior to the crista supraventricularis and inferior to the pulmonary valve, encompassing the infundibular area.

Any or all of these areas may be totally absent or hypoplastic. Even when only one area is atretic, the other two are generally hypoplastic and diminished in size to some degree. From a clinical standpoint, it is necessary to describe the size and position of the atretic portion(s), the atrioventricular connections, the size of the segments that remain, and the ventriculoarterial connections. For the purposes of this discussion all hypoplastic chambers, even if the inlet portion is atretic, will be referred to as ventricles. When both inlets or atrioventricular valves connect to the same ventricle and a second small chamber is present, such hypoplastic chambers are referred to as rudimentary chambers. Rudimentary chambers that give rise to a great vessel are termed outlet chambers while those that have neither inlet or outflow portions are termed trabecular pouches.[1]

Atresia of the right ventricular inlet portion results in the classic picture of tricuspid atresia. Characteristically, there is a fat-filled sulcus separating the floor of the right atrium from the remaining small right ventricular cavity[2, 3]; on occasion, however, only a very thin membrane separates the right atrium from the small right ventricle.[4] In the first situation, there is complete absence of the right ventricular inlet portion; in the second situation the right ventricular inlet portion exists but lacks a patent atrioventricular orifice. From a clinical standpoint, there is no difference in the hemodynamic effects of either of these two entities, and the surgical treatment is identical.

In certain cases the inlet portion may, in fact, be present but markedly hypoplastic. In this situation, definite

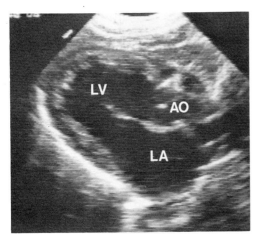

FIG 7–1.
Parasternal long-axis view from an infant with tricuspid atresia, a tiny ventricular defect, and a very tiny right ventricle. Virtually no evidence of the right ventricle can be seen. AO = aorta; LA = left atrium; LV = left ventricle.

valve tissue and tensor apparatus are present, but their size is quite diminutive.

The apical portion of the right ventricle is usually preserved, and primary atresia of this portion of the right ventricle is rare. The apical portion is generally affected secondary to atresia of either the inlet or outlet portions. When primary atresia of this segment does exist, there is usually direct communication from the inlet to the outlet portion, so that flow from the right atrium to the pulmonary artery is preserved. However, the functional size of the chamber can be markedly diminished to a point where it may not support the entire cardiac output.

Finally, atresia of the outlet portion with resultant pulmonary atresia or severe, critical pulmonic stenosis can also be seen. This is usually accompanied by marked underdevelopment of both the inlet and the apical portions of the right ventricle, except when there has been flow through the right ventricle, either as a consequence of a ventricular septal defect or of severe tricuspid regurgitation in utero. Both of these latter two entities may result in preservation of normal right ventricular size. In most situations, the infundibulum is markedly hypoplastic, ending in a blind pouch with no pulmonary valve tissue. There may be only a thin membrane separating the infundibulum from the main pulmonary artery, or there may be marked atresia of this area with a long gap separating the right ventricular cavity from the pulmonary arterial tree.

Inlet Atresia

Parasternal Long-Axis View

The echocardiographic examination begins from the parasternal long-axis view, where the relative increase in the size of the left ventricle, together with the diminutive size of the right ventricular cavity, are immediately apparent (Fig 7–1). However, as only portions of the apical and outlet segments are imaged, isolated hypoplasia of the

inlet region will not be appreciated. There is often muscular hyperplasia of the apical portion of the right ventricle that further impinges upon the remnants of the right ventricular cavity.

The ventricular septum must be carefully examined for the presence of ventricular septal defects. Defects may occur in any segment of the ventricular septum, most commonly in the membranous septum (Figs 7–2 and 7–3). In addition, the location of the posterior great vessel must be noted, as the aorta and pulmonary artery may both arise from the hypoplastic right ventricle, so that both systemic and pulmonary flow depend upon the size of the ventric-

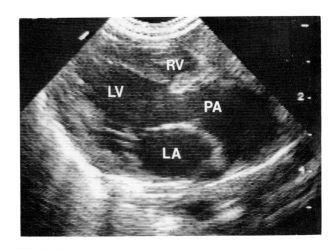

FIG 7–2.
Parasternal long-axis view from an infant with tricuspid atresia, d-transposition of the great arteries, a small membranous ventricular septal defect, and an interrupted aortic arch. The tiny membranous septal defect can be seen. The posterior great artery sweeps posteriorly and bifurcates, which indicates that it is a pulmonary artery (PA). A small right ventricle (RV) can be seen anteriorly. LA = left atrium; LV = left ventricle.

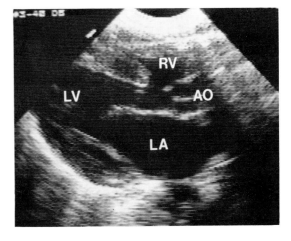

FIG 7–3.
Parasternal long-axis view from a patient with tricuspid atresia, normally related great vessels, and a large ventricular septal defect. The large ventricular septal defect and a sizeable right ventricle (RV) are visible. AO = aorta; LA = left atrium; LV = left ventricle.

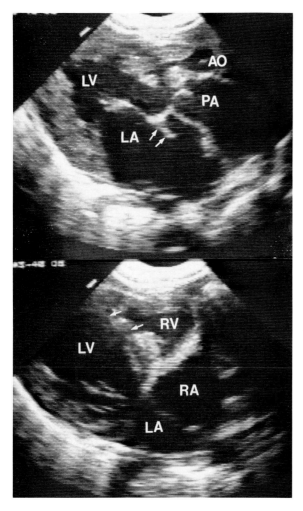

FIG 7–4.
Parasternal long-axis views from an infant with tricuspid atresia and transposition of the great arteries. In the standard parasternal long-axis view (*top*), the aorta (AO) and the pulmonary artery (PA) can be seen arising from the heart in a parallel fashion. The pulmonary artery has a posterior sweep. These findings are highly suggestive of transposition of the great arteries. The subaortic region is markedly narrowed by prominent infundibular muscle bundles. In addition, the conal septum between the AO and PA protrudes under the pulmonary valve, causing subpulmonary obstruction. An outlet ventricular septal defect is present, and there is the suggestion of a more inferior muscular septal defect. A portion of the atrial septum (*arrows*) can be seen in an unusual orientation. The appearance of the atrial septum in the parasternal long-axis view is highly suggestive of juxtaposition of the atrial appendages. This patient did have left juxtaposition of the right atrial appendage, as confirmed in other views. In the parasternal long-axis view through the right ventricular inflow tract (*bottom*) a thick membrane occupies the position that would normally have been occupied by the tricuspid valve. In addition, the multiple muscular ventricular septal defects (*arrows*) are seen more clearly in this view. LA = left atrium; LV = left ventricle; RA = right atrium; RV = right ventricle.

ular septal defect. Or, the great arteries may be transposed so that the aorta arises from the hypoplastic right ventricle (Figs 7–4 and 7–5). Any ventriculoarterial connection is possible, and the long-axis view provides important in-

formation about which type of connection is present.

The position of the outlet ventricular septum should be noted, especially when a ventricular septal defect is present. The septum can be deviated anteriorly or posteriorly, impinging upon either the right or left ventricular outflow tract (see Fig 7–4). Anterior deviation is common with normally related great vessels, and posterior deviation is common in the presence of transposition of the great arteries.[5] The left ventricular outflow tract can also be obstructed by muscular ridges or membranes.

Finally, in this view careful attention must be paid to the posterior atrioventricular groove, to find evidence of a large coronary sinus that suggests the presence of a left superior vena cava. Also, if the atrial septum is seen aligned perpendicular to the posterior great artery, juxtaposition of the atrial appendages should be suspected and sought using additional views (see Fig 7–4).

Parasternal Short-Axis View

The parasternal short-axis view at the level of the left ventricular papillary muscles shows the small size of the right ventricle and can be useful in delineating the size, number, and location of any ventricular septal defects that may be present, particularly in the trabecular septum. This view also permits assessment of the function of the left ventricle.[6, 7]

Scanning superiorly to the level of the great vessels allows evaluation of the small right ventricular outflow tract, as well as evaluation of the presence or absence of coexisting pulmonary atresia. In addition, the size of the main pulmonary artery and the proximal right pulmonary artery can be assessed. In many cases, the proximal left pulmonary artery can also be evaluated. A large pulmonary root implies the presence of a large ventricular septal defect with significant antegrade flow from the right ventricle into the pulmonary arterial tree. The size of the proximal pul-

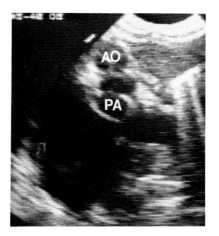

FIG 7–5.
Parasternal short-axis view at the base of the heart of the same patient as in Figure 7–4. Both great vessels are seen together in cross-section, suggesting transposition of the great arteries. The pulmonary valve is thickened and bicuspid. AO = aorta; PA = pulmonary artery.

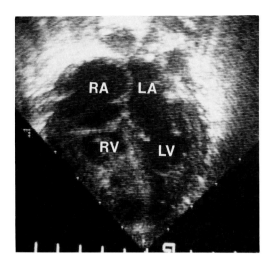

FIG 7–6.
Apical four-chamber view from a patient with a hypoplastic right heart. In this patient, a tiny tricuspid orifice with diminutive leaflets was present. Functionally, however, this patient had tricuspid atresia with a very small and hypertrophic right ventricular (RV) cavity. LA = left atrium; LV = left ventricle; RA = right atrium.

monary artery system is important in planning initial palliation as well as later, definitive repair. If the proximal pulmonary arteries are not well seen in this view, subsequent views must be inspected carefully to establish their presence or absence. Finally, the proximal portion of the ductus arteriosus, and often the entire ductus arteriosus to its insertion into the descending aorta, can be visualized.

Careful Doppler flow studies of the main pulmonary artery can also be performed using this view. Such studies are useful for confirming the presence of antegrade flow, for evaluating the pulmonary valve and subvalvar region for stenosis, and for confirming the presence of ductal flow. In the presence of a ductus arteriosus, it is important not to mistake swirling systolic flow that comes from the ductus for antegrade flow that comes out of the heart. In cases where there is significant pulmonary stenosis as well as tricuspid atresia, this distinction can be difficult to discern.

Finally, careful inspection of the ventricular septum, particularly the membranous septum just inferior to the aortic root, can be performed with Doppler echocardiography to confirm or exclude the presence of an associated ventricular septal defect. If there is any question that the tricuspid valve may be patent, careful Doppler inspection of this region can also be performed from this view.

Apical Four-Chamber View

The apical four-chamber view obtained from the cardiac apex also permits careful inspection of the right ventricular inlet region[8] (Figs 7–6 to 7–8). Remnants of the tricuspid valve apparatus, particularly leaflet and tensor apparatus, should be carefully sought, as severe tricuspid hypoplasia without complete atresia can mimic tricuspid atresia and can only be distinguished from it by visualization of the tricuspid valve remnants. In addition, distinction can be made between tricuspid atresia caused by a

membrane and the more classic form in which a fat-filled sulcus separates the floor of the right atrium from the right ventricle. If juxtaposition of the atrial appendages is present, the orientation of the atrial septum will be changed in this view. Angling the scan plane more posteriorly, the coronary sinus is imaged. Enlargement may indicate the presence of a left superior vena cava.

Scanning superiorly allows evaluation of the outlet ventricular septum for the presence of potential defects and also allows characterization of the overall size of the

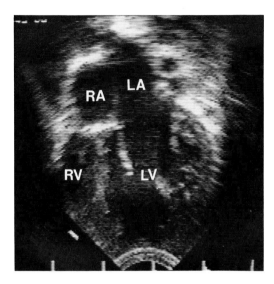

FIG 7–7.
Apical four-chamber view from a patient with tricuspid atresia, normally related great arteries, a small ventricular septal defect, and a tiny right ventricular (RV) cavity. LA = left atrium; LV = left ventricle; RA = right atrium.

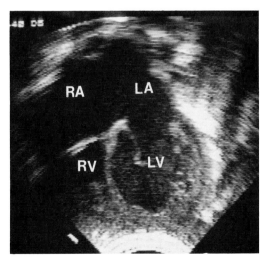

FIG 7–8.
Apical four-chamber view from a patient with tricuspid atresia, normally related great vessels, a large ventricular defect (seen in another plane), and a fair-sized right ventricular (RV) chamber. LA = left atrium; LV = left ventricle; RA = right atrium.

remaining right ventricle. If it is possible to angle significantly anteriorly, the anterior great vessel can be visualized. This view also allows evaluation of the left ventricular outflow tract. When transposition of the great arteries is present, there may be significant deviation of the remainder of the outlet septum, causing subpulmonic obstruction. In fact, any form of left ventricular outflow obstruction can occur.

Finally, the mitral valve apparatus must be carefully inspected for any accompanying anomalies. Doppler evaluation from this view should be performed to rule out mitral regurgitation.

Subcostal Views

The subcostal views, both coronal and sagittal, again permit careful inspection of the inlet region and identification of remnants of the tricuspid valve.[9] In addition, the atrial septum can be carefully inspected, particularly to determine the size and location of the atrial septal defect. A small defect that impedes flow of blood from the right atrium to the left atrium can significantly limit cardiac output and can be extremely important clinically.[10] Bowing of the atrial septum into the left atrium with marked dilatation of the right atrium often suggests a restrictive atrial septal defect. Doppler evaluation of the right-to-left atrial flow is also helpful for defining the presence of restrictive defects. Nevertheless, assessment of defect size by direct imaging remains the most useful technique, as altered flow states can affect the Doppler-determined gradient. The location of the atrial septal defect is equally important, as coronary sinus defects can be missed.[11] Defects of the atrioventricular septum can mimic tricuspid atresia, particularly if the atrioventricular region is unbalanced in favor of the left ventricle.[12-14]

The presence and location of the pulmonary veins must also be evaluated. When pulmonary blood flow is low, clinical evidence and Doppler evidence of pulmonary vein obstruction may be lacking. Imaging of the entrance of the veins into the left atrium may be the only way to diagnose pulmonary venous obstruction.

The subcostal coronal view is an excellent method for assessing the ventriculoarterial connections (see Chapter 6) and the size of the right ventricle (Figs 7–9 and 7–10). This view is also useful for detecting left juxtaposition of the right atrial appendage. When the scan plane is tilted far posteriorly in the presence of this defect (Fig 7–11), the atrial septum has a bizarre curvature, with the convexity toward the left atrium. As the scan plane is tilted anteriorly, the atrial septum in the region of the fossa ovalis is oriented more normally. As the scan plane is tilted even more anteriorly, the communication between the right atrium on the right and its appendage on the left is seen. It is important not to mistake this communication for a large atrial septal defect.

Turning to the sagittal view, the right ventricular outflow tract can again be assessed for any potential narrowing. This region must be carefully assessed, as obstruction is often present. The presence of significant cristal hyper-

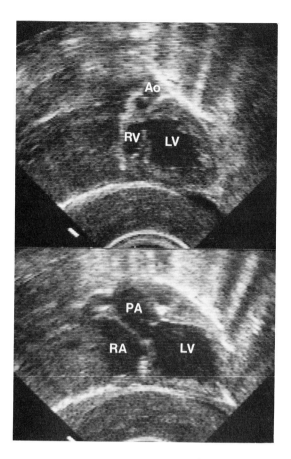

FIG 7–9.
Subcostal views from a patient with tricuspid atresia, transposition of the great arteries, a small right ventricular chamber, and an interrupted aortic arch. The *top frame* is a subcostal coronal view, with the plane of sound tilted far anteriorly. The aorta (Ao) can be seen arising from a diminutive right ventricle (RV). A prominent muscle bundle is present in the subaortic region, causing obstruction to forward flow out from the Ao. A small ventricular septal defect is also seen. In the *bottom frame,* the plane of sound has been tilted posteriorly. The pulmonary artery (PA) with its bifurcation is seen arising from the left ventricle (LV). RA = right atrium.

trophy, anterior deviation of the outlet septum, and anomalous muscle bundles can all be seen, and all can significantly obstruct flow into the anterior great vessel. In addition, the size and position of the anterior great vessel itself can be assessed as it arises from the heart.

Scanning rightward, the right atrium and the region of the tricuspid valve are seen. This is an excellent view for determining whether there is a tricuspid valve present or simply an imperforate membrane, which in many instances can move as a valve would move. Doppler interrogation of this region, especially with color Doppler mapping, is helpful in making this distinction.

Suprasternal Notch Views

The echocardiographic examination should conclude with the suprasternal notch views, beginning with the long-axis view of the aortic arch. Careful note must be made of the position of the arch relative to the tracheal air column. This can only be assessed by the examiner and not from review of the videotape. A ductus arteriosus is easily seen joining the descending aorta to the main pulmonary artery. If, however, the aortic arch is right-sided, the ductus may originate from the left innominate artery and will not be seen in the same plane as the aortic arch. The ductus arteriosus is often oriented in the reverse direction from normal, going superior and posterior from the main pulmonary artery to the aorta rather than inferior and posterior, as is the usual situation. In the normal heart, intrauterine flow patterns result in predominant flow from the main pulmonary artery into the descending aorta. However, in the presence of right ventricular hypoplasia, flow is predominantly from the aorta into the pulmonary artery, which accounts for the abnormal orientation. The ductus arteriosus often is quite long and narrow. In addition, with

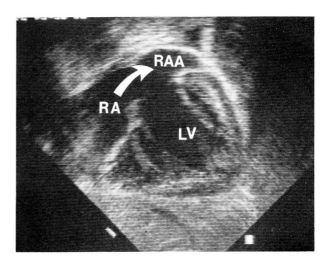

FIG 7–11.
Subcostal view from the same patient as in Figure 7–4 and Figure 7–10. This patient had left juxtaposition of the right atrial appendage. The communication between the right atrium (RA) on the right and the right atrial appendage (RAA) on the left is seen. LV = left ventricle.

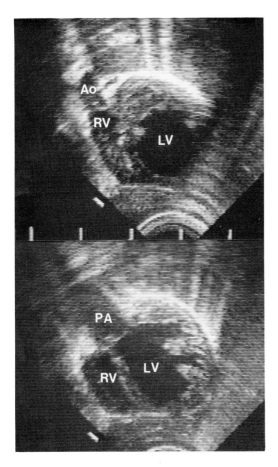

FIG 7–10.
Subcostal views from the same patient in Figure 7–4. In the *top frame,* the plane of sound has been tilted far anteriorly to image the aorta (Ao) arising from the right ventricle (RV). The RV is very small, and multiple muscular ventricular septal defects are seen. The *bottom frame* was obtained by tilting the plane of sound further posteriorly. The pulmonary artery (PA) is seen arising from the left ventricle (LV). An additional outlet ventricular septal defect is also seen.

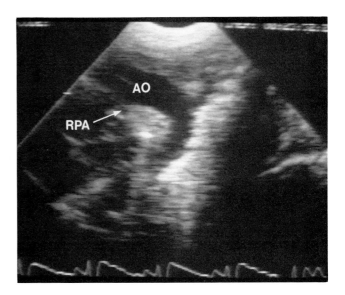

FIG 7–12.
Suprasternal long-axis view from a patient with tricuspid atresia, a small ventricular septal defect, and severe pulmonary stenosis. In the suprasternal notch view a tiny right pulmonary artery (RPA) is seen underneath the aortic (AO) arch. There is no evidence of isthmus narrowing of the aorta, indicating altered fetal flow patterns, caused by severe right ventricular outflow obstruction.

severe right ventricular hypoplasia, the isthmus narrowing that is normally present in the aortic arch disappears and the arch has a strikingly uniform diameter throughout (Fig 7–12). The loss of isthmus narrowing is also caused by altered fetal flow patterns, with the majority of flow ejected by the left ventricle into the aortic arch rather than into the main pulmonary artery and subsequently into the descending aorta.

Angling slightly leftward, the left pulmonary artery can be seen and should be traced back to the main pulmonary artery, establishing continuity between the main and left pulmonary artery.

Turning the transducer into the short-axis view permits evaluation of both the main and right pulmonary arteries for the presence of pulmonary arterial continuity.

Outflow Atresia

The same basic views are used to evaluate right ventricular outflow atresia as were used to assess right ventricular inflow atresia[15-19] (Fig 7–13). In the presence of a ventricular septal defect and a normal-sized inlet region, the right ventricle may be well developed and, in fact, may be larger than normal. This condition is distinguished from tetralogy of Fallot by the presence of complete atresia of the pulmonary valve with no detectable antegrade flow into the main pulmonary artery by Doppler examination. Imaging of the region of the valve to see if cusp opening occurs and Doppler detection of antegrade flow are both needed. A thin imperforate membrane can mimic the appearance of a perforate valve and may even have motion similar to that of a valve. Doppler examination is extremely useful for detection of antegrade pulmonary blood flow; however, in the presence of tricuspid atresia or pulmonary hypertension, Doppler examination may show no antegrade flow even when the pulmonary valve is patent.[20] Practically speaking, however, if the right ventricular outflow tract and valve annulus are of good size and only an imperforate membrane is present, the surgical approach is similar to that of tetralogy of Fallot.

With outflow atresia, careful attention must be paid

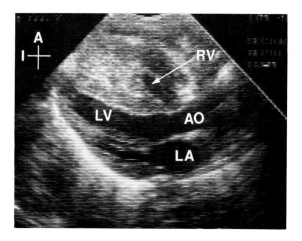

FIG 7–13.
Parasternal long-axis view from a patient with pulmonary atresia and a diminutive right ventricle (RV). The RV is heavily trabeculated and has a tiny cavity. A = anterior; AO = aorta; I = inferior; LA = left atrium; LV = left ventricle.

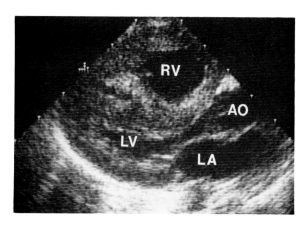

FIG 7–14.
Parasternal long-axis view in a patient with pulmonary atresia and a good-sized tricuspid valve. The right ventricle (RV) is heavily trabeculated but has a sizeable chamber. This patient also had suprasystemic RV pressure. AO = aorta; LA = left atrium; LV = left ventricle.

to the anatomy of the main, right, and left pulmonary arteries.[21, 22] Depending upon the degree of in utero ductal flow, the main pulmonary artery may be totally absent or of good size. Angiographically, it may be difficult to demonstrate the proximal pulmonary artery system. Echocardiography provides a better evaluation of this area. The parasternal short-axis view and the suprasternal notch views offer the best imaging of the proximal pulmonary arteries and the best information about whether or not they are confluent.

In the presence of an intact ventricular septum and severe tricuspid regurgitation, the right ventricle may be of considerable size, although in general it is still less well developed than it is in the presence of a ventricular septal defect[14, 23] (Figs 7–14 to 7–16). In this situation the inlet portion of the ventricle is large, although frequently the apical and outlet portions are markedly hypoplastic. This condition is readily apparent in the apical four-chamber view, where both the inlet and apical portions can be easily seen (Fig 7–17). In this view, there is marked muscular hypertrophy of the apical portion with enlargement confined mostly to the inlet region. The size of the tricuspid annulus is critical in planning future surgery, and its diameter should be compared to normal data if doubt about its adequacy exists.

In the absence of tricuspid insufficiency or a ventricular septal defect, the right ventricle is quite small. The inlet region is markedly hypoplastic, often with a small tricuspid annulus and diminutive tricuspid valve apparatus. The apical portion is markedly hypertrophic. Cavity size is best evaluated from the apical four-chamber view and the subcostal coronal views (Figs 7–18 to 7–20). Also in this condition, the right ventricular pressure may be exceedingly high. If a tricuspid insufficiency jet is present, Doppler recordings can often be used to indicate right ventricular hypertension. If significant hypertension does exist, the possibility of sinusoids connecting the right

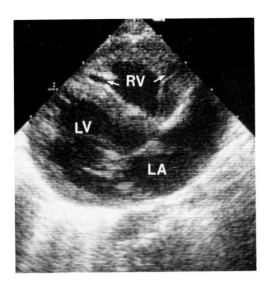

FIG 7–15.
Parasternal long-axis view through the right ventricular (RV) inflow tract of a patient with pulmonary atresia and multiple sinusoids connecting the coronary arteries and RV cavity (*arrows*). LA = left atrium; LV = left ventricle.

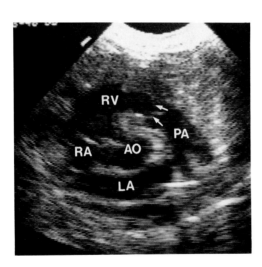

FIG 7–16.
Parasternal short-axis view at the base of the heart from the same patient as in Figure 7–15. An imperforate membrane (*arrows*) can be seen in the area normally occupied by the pulmonary valve. In systole and diastole, there was no evidence of any antegrade flow across this membrane. The pulmonary artery (PA) branches are considerably smaller than normal. AO = aorta; LA = left atrium; RA = right atrium; RV = right ventricle.

ventricular cavity to the coronary arterial system exists. Although there is much discussion about the clinical significance of these sinusoids, it is felt that their presence indicates the potential for myocardial ischemia. Sinusoids are best visualized from the apical four-chamber view and the subcostal views (see Fig 7–18).

LEFT VENTRICULAR HYPOPLASIA

Anatomy

Like the right ventricle, the left ventricle consists of three components, although they are less well defined than in the right ventricle. The left ventricular inflow region is composed of the mitral valve and its support structures. The left ventricular apical region makes up the majority of the ventricle. The outflow region is relatively small, giving rise almost immediately to the aorta. In the presence of left

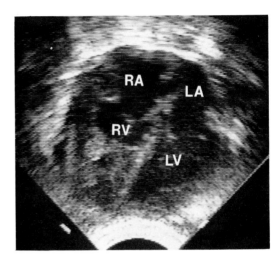

FIG 7–17.
Apical four-chamber view from a patient with pulmonary atresia and an intact ventricular septum. The tricuspid valve annulus is of good size; however, the tricuspid valve leaflets moved in a stenotic and domed fashion. The right ventricle (RV) is heavily trabeculated and its cavity is markedly diminished. LA = left atrium; LV = left ventricle; RA = right atrium.

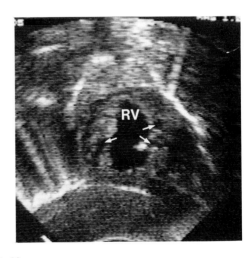

FIG 7–18.
Subcostal coronal view of the right ventricle (RV) from the same patient as in Figure 7–15. This patient had pulmonary atresia and an intact ventricular septum with multiple sinusoidal connections (*arrows*) between the RV and coronary arteries.

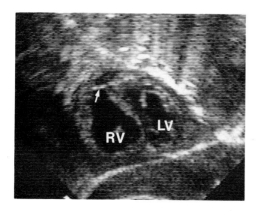

FIG 7–19.
Subcostal coronal view of the right ventricle (RV) from a patient with pulmonary atresia and an intact ventricular septum. An imperforate, echodense membrane (*arrow*) is seen in the position normally occupied by the pulmonary valve. The RV chamber is smooth-walled and diminished in size. In real time, this chamber did not change dimensions between systole and diastole. LV = left ventricle.

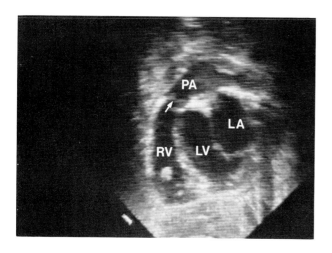

FIG 7–20.
Subcostal sagittal view of the right ventricle (RV) from a patient with pulmonary atresia and an intact ventricular septum. In this patient, an imperforate membrane (*arrow*) occupied the position normally occupied by the pulmonary valve. In real time, the membrane bowed toward the pulmonary artery (PA) in systole and away from the PA in diastole; however, Doppler studies showed no evidence of antegrade flow across the membrane. The RV chamber is small and hypertrophic. LA = left atrium; LV = left ventricle.

ventricular hypoplasia, all three segments are usually poorly developed. In most cases there is either severe hypoplasia or total atresia of both the aortic and mitral valves. Although either can be normal in the presence of hypoplasia of the other, both are usually affected. With hypoplasia of the left ventricle, endocardial thickening of both the left ventricle and the left atrium can usually be seen. In addition, the left atrium is often quite small, and the atrial

septum frequently possesses only a small defect. The mitral valve ring may be quite small, if not totally atretic, and the cusps may be thickened and attached directly to the papillary musculature with no well-defined chordae present. The aortic valve may be atretic or dysplastic, with thickened small leaflets, although the valve often is tricuspid. In most instances, the ventricular septum is intact, particularly when there is atresia of the aortic valve. However, when there is atresia only of the mitral valve, there may be a ventricular septal defect. In the presence of a large septal defect, the left ventricular cavity may be of normal size, even though there is no left ventricular inflow present.

In cases of aortic atresia or severe hypoplasia, the ascending aorta is quite small, being essentially an extension of the coronary arteries. At the origin of the first arch vessel, the aorta becomes larger because of retrograde flow from the ductus arteriosus. The aortic arch diameter increases around the arch but does not reach a normal diameter until it is distal to the insertion of the ductus arteriosus. At the insertion of the ductus arteriosus, it is often possible to find a posterior shelf that creates an area of coarctation that further limits blood flow to the upper extremities and the coronary arteries. The ductus arteriosus is large and forms an inferior arch from the main pulmonary artery to the descending aorta. Finally, the right ventricle is frequently quite large but otherwise normal. Associated lesions of the right ventricle, specifically pulmonary stenosis, may be present.

Echocardiographic Views

Parasternal Long-Axis View

The echocardiographic examination begins with the parasternal long-axis view.[24] In this view, the large size of the right ventricle and the small size of the left ventricular cavity are immediately apparent (Fig 7–21). At first, it is possible to mistake this defect for a single ventricle; on closer examination, however, a definite ventricular septum with a small posterior chamber is seen. It is important to note the appearance of the mitral valve and to describe the remaining portions of that valve. The aorta may also be seen arising from the small left ventricle. This vessel is usually a very small structure with or without a patent valve. An ascending aorta with a diameter of less than 5 mm is considered hypoplastic.[25, 26]

The size of the left atrium must also be described. The left atrium may be small or large.[25] Echo-bright areas in the endocardial surface of the left atrium as well as the left ventricle are often present, implying endocardial fibrotic changes.

Finally, the ventricular septum must be carefully inspected for the presence of a ventricular septal defect. A ventricular septal defect is rare in the presence of aortic atresia, but, in the presence of mitral atresia with a patent aortic valve is much more common. This is relevant clinically, as a ventricular septal defect may be associated with a normal-sized aortic annulus and ascending aorta, even in the presence of left ventricular hypoplasia.

Parasternal Short-Axis View

The parasternal short-axis view at the level of the ventricles allows assessment of the overall size of the left ventricle in a view orthogonal to the previous projection (Figs 7–22 and 7–23). The presence or absence of two papillary muscles can easily be ascertained, and the endocardial changes of the left ventricle can again be seen as echo-bright areas.

Scanning superiorly to the base of the heart, the great vessels are clearly seen. This view is particularly important, as it allows definite assessment of aortic root size and position (see Fig 7–22). The aortic root is usually quite small (<5 mm) and the main pulmonary artery is usually quite dilated. The main pulmonary artery connects to a prominent ductus arteriosus, which may be larger than either branch of the pulmonary artery. The ductus arteriosus then sweeps around to the descending aorta.

Apical Four-Chamber View

The apical four-chamber view shows the small size of the left ventricle and allows close inspection of the remnants of the left ventricular inflow region (Fig 7–24).[27] If any mitral valve tissue is present, Doppler examination can be used to assess flow from the left atrium to the left ventricle.

Scanning anteriorly, the left ventricular outflow tract is easily seen, and the aortic valve can again be inspected to determine the degree of hypoplasia present. Doppler interrogation of the ascending aorta can provide information about the patency or total atresia of the valve. When the ascending aorta is small, valve patency is of little clinical relevance. The ventricular septum should also be carefully inspected for any defects.

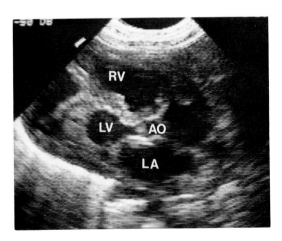

FIG 7–21.
Parasternal long-axis view from a patient with a hypoplastic left heart. Diminutive mitral and aortic valve leaflets are present. The left ventricular (LV) chamber is muscle-bound and exhibited no contractility in real time. This chamber has a very smooth endocardial surface, suggesting extensive endocardial fibroelastosis. The ascending aorta (AO) is also hypoplastic. The right ventricular (RV) apex makes up the apex of the heart. LA = left atrium.

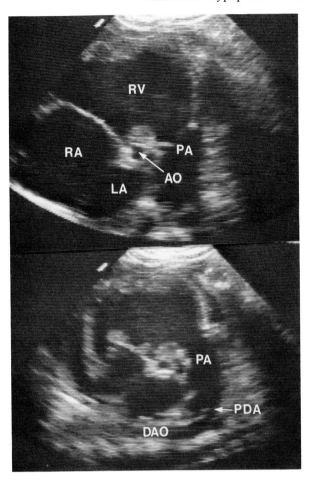

FIG 7–22.
Parasternal short-axis views at the base of the heart from a patient with hypoplastic left heart syndrome. The *top frame,* a standard parasternal short-axis view, shows a tiny aortic root in cross-section. In the *bottom frame,* the plane of sound has been rotated back toward the long-axis view. With this transducer orientation, a patent ductus arteriosus (PDA) can be seen connecting the pulmonary artery (PA) and descending aorta (DAO). AO = aorta; LA = left atrium; RA = right atrium; RV = right ventricle.

Subcostal Views

Subcostal views are helpful in assessing the degree of atrial septal patency[9] and left atrial size (Fig 7–25). These views are useful for detecting anomalies of the pulmonary veins and their drainage as well. The nature of the atrial septum is also important. Atrial septal aneurysms may be present and bow into the right atrium. As pulmonary flow may be high and the atrial septal defect may be the only outlet from the left atrium, left atrial pressure may be elevated. Doppler flow studies of the foramen ovale can indicate the degree of left atrial hypertension (Plate 18).

The sagittal view usually confirms the findings of the subcostal view and in general does not provide significant additional information.

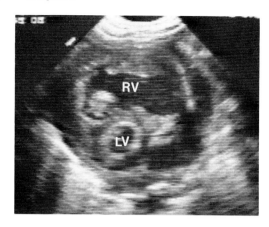

FIG 7–23.
Parasternal short-axis view at the level of the papillary muscles in the same patient as in Figure 7–22. A tiny, muscle-bound left ventricle (LV) is seen. RV = right ventricle.

Suprasternal Notch Views

These views are critical in the clinical management of children with hypoplastic left heart, particularly because palliative procedures for the treatment of this entity have been developed. Of importance to the surgeon is the precise anatomy of the aortic arch, particularly at the area of the ductal insertion.[28] The size of the ascending aorta is easily assessed, but the important surgical questions are the size of the transverse aorta and whether or not there is a posterior shelf at the insertion of the ductus arteriosus, producing a coarctation (Fig 7–26). Such an obstruction requires the surgeon to extend reconstruction of the arch around to the descending aorta beyond the level of any potential obstruction. The suprasternal long-axis view of the aortic arch is therefore critically important for defining the arch anatomy. In addition, this view allows assessment of the presence or absence of aortic interruption, which may accompany hypoplastic left heart. Although Doppler assessment of flow in the descending aorta is useful, it does not rule out the presence of a coarctation. Care must be taken not to confuse the ductus arteriosus arch from the main

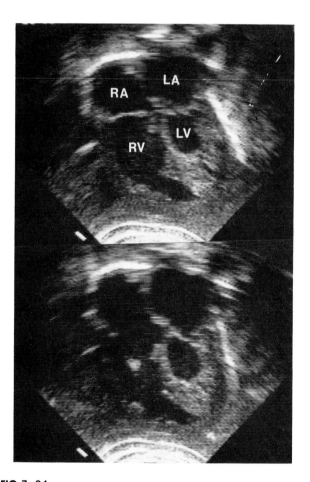

FIG 7–24.
Apical four-chamber views in systole (above) and diastole (below) from a patient with a hypoplastic left heart. The left ventricular (LV) chamber is small and muscle-bound and in real time moved passively, almost as an appendage to the right ventricle (RV). In the diastolic frame, a small, dysplastic mitral valve with a patent orifice can be seen. LA = left atrium; RA = right atrium.

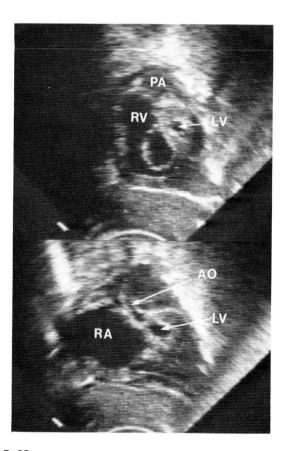

FIG 7–25.
Subcostal views from a patient with hypoplastic left heart syndrome. The top frame, a subcostal sagittal view, shows a diminutive muscle-bound left ventricle (LV) and a large anterior right ventricle (RV). The bottom frame, a subcostal coronal view, shows a hypoplastic ascending aorta (AO) arising from the tiny LV. RA = right atrium; PA = pulmonary artery.

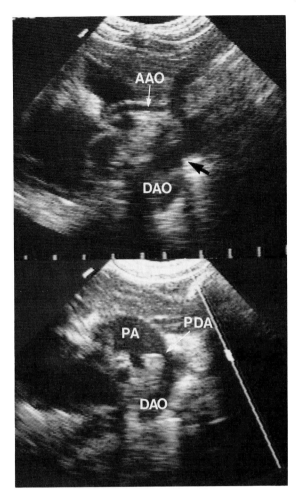

FIG 7–26.
Suprasternal long-axis view from a patient with aortic atresia. In the standard suprasternal long-axis view (*top frame*), the ascending aorta, from the level of the valve leaflets to the origin of the in-nominate artery, is hypoplastic. The innominate artery and trans-verse aorta are of fair size. A prominent coarctation of the descending aorta (*arrow*) is seen. When the plane of sound is tilted toward the left (*bottom frame*), it is possible to see the arch formed by the pulmonary artery (PA) and its connection to the patent ductus ar-teriosus (PDA) and descending aorta (DAO). AAO = ascending aorta.

pulmonary artery to the descending aorta for a normal aortic arch.

Special Considerations Relative to Surgical Palliation

With the development of surgical approaches to palliation in children with left ventricular hypoplasia, the potential for salvage of children with this heretofore lethal lesion becomes possible. Although it has been difficult to provide definitive prognostic indicators,[29] several issues need to be addressed with echocardiography to determine the suitability of the patient for surgery.

Of critical importance is the function and integrity of the right ventricle. Clearly, the left ventricle is of little usefulness, and therefore the child must rely solely upon the right ventricle. Right ventricular function is assessed in a qualitative manner; quantitative tests of right ventricular function remain unproven. In particular, the apical and subcostal four-chamber views provide good overall appraisal of right ventricular motion. Also, careful inspection of the right ventricle for echogenic areas that suggest endocardial fibrotic changes must also be made. The presence of such changes is ominous and markedly increases surgical risk.

The presence of severe tricuspid regurgitation is also a relative contraindication for surgery; therefore, the tricuspid valve must be carefully interrogated for the presence of regurgitation. With a large dilated right ventricle, tricuspid regurgitation can often exist. Doppler color-flow mapping is quite helpful, as the jet orientation may be unusual and can be missed with pulsed Doppler mapping. The apical four-chamber view provides the best orientation for tricuspid Doppler examination.

Next, the atrial septum and particularly the pulmonary venous drainage should be examined. Although pulmonary venous drainage usually is normal, anomalies of the pulmonary veins do occur. The atrial septum generally has only a small defect present, which may be advantageous because it raises left atrial pressure and limits pulmonary flow to some degree, thus providing more systemic flow preoperatively.

Finally, careful attention must be paid to the aortic arch as described above. The anatomy of the ascending aorta is less important, although its size does affect surgical complexity. The anatomy of the transverse arch and the region of ductal insertion are of prime importance, as they determine how far around the arch the surgeon must extend the repair. Because the distal arch is a difficult region for the surgeon to approach from a median sternotomy incision, the anatomy of this region must be clearly described.

Echocardiographic Assessment Following Palliative Surgery (Norwood Procedure)

The aims of the initial palliative surgery (Norwood stage I procedure) are: (1) to establish permanent unobstructed blood flow from the right ventricle to the systemic arterial circulation; (2) to limit pulmonary blood flow and pressure to normal levels with the use of a systemic-to-pulmonary artery shunt as the sole source of pulmonary blood flow; and (3) to relieve pulmonary venous hypertension by creating a large interatrial communication. This will produce a circulatory state that will eventually be suitable for a modified Fontan procedure as a second-stage operation.[30, 31]

In the Norwood stage I procedure,[31] the main pulmonary artery is transected and an incision is made in the ascending aorta and extended around the aortic arch, past the area where a coarctation may occur at the entrance of the ductus arteriosus (Fig 7–27). The distal main pulmonary artery is oversewn and a systemic-to-pulmonary artery shunt is created. The proximal main pulmonary artery is anastomosed to the ascending aorta, and a graft is placed to enlarge the aortic arch from the anastomosis to the descending aorta. Finally, the atrial septum is excised almost completely.

The three most important complications that can limit the suitability of a patient for the Fontan procedure are (1) an inadequate atrial defect; (2) any obstruction in the newly created aortic arch; and (3) distortion of the branch pulmonary arteries. The diagnosis of a restrictive atrial septal defect is based on imaging a defect with a diameter less than one-half the length of the atrial septum in the subcostal view (Figs 7–28 and 7–29). When a restrictive atrial defect is present, Doppler interrogation usually shows a peak flow velocity greater than 2 m/sec, and the pulmonary veins become engorged as a result of pulmonary venous hypertension. The degree of hypertension, which influences the detected Doppler peak flow velocity, and the degree of venous distension are affected by the size of the systemic-to-pulmonary artery shunt. A low-flow shunt may mask features of a restrictive atrial septal defect, and as-

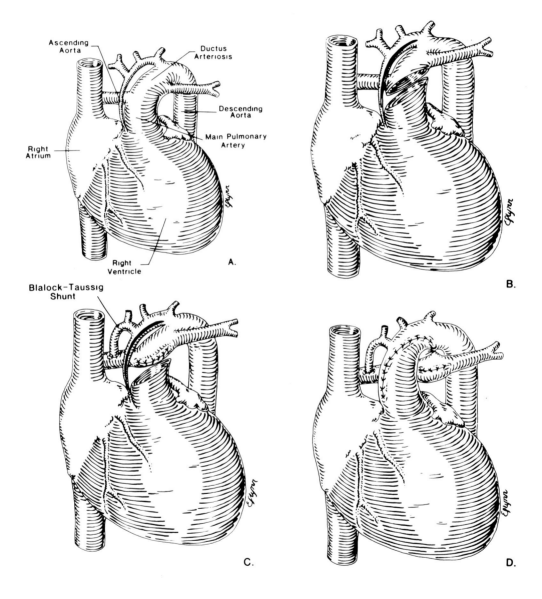

FIG 7–27.
Diagrammatic respresentation of the Norwood stage I procedure. **A**, the heart with aortic atresia and a hypoplastic ascending aorta and aortic arch are seen. **B**, the main pulmonary artery is transected and an incision is made in the ascending aorta that extends around the aortic arch. **C**, the distal main pulmonary artery is oversewn and a right Blalock-Taussig shunt is created as the sole source of pulmonary blood flow. **D**, the main pulmonary artery is anastomosed to the ascending aorta and aortic arch and the ductus arteriosus is ligated. Not shown in this figure is the nearly complete excision of the atrial septum. (From Lang P, Norwood WI: *Circulation* 1983; 68:107. Used by permission.)

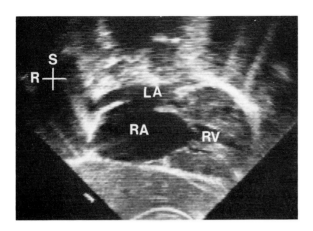

FIG 7–28.
Subcostal four-chamber view from an infant after Norwood I procedure for hypoplastic left ventricle. In this infant, the atrial septal defect became progressively more restrictive on serial postoperative echocardiographic examinations. The left atrial (LA) cavity is small but the pulmonary veins are engorged and distended, suggesting pulmonary venous hypertension. R = right; RA = right atrium; RV = right ventricle; S = superior.

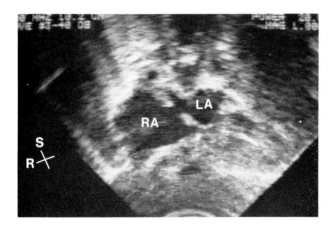

FIG 7–29.
Subcostal four-chamber view from an infant with hypoplastic left heart syndrome following Norwood stage I procedure. An inadequate atrial septal defect is seen. Following the echocardiogram, this infant required a repeat atrial septectomy. Anatomically, the defect is very small and the right upper pulmonary vein is sandwiched in between the superior limbic portion of the atrial septum and the descending aorta. At cardiac catheterization, this patient had significant gradients across the origin of the right upper pulmonary vein and across the atrial septal defect. LA = left atrium; R = right; RA = right atrium; S = superior.

sessment of the defect size by direct imaging is therefore the most useful technique.

Aortic arch obstruction can occur at various levels, including the proximal suture line, the distal suture line, or obstruction distal to the area of arch reconstruction. Aortic arch obstruction can be imaged from either the suprasternal or the subcostal views (Fig 7–30). Proximal ob-

struction is suggested by a narrowed and distorted proximal anastomosis generally associated with a Doppler gradient of >50 mm Hg (Figs 7–31 and 7–32). Distal suture line obstruction is marked by a distal narrowed area and usually by an aneurysmal dilatation of the proximal neoaorta presumably secondary to elevated proximal pressures (Fig 7–33). When such aneurysmal dilatation occurs, compression of adjacent structures must be excluded. Such compression can affect the pulmonary arteries (to be discussed below) or the superior vena cava (Fig 7–34). Caval compression

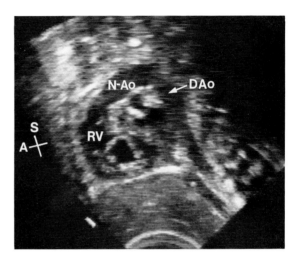

FIG 7–30.
Subcostal sagittal view of the right ventricle (RV) from an infant following Norwood stage I procedure. The neoaortic arch (N-Ao) is well seen, and there is no evidence of an aortic arch obstruction. A = anterior; DAo = descending aorta; S = superior.

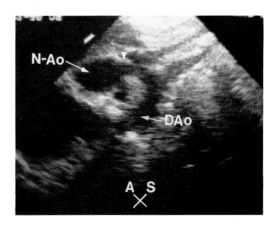

FIG 7–31.
Suprasternal long-axis view of the neoaortic (N-Ao) arch created by the Norwood stage I procedure in an infant with hypoplastic left heart. There is a mild narrowing in the proximal portion of the anastomosis (*arrow*), with mild dilatation of the neoaorta. A = anterior; DAo = descending aorta; S = superior.

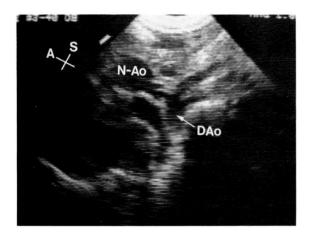

FIG 7–32.
Suprasternal long-axis view of the neoaortic arch (N-Ao) created by the Norwood stage I procedure in an infant with hypoplastic left heart syndrome. A narrow and distorted proximal suture line is seen. This patient had a 90 mm gradient across the proximal obstruction. A = anterior; DAo = descending aorta; S = superior.

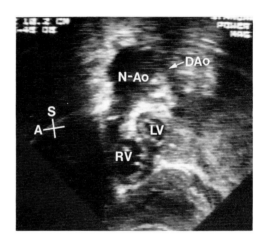

FIG 7–33.
Subcostal sagittal view of the right ventricle (RV) from an infant with hypoplastic left ventricle (LV) after Norwood stage I operation. There is a marked narrowing in the distal suture line of the neoaortic (N-Ao) arch. This narrowing required reoperation. The neoaorta has a marked aneurysmal dilatation, presumably caused by high aortic pressures proximal to the obstruction. A = anterior; DAo = descending aorta; S = superior.

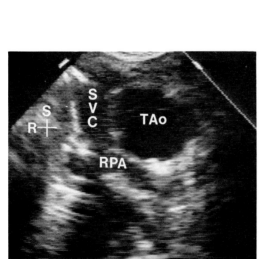

FIG 7–34.
Suprasternal short-axis view from an infant with Norwood stage I procedure who developed a distal aortic arch obstruction and a huge aneurysm of the proximal and transverse aorta (TAo), which compressed the adjacent superior vena cava (SVC) and right pulmonary artery (RPA). R = right; S = superior.

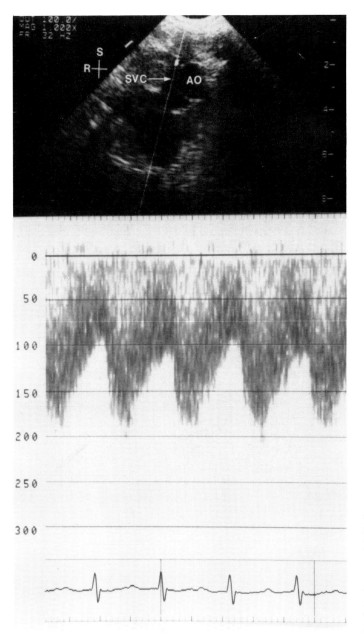

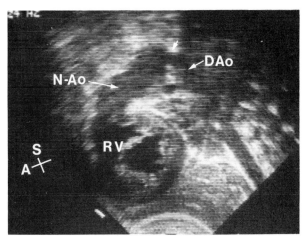

FIG 7–36.
Subcostal sagittal view of the right ventricle (RV) from a patient with hypoplastic left heart following Norwood stage I procedure. This patient developed a severe distal arch obstruction (*arrow*) and marked aneurysmal dilatation of the neoaorta (N-Ao). The aneurysmal anastomosis caused compression of the adjacent right pulmonary artery. A = anterior; DAo = descending aorta; S = superior.

FIG 7–35.
Doppler spectral recording (*bottom*) from the superior vena cava (SVC) of a patient with SVC obstruction following Norwood stage I procedure for hypoplastic left heart. Aneurysmal dilatation of the aorta (AO) compressed the adjacent SVC and created the obstruction. The freeze-frame image (*top*) is a suprasternal short-axis view. The Doppler sample volume was actually lower in the SVC at the time of the Doppler spectral tracing. The Doppler spectral tracing shows a continuous disturbed flow below the baseline, indicating flow away from the transducer. The biphasic flow normally present in the SVC has disappeared. Instead, there is a single peak velocity in late systole. In this patient, the peak velocity is 2 m/sec, which indicates a significant degree of SVC obstruction. R = right; S = superior.

should be evaluated in multiple projections, with the subcostal sagittal and suprasternal views the most helpful. Pulsed and color-flow Doppler are helpful (Fig 7–35).

The third major problem that must be evaluated is distortion of the branch pulmonary arteries secondary to either the systemic-to-pulmonary artery shunt or compression from an adjacent aneurysm of the neoaorta (Fig 7–36). The suprasternal notch long-axis view is helpful for evaluating the right pulmonary artery.

Other problems that require evaluation are aneurysms of the neoaorta (Figs 7–37 to 7–39), tricuspid regurgitation, pulmonary valve (neoaorta) regurgitation (Fig 7–40), diminished right ventricular function, shunt patency, and intracardiac thrombi (Fig 7–41). The low systemic flow and dilated right heart chambers place the patient after the Norwood stage I procedure at risk of developing intracardiac thrombi.

Echocardiographic evaluation of the patient after the Norwood stage I procedure requires an understanding of the goals of the procedure, the factors that limit the patient's suitability for a second-stage procedure, and knowledge of the complications that can arise.

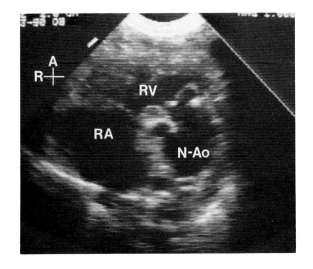

FIG 7–37.
Parasternal short-axis view from a patient with hypoplastic left heart following Norwood stage I procedure. The anastomosis between the aorta and the main pulmonary artery can be seen. In this patient, the neoaortic arch (N-Ao) is of normal size. A = anterior; R = right; RA = right atrium; RV = right ventricle.

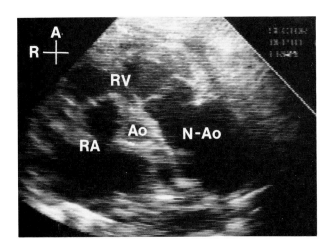

FIG 7–38.
Parasternal short-axis view from an infant after Norwood stage I procedure who developed a large aneurysm of the neoaorta (N-Ao). A = anterior; Ao = aorta; R = right; RA = right atrium; RV = right ventricle.

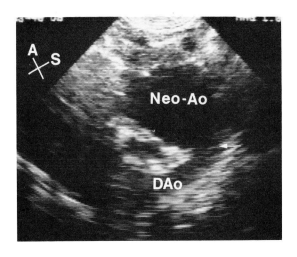

FIG 7–39.
Suprasternal long-axis view from an infant following Norwood stage I procedure who developed a massive aneurysm of the neoaortic arch (Neo-Ao). A = anterior; DAo = descending aorta; S = superior.

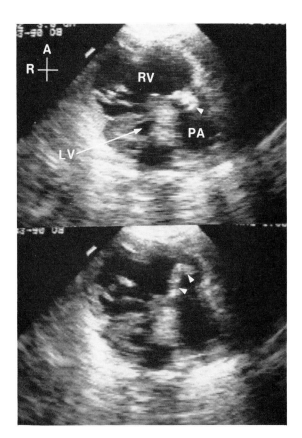

FIG 7–40.
Parasternal long-axis views of the right ventricular (RV) outflow tract from an infant with hypoplastic left ventricle (LV) who developed bacterial endocarditis following Norwood stage I operation. In the systolic frame (*top*), a large vegetation (*arrow*), seen attached to the pulmonary valve (neoaortic valve), was associated with severe pulmonary regurgitation (neoaortic regurgitation). A = anterior; PA = pulmonary artery; R = right.

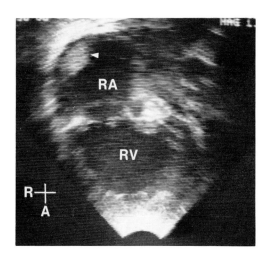

FIG 7–41.
Apical four-chamber view from an infant following Norwood stage I procedure. A large thrombus (*arrow*) is seen in the right atrium (RA). Because of low systemic flow and dilated right heart chambers, patients who have had the Norwood operation are at risk for developing intracardiac thrombi. A = anterior; R = right; RV = right ventricle.

REFERENCES

1. Anderson RH, Becker AE, Tynan M, et al: The univentricular atrioventricular connection: Getting to the root of a thorny problem. *Am J Cardiol* 1984; 54:822–828.
2. Wenick ACG, Ottenkorp J: Tricuspid atresia. Microscopic findings in relation to absence of the atrioventricular connexion. *Int J Cardiol* 1987; 16:57–73.
3. Anderson RH, Wilkinson JC, Gerlis M, et al: Atresia of the right ventricular orifice. *Br Heart J* 1977; 39:414–428.
4. Ottenkamp J, Wenink AC, Rohmer J, et al: Tricuspid atresia with overriding imperforate tricuspid membrane: An anatomic variant. *Int J Cardiol* 1984; 6:599–613.
5. Ottenkamp J, Wenink AC, Quaegebeur JM, et al: Tricuspid atresia. Morphology of the outlet chamber with special emphasis on surgical implications. *J Thorac Cardiovasc Surg* 1985; 89:597–603.
6. Graham TP Jr, Franklin RC, Wyse RK, et al: Left ventricular wall stress and contractile function in childhood: Normal values and comparison of Fontan repair v. palliation only in patients with tricuspid atresia. *Circulation* 1986; 74(suppl 1):161–169.
7. Hurwitz RA, Caldwell RL, Girod DA, et al: Left ventricular function in tricuspid atresia: A radionuclide study. *J Am Coll Cardiol* 1986; 8:916–921.
8. Silverman NH, Schiller NB: Apex echocardiography: A two-dimensional technique for evaluation of congenital heart disease. *Circulation* 1978; 57:503–511.
9. Gutgesell HP, Cheatham J, Latson LA, et al: Atrioventricular valve abnormalities in infancy: Two-dimensional echocardiographic and angiocardiographic comparison. *J Am Coll Cardiol* 1983; 2:531–537.
10. Fyfe DA, Taylor AB, Gillette PC, et al: Doppler echocardiographic confirmation of recurrent atrial septal defect stenosis in infants with mitral valve atresia. *Am J Cardiol* 1987; 60:410–411.
11. Rumisek JD, Pigott JD, Weinberg PM, et al: Coronary sinus septal defect associated with tricuspid atresia. *J Thorac Cardiovasc Surg* 1986; 92:142–145.
12. Rao PS: Atrioventricular canal mimicking tricuspid atresia: Echocardiographic and angiographic features. *Br Heart J* 1987; 58:409–412.
13. Magherini A, Azzolina G, Careri J: Anatomy of the echocardiographic crux cordis in the evaluation of the spectrum of atrioventricular valve atresia. *Int J Cardiol* 1984; 5:163–174.
14. Kurosawa H, Yagi Y, Imamura E, et al: A problem in Fontan's operation: Sinus septal defect complicating tricuspid atresia. *Heart Vessels* 1985; 1:48–50.
15. Silove ED, de Giovanni JV, Shiu MF, et al: Diagnosis of right ventricular outflow obstruction in infants by cross sectional echocardiography. *Br Heart J* 1983; 50:416–420.
16. Hagler DJ, Tajik AS, Seward JB, et al: Wide-angle two-dimensional echocardiographic profiles of conotruncal abnormalities. *Mayo Clin Proc* 1980; 55:73–82.
17. Sanders SP, Bierman FZ, Williams RG: Conotruncal malformations: Diagnosis in infancy using subxiphoid two-dimensional echocardiography. *Am J Cardiol* 1982; 50:1361–1362.
18. Marino B, Franceschini E, Ballerini L, et al: Anatomical-echocardiographic correlations in pulmonary atresia with intact ventricular septum. Use of subcostal cross-sectional views. *Int J Cardiol* 1986; 11:103–109.
19. Silove ED, deGiovani JV, Shiu MF, et al: Diagnosis of right ventricular obstruction in infants by cross sectional echocardiography. *Br Heart J* 1983; 50:416–420.
20. Smallhorn JF, Izukawa T, Benson L, et al: Noninvasive recognition of functional pulmonary atresia by echocardiography. *Am J Cardiol* 1984; 54:925–926.
21. Vargas Barron J, Sahn DJ, Attie F, et al: Two-dimensional echocardiographic study of right ventricular outflow and great artery anatomy in pulmonary atresia with ventricular septal defects and in truncus arteriosus. *Am Heart J* 1983; 105:281–286.
22. Huhta JC, Piehler JM, Tajik AJ, et al: Two-dimensional echocardiographic detection and measurement of the right pulmonary artery in pulmonary atresia-ventricular septal defect. Angiographic and surgical correlation. *Am J Cardiol* 1982; 49:1235–1240.
23. Andrade JL, Serino W, de Leval M, et al: Two-dimensional echocardiographic evaluation of tricuspid hypoplasia in pulmonary atresia. *Am J Cardiol* 1984; 53:387–388.
24. Lange LW, Sahn DJ, Allen HD, et al: Cross-sectional echocardiography in hypoplastic left ventricle: Echocardiographic-angiographic-anatomic correlations. *Pediatr Cardiol* 1980; 2:287–299.
25. Farooki ZQ, Henry JG, Green EW: Echocardiographic spectrum of the hypoplastic left heart syndrome. *Am J Cardiol* 1976; 38:337–343.
26. Van der Horst RC, Hastreiter AR, DuBrow IW, et al:

Pathologic measurements in aortic atresia. *Am Heart J* 1983; 108:1411–1415.

27. Rigby ML, Gibson DG, Joseph MC, et al: Recognition of imperforate atrioventricular valves by two-dimensional echocardiography. *Br Heart J* 1982; 47:329–336.

28. Bash SE, Huhta JC, Vick GW III, et al: Hypoplastic left heart syndrome: Is echocardiography accurate enough to guide surgical palliation? *J Am Coll Cardiol* 1986; 7:610–616.

29. Helton JG, Aglira BA, Chin AJ, et al: Analysis of potential anatomic or physiologic determinants of outcome of palliative surgery for hypoplastic left heart syndrome. *Circulation* 1986; 74:170–176.

30. Norwood WI, Lang P, Hansen D: Physiologic repair of aortic atresia: Hypoplastic left heart syndrome. *N Eng J Med* 1983; 308:23–26.

31. Lang P, Norwood WI: Hemodynamic assessment after palliative surgery for hypoplastic left heart syndrome. *Circulation* 1983; 68:104–108.

8

Abnormalities of Ventricular Inflow

This chapter examines abnormalites of both the right and left ventricular inflow in cases where there are two distinct atria and two distinct atrioventricular valves. Situations in which there is complete atresia of one valve or a common atrioventricular valve have been discussed in other chapters. The discussion in this chapter focuses on isolated tricuspid and mitral valve abnormalites as well as abnormalities of the atria that affect flow through the valves. Discussion is confined to cases in which there is levocardia with concordant visceral-atrial situs.

ABNORMALITIES OF RIGHT VENTRICULAR INFLOW

Isolated Tricuspid Valve Abnormalities

Although isolated tricuspid valve abnormalities are usually of little hemodynamic consequence, they do exist and may be significant from a clinical standpoint. Every echocardiographic examination should include a careful examination of the tricuspid valve for both structural and functional abnormalities. This discussion begins with a review of functional abnormalities of the tricuspid valve such as tricuspid regurgitation, stenosis, and prolapse; the more severe structural abnormalities such as Ebstein anomaly of the tricuspid valve will then be considered. The chapter concludes with a discussion of obstructions that exist within the right atrium such as cor triatriatum dexter.

Parasternal Long-Axis View

From the standard parasternal long-axis view, the right ventricular inflow is not imaged. However, by angling the scan plane rightward, the tricuspid valve, the right atrium, and the right ventricular inflow region are clearly seen. From this view, the septal and anterior leaflets are imaged. It is important to note the appearance of the leaflets and to determine if any myxomatous changes are present. This is a particularly good view for evaluating tricuspid valve prolapse. Systolic bulging of either leaflet superior to a line

drawn through the tricuspid valve annulus is diagnostic of prolapse (Fig 8–1).[1, 2] Color Doppler examination clearly shows the presence or absence of associated regurgitation (Plate 19). Incomplete closure of the leaflets may also be seen, particularly in the context of a dilated right ventricle.[3] However, this view does not permit evaluation of the posterior leaflet, making other views necessary.

Parasternal Short-Axis View

This view permits evaluation of the anterior and septal leaflets of the tricuspid valve and provides another window for evaluating the tricuspid regurgitant jet with Doppler color-flow mapping. The presence of any leaflet thickening, which may indicate myxomatous changes, should be carefully noted, particularly in patients with tricuspid valve prolapse.

Apical Four-Chamber View

In this view, which permits simultaneous visualization of the right atrium and inlet of the right ventricle, the septal and anterior leaflets are visualized. As will be discussed below, this is a particularly excellent view for the evaluation of Ebstein anomaly. It also permits assessment of the chordal attachments of the septal leaflet to the septum, which is helpful in assessing malformations of the tricuspid valve. Shortening of such attachments may limit closure, preventing the proper mobility of the leaflet (Fig 8–2).

In the newborn, a small amount of tricuspid regurgitation is commonly seen.[4, 5] With the enhanced sensitivity of color-flow mapping, tricuspid regurgitation may be found in a large percentage of normal newborns; small degrees of regurgitation are not pathologic (Plate 20). In the context of elevated pulmonary artery pressure, with the extreme state being persistence of the fetal circulation, right ventricular dilatation with subsequent tricuspid regurgitation may occur. In this view, dilatation of the tricuspid valve, with subsequent stretching of the chordal attachments, in-

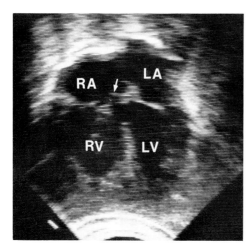

FIG 8–1.
Apical four-chamber view from a patient with a large inlet ventricular septal defect and tricuspid valve prolapse (*arrow*). LA = left atrium; LV = left ventricle; RA = right atrium; RV = right ventricle.

complete valve closure, and resultant tricuspid regurgitation can be assessed.

As flow through the tricuspid valve occurs at an angle of nearly zero degrees to the transducer, this view is useful for assessing the peak velocity of the regurgitant tricuspid jet (Figs 8–3 and 8–4). The peak velocity of the regurgitant jet is indicative of the systolic right ventricular to right atrial peak pressure gradient and is quite helpful in assessing the degree of right ventricular hypertension.[6, 7] However, it is important to be sure that the entire jet is visualized so that the peak velocity is accurately estimated. From the peak velocity and the simplified Bernoulli equation (pressure gradient = $4 \times$ peak velocity[2]), the systolic pressure gradient across the tricuspid valve can be calculated (see Chapter 4). To arrive at right ventricular systolic pressure itself, the right atrial pressure must be estimated, which may be difficult. It is best to report the pressure gradient only when the right atrial pressure cannot be measured directly. A high gradient indicates elevated right ventricular systolic pressure.

Subcostal Views

Both the sagittal and coronal subcostal views are helpful for evaluating the tricuspid valve from multiple angles. The subcostal coronal view allows visualization of the anterior and septal leaflets, whereas the sagittal view allows visualization of the anterior and posterior leaflets. In addition, angulation to the left while in the subcostal sagittal view allows visualization of the tricuspid valve en face, permitting simultaneous visualization of all three leaflets. This is the only view in which this is possible, and it is particularly important for evaluating the degree of coaptation of all three leaflets. In situations of isolated tricuspid valve abnormalites caused by abnormal partitioning of the atrioventricular canal, this is a particularly useful view for evaluating the degree of deficiency of the septal leaflet. Abnormal fusion between the septal and anterior leaflets

producing congenital tricuspid stenosis is also readily apparent in this view.

Although congenital tricuspid regurgitation and congenital tricuspid stenosis are rare entities, they do exist and their presence must be carefully assessed. Doppler evaluation of tricuspid valve flow from multiple views is mandatory (Fig 8–5). The chordal attachments of the tricuspid valve must be carefully examined. In the normal tricuspid valve, there are multiple chordal attachments to the septum, clearly distinguishing the tricuspid valve from the mitral valve in which all of the normal chordal attach-

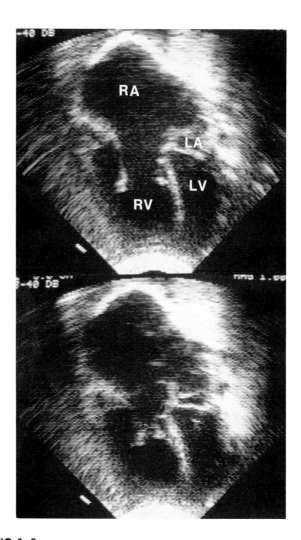

FIG 8–2.
Apical four-chamber view from a patient with an abnormal septal leaflet of the tricuspid valve. In the diastolic frame (*top*), the septal leaflet appears to arise normally from the fibrous annulus at about the same level as the mitral valve leaflets. In systole (*bottom*), the tricuspid valve septal leaflet is tethered to the ventricular septum and cannot close to meet the anterior tricuspid valve leaflet. The regurgitation through this orifice is severe, as evidenced by the enormous size of the right atrium (RA). LA = left atrium; LV = left ventricle; RV = right ventricle.

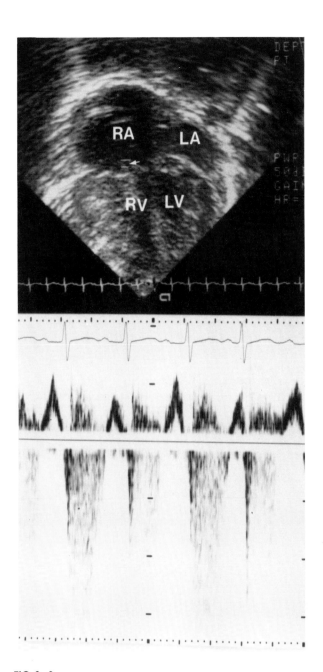

FIG 8–3.
Doppler recording (*bottom*) from the apical four-chamber view (*top*) of a child with tricuspid regurgitation. The top frame shows the position of the sample volume (*arrow*) at the inlet of the tricuspid valve at the time of the Doppler recording. The Doppler tracing shows forward flow toward the transducer in diastole from the right atrium (RA) through the tricuspid valve to the right ventricle (RV). In systole, the flow signals below the baseline indicate flow away from the transducer from the RV to the RA. These flow signals represent tricuspid insufficiency. LA = left atrium; LV = left ventricle.

ments are to the papillary muscles. In cases of heterotaxy, as will be discussed later, this may become an important distinction when determining which valve is the morphologic tricuspid valve.

Ebstein Malformation

Ebstein anomaly of the tricuspid valve consists of a downward displacement of the septal and posterior leaflets away from the annulus fibrosus. This displacement results in atrialization of the proximal portion of the right ventricle, a reduction in size of the functioning right ventricle, and tricuspid regurgitation. The anterior tricuspid valve leaflet is usually thickened and redundant and can cause right ventricular outflow obstruction. Variations in the degree of downward displacement of the tricuspid valve lead to a wide spectrum of anatomic abnormalities in patients with Ebstein anomaly.

Parasternal Long-Axis View

The diagnosis of Ebstein anomaly cannot be made from the standard parasternal long-axis view because this view does not allow imaging of the tricuspid valve fibrous annulus or the origins of the tricuspid valve leaflets. Usually, this view shows evidence of marked right ventricular volume overload and paradoxical septal motion. In patients with Ebstein anomaly, the free edges of the tricuspid leaflets can be seen in the right ventricle in this view (Fig 8–6); however, this appearance can be seen in any defect with severe right ventricular volume overload and rotation of the enlarged right ventricle toward the left. The diagnosis of Ebstein anomaly depends upon visualization of the displaced *origins* of the valve leaflets, not the free edges.

In the parasternal long-axis view through the right ventricle, the inferior displacement of the septal leaflet into the right ventricle can be seen. It is important to distinguish between the anatomic annulus, which is not displaced, and the functional annulus, marked by the beginning of the attachments of the leaflets. The chordal attachments of these leaflets, particularly the anterior leaflet, can also be appreciated. These attachments are exceedingly important in surgical decisions about valve replacement or valvuloplasty in the more severely deformed valves. Short, thickened chordal attachments of this leaflet may not lend themselves to valvuloplasty but instead may require valve replacement.[8]

Because the angle of incidence to flow through the tricuspid valve is nearly zero degrees, this view is particularly useful for Doppler assessment of the valve. Pulsed and color-flow Doppler should be performed above and below the valve, evaluating its competency as well as stenosis. However, even when flow abnormalities are not seen in this view, it cannot be assumed that they do not exist.

Parasternal Short-Axis View

In this view, the septal and anterior leaflets of the tricuspid valve are seen. The septal leaflet is usually adherent to the septal surfaces and, in more severe forms, may be functionally absent with essentially no free margin. Again, the length of the anterior leaflet, together with its mobility, can be further assessed, as in the prior view. Excessive size of the anterior leaflet may result in systolic obstruction of the right ventricular outflow tract.[9] Because of the orthogonal nature of this view compared with the previous view, the Doppler flow study should be repeated to assess the degree of insufficiency and/or obstruction, as well as the effect upon the right ventricular outflow tract.

In the most severe form of Ebstein anomaly, the anterior tricuspid valve leaflet can completely obstruct forward flow out the right ventricle causing functional and, in many cases, anatomical pulmonary atresia. In neonates with severe Ebstein deformity, the pulmonary valve annulus and branches are small (Fig 8–7), and pulmonary blood flow is dependent upon patency of the ductus arteriosus. In the parasternal short-axis view, a bright linear echo often occupies the position of a normal pulmonary valve. It may be extremely difficult to determine if this echo represents an imperforate membrane (anatomical pulmonary atresia) or a pulmonary valve that is not opening (functional pulmonary atresia) because of lack of forward flow in the right ventricle.

Apical Four-Chamber View

This is the best view for making the diagnosis of Ebstein anomaly because it permits visualization of both the septal and anterior leaflets and detailed assessment of the degree of atrialized right ventricle present (Figs 8–8 and 8–9).[10–12] The true functional size of the right ventricular inflow region can be assessed. Doppler flow studies should be repeated here to further define the degree of regurgitation and/or stenosis. The mitral valve should be carefully examined, as mitral valve prolapse can coexist and the left ventricle may be smaller than normal.[13, 14]

In the apical four-chamber view, bright echoes can often be seen arising from the true annulus fibrosus. These echoes should not be mistaken for valve leaflets. Any structure identified as a valve leaflet should exhibit the pattern of motion characteristic of an atrioventricular valve. Similarly, care must be taken not to mistake the moderator band (or other septal-parietal muscle bundles) for the displaced septal leaflet. With marked displacement of the sep-

tal leaflet into the right ventricular apex, it may be very difficult to differentiate the septal leaflet from the right ventricular trabeculations. Finally, because of the marked right atrial and right ventricular enlargement present in most patients with Ebstein anomaly, obtaining the apical four-chamber view can be very difficult. Because the apex is displaced inferiorly and posteriorly, the patient must usually be placed in a steep, left lateral decubitus position.

Subcostal Views

The subcostal coronal view allows evaluation of the anterior and septal leaflets, again permitting evaluation of the degree of adherence of the septal leaflet to the ventricular myocardium and the degree of elongation of the anterior leaflet (Fig 8–10). More important, when the transducer is angled superiorly to visualize the right ventricular outflow tract, the degree of encroachment of the anterior leaflet upon the right ventricular outflow tract can be assessed. When this leaflet becomes extremely elongated, it can encroach upon the right ventricular outflow tract, resulting in obstruction.[9] In addition, the size of the right ventricular outflow tract can be assessed, and it is therefore possible to describe more accurately the size of the entire right ventricular cavity.

The subcostal coronal view of the right ventricular outflow tract also allows imaging of the displaced origin of the septal leaflet. This leaflet is not only displaced downward in the right ventricle but also outward into the infundibulum. The subcostal sagittal view is also useful for visualizing the sail-like anterior leaflet and the abnormal posterior leaflet.

Associated Anomalies

While Ebstein anomaly may exist as an isolated entity, it is often associated with other problems. Atrial septal defects with right-to-left atrial shunting are commonly associated with Ebstein anomaly. Pulsed and color-flow Dop-

FIG 8–4.
Continuous-wave Doppler tracing of the tricuspid valve from the cardiac apex of a patient with severe tricuspid regurgitation (TR). The signals arising from the TR jet are displayed below the baseline in systole, indicating flow away from the transducer. The forward flow signals through the tricuspid valve are displayed above the baseline in diastole, indicating flow toward the transducer. With severe tricuspid regurgitation, a notch (*black arrow*), seen on the deceleration flow of the TR jet, indicates a severe amount of TR.

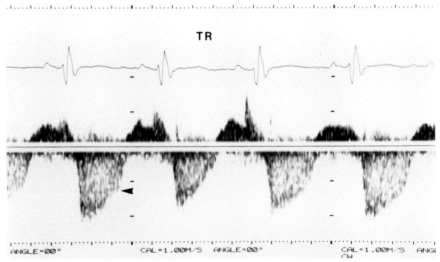

etry, although this is not fully understood. Left ventricular function may be very important in the long-term management of the patient with Ebstein anomaly, and therefore it must be carefully assessed with each examination.

Finally, abnormalities of septal motion and abnormalities of the timing of tricuspid and mitral valve closure

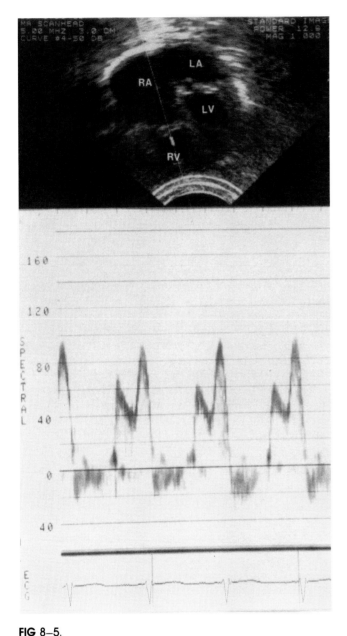

FIG 8–5.
Doppler spectral tracing (*bottom*) from the apical four-chamber view (*top*) of a patient with critical pulmonary stenosis and tricuspid stenosis. The apical four-chamber view shows the position of the sample volume on the right ventricular (RV) side of the tricuspid valve at the time of the Doppler recording. The Doppler recording shows a low peak E velocity, a prolonged deceleration time from peak E velocity, and a markedly elevated peak A velocity. These findings are consistent with tricuspid valve stenosis.

pler are particularly useful for detecting these defects (Plates 21 and 22). Mitral valve prolapse and left ventricular functional abnormalities have been associated with Ebstein anomaly.[13, 14] Careful assessment of right ventricular function must be performed, and the size of the left ventricle must be assessed, as it may be small. The abnormal shape, size, and function of the left ventricle may be a consequence of the abnormality of the right ventricular geom-

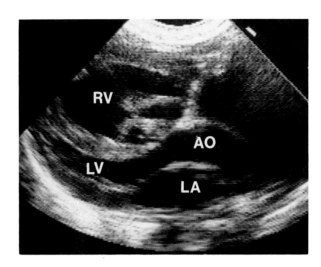

FIG 8–6.
Parasternal long-axis view from an infant with Ebstein anomaly of the tricuspid valve. In this view, the right ventricle (RV) is massively enlarged as a result of severe tricuspid regurgitation. The RV volume overload causes the ventricular septum to be displaced into the left ventricle (LV). With RV dilatation, the RV is rotated leftward and anteriorly, so that portions of the tricuspid valve leaflets are seen in the body of the RV in the long-axis view. The origins of the leaflets, however, cannot be seen. AO = aorta; LA = left atrium.

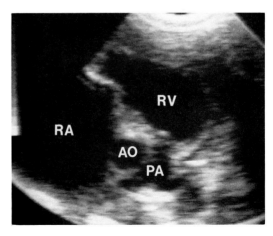

FIG 8–7.
Parasternal short-axis view from a neonate with Ebstein malformation of the tricuspid valve. Because of Ebstein malformation and severe tricuspid regurgitation, this patient developed severe pulmonary stenosis with a small pulmonary valve annulus. Note the marked dilatation of the right ventricular (RV) outflow tract proximal to the pulmonary valve. AO = aorta; PA = pulmonary artery; RA = right atrium.

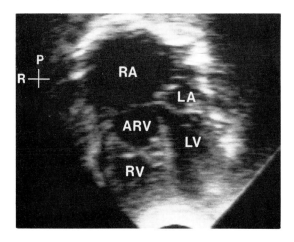

FIG 8–8.
Apical four-chamber view from a neonate with Ebstein malformation of the tricuspid valve. Bright echoes are seen arising from the area of the fibrous annulus of the tricuspid valve; however, the tricuspid valve septal leaflet is displaced downward and arises from the lower portion of the right ventricle. Between the tricuspid valve and the fibrous annulus is the atrialized right ventricle (ARV). The remaining functional right ventricle (RV) is small. The right atrium (RA) is massively enlarged because of tricuspid insufficiency. LA = left atrium; LV = left ventricle; P = posterior; R = right.

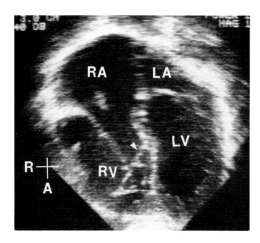

FIG 8–9.
Apical four-chamber view from a patient with Ebstein malformation of the tricuspid valve. The septal leaflet of the tricuspid valve is displaced downward (arrow) and arises from the lower portion of the ventricular septum, away from the fibrous annulus. The anterior leaflet of the tricuspid valve is large and sail-like but arises normally from the fibrous annulus. A = anterior; LA = left atrium; LV = left ventricle; R = right; RA = right atrium; RV = right ventricle.

have been described. Clearly, there is a high incidence of pre-excitation syndrome with Ebstein anomaly; but even when this is absent, the activation time of the two ventricles is often altered as a result of the increased distance the right ventricular excitation wavefront must travel. This may result in abnormal septal motion or an increase in the time between the C points of the tricuspid and the mitral valve.[15] Simultaneous M-mode tracings from both the tricuspid and mitral valve can often show this increase. Before two-dimensional echocardiography was developed, this timing difference was often used as a diagnostic criterion for Ebstein anomaly.

Cor Triatriatum Dexter

In the fetus, the inferior sinus venosus valve is responsible for directing blood toward the atrial septum, which accounts for the fact that a significant portion of the inferior vena caval return crosses the atrial septum to the left atrium. In the mature heart, this valve becomes the eustachian valve and the thebesian valve of the coronary sinus. Abnormal persistence of this structure, which may run from the inferior vena cava to the superior vena cava, may result in division of the right atrial chamber into two chambers, with the upstream chamber receiving the superior and inferior vena caval flow and the downstream chamber incorporating the right atrial appendage and the tricuspid valve. When this double-chambered right atrium exists, the condition is known as cor triatriatum dexter. In this situation, venous return to the heart is directed to the upstream chamber and subsequently across an atrial septal defect to the left atrium, resulting in a right-to-left shunt. As this membrane is usually perforate, there is also some flow across the membrane into the more downstream chamber and through the tricuspid orifice into the right ventricle. Physiologically, this situation is similar to tricuspid atresia. As it may clinically mimic tricuspid atresia, careful distinction between these entities on the echocardiographic examination is necessary, especially because this lesion is easily amenable to surgery, even in the newborn. This condition is best imaged from the subcostal

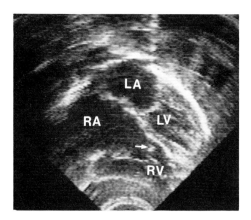

FIG 8–10.
Subcostal four-chamber view from a patient with Ebstein malformation of the tricuspid valve. The anterior tricuspid valve leaflet is seen arising normally from the fibrous annulus. The tricuspid valve septal leaflet (arrow) is displaced inferiorly in the right ventricle (RV) and arises from the inferior portion of the ventricular septum. LA = left atrium; LV = left ventricle; RA = right atrium; RV = right ventricle.

views in both the coronal and sagittal planes.[16] In the sagittal plane, a prominent membrane is seen running from the inferior vena cava toward the superior vena cava, clearly separating the right atrial appendage and tricuspid valve from the inferior and superior venae cavae. The coronary sinus usually empties into the upstream chamber, but may empty into the downstream chamber. An atrial septal defect is also seen, and color-flow mapping clearly indicates a right-to-left atrial level shunt. In addition, flow is seen traversing this membrane into the lower chamber and through the tricuspid orifice to the right ventricle. A normally formed tricuspid orifice and normal-sized right ventricle are seen, clearly distinguishing this defect from tricuspid atresia. Normal motion of the tricuspid valve also should distinguish this entity from tricuspid valve stenosis.

This condition must also be differentiated from the normal but prominent eustachian valve. This distinction is made by tracing the membrane from its inferior margin at the entrance of the inferior vena cava into the right atrium to its superior margin, clearly demonstrating a dual-chambered right atrium. This lesion must also be differentiated from a prominent Chiari's network, which also may be seen within the right atrial cavity. Chiari's network has multiple fenestrations and does not obstruct flow into the right ventricle, unlike the membrane of cor triatriatum dexter.

ABNORMALITIES OF LEFT VENTRICULAR INFLOW

This section will examine abnormalities of left ventricular inflow in the context of normal connection of the pulmonary veins to the left atrium. Total anomalous pulmonary venous return will be discussed in a subsequent chapter, as will abnormalities of left ventricular inflow as a consequence of prior cardiac surgery. The lesions that will be discussed here are pulmonary vein stenosis, cor triatriatum, supravalvular mitral stenosis, and abnormalities of the mitral apparatus itself, such as parachute mitral valve.

Pulmonary Vein Stenosis

Because of the geometry of pulmonary venous inflow and pulmonary venous attachment to the posterior wall of the left atrium, there are limited views in which the pulmonary veins can be adequately visualized. In addition, there are few views in which adequate Doppler flow interrogation can be performed because of the poor angle of incidence of the Doppler beam with pulmonary venous flow.[17-19] The parasternal long-axis view may in some patients permit imaging of the entrance of the left pulmonary veins, particularly the left lower lobe pulmonary vein, into the posterior wall of the left atrium. Color-flow Doppler mapping is sometimes quite helpful for visualizing this entrance. Pulmonary venous flow seen coming toward the

transducer may be traced backward to the orifice of the left-sided pulmonary veins.

The apical four-chamber view is quite useful for evaluating the entrance of the right upper pulmonary vein into the left atrium just leftward of the atrial septum (see Chapter 3).[18] This is also the best view for Doppler evaluation fo venous inflow, as the angle of incidence is the closest to zero of any position. From this view, it is possible to evaluate the orifice size and properly position the Doppler sample volume for characterization of flow patterns, as will be discussed below.

The subcostal four-chamber view is also extremely helpful for visualizing not only the entrance of the right upper pulmonary vein but also the left upper pulmonary vein (see Chapter 3). This view may, in fact, give the examiner the best view of the pulmonary venous entrance. A word of caution is necessary. The pulmonary veins may come posterior to the left atrium and yet not connect directly with it. Careful attention must be paid to tracing the pulmonary veins all the way into the left atrial cavity to be sure that a direct communication exists. Stenosis at the orifice of the pulmonary veins may be visualized, but this can be quite difficult. The diagnosis of pulmonary venous obstruction truly rests with Doppler studies.

Characterization of a Doppler-determined flow pattern within the pulmonary veins is critical for establishing the presence or absence of pulmonary venous obstruction. Normal pulmonary vein flow is best sampled from the apical four-chamber view by placing the Doppler sample volume at the orifice of the right upper pulmonary vein. Color-flow mapping should be performed first to establish the position of the pulmonary vein jet and to best align the Doppler sample volume with the jet (Plate 23). Flow at the orifice is normally a biphasic antegrade flow, occurring during ventricular systole and early ventricular diastole. At low heart rates, retrograde flow may be seen during atrial systole. As the Doppler sample volume is moved farther distally out the pulmonary vein, the retrograde component is lost and flow is more continuous with loss of the distinct peaks seen more proximally. Only minor changes in the velocity profile are observed during normal respiration, and the biphasic nature of such flow is also maintained in situations where pulmonary artery flow is no longer phasic, such as after a Fontan procedure. In the presence of pulmonary vein obstruction or stenosis, the maximal velocity is increased, with severe obstruction present when flow velocity exceeds 2 m/sec.[17] This number assumes a very shallow angle of incidence, which usually is only observed when sampling flow in the right upper pulmonary vein from an apical four-chamber view. Left upper pulmonary vein flow from a subcostal view may also be interrogated with a fairly low angle of incidence. However, interrogation of flow in other pulmonary veins may not show velocities greater than 2 m/sec even when obstruction exists because of the poor intercept angle. The examiner must bear in mind the effect of the angle of sampling upon the recorded velocity.

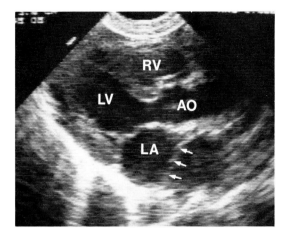

FIG 8–11.
Parasternal long-axis view from a patient with cor triatriatum (*arrows*). The membrane of cor triatriatum is seen stretching across the midportion of the left atrium (LA). AO = aorta; LV = left ventricle; RV = right ventricle.

Abnormalities Within the Left Atrium

Abnormal membranes may exist within the left atrial cavity. These membranes can subdivide the left atrial cavity into two chambers (cor triatriatum) or be adherent to the mitral valve, creating supravalvular mitral stenosis. It is therefore essential that the left atrial cavity be closely inspected from multiple views. The region superior to the mitral valve must be inspected especially closely. Left atrial dilatation and/or pulmonary vein dilatation may or may not be present, depending upon the presence or absence of an atrial septal defect. An atrial septal defect may decompress the distal chamber and prevent dilatation of either the left atrium or pulmonary veins.

The most useful views for detecting membranes in the left atrium are the parasternal long-axis, apical four-chamber, and subcostal four-chamber views.[20, 21] In cor triatriatum in the long-axis view, the membrane stretches obliquely across the left atrium, with extensions anterosuperiorly to the posterior aortic root and posteroinferiorly to the posterior left atrial wall (Figs 8–11 and 8–12). In the four-chamber views, the membrane is situated in a horizontal plane extending on the right to the atrial septum and on the left to the lateral wall of the left atrium (Figs 8–13 and 8–14). In real time, the membrane moves toward the mitral valve in diastole and away from the valve in systole. In cor triatriatum, the membrane divides the left atrium into two chambers—a posterior, superior chamber that usually receives the pulmonary veins and an anterior, inferior chamber that gives rise to the left atrial appendage and communicates with the mitral valve. In some cases, however, pulmonary veins drain to both chambers. Usually, an atrial septal defect is present, and this defect can communicate with either or both chambers. The mitral valve is usually normal.

The peak diastolic pressure gradient across the mem-

brane can be calculated from a Doppler recording of the peak velocity of the jet flow across the membrane and the simplified Bernoulli equation (see Chapter 4) (Fig 8–15). Doppler color-flow mapping shows a high-velocity (usually over 2 m/sec), mosaic jet just beyond the membrane in the inferior chamber (Plate 24). Color-flow Doppler is useful for aligning the pulsed or continuous-wave Doppler beam with the jet flow. It should be noted that in cor tria-

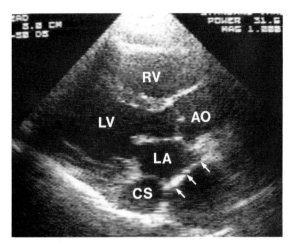

FIG 8–12.
Parasternal long-axis view from a patient with cor triatriatum (*arrows*) and persistent left superior vena cava draining to the coronary sinus (CS). The membrane of the cor triatriatum is seen stretching obliquely across the midportion of the left atrium (LA). AO = aorta; LV = left ventricle; RV = right ventricle.

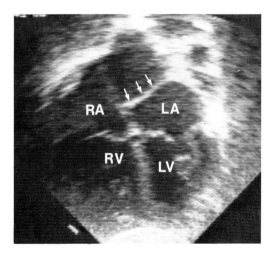

FIG 8–13.
Apical four-chamber view from a patient with cor triatriatum (*arrows*). The membrane of the cor triatriatum divides the left atrium (LA) into two chambers. The upper chamber usually receives the pulmonary veins. The lower chamber usually receives the left atrial appendage and communicates with the mitral valve. LV = left ventricle; RA = right atrium; RV = right ventricle.

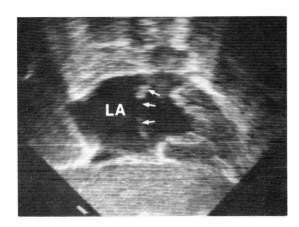

FIG 8–14.
Subcostal four-chamber view from a patient with cor triatriatum (*arrows*). The membrane of the cor triatriatum divides the left atrium (LA) into two chambers. In this view, the pulmonary veins can be seen draining to the superior chamber, and the left atrial appendage can be seen communicating with the inferior chamber.

triatum the mosaic jet forms in the left atrium; with mitral valve stenosis or supravalvular mitral ring, the mosaic jet is downstream from the mitral valve in the left ventricle.

Although the membrane of a supravalvular mitral stenosing ring may appear similar to that present in cor triatriatum, it is located much closer to the mitral valve, between the left atrial appendage and the mitral valve. The membrane may lie just above the valve or be adherent to the valve leaflets (Figs 8–16 and 8–17). This membrane may be extremely close to the mitral valve, with no discernible separation during ventricular systole. Diagnosis of this lesion requires careful examination of the diastolic frames for a membrane that is just superior to the mitral valve leaflets or adherent to the mitral valve leaflets but that separates from them slightly during diastole.[22] When the membrane is adherent to the leaflets, a "hinging" phenomenon has been described, whereby the leaflets appear to move during diastole from a hinge point separate from the mitral annulus. Care must be taken not to mistake echoes that arise from the mitral valve fibrous annulus or a thickened mitral valve for supravalvular mitral ring. Examination of the mitral funnel in multiple planes will usually make it possible to distinguish these entities. The proximity of the membrane to the mitral valve in patients with supravalvular mitral ring often leads to damage to the mitral valve leaflets, caused by the jet flow across the membrane. The leaflets may appear thickened and myxomatous. Doppler studies of flow across the mitral orifice may show elevated peak velocity and a persistent gradient throughout diastole or may be normal, particularly if a large atrial septal defect is present. The presence of an atrial septal defect may lower left atrial pressures, resulting in little detectable or measurable gradient across the mitral valve. In this situation, there is usually a large left-to-right shunt with marked right atrial and right ventricular dilatation. The left atrial cavity itself may in fact be small.

Associated lesions commonly occur. The lesion most commonly associated with either cor triatriatum or supravalvular mitral stenosis, aside from an atrial septal defect, is a left superior vena cava draining to the coronary sinus.

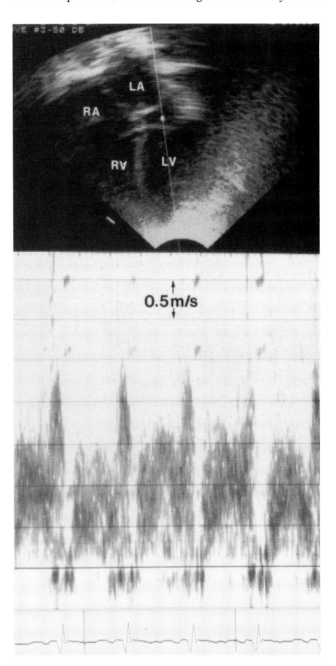

FIG 8–15.
Pulsed Doppler recording (*bottom*) from the apical four-chamber view (*top*) of a patient with cor triatriatum. The freeze-frame image on the top shows the position of the sample volume just distal to the membrane of the cor triatriatum and proximal to the mitral valve at the time of the Doppler tracing. The Doppler tracing on the bottom shows a high-velocity jet whose peak velocity is 2.5 m/sec above the baseline throughout systole and diastole. This jet indicates obstruction to forward flow across the membrane.

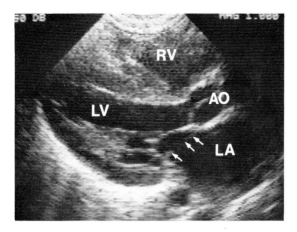

FIG 8–16.
Parasternal long-axis view from a patient with a supravalvular mitral ring (*arrows*). The supravalvular mitral ring is positioned close to the mitral valve leaflets between the left atrial appendage and the mitral valve. In the parasternal long-axis view, the ring is aligned nearly parallel to the ultrasound beam and is difficult to image directly. AO = aorta; LA = left atrium; LV = left ventricle; RV = right ventricle.

Other defects that have been described include coarctation of the aorta, ventricular septal defect, and multiple left heart obstructive lesions.[22]

Abnormalities of the Mitral Valve

This section will discuss primary abnormalities of the mitral valve leaflets themselves. These abnormalities may exist in isolation or in combination with other congenital anomalies of the heart. Here, they will be discussed as they exist in isolation. Entities to be considered are mitral valve prolapse, mitral valve stenosis, isolated clefts of the mitral valve, double-orifice mitral valve, and ruptured mitral valve chordae.

Before proceeding to the echocardiographic description of these entities, some generalities and definitions need to be discussed. Foremost among these is mitral valve prolapse. This has been defined using numerous criteria, with the overall incidence of mitral valve prolapse among the general population greatly affected by the manner in which it is described.[23–27] Strict definitions limiting the diagnosis to only those valves with definite prolapse of the leaflets posterior to the mitral annulus observed in several echocardiographic views and with thickening of the valve leaflets results in a very low incidence of approximately 5%. When the definition is broadened to include those valves where prolapse is noted in only one view with no thickening of the mitral valve leaflets, the incidence increases to approximately 35% of the general population. As the mitral annulus plane is not necessarily euclidian (i.e., flat during ventricular systole), the appearance of leaflet prolapse is greatly affected by the manner in which the leaflets are imaged.[28] Changes in angulation produce changes in the appearance of the valve leaflets. Because of this, it is felt that true mitral valve prolapse must result

in definite prolapse of the leaflets observed in at least two echocardiographic planes or in only one echocardiographic plane if definite mitral regurgitation is present. Whether or not leaflet thickening is present often depends upon the underlying etiology of the prolapse. Mitral valve prolapse is felt to be a multietiologic entity that is a result of connective tissue disorders, abnormal chordal attachments, rheumatic fever, or papillary muscle dysfunction.[29–32] This multietiologic nature of the disease is in part responsible for the differing definitions and the widely divergent incidence of this abnormality within the general population. For the purpose of this chapter, mitral valve prolapse will be defined as prolapse during systole of the mitral valve leaflets posterior and superior to the plane of the mitral annulus in at least two echocardiographic views or in only one view when associated mitral regurgitation or myxomatous changes of the mitral valve are present.

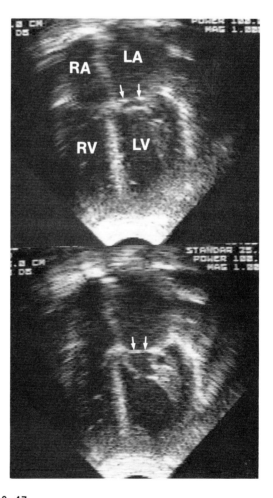

FIG 8–17.
Apical four-chamber views in systole (*above*) and diastole (*below*) from the same patient as in Figure 8–16. The membrane of a supravalvular mitral ring (*arrows*) can be seen stretching across the mitral valve funnel. This membrane is closely applied to the mitral valve. LA = left atrium; LV = left ventricle; RA = right atrium; RV = right ventricle.

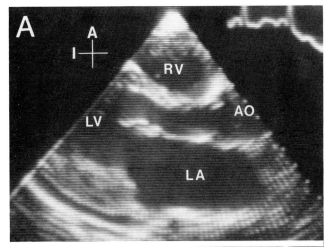

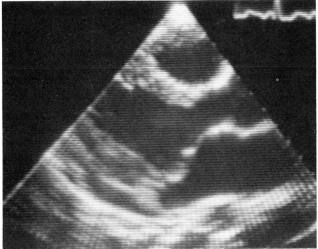

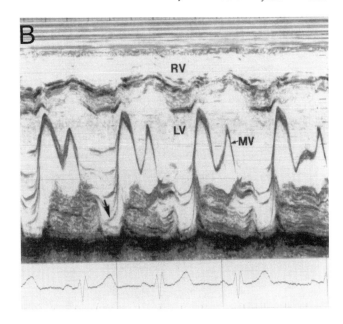

FIG 8–18.
A, parasternal long-axis views in diastole (*above*) and systole (*below*) from a patient with myxomatous thickening and prolapse of the mitral valve. **B,** M-mode echocardiogram of the left ventricle (LV) from a patient with prolapse of the mitral valve (MV). The prolapse of the anterior mitral valve leaflet (*arrow*) toward the left atrium is easily seen on this echocardiogram. A = anterior; AO = aorta; I = inferior; LA = left atrium; LV = left ventricle; RV = right ventricle.

Isolated cleft of the mitral valve is defined as a cleft in the anterior leaflet of the mitral valve unassociated with any defect of the atrioventricular septum.[33, 34] While this defect is still embryologically related to an abnormality in partitioning of the atrioventricular canal, it is distinct clinically from an atrioventricular septal defect in that the mitral valve position within the heart is normal and there are no other associated cardiac abnormalities. Finally, double-orifice mitral valve is defined as the presence of two orifices through the mitral valve as a consequence of bridging tissue that connects the mitral valve leaflets. This bridging tissue may be only a small strand of tissue that connects the leaflets at their edges or a thickened fibrous bridge that divides the left atrioventricular orifice into equal or unequal parts. In addition, double-orifice mitral valve may occur as a result of fusion of the subvalvular chordal apparatus, prohibiting complete opening of the valve with a resultant double-orifice appearance in diastole.[35]

Parasternal Long-Axis View

In this view, the mitral valve is imaged in the anterior-posterior direction, with excellent visualization of both the anterior and posterior leaflets. Prolapse of the mitral valve may be evident during systole (Fig 8–18 A and B). In this view, superior prolapse of the mitral valve leaflets into the left atrium can be detected. Since superior prolapse often precedes posterior prolapse, this view is especially sensitive for the early detection of minor degrees of valve prolapse. The mitral valve leaflets can be inspected for myxomatous thickening that may be present as well. Abnormal chordal attachments may not be evident in this view. Likewise, congenital anomalies of the leaflets themselves, such as isolated clefts and double-orifice mitral valve, cannot be seen in this view. When ruptured chordae occur, they are seen easily in this view, as evidenced by a rapid, whiplike motion of the valve during both systole and diastole.[36, 37]

Color-flow imaging of the mitral valve in this view is quite helpful in detecting mitral regurgitation, particularly when there is a posteriorly oriented regurgitant jet (Plate 25).

Parasternal Short-Axis View

The parasternal short-axis view at the level of the papillary muscles is quite helpful in discerning the orientation and number of the papillary muscles. In parachute mitral

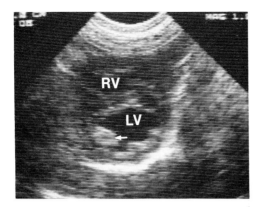

FIG 8–19.
Parasternal short-axis view at the level of the left ventricular (LV) papillary muscles in a patient with mitral stenosis and a single LV papillary muscle (*arrow*). This patient had a Shone complex and parachute mitral valve deformity. RV = right ventricle.

valve where all of the chordae attach to a single large papillary muscle, this view shows a single large papillary muscle rather than two separate papillary muscles (Fig 8–19).[38, 39] As the examiner then scans superiorly to the base of the heart, abnormal attachments of either mitral valve leaflet is evident, even in the presence of two papillary muscles; subvalvular chordal fusion, which may be present in double-orifice mitral valve, is also seen (Fig 8–20).[35] In addition, as the plane of sound is tilted to the level of the anterior mitral valve leaflet, clefts in this leaflet can easily be seen as a split in the leaflet in diastole.

This view is particularly advantageous for detecting double-orifice mitral valve (Fig 8–21). Careful scans from the cardiac apex to the base clearly show fusion of the mitral leaflets, and it is possible to distinguish the level at which fusion occurs. In addition, abnormal orientation of the papillary muscles, which may accompany this disorder, is easily seen. It should be noted that in double-orifice mitral valve all chordal attachments from the same orifice attach to the same papillary muscle, and in a sense this lesion can be thought of as a double parachute mitral valve.

Apical Four-Chamber View

This view presents an image of the mitral valve in a plane orthogonal to that found in the parasternal long-axis view. As the plane of the mitral valve is not euclidian but saddle-shaped, the level of the annulus seen in this view relative to the point of leaflet coaptation may not be the same as that seen in the parasternal long-axis view. Because of this, mitral valve prolapse seen in one view may not be seen in the other. However, when prolapse is seen in both views, the degree of mitral valve prolapse can be considered to be significant.

The mitral valve opening is easily seen in this view, and valves with abnormal opening are readily apparent. It is easy to discern if this is the result of abnormal chordal attachments, such as in parachute mitral valve, or due to valve thickening, as in rheumatic mitral stenosis (Fig 8–22).

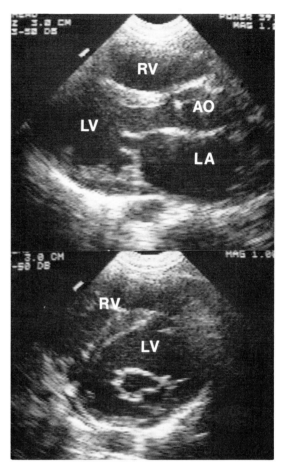

FIG 8–20.
Parasternal long- (*top*) and short- (*bottom*) axis views from a patient with severe mitral valve stenosis and two papillary muscles. These frames were both taken at the time of maximum diastolic excursion of the mitral valve. The mitral valve orifice, as shown in both views, is extremely small. AO = aorta, LA = left atrium; LV = left ventricle; RV = right ventricle.

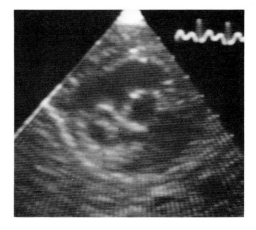

FIG 8–21.
Parasternal short-axis view of the left ventricle from a patient with double-orifice mitral valve. This patient also had a coarctation of the aorta. The two orifices of the mitral valve can be seen and give the mitral valve the appearance of a figure-of-eight.

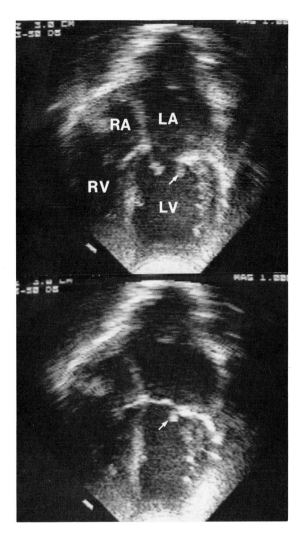

FIG 8–22.
Apical four-chamber views in diastole (*above*) and systole (*below*) from a patient with severe mitral valve stenosis and a thickened, tethered mitral valve leaflet (*arrow*). The lack of mobility of this leaflet causes a marked reduction in the diameter of the orifice. Note the severe enlargement of the left atrium (LA). LV = left ventricle; RA = right atrium; RV = right ventricle.

Doppler flow studies using both pulsed and color-flow mapping methods are optimal from this view, as the angle of incidence of the Doppler beam to the flow is near zero degrees. Color-flow Doppler clearly shows the presence of both stenotic as well as regurgitant jets (Fig 8–23 and Plate 26). However, it is necessary to interrogate carefully all aspects of the mitral valve by sweeping the scan plane from posterior to anterior. If only one area is examined, a regurgitant jet may be missed.

Pulsed Doppler recordings should be obtained both above and below the mitral valve leaflets. Positioning the sample volume within the left atrium is useful for assessing the presence of regurgitation and is particularly useful in confirming the presence of regurgitant jets initially seen on color-flow Doppler (Fig 8–24). Our current practice is

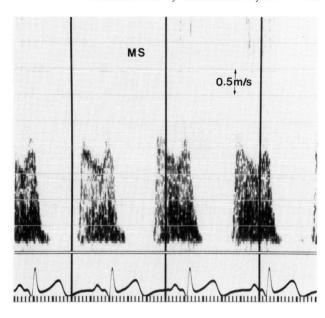

FIG 8–23.
Continuous-wave Doppler examination of the mitral valve from the cardiac apex of a patient with mitral stenosis (MS). In diastole, a high-velocity jet is displayed above the baseline. The contour of the Doppler recording is very suggestive of significant mitral stenosis. The pressure half-time is prolonged.

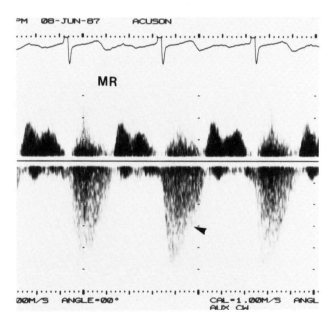

FIG 8–24.
Continuous-wave Doppler examination of the mitral valve from the cardiac apex of a patient with severe mitral regurgitation (MR). Note the notched contour of the deceleration portion of the MR jet (*arrow*). This notch is present when the regurgitant volume is large.

to examine the valve using color-flow Doppler and then to confirm the presence of regurgitant jets using color-flow directed pulsed and continuous-wave Doppler.

The sample volume should then be positioned on the ventricular side of the valve to assess the presence of stenotic jets. Quantitation of the degree of mitral stenosis has been done in several ways. The area of the mitral valve orifice as seen from the parasternal short-axis view has been imaged and then planimetered to obtain the valve cross-sectional area.[40] However, this requires careful imaging of the mitral valve in the parasternal short-axis view and careful digitizing of the orifice area.

Doppler methods for calculation of mitral valve gradients and areas are easier to perform and have been highly successful.[41–45] Calculation of the mean gradient by tracing the Doppler envelope during diastole and measurement of the pressure half-time have been particularly useful. From the pressure half-time or the continuity equation, the mitral valve cross-sectional area can be calculated (see Chapter 4). In general, Doppler methods for calculation of mean gradient, pressure half-time, and valve area are felt to be more indicative of the true physiologic state than is direct measurement of the two-dimensional orifice area. This is because of the irregular orifice shape of most stenotic valves and the difficulty in truly imaging the most restrictive orifice. Thus, for mitral stenosis, Doppler pressure gradients, half-time data, and valve areas are felt to provide a better indication of the true physiologic or functional status of the valve. Imaging, on the other hand, provides complementary anatomic data about the type of mitral valve lesion that is producing the functional changes detected by the Doppler technique.

Subcostal Views

The subcostal coronal view provides an image similar to the apical four-chamber view. However, because the angle of incidence with the mitral valve is now closer to 90°, imaging of the mitral valve apparatus is superior but Doppler studies are less satisfactory. Therefore, this view should be used to evaluate the anatomic detail of the mitral valve itself rather than for Doppler flow studies (Fig 8–25). Specifically, in this view ruptured chordae can easily be seen as structures whipping around within the left ventricular cavity. In older adult patients, ruptured chordae can be seen with a somewhat increased degree of frequency, whereas they are fairly uncommon in pediatric patients. They may relate to mitral insufficiency or may be a totally incidental finding.

Turning into the sagittal plane and angling the transducer slightly toward the left produces a short-axis image similar to that obtained from the parasternal view. This allows imaging of the mitral valve en face, which can be quite useful in diagnosing isolated clefts of the mitral valve and double-orifice mitral valve. Isolated clefts of the mitral valve are usually clefts of the anterior leaflet rather than a cleft between the posterior and anterior bridging leaflets, as occurs in atrioventricular septal defect (Fig 8–26). The degree of regurgitation through these isolated clefts can be

minimal or significant, depending upon the degree of deformity present. The mitral valve position within the heart is normal, not being inferiorly displaced as in an atrioventricular septal defect. However, when cleft mitral valve occurs, it is necessary to inspect totally all regions of the heart, particularly the atrial and inlet ventricular septa to make certain that no septal defects exist.

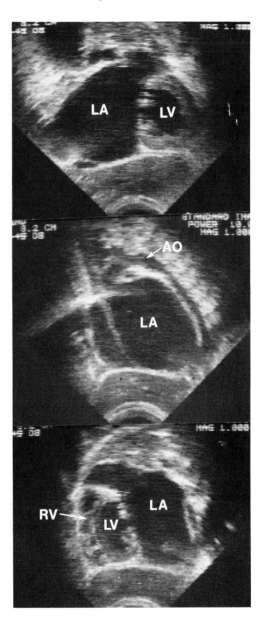

FIG 8–25.
Subcostal views from a patient with an isolated cleft of the anterior mitral valve leaflet and severe mitral regurgitation. The *top frame* is a subcostal coronal view of the left atrium (LA) and left ventricle (LV). The *middle frame* is a subcostal sagittal view of the aortic (AO) arch. The *bottom frame* is a subcostal sagittal view of the LV. All frames show massive enlargement of the left atrium. Note also the massive enlargement of the left atrial appendage in the top and bottom frames. RV = right ventricle.

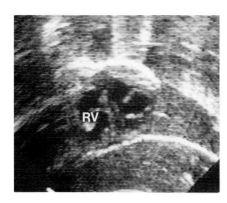

FIG 8–26.
Subcostal short-axis view of the right ventricle (RV) and left ventricle.
Note the cleft in the anterior mitral valve leaflet.

REFERENCES

1. Ogawa S, Hayashi J, Sasaki H, et al: Evaluation of combined valvular prolapse syndrome by two-dimensional echocardiography. *Circulation* 1982; 65:174–180.
2. Morganroth J, Jones RH, Chen CC, et al: Two-dimensional echocardiography in mitral, aortic and tricuspid valve prolapse. The clinical problem, cardiac nuclear imaging considerations and a proposed standard for diagnosis. *Am J Cardiol* 1980; 46:1164–1177.
3. Gibson TC, Foale RA, Guyer DE, et al: Clinical significance of incomplete tricuspid valve closure seen on two-dimensional echocardiography. *J Am Coll Cardiol* 1984; 4:1052–1057.
4. Mahoney LT, Coryell KG, Lauer RM: The newborn transitional circulation: A two-dimensional Doppler echocardiographic study. *J Am Coll Cardiol* 1985; 6:623–629.
5. Reller MD, Rice MJ, McDonald RW: Tricuspid regurgitation in newborn infants with respiratory distress: Echo-Doppler study. *J Pediatr* 1987; 110:760–764.
6. Currie PJ, Seward JB, Chan KL, et al: Continuous wave Doppler determination of right ventricular pressure: A simultaneous Doppler-catheterization study in 127 patients. *J Am Coll Cardiol* 1985; 6:750–756.
7. Yock PG, Popp RL: Noninvasive estimation of right ventricular systolic pressure by Doppler ultrasound in patients with tricuspid regurgitation. *Circulation* 1984; 70:657–662.
8. Shiina A, Seward JB, Tajik AJ, et al: Two-dimensional echocardiographic-surgical correlation in Ebstein anomaly: Preoperative determination of patients requiring tricuspid valve plication v. replacement. *Circulation* 1983; 68:534–544.
9. Sealy WC: The cause of the hemodynamic disturbances in Ebstein anomaly based on observations at operation. *Ann Thorac Surg* 1979; 27:536–546.
10. Ports TA, Silverman NH, Schiller NB: Two-dimensional echocardiographic assessment of Ebstein anomaly. *Circulation* 1978; 58:336–343.
11. Shiina A, Seward JB, Edwards WD, et al: Two-dimensional echocardiographic spectrum of Ebstein anomaly: Detailed anatomic assessment. *J Am Coll Cardiol* 1984; 3:356–370.
12. Nihoyannopoulos P, McKenna WJ, Smith G, et al: Echocardiographic assessment of the right ventricle in Ebstein anomaly: Relation to clinical outcome. *J Am Coll Cardiol* 1986; 8:627–635.
13. Matsumoto M, Matsuo H, Nagata S, et al: Visualization of Ebstein anomaly of the tricuspid valve by two-dimensional and standard echocardiography. *Circulation* 1976; 53:59–79.
14. Benson LN, Child JS, Schwaiger M, et al: Left ventricular geometry and function in adults with Ebstein anomaly of the tricuspid valve. *Circulation* 1987; 75:353–359.
15. Farooki ZQ, Henry JG, Green EW: Echocardiographic spectrum of Ebstein anomaly of the tricuspid valve. *Circulation* 1976; 53:63–68.
16. Burton DA, Chin A, Weinberg PM, et al: Identification of cor triatriatum dexter by two-dimensional echocardiography. *Am J Cardiol* 1987; 60:409–410.
17. Vick GW III, Murphy DJ Jr, Ludomirsky A, et al: Pulmonary venous and systemic ventricular inflow obstruction in patients with congenital heart disease: Detection by combined two-dimensional and Doppler echocardiography. *J Am Coll Cardiol* 1987; 9:580–587.
18. Smallhorn JF, Freedom RM, Olley PM: Pulsed Doppler echocardiographic assessment of extraparenchymal pulmonary vein flow. *J Am Coll Cardiol* 1987; 9:573–579.
19. Smallhorn JF, Pauperio IT, Benson L, et al: Pulsed Doppler assessment of pulmonary vein obstruction. *Am Heart J* 1985; 110:483–485.
20. Ostman-Smith I, Silverman NH, Oldershaw P, et al: Cor triatriatum sinestrum. Diagnostic features in cross-sectional echocardiography. *Br Heart J* 1984; 51:211–219.
21. Jacobstein MD, Hirschfeld SS: Concealed left atrial membrane: Pitfalls in the diagnosis of cor triatriatum and supravalve mitral ring. *Am J Cardiol* 1982; 49:780–786.
22. Sullivan ID, Robinson PJ, de Leval M, et al: Membranous supravalvular mitral stenosis: A treatable form of congenital heart disease. *J Am Coll Cardiol* 1986; 8:159–164.
23. Warth DC, King ME, Cohen JM, et al: Prevalence of mitral valve prolapse in normal children. *J Am Coll Cardiol* 1985; 5:1173–1177.
24. Alpert MA, Carney RJ, Flaker GC, et al: Sensitivity and specificity of two-dimensional echocardiographic signs of mitral valve prolapse. *Am J Cardiol* 1984; 54:792–796.
25. Krivokapich J, Child JS, Dadourian BJ, et al: Reassessment of echocardiographic criteria for diagnosis of mitral valve prolapse. *Am J Cardiol* 1988; 61:131–135.
26. Perloff JK, Child JS, Edwards JE: New guidelines for the clinical diagnosis of mitral valve prolapse. *Am J Cardiol* 1986; 57:1124–1129.
27. Wann LS, Grove JR, Hess TR, et al: Prevalence of mitral prolapse by two-dimensional echocardiogra-

phy in healthy young women. *Br Heart J* 1983; 49:334–340.

28. Levine RA, Triulzi MO, Harrigan P, et al: The relationship of mitral annular shape to the diagnosis of mitral valve prolapse. *Circulation* 1987; 75:756–767.

29. Jaffe AS, Geltman EM, Rodey GE, et al: Mitral valve prolapse: A consistent manifestation of type IV Ehlers-Danlos syndrome. The pathogenetic role of the abnormal production of type III collagen. *Circulation* 1981; 64:121–125.

30. Virmani R, Atkinson JB, Byrd BF III, et al: Abnormal chordal insertion: A cause of mitral valve prolapse. *Am Heart J* 1987; 113:851–858.

31. Naito M, Morganroth J, Mardelli TJ, et al: Rheumatic mitral stenosis: Cross-sectional echocardiographic analysis. *Am Heart J* 1980; 100:34–40.

32. Lembo NJ, DellItalia LJ, Crawford MH, et al: Mitral valve prolapse in patients with prior rheumatic fever. *Circulation* 1988; 77:830–836.

33. Di Segni E, Bass JL, Lucas RV Jr, et al: Isolated cleft mitral valve: A variety of congenital mitral regurgitation identified by 2-dimensional echocardiography. *Am J Cardiol* 1983; 51:927–931.

34. Smallhorn JF, de Leval M, Stark J, et al: Isolated anterior mitral cleft. Two-dimensional echocardiographic assessment and differentiation from "clefts" associated with atrioventricular septal defect. *Br Heart J* 1982; 48:109–116.

35. Trowitzsch E, Bano-Rodrigo A, Burger BM, et al: Two-dimensional echocardiographic findings in double orifice mitral valve. *J Am Coll Cardiol* 1985; 6:383–387.

36. Jeresaty RM, Edwards JE, Chawla SK: Mitral valve prolapse and ruptured chordae tendineae. *Am J Cardiol* 1985; 55:138–142.

37. Boxer RA, Singh S, Goldman M, et al: Flail posterior mitral leaflet: An unusual cause of mitral regurgitation in childhood. *Am Heart J* 1986; 111:604–606.

38. Grenadier E, Sahn DJ, Valdes-Cruz LM, et al: Two-dimensional echo Doppler study of congenital disorders of the mitral valve. *Am Heart J* 1984; 107:319–325.

39. Snider AR, Roge CL, Schiller NB, et al: Congenital left ventricular inflow obstruction evaluated by two-dimensional echocardiography. *Circulation* 1980; 61:848–855.

40. Riggs TW, Lapin GD, Paul MH, et al: Measurement of mitral valve orifice area in infants and children by two-dimensional echocardiography. *J Am Coll Cardiol* 1983; 1:873–878.

41. Richards KL, Cannon SR, Crawford MH, et al: Non-invasive diagnosis of aortic and mitral valve disease with pulsed-Doppler spectral analysis. *Am J Cardiol* 1983; 51:1122–1127.

42. Gonzalez MA, Child JS, Krivokapich J: Comparison of two-dimensional and Doppler echocardiography and intracardiac hemodynamics for quantification of mitral stenosis. *Am J Cardiol* 1987; 60:327–332.

43. Jaffe WM, Roche AH, Coverdale HA, et al: Clinical evaluation v. Doppler echocardiography in the quantitative assessment of valvular heart disease. *Circulation* 1988; 78:267–275.

44. Smith MD, Handshoe R, Handshoe S, et al: Comparative accuracy of two-dimensional echocardiography and Doppler pressure half-time methods in assessing severity of mitral stenosis in patients with and without prior commissurotomy. *Circulation* 1986; 73:100–107.

45. Hatle L, Angelsen B, Tromsdal A: Noninvasive assessment of atrioventricular pressure half-time by Doppler ultrasound. *Circulation* 1979; 60:1096–1104.

Abnormalities of Ventricular Outflow

ABNORMALITIES OF THE RIGHT VENTRICULAR OUTFLOW

Valvular Pulmonary Stenosis

Pulmonary valve stenosis can occur as an isolated defect or as part of a more complex malformation, such as tetralogy of Fallot or transposition complexes. This chapter reviews the echocardiographic features of isolated pulmonary valve stenosis—a primary lesion of the pulmonary valve in an otherwise normal heart. Isolated pulmonary valve stenosis occurs in three anatomic forms: (1) valvular stenosis caused by cusp fusion, (2) valvular and infundibular stenosis, and (3) hypoplastic valve annulus and pulmonary conus.[1]

Anatomic Features

Isolated pulmonary valve stenosis resulting from cusp fusion.—In isolated pulmonary valve stenosis resulting from cusp fusion, there is usually a normal-sized pulmonary valve annulus and three well-developed valve sinuses and commissures. Obstruction to forward flow out the right ventricle is caused by partial fusion of the commissures. In isolated pulmonary valve stenosis, unicuspid and bicuspid pulmonary valves are rare. This is in contrast to tetralogy of Fallot, where unicuspid and bicuspid valves are fairly common.[1] On the two-dimensional echocardiogram, the motion of the pulmonary valve leaflets can easily be observed in the parasternal short-axis view at the base of the heart, in the parasternal long-axis view through the right ventricular outflow tract, and in the subcostal four-chamber and sagittal views of the right ventricle. In these views, the pulmonary valve annulus is of normal size. The pulmonary valve leaflets are thickened and domed in systole.[2, 3] In some cases, the leaflets prolapse into the right ventricular outflow tract in diastole (Figs 9–1 and 9–2). The jet flow through the stenotic orifice of the pulmonary valve creates poststenotic dilatation usually involving the main and left pulmonary arteries (see Figs 9–1 and 9–2). The degree of poststenotic dilatation does not correlate with the severity of the obstruction, so that very marked

dilatation of the main pulmonary artery is frequently found in children with mild pulmonary stenosis. In the parasternal short-axis view in patients with marked poststenotic dilatation of the main pulmonary artery, the pulmonary valve may be pushed into a more anterior position than usual. In some patients, the pulmonary valve can be imaged in cross-section in a standard parasternal long-axis view. This abnormal rotation of the valve is also caused by enlargement of the main pulmonary artery segment.

On the two-dimensional echocardiogram, the right ventricle is of normal size, and if the stenosis is severe, the right ventricle is concentrically hypertrophied. The infundibulum of the right ventricle is also of normal size or slightly narrowed as a result of the hypertrophic changes. In the four-chamber views in patients with very severe obstruction, the right atrium is dilated and the atrial septum bows toward the left atrium. These echocardiographic features are caused by a noncompliant right ventricle with an elevated right atrial pressure.

In the neonatal period, the echocardiographic diagnosis of pulmonary valve stenosis should not be based solely on the findings of right ventricular hypertrophy and thickened pulmonary valve leaflets. Infants with severe pulmonary artery hypertension can also have echo-bright pulmonary valve leaflets and right ventricular hypertrophy on the two-dimensional echocardiogram. Doppler echocardiography (see below) is useful for distinguishing these two disorders.

In patients with isolated pulmonary valve stenosis and Noonan's syndrome, the pulmonary valve leaflets appear especially thickened and myxomatous on the two-dimensional echocardiogram. These myxomatous changes may be so severe that it is difficult to image the movement of any individual valve leaflet separate from the myxomatous mass. In these patients, we have frequently observed an associated long-segment muscular subaortic stenosis that resembles hypertrophic cardiomyopathy.

Valvular and infundibular stenosis.—In these patients, the pulmonary valve has the same anatomy and

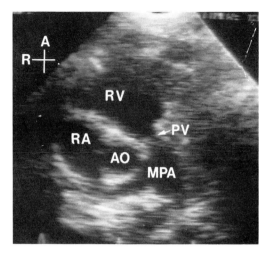

FIG 9–1.
Parasternal short-axis view from a child with pulmonary valve (PV) stenosis. Note the marked poststenotic dilatation of the main pulmonary artery (MPA). In this child, the PV annulus was nearly the same diameter as the aortic (AO) annulus; the right ventricular (RV) cavity size was normal. A = anterior; R = right; RA = right atrium.

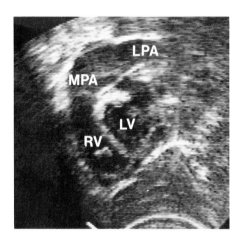

FIG 9–2.
Subcostal sagittal view of the right ventricle (RV) and main pulmonary artery (MPA) from a patient with pulmonary valve stenosis. This patient has a normal-sized pulmonary valve annulus and stenosis caused by cusp fusion. Note the marked poststenotic dilatation of the MPA and left pulmonary artery (LPA). LV = left ventricle.

echocardiographic appearance as it does in the preceding group. The lumen of the subpulmonary conus, however, is significantly narrowed because of abnormal hypertrophy of the muscular walls of the right ventricle and the surrounding conus musculature.[1] The valve annulus is of normal size; however, there is usually no poststenotic dilatation of the main pulmonary artery. The size of the right ventricular infundibulum can be assessed from a combination of parasternal and subcostal views (Fig 9–3). Many of the patients in this group have critical pulmonary stenosis (su-

prasystemic right ventricular pressure, with a normal-sized valve annulus and right ventricular chamber).

Hypoplastic pulmonary valve annulus and conus.— In this group of patients, the pulmonary valve is thickened, domed, and stenotic; in addition, the valve annulus is narrowed or hypoplastic (Fig 9–4).[1] The pulmonary conus is short and narrow, exhibiting the anatomic features of hypoplasia. The right ventricle is heavily trabeculated and usually has decreased cavity dimensions (Fig 9–5). Children with this disorder often develop symptoms in the newborn period and their pulmonary blood supply may

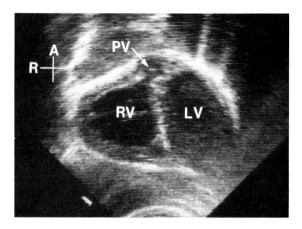

FIG 9–3.
Subcostal coronal view of the right ventricle (RV) from a patient with pulmonary valvular (PV) stenosis. This patient has infundibular stenosis with a normal-sized valve annulus and therefore no poststenotic dilatation of the main pulmonary artery. Although this patient had critical pulmonary stenosis, the RV chamber is of normal size. A = anterior; LV = left ventricle; R = right.

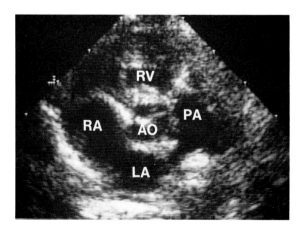

FIG 9–4.
Parasternal short-axis view from an infant with critical pulmonary valve stenosis. This patient has a hypoplastic pulmonary valve annulus and conus. The right ventricle (RV) is heavily trabeculated and has decreased cavity dimensions. AO = aorta; LA = left atrium; PA = pulmonary artery; RA = right atrium.

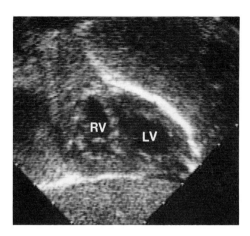

FIG 9–5.
Subcostal coronal view of the right ventricle (RV) from the same infant as in Figure 9–4. Note the heavy trabeculations and small size of the RV. LV = left ventricle.

be dependent on patency of the ductus arteriosus or, rarely, systemic-to-pulmonary collateral vessels. This defect, also known as critical pulmonary stenosis, is part of a continuum of defects that runs the spectrum from severe valvular pulmonary stenosis with a normal-sized right ventricle to critical pulmonary stenosis with a normal or small right ventricle to pulmonary atresia with an intact ventricular septum and ventricular hypoplasia.

On the two-dimensional echocardiogram in infants with critical pulmonary stenosis and a hypoplastic valve annulus, the right ventricular dimensions and volume are usually smaller than normal and the right ventricle is heavily trabeculated. Echo-bright areas of endocardial fibroelastosis may be seen in a patchy distribution throughout the right ventricle, especially near the bases of the papillary muscles. If the right ventricular systolic pressure is suprasystemic, the ventricular septum can be seen bowing in the parasternal long-axis view into the left ventricular outflow tract in systole (Fig 9–6). In real time, the shortening fraction of the right ventricle is markedly reduced because of the high afterload. In the parasternal and suprasternal views, a patent ductus arteriosus can usually be identified. With pulsed and color-flow Doppler examinations, a continuous left-to-right shunt is present across the ductus arteriosus (see Chapter 10).

Tricuspid valve abnormalities are frequently present in infants with critical pulmonary stenosis and a small valve annulus. The tricuspid valve can be thickened and domed with fused leaflets or mildly plastered to the ventricular walls with resultant regurgitation (Ebstein-like deformity). The tricuspid valve annulus can have a normal or decreased diameter.[4] The diameter can be measured in apical or subcostal four-chamber views and compared to normal values for different body surface areas (see Chapter 3).

In infants with severe pulmonary stenosis, the elevated right atrial pressure prevents closure of the flap valve

of the foramen ovale after birth. As a result, there is a large right-to-left shunt through the wide-open foramen ovale. On the two-dimensional echocardiogram, the flap valve can be seen flicking rapidly back and forth across the atrial septum, with phasic changes in pressure between the two atria. The predominantly right-to-left atrial shunt can be detected with pulsed and color-flow Doppler techniques (Plate 27).

Assessment of the Severity of the Obstruction

Before the introduction of Doppler echocardiography, M-mode and two-dimensional echocardiography were used to assess the severity of pulmonary stenosis. For example, in patients with pulmonary valve stenosis, the M-mode echocardiogram of the pulmonary valve frequently shows a premature opening at the time of atrial contraction. This "a" wave opening is probably caused by decreased right ventricular compliance, augmented atrial systole, and a resultant right ventricular-pulmonary artery pressure gradient at the end of diastole. In one study, patients with catheterization peak-to-peak gradients greater than 50 mm Hg had "a" waves measuring on average 9.9 mm (range 6 to 18 mm), while patients with gradients less than 50 mm Hg had "a" wave depths averaging 6 mm (range 2 to 10 mm).[5] In the clinical setting, the increased "a" wave depth was neither a sensitive nor a specific indicator of severe pulmonary stenosis (increased "a" waves occur with pulmonary hypertension, Uhl's anomaly, etc.).

Right ventricular hypertrophy (measured as the right ventricular anterior wall thickness from the M-mode echocardiogram or assessed by two-dimensional echocardiography) is not a sensitive indicator of the severity of pulmonary stenosis. The right ventricular anterior wall thickness does not correlate with the pulmonary valve systolic pressure gradient. This is particularly true in patients who have had pulmonary valvotomy or balloon valvulo-

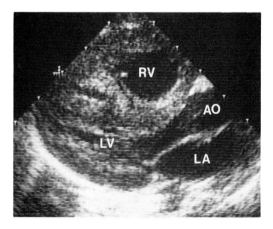

FIG 9–6.
Parasternal long-axis view from an infant with critical pulmonary valve stenosis. Because of suprasystemic pressures in the right ventricle (RV), the ventricular septum bows prominently into the left ventricle (LV). AO = aorta; LA = left atrium.

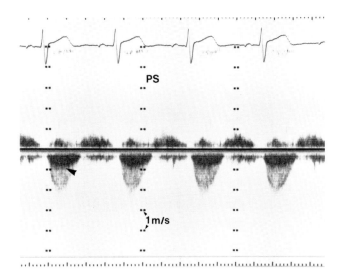

FIG 9–7.
Continuous-wave Doppler examination of the pulmonary artery of a child with pulmonary stenosis (PS). The Doppler tracing was obtained with the transducer in the second left intercostal space. For this location, the jet flow across the pulmonary valve is directed away from the transducer and is therefore displayed below the baseline in systole. The peak velocity of the systolic jet is 2 m/sec. The higher amplitude, lower velocity signals (*arrow*) from the right ventricular outflow tract proximal to the pulmonary valve are seen superimposed on the flow signals from the PS jet.

plasty. Even after successful relief of the outflow tract obstruction, regression of right ventricular hypertrophy may not occur for years, if at all.

The introduction of Doppler echocardiography provided a technique for direct quantification of the severity of the pulmonary valve stenosis. On the Doppler examination, an increased peak systolic flow velocity in the main pulmonary artery can indicate either pulmonary stenosis or increased flow (i.e., left-to-right shunt, pulmonary insufficiency). If the increased velocity is the result of increased flow, both the right ventricular outflow tract and pulmonary artery Doppler recordings will have a high velocity; if the increased velocity is the result of pulmonary valve stenosis, however, the right ventricular outflow will have a normal velocity.[6–8]

Doppler recordings of the flow velocities across the pulmonary valve are best obtained from the parasternal short-axis view, the parasternal long-axis view of the right ventricular outflow tract, and the subcostal views of the right ventricle (Fig 9–7). With the pulsed Doppler instrument, the sample volume is placed in the right ventricular outflow tract proximal to the pulmonary valve. The sample volume is then gradually moved across the valve into the main pulmonary artery. With this technique, the examiner can record the peak velocity of flow in the right ventricular outflow tract and can determine the precise level at which the increased flow velocity occurs. With pulmonary valve stenosis, a dramatic increase in peak systolic velocity occurs as the sample volume is moved into the main pul-

monary artery.[6] Multiple sample volume locations and beam angulations are attempted so that the best alignment between the Doppler ultrasound beam and the jet flow through the pulmonary valve can be obtained. In most cases of valvular pulmonary stenosis, the jet flow is directed toward the left lateral border of the main pulmonary artery or the origin of the left pulmonary artery. In the parasternal short-axis view, we have found it helpful to move the transducer an interspace lower than the standard parasternal position. From this lower position, it is possible to aim the transducer very superiorly so that the Doppler beam is better aligned with flow in the main pulmonary artery. In patients with anterior rotation of the main pulmonary artery caused by marked poststenotic dilatation, it is extremely difficult to obtain an acceptable alignment between the Doppler beam and jet flow from a parasternal short-axis location. In these patients, the best alignment between the Doppler beam and flow through the anteriorly-rotated main pulmonary artery is obtained from the subcostal four-chamber view of the right ventricle.

In each patient, the jet flow across the pulmonary valve should be recorded from every possible echocardiographic window.[9] The highest value for the peak velocity is then used to calculate the peak instantaneous pressure gradient across the pulmonary valve. If aliasing occurs on the pulsed Doppler examination, high pulse repetition frequency or continuous-wave Doppler should be used to display the peak velocities unambiguously (see Chapter 1).

The peak velocity of the jet is used in the simplified Bernoulli equation ($4V^2$) to calculate the peak gradient across the pulmonary valve.[6–11] Figure 9–8 is a pulmonary artery Doppler tracing obtained from a child with pulmonary valve stenosis. The continuous-wave Doppler recording shows the lower right ventricular outflow velocities superimposed on the high velocities of the jet. The peak systolic velocity of 4 m/sec predicts a peak gradient of 64 mm Hg (4×4^2). If the velocities proximal to the valve are greater than 1.0 m/sec, the expanded Bernoulli equation should be used to minimize errors in predicting the peak gradient (see Chapter 4). The peak velocity proximal to the valve can be recorded with the pulsed Doppler system or, in cases such as the one shown in Figure 9–7, can be measured from the continuous-wave Doppler recording of the pulmonary stenosis jet.

Using the Doppler techniques outlined in Chapter 4, the mean gradient across the pulmonary valve and the pulmonary valve area can be calculated. In the clinical setting, these measurements are seldom used because most clinicians base the decision for therapeutic intervention on the catheterization-measured peak-to-peak gradient or the severity of the symptoms.

Color-flow Doppler examination of the pulmonary valve can be performed from parasternal or subcostal transducer positions. Systolic flow in the right ventricular outflow tract and main pulmonary artery is directed away from the transducer and is therefore blue. Often, a small red flow area is seen in systole just proximal to the pulmonary valve (Plate 28). These flow signals represent an area of increased flow velocity with aliasing or color reversal. The proximal flow acceleration probably occurs because of a decrease in flow area before the valve (i.e., because of muscle hypertrophy).[12] Distal to the valve, a high-velocity mosaic jet is seen. The color Doppler examination provides a spatial display of the jet and is therefore useful for obtaining the best alignment between the pulsed or continuous-wave Doppler beam and the jet flow.

In children with valvular pulmonary stenosis, excellent correlation has been found between catheterization-measured peak-to-peak pressure gradients and Doppler-derived peak instantaneous pressure gradients across the valve.[7-11] For pulmonary valve stenosis, the discrepancy between peak instantaneous and peak-to-peak pressure gradients is far less than it is for aortic valve stenosis; hence, correlations between Doppler and catheterization estimates of the pressure gradient are exceptionally close in children with pulmonary valve stenosis. After surgical valvotomy or balloon angioplasty, correlations between the two techniques continue to be excellent.[11, 13] In the postoperative patient, pulmonary insufficiency may be signif-

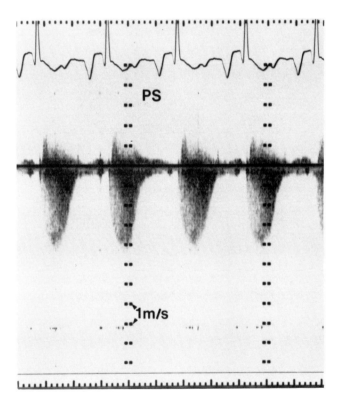

FIG 9–8.
Continuous-wave Doppler tracing from a child with severe pulmonary valve stenosis (PS). This tracing was also obtained from the second left intercostal space. The jet flow across the pulmonary valve is seen below the baseline in systole, indicating flow away from the transducer. The peak velocity of the jet is 4 m/sec. From the simplified Bernoulli equation, this predicts a peak pressure gradient across the valve of 4×4^2 or 64 mm Hg.

icant enough to increase the flow velocities proximal to the valve, in which case an expanded Bernoulli equation should be used to estimate the peak gradient. Figure 9–9 is a continuous-wave Doppler recording from a small child after surgical pulmonary valvotomy. The Doppler tracing shows an increased velocity in the pulmonary artery (peak velocity = 2.4 m/sec), as well as diastolic flow toward the transducer or pulmonary insufficiency. The increased velocity in the pulmonary artery could be the result of residual mild stenosis or increased flow across the valve (pulmonary insufficiency). The recording of a low right-ventricular outflow tract velocity superimposed on the systolic jet suggests that the increase in pulmonary artery velocity is caused by residual obstruction rather than increased flow.

In patients with severe infundibular and valvular pulmonary stenosis, the Doppler-predicted peak gradient may overestimate the catheterization-measured peak-to-peak gradient.[14-16] In serial obstructions, such as tunnel subvalvular and valvular stenosis, continuous-wave Doppler predicts the decrease in pressure to the point of the maximum gradient. This point is known as the vena contracta and is usually located just distal to the subvalvular obstruction and proximal to the valve.[16] Downstream, relaminarization and pressure recovery occur, so that the pressure drop across the valve itself is less. In fact, the maximum pressure drop predicted by the continuous-wave Doppler examination is not the sum of the pressure drops across the two obstructions. The catheter-measured pressure gradient will be lower than the true maximum gradient if the catheter is not positioned in the vena contracta at the time of the pressure recording. In the clinical setting, the catheter peak-to-peak pressure gradient is obtained by withdrawing the catheter across both areas of obstruction and determining the differences in peak systolic pressure between the right ventricle and the main pulmonary artery. This gradient will be smaller than the true maximal gradient, which is the gradient predicted by the continuous-wave Doppler technique that occurs just distal to the subvalvular obstruction and proximal to the valve.

In evaluating children with pulmonary stenosis, especially infants with critical pulmonary stenosis, it is necessary to keep in mind that the pressure gradient depends upon the flow across the valve and is therefore not always a reliable indicator of the severity of the stenosis. For example, infants with critical pulmonary stenosis may have poor right ventricular function, decreased right ventricular stroke volume, and atrial right-to-left shunting. The decreased forward flow out of the right ventricle may cause the peak systolic velocity in the pulmonary artery to be low, even in the presence of severe valvular stenosis. Similarly, if the ductus arteriosis is widely patent, pulmonary artery pressure will be elevated. In this case, the right ventricular pulmonary artery systolic pressure gradient and the peak velocity of the pulmonary stenosis jet will be low, even in the presence of severe valvular stenosis. In cases such as these, the examiner must rely on combined information derived from both the two-dimensional echocar-

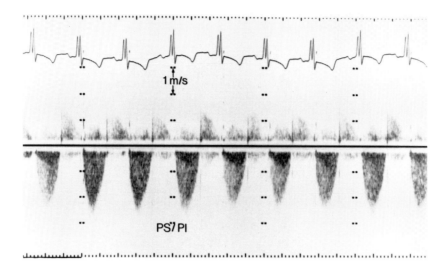

FIG 9–9.
Continuous-wave Doppler recording taken from the left parasternal region of an infant following pulmonary valvotomy. Systolic forward flow is seen away from the transducer and below the baseline. The peak velocity of the systolic jet is 2.4 m/sec, which predicts a mild residual gradient. Diastolic flow signals are also seen above the baseline, indicating diastolic flow toward the transducer or pul-monary insufficiency (PI). The increased velocity in the pulmonary artery could be the result of residual mild pulmonary stenosis (PS) or increased flow across the valve. The recording of low right ven-tricular outflow velocities superimposed on the jet suggests that the increase in pulmonary artery velocity is caused by residual obstruc-tion and not by increased flow.

diogram and the Doppler examination to assess the severity of the stenosis. The morphology of the valve leaflets, the size of the valve annulus, the thickness of the right ven-tricle, and the position of the ventricular septum are help-ful clues for this evaluation.

Subvalvular Pulmonary Stenosis

Subvalvular pulmonary stenosis includes defects in which the obstruction occurs between the right ventricle and the pulmonary conus. The pulmonary infundibulum or conus and valve are not obstructed. Two types of sub-valvular pulmonary stenosis occur: (1) discrete stenosis of the infundibular ostium and (2) double-chambered right ventricle.[1]

Stenosis of the Infundibular Ostium

Discrete subpulmonary stenosis rarely occurs as an isolated defect. The right ventricle proximal to the obstruc-tion is hypertrophic but otherwise normal. Above the pap-illary muscle of the conus, the orifice between the right ventricle and its infundibulum is severely narrowed by the presence of a fibromuscular ring at that level. The infun-dibular chamber and pulmonary valve are usually normal.[1] Some investigators have referred to this defect as a "napkin ring" deformity or a "high" type of double-chambered right ventricle.

The right ventricle, the infundibulum, and the pul-monary valve are well imaged in the subcostal four-cham-ber view of the right ventricle. In patients with discrete subpulmonary stenosis, a thick, rigid muscular collar is seen protruding into the lumen of the ventricle at the level of the infundibular ostium (Fig 9–10). The fibromuscular ring can also be visualized in the subcostal sagittal view of the right ventricle.

Doppler examination is useful for determining the pressure gradient across the obstruction, and the subcostal views provide the best alignment between the Doppler beam

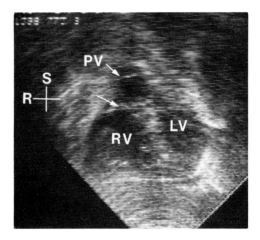

FIG 9–10.
Subcostal coronal view of the right ventricle (RV) from a child with discrete subpulmonary stenosis. A thick, rigid muscular collar (*arrow*) is seen at the level of the infundibular ostium below the pulmonary valve (PV). This type of double-chambered right ventricle has been called a napkin-ring deformity. LV = left ventricle; R = right; S = superior.

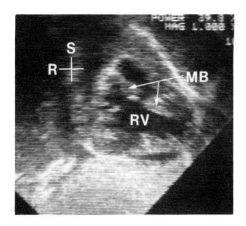

FIG 9–11.
Subcostal coronal view of the right ventricle (RV) from a patient with a double-chambered right ventricle. An anomalous muscle bundle (MB) is seen crossing the body of the RV and connecting to the apical portion of the RV. R = right; S = superior.

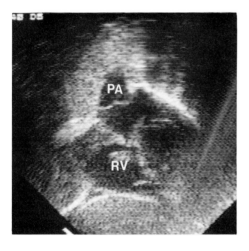

FIG 9–12.
Subcostal coronal view of the right ventricle (RV) from a child with a double-chambered right ventricle. An anomalous muscle bundle is seen crossing the midsection of the RV. PA = pulmonary artery.

and jet flow across the subvalvular stenosis. With color-flow mapping techniques, a mosaic jet can be seen originating below the pulmonary valve.

Double-Chambered Right Ventricle

In double-chambered right ventricle, an anomalous muscle bundle crosses the right ventricle perpendicular to the ventricular septum and inserts into the parietal wall of the right ventricle. Some believe that this muscle represents an abnormally hypertrophic moderator band.[1, 17] The anomalous muscle bundle may be located anywhere from the apex of the right ventricle to the conoventricular junction, although it usually does not traverse the sinus portion of the ventricle.

As with discrete subpulmonary stenosis, double-

chambered right ventricle is best evaluated by two-dimensional and Doppler echocardiographic examination from subcostal transducer positions (Figs 9–11 to 9–13).[18]

Associated cardiac anomalies are common in patients with double-chambered right ventricle. Ventricular septal defect is the most commonly associated lesion, occurring in 80% to 90% of cases (Fig 9–14).[17, 18] The ventricular septal defect is usually in the membranous septum but can be located anywhere. Frequently, an aneurysm of the membranous septum is present, with or without the ventricular septal defect. Valvular pulmonary stenosis is the second most commonly occurring defect. Other associated

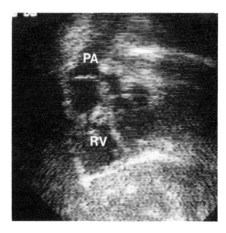

FIG 9–13.
Subcostal sagittal view of the right ventricle (RV) from the same patient as in Figure 9–12. The anomalous muscle bundle is seen traversing the midsection of the RV. PA = pulmonary artery.

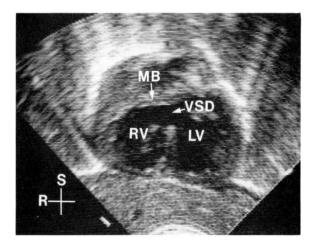

FIG 9–14.
Subcostal coronal view from a patient with a double-chambered right ventricle (RV) and a large ventricular septal defect (VSD). An anomalous muscle bundle (MB) is seen traversing the RV superior to the VSD. RV = right ventricle; R = right; S = superior.

defects include discrete subaortic membrane,[19] patent ductus arteriosus, and right aortic arch.

The severity of the stenosis can be assessed with Doppler echocardiography. If a nonimaging Doppler transducer is used, care must be taken not to mistake the systolic jet of a ventricular septal defect for that of the anomalous muscle bundle. The use of equipment such as high pulse repetition frequency Doppler or probes that perform two-dimensional imaging and continuous-wave Doppler simultaneously will help prevent this type of error.

Supravalvular Pulmonary Stenosis

Supravalvular pulmonary stenosis is distal to the pulmonary valve and may involve the main pulmonary artery, the two pulmonary artery branches, or the segmental branches. The stenosis may be a discrete membranelike stenosis or a tubular hypoplasia.[1] Most patients with supravalvular pulmonary stenosis have numerous areas of stenosis.

Main Pulmonary Artery Stenosis

Discrete fibrous diaphragm.—Several investigators have described discrete supravalvular pulmonary stenosis caused by a thick, fibrous ring or diaphragm in the main pulmonary artery just above the pulmonary valve sinuses.[20, 21] This type of stenosis has been described in children with characteristic facial features different from those of Williams syndrome.[21] Unlike children with Williams syndrome, those with a discrete supravalvular diaphragm do not have numerous associated stenoses in the pulmonary artery branches.

On the two-dimensional echocardiogram, a discrete diaphragm in the main pulmonary artery can best be visualized from the parasternal long-axis view of the right ventricle, the parasternal short-axis view, and subcostal views of the right ventricle (Fig 9–15). Pulmonary valve stenosis is frequently associated with the membrane.

The peak velocity of the jet through the discrete membrane can be recorded from parasternal, subcostal, or suprasternal notch locations.

Tubular hypoplasia of the main pulmonary artery.— Supravalvular pulmonary stenosis can occur as a long tubular hypoplasia of the main pulmonary artery segment. This defect can be seen in children with rubella syndrome and in those with Williams syndrome.

Tubular hypoplasia can be imaged from parasternal or subcostal views of the right ventricle, and Doppler estimates of the severity of the obstruction can be derived from the peak velocity of the jet flow in these views. With a very long, narrow lumen, however, the Doppler technique can underestimate the catheterization-measured pressure gradient. In this situation, the pressure drop caused by viscous friction along the flow path may be quite large; ignoring this pressure drop in the simplified Bernoulli equation can lead to underestimation of the total pressure gradient.

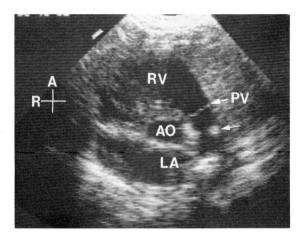

FIG 9–15.
Parasternal short-axis view from a child with supravalvular pulmonary stenosis caused by a discrete diaphragm (*arrow*) in the main pulmonary artery. A = anterior; AO = aorta; LA = left atrium; PV = pulmonary valve; R = right; RV = right ventricle.

Branch Pulmonary Artery Stenosis

Branch pulmonary artery stenosis can occur as discrete membranelike stenosis or as tubular hypoplasia or stricture. Because of the fetal circulatory patterns, the pulmonary artery branches are considerably smaller in diameter than the main pulmonary artery at birth. This normal discrepancy in size between the main and branch pulmonary arteries should not be mistaken for pathologic peripheral pulmonary stenosis. When there is uniform hypoplasia of both pulmonary artery branches, the diagnosis depends on accurate measurement of the branch pulmonary artery diameter from the two-dimensional echocardiogram and comparison of this measurement with normal values for the branch pulmonary artery diameter at various body surface areas.[22] Localized areas of branch stenosis are more easily diagnosed by two-dimensional echocardiography because they appear as discrete areas of narrowing in the pulmonary artery branch followed distally by poststenotic dilatation.

On the two-dimensional echocardiogram, the entire length of the right pulmonary artery (from its origin from the main pulmonary artery to its entry into the hilum of the right lung) is easily imaged. Longitudinal sections of the right pulmonary artery can be obtained from the parasternal short-axis view (Fig 9–16), the suprasternal short-axis view (Fig 9–17), and the subcostal four-chamber view (Fig 9–18). Cross-sectional images of the right pulmonary artery can be obtained from the suprasternal long-axis view and the subcostal sagittal view of the aortic arch. In most patients, the left pulmonary artery can be seen for only a short distance before it dives posteriorly toward the left lung. Longitudinal sections through the junction of the main and left pulmonary arteries and through a segment of the left pulmonary artery can be obtained from the su-

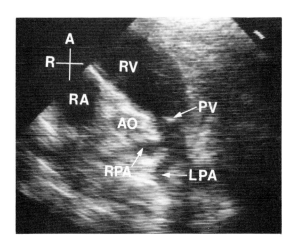

FIG 9–16.
Parasternal short-axis view from a patient with severe bilateral peripheral pulmonary artery stenosis. Both the right pulmonary artery (RPA) and the left pulmonary artery (LPA) are narrowed throughout their lengths. A = anterior; AO = aorta; PV = pulmonary valve; R = right; RA = right atrium; RV = right ventricle.

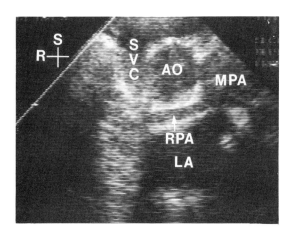

FIG 9–17.
Suprasternal short-axis view from a child who had undergone previous repair of tetralogy of Fallot. In this patient, there is a tubular hypoplasia of the entire right pulmonary artery (RPA). AO = aorta; LA = left atrium; MPA = main pulmonary artery; R = right; S = superior; SVC = superior vena cava.

prasternal long-axis view and the subcostal sagittal view of the right ventricle (Fig 9–19). In infants, long segments of both pulmonary artery branches can be visualized from a high left parasternal position (Fig 9–20). Using all of these views, it is possible to visualize areas of pulmonary artery branch stenosis in a sizeable percentage of patients.

Several two-dimensional echocardiographic findings suggest the existence of severe peripheral pulmonary artery stenosis, even when it cannot be imaged directly. Unexplained severe right ventricular hypertrophy and marked pulsatility of the proximal pulmonary artery branches

should suggest severe peripheral pulmonary artery stenosis. Exaggerated pulsatility of the proximal pulmonary arteries is caused by the continued runoff of blood into the peripheral pulmonary circulation into diastole which, in turn, causes a low pulmonary artery diastolic pressure, wide pulse pressure, and bounding pulmonary artery pulsations.

Doppler echocardiography can be useful for estimating the severity of supravalvular pulmonary stenosis. In newborns, it is common to record a slight increase in velocity as the sample volume is moved from the main pulmonary artery to the branch pulmonary artery. This is probably caused by the discrepancy in size between the main pulmonary artery and the pulmonary artery branches that exists at birth and is a normal finding (physiologic pe-

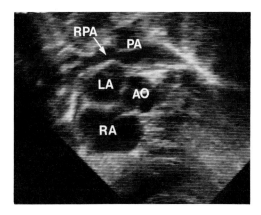

FIG 9–18.
Subcostal four-chamber view from a patient with multiple discrete areas of stenosis in the right pulmonary artery (RPA). The areas of narrowing in the RPA are followed by areas of poststenotic dilatation. AO = aorta; LA = left atrium; PA = pulmonary artery; RA = right atrium.

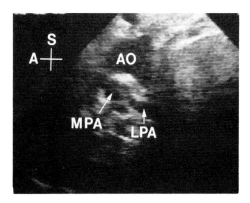

FIG 9–19.
Suprasternal long-axis view from a patient with a discrete area of stenosis at the origin of the left pulmonary artery (LPA). Beyond the area of stenosis, there is poststenotic dilatation of the LPA. A = anterior; AO = aorta; MPA = main pulmonary artery; S = superior.

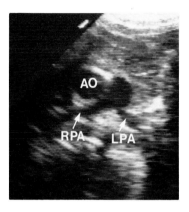

FIG 9–20.
High left parasternal view from an infant with stenosis of the origin of the left pulmonary artery (LPA). Note the poststenotic dilatation of the LPA beyond the area of stenosis. AO = aorta; RPA = right pulmonary artery.

ripheral pulmonary stenosis). In children with multiple levels of right ventricular/pulmonary artery obstruction or multiple associated obstructive lesions (i.e., supravalvular pulmonary stenosis and supravalvular aortic stenosis in children with Williams syndrome), the nonimaging Doppler probe may not be helpful in separating the various systolic jets or determining the severity of each level of obstruction. In these situations, combined imaging and Doppler probes are extremely helpful.

Often, the suprasternal notch provides the best echocardiographic window for alignment of the Doppler beam parallel with flow in the left pulmonary artery. Because of its orientation perpendicular to the aortic arch, the right pulmonary artery is difficult to interrogate from any of the echocardiographic views. With severe obstruction in a peripheral artery, the jet peaks in systole but extends into diastole because of a persistent pressure gradient into diastole (Fig 9–21).

With color-flow Doppler mapping techniques, peripheral pulmonary artery stenosis causes a mosaic, high-velocity jet directed away from the transducer (Plate 29). In this regard, the color Doppler examination is very useful for detecting mild degrees of supravalvular stenosis that cannot be clearly visualized by two-dimensional echocardiography. The color Doppler examination is also helpful for obtaining the best alignment of the single crystal Doppler beam with the jet flow. With very severe peripheral pulmonary artery stenosis, backflow of blood from the branch pulmonary artery to the main pulmonary artery can be seen in diastole on the color Doppler examination (Plate 30). The diastolic backflow of blood should not be mistaken for flow through a patent ductus arteriosus. The diastolic backflow usually is a low-velocity, laminar flow and produces a pure red color on the Doppler examination; the diastolic flow through a patent ductus arteriosus, however, is usually higher velocity, disturbed flow which produces a multilayered, multicolored jet on the velocity/variance display.

Pulmonary Insufficiency

Pulmonary insufficiency occurs in a large percentage of children with congenital heart disease (i.e., valvular pulmonary stenosis, pulmonary artery hypertension) and is a frequent finding following surgical procedures to relieve right ventricular outflow obstruction (i.e., repair of tetralogy of Fallot, pulmonary valvotomy). In addition, Doppler evidence of physiologic amounts of pulmonary insufficiency is present in large percentages of normal children, as high as 92% in some studies.[23, 24] Isolated pulmonary insufficiency, however, is rare, although it has been reported to occur in children with idiopathic dilatation of the main pulmonary artery, pulmonary valve prolapse (usually as part of a generalized connective tissue disorder), and myxomatous degeneration of the pulmonary valve (usually as part of a syndrome of multivalvular disease).

In patients with a significant amount of pulmonary insufficiency, the M-mode and two-dimensional echocardiograms show evidence of right ventricular volume overload (dilated right ventricle with vigorous ejection, paradoxical septal motion). In the parasternal long-axis view, the dilated right ventricular outflow tract can be seen rocking vigorously back and forth. With very severe pulmonary insufficiency and a large runoff of blood in diastole from the pulmonary artery to the right ventricle, the pulmonary artery diastolic pressure is lower, the pulse pressure is wider, and vigorous pulsations of the main

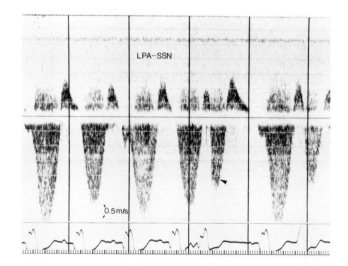

FIG 9–21.
Continuous-wave Doppler recording from the suprasternal notch (SSN) of a child with previous repair of tetralogy of Fallot. With the Doppler transducer aimed leftward and posterior, a systolic jet was recorded in the left pulmonary artery (LPA), indicating stenosis of the LPA. Note that the jet peaks in systole but extends into diastole because of a persistent pressure gradient into diastole. This flow pattern is characteristic of severe obstruction in a peripheral artery. This figure also demonstrates the effect of an ectopic beat (*arrow*) on the Doppler peak velocities. The peak velocity of the early ectopic beat is decreased due to decreased ventricular filling, and the peak velocity of the postectopic beat is increased as a result of increased ventricular stroke volume.

pulmonary artery and its branches are seen on the two-dimensional echocardiogram (especially in the suprasternal long-axis view).

In patients with pulmonary insufficiency, the Doppler examination of the right ventricular outflow tract from the parasternal short-axis view shows normal forward flow in systole below the baseline (away from the transducer) and reverse flow in diastole above the baseline (toward the transducer) (Fig 9–22). The pulsed Doppler can be used to map the extension of the regurgitant jet into the right ventricle and thus obtain an estimate of the severity of the pulmonary insufficiency (see Chapter 4). In some patients, reverse flow can be recorded in the main pulmonary artery as well as proximal to the pulmonary valve (Fig 9–23). The finding of a reverse diastolic flow pattern in the main pulmonary artery usually indicates a more severe degree of pulmonary insufficiency. Thus, an estimation of the severity of the pulmonary insufficiency is made based on the extension of the regurgitant jet into the right ventricle, the intensity of the diastolic signals, and the detection of reverse diastolic flow in the main pulmonary artery.

In most cases, the peak velocity of a pulmonary insufficiency jet is lower than the peak velocity of an aortic insufficiency jet because the pulmonary artery-right ventricular diastolic pressure difference is usually less than the aorta-left ventricular diastolic pressure difference. The exceptions to this finding are patients with pulmonary hypertension in whom large pressure differences can occur between the pulmonary artery and the right ventricle in diastole. In these patients, the peak velocity of the regurgitant jet is very high. In most patients with pulmonary insufficiency, the regurgitant velocities peak early in diastole and decrease rapidly throughout diastole as the pulmonary artery-right ventricular pressure difference decreases. In fact, if the pulmonary artery diastolic pressure is low, the regurgitant signals return to the baseline before the end of diastole, indicating an equalization of right ventricular and pulmonary artery pressures before end-diastole (see Fig 9–22). The finding of a high-velocity regurgitant signal at end-diastole suggests a large difference between the pulmonary artery diastolic pressure and right ventricular end-diastolic pressure, as is found in pulmonary hypertension. To avoid false-positive diagnoses, the regurgitant diastolic flow signals should occupy more than 50% of diastole before the diagnosis of pulmonary insufficiency is made.[25, 26]

On the Doppler color-flow mapping examination (from parasternal or subcostal views), normal systolic flow out the right ventricle is displayed as a blue flow area. Pulmonary insufficiency is seen as a red flow area (flow toward the transducer) in diastole (Plates 31 and 32). Methods for quantification of the amount of regurgitation from the color-flow mapping examination are discussed in Chapter 4.

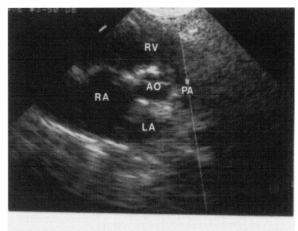
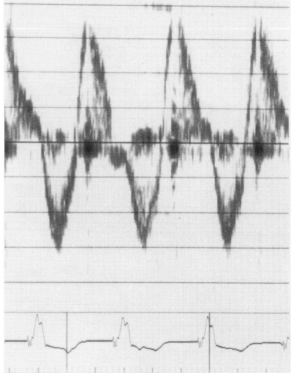

FIG 9–22.
Pulsed Doppler recording (*bottom*) from the parasternal short-axis view (*top*) of a patient with pulmonary insufficiency. At the time of the Doppler recording, the Doppler sample volume was proximal to the pulmonary valve rather than distal to the valve, as is shown on the still frame. The Doppler signals above the baseline in diastole represent flow toward the transducer from the pulmonary artery (PA) to the right ventricle (RV) in diastole (pulmonary insufficiency). The pulmonary insufficiency signals return to the baseline at the end of diastole, indicating normal RV end-diastolic pressure, low PA diastolic pressure, and mild PI. AO = aorta; LA = left atrium; RA = right atrium.

ABNORMALITIES OF THE LEFT VENTRICULAR OUTFLOW

Valvular Aortic Stenosis

Aortic valvular stenosis is a common form of congenital heart disease that can occur as an isolated defect or in combination with multiple left-sided obstructive lesions (see the section on subvalvular aortic stenosis). Aortic valvular stenosis is caused by cusp deformities, either with or without narrowing of the aortic valve fibrous annulus. The anatomic types of aortic valvular stenosis include unicuspid, bicuspid, tricuspid, quadricuspid, and undifferentiated aortic valves.[1]

Two-Dimensional Echocardiographic Features

Number and morphology of the aortic valve cusps.— The number and morphology of the aortic valve cusps is best determined from the parasternal short-axis view at the base of the heart. In cross-section, the commissures of the normal aortic valve form a Y-shaped pattern in diastole. In systole, the normal aortic valve leaflets open all the way to the valve annulus and thus create a wide-open circular orifice. In congenitally stenotic aortic valves, fused commissures or shallow ridges called raphae, representing abortive commissures are often present. When the abnormal aortic valve is in the closed position, these ridges re-

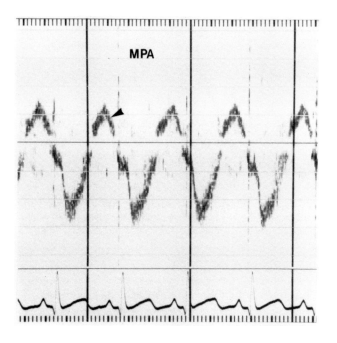

FIG 9–23.
Postoperative recording from the main pulmonary artery (MPA) of a patient with pulmonary insufficiency. There is normal forward flow in systole away from the transducer and below the baseline. The Doppler signals recorded above the baseline (*arrow*) indicate reverse flow in the pulmonary artery toward the right ventricle in diastole. The finding of a reverse diastolic flow pattern in the MPA usually indicates a severe degree of pulmonary insufficiency.

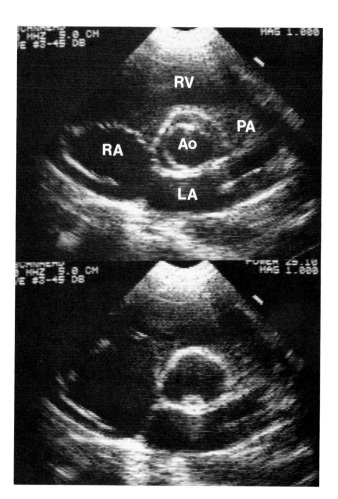

FIG 9–24.
Parasternal short-axis view in systole (*above*) and diastole (*below*) from a patient with a unicuspid aortic valve and aortic valve stenosis. When the unicuspid valve opens in systole, the orifice appears circular. In diastole, no raphae can be seen; instead, an eccentrically located valve closure is present. Ao = aorta; LA = left atrium; PA = pulmonary artery; RA = right atrium; RV = right ventricle.

flect ultrasound and have the appearance of a normal commissure. The echo-bright line that arises from a raphe can only be distinguished from a true commissure when the valve opens in systole. If the echo-bright line is a true commissure, the valve leaflets will separate along this line as they open back to the valve annulus. Thus, to determine the number of valve cusps, the movement of the aortic valve leaflets from diastole to systole should be carefully examined, preferably in a slow-motion playback mode.

In cross-sectional views, the unicuspid aortic valve has a single, slitlike commissure. One or two raphae representing abortive commissures may be present. When the unicuspid valve opens in systole, the orifice frequently appears circular or oval and is located eccentrically in the valve annulus (Fig 9–24). Most children with severe or critical aortic stenosis requiring intervention in the first year of life have a unicuspid aortic valve.

Congenital bicuspid aortic valve occurs in about 2%

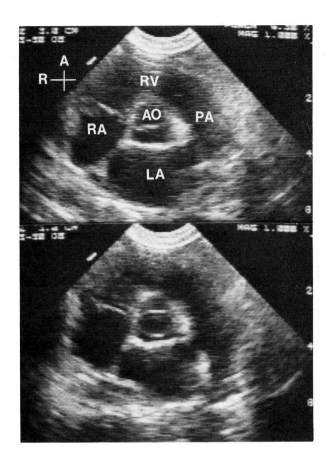

FIG 9–25.
Parasternal short-axis views in diastole (*above*) and systole (*below*) from a child with a bicuspid aortic valve. In this patient, the two cusps are equal in size and the single diastolic closure line is located in the center of the aorta (AO). In systole, the valve has a fish-mouth shape. A = anterior; LA = left atrium; PA = pulmonary artery; R = right; RA = right atrium; RV = right ventricle.

aortic wall in diastole. Thus, normal patients with a central aortic closure line had indexes of 1.0 to 1.25; an index of 1.3 or greater was interpreted as a bicuspid aortic valve.[27, 29] The use of this index in the clinical setting led to many false-positive and false-negative diagnoses. The reason for these diagnostic failures was readily apparent with the introduction of two-dimensional echocardiography.[28] As is apparent from Figures 9–25 to 9–28, nearly any value for the eccentricity index can be obtained, depending on the angle between the M-mode echocardiographic beam and the diastolic closure line. For this reason, the eccentricity index is no longer used in most laboratories.

The congenitally stenotic tricuspid aortic valve has three aortic cusps. In some instances, the cusps are incompletely developed lumps of fibrous tissue.[1] The edges of the cusps are rolled and gnarled, and there are varying degrees of commissural fusion. This type of valve morphology tends to occur with a narrowed aortic annulus and tends to cause symptoms in the newborn period. In other instances, three well-developed aortic cusps with very thickened edges are present. The thickening of the edges of the valve leaflets makes the diastolic Y pattern easier to visualize in the parasternal short-axis view (Fig 9–29). In systole, a distinct, restrictive triangular valve orifice is seen.

Congenitally quadricuspid aortic valves are extremely rare. These valves usually have three normal-sized cusps and one small accessory cusp.[30] In the parasternal short-axis view, four diastolic closure lines are present.[31]

In some newborn infants with critical aortic stenosis, the aortic valve cusps are not differentiated. Instead, a fibrous diaphragm or an immobile lump of tissue occupies the position of the normal valve leaflets. In the parasternal long- or short-axis views, it is usually not possible to discern individual valve leaflets or a clear valve orifice.

of the population.[27] In the parasternal short-axis view, the two cusps are usually equal or nearly equal in size (Fig 9–25); in rare cases, however, there is one large and one small cusp (Fig 9–26). In diastole, a raphe may or may not be present. When a raphe is not present, the valve has a single closure line in diastole. In the parasternal short-axis view, the closure line can be oriented directly anteroposteriorly, directly right to left, or in any rotation in between (Fig 9–27).[28] When a raphe is present, the valve appears to have three distinct closure lines in diastole (Fig 9–28). In systole, however, the valve cusps separate only along two of the closure lines and the valve orifice has a fish-mouth shape (much like the shape of the normal mitral valve orifice).

Before the advent of two-dimensional echocardiography, one of the criteria for diagnosis of a bicuspid aortic valve on M-mode echocardiography was eccentricity of the diastolic closure line in the aortic root. One index of eccentricity, the eccentricity index, was measured as one-half the aortic root diameter in diastole divided by the smallest distance between the cusp echo and the nearest

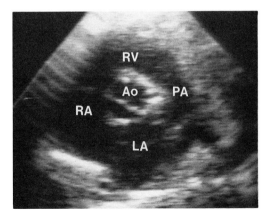

FIG 9–26.
Parasternal short-axis view from a patient with a bicuspid aortic valve. In this patient, the cusps are not of equal size and the single diastolic closure line is located eccentrically in the aortic root. AO = aorta; LA = left atrium; PA = pulmonary artery; RA = right atrium; RV = right ventricle.

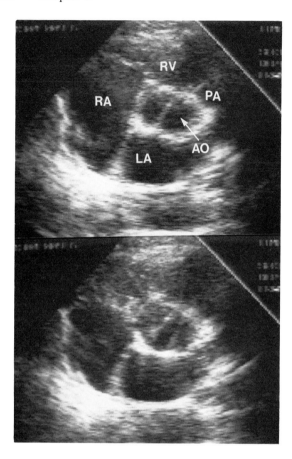

FIG 9–27.
Parasternal short-axis views in diastole (*above*) and systole (*below*) from a patient with a bicuspid aortic valve. In this patient, the diastolic closure line is oriented in a more vertical direction in the aortic (AO) root than in the patient in Figure 9–25. In systole, the valve has a fish-mouth shape as it opens. LA = left atrium; PA = pulmonary artery; RA = right atrium; RV = right ventricle.

Hemodynamic effects.—In real time, the normal aortic valve leaflets are thin structures with rapid, unrestricted mobility. In aortic valvular stenosis, the aortic valve cusps are thickened and restricted in lateral mobility.[32] This diminished cusp separation creates the appearance of a valve that is dome-shaped in systole (Fig 9–30).[32, 33] The parasternal and apical long-axis views and the subcostal views of the left ventricular outflow tract are particularly useful for evaluating aortic valve motion. The size of the aortic valve annulus can also be assessed in these views.

The jet through the stenotic aortic valve orifice may create poststenotic dilatation of the ascending aorta. This dilatation usually occurs along the right lateral or anterior borders of the ascending aorta and can be well visualized in the parasternal long-axis view, the suprasternal long- or short-axis views, or the subcostal long- or short-axis views of the left ventricle (Figs 9–31 and 9–32). The location of the poststenotic dilatation provides a valuable clue about the direction of the aortic stenosis jet and thus the best

echocardiographic view for performing the Doppler examination.

Patients with moderate-to-severe aortic valvular stenosis usually develop concentric left ventricular hypertrophy that can be detected on the M-mode and two-dimensional echocardiogram. The thickness of the left ventricular posterior wall, however, does not correlate well with the aortic valve peak-to-peak gradient measured at cardiac catheterization. This is particularly true in post-operative patients in whom left ventricular hypertrophy may persist for years, even after successful relief of the outflow gradient. In patients with left ventricular hypertrophy, left atrial enlargement may occur and usually is an early sign of decreased left ventricular compliance.

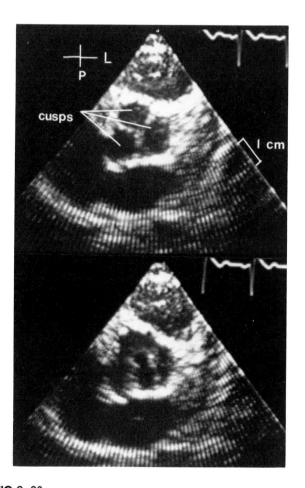

FIG 9–28.
Parasternal short-axis views in diastole (*above*) and systole (*below*) from a patient with a bicuspid aortic valve and a fused raphe. When the valve is closed in diastole, the valve appears to have three distinct closure lines and three distinct cusps. However, when the valve opens in systole, the valve cusps separate only along two of the closure lines and the valve orifice has a fish-mouth shape. LT = left; P = posterior. (From Silverman NH, Snider AR: *Two-Dimensional Echocardiography In Congenital Heart Disease.* Norwalk, Appleton-Century-Crofts, 1982, p 103. Used by permission.)

mobile and a clear systolic opening cannot be visualized. The annulus is usually 5 to 8 mm in diameter. Second, there is usually poststenotic dilatation of the ascending aorta. Third, the left ventricle is thickened and has a cross-sectional area in the parasternal long-axis view of 1.7 cm² or greater (this is the normal-term newborn value compatible with perinatal survival).[37, 38] Often, dense echoes arising from areas of endocardial fibroelastosis can be seen in the bases of the papillary muscles or throughout the endocardium (Fig 9–33). In some infants, the left ventricular shortening fraction is depressed and the ventricle is dilated (Fig 9–34). In others, the shortening fraction is normal. Fourth, because of redirection of fetal flow patterns in utero, the right ventricle and main pulmonary artery are enlarged. The ventricular septum may even be pushed into the left ventricle, giving it a somewhat crescent shape in cross-section.[36, 37] Finally, Doppler echocardiography shows evidence of disturbed systolic flow in the ascending aorta.

In infants with valvular aortic stenosis and a dilated, poorly contractile left ventricle, the distinction between

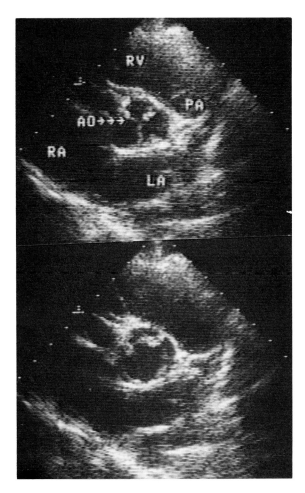

FIG 9–29.
Parasternal short-axis views in diastole (*top*) and systole (*bottom*) from a patient with aortic stenosis and a tricuspid aortic (AO) valve. In diastole, three distinct valve closure lines are seen. In systole, the valve has a triangular shape as it opens. LA = left atrium; RA = right atrium; RV = right ventricle.

Two-dimensional echocardiography in critical aortic stenosis.—Aortic valvular stenosis that causes symptoms in the neonatal period is usually hemodynamically severe, and infants with this defect are critically ill. Two-dimensional and Doppler echocardiography provide a technique for the rapid, noninvasive diagnosis of the anatomic type of obstruction and its severity. In many instances, the non-invasive techniques have replaced diagnostic cardiac catheterization prior to surgical therapy in these very sick newborns.[34, 35] This approach has been especially useful in the care of infants with severe left ventricular obstruction in whom dye injections at the time of cardiac catheterization may be poorly tolerated because of low systemic output and poor renal perfusion.

Several two-dimensional echocardiographic features are especially useful in the diagnosis of critical aortic valvular stenosis.[36, 37] First, the aortic valve leaflets are usually thickened and domed. In many cases, the leaflets are im-

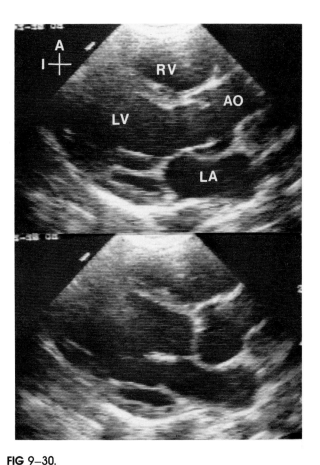

FIG 9–30.
Parasternal long-axis views in systole (*top*) and diastole (*bottom*) from a patient with a bicuspid aortic valve and aortic stenosis. The diminished cusp separation creates the appearance of a valve that is dome-shaped in systole. In diastole, the valve closure is eccentrically located in the aortic (AO) root. A = anterior; I = inferior; LA = left atrium; LV = left ventricle; RV = right ventricle.

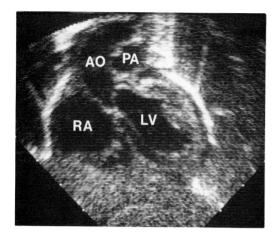

FIG 9–31.
Subcostal four-chamber view of the left ventricular (LV) outflow tract in a patient with aortic valve stenosis. The aortic valve is domed and there is marked poststenotic dilatation of the ascending aorta (AO). PA = pulmonary artery; RA = right atrium.

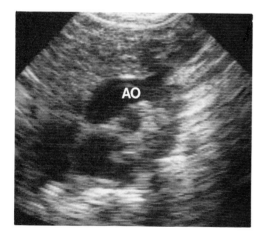

FIG 9–32.
Suprasternal long-axis view from a patient with aortic valvular stenosis and marked poststenotic dilatation of the ascending aorta (AO).

aortic stenosis and cardiomyopathy may not be readily apparent. Usually, infants with cardiomyopathy have a normal aortic valve, no poststenotic dilatation, and no systolic flow disturbance in the ascending aorta.

In infants with severe aortic stenosis, dilatation of the right ventricle may give the hypertrophic left ventricle the appearance of being small or even hypoplastic. Difficulty may then arise in distinguishing aortic stenosis from a hypoplastic left ventricle. Usually, infants with critical aortic stenosis have a left ventricular cross-sectional area of ≥ 1.7 cm^2 in the parasternal long-axis view and an aortic annulus of 5 mm or more.[38] In the presence of severe right ventricular dilatation, the shape of the left ventricle may

be useful. In critical aortic stenosis, the left ventricle is ellipsoid and extends to the cardiac apex in the four-chamber views. The hypoplastic left ventricle is a muscle-bound, globular chamber that usually does not extend to the cardiac apex.[37]

Doppler Echocardiographic Features

Direct quantitative assessment of the severity of aortic valvular stenosis can be obtained using Doppler echocardiography. On the Doppler examination, an increased peak systolic flow velocity in the ascending aorta can indicate either aortic stenosis or increased flow (i.e., aortic insufficiency). If the increased velocity is caused by increased flow, the left ventricular outflow tract and ascending aorta will both have a high velocity. On the other hand, if the increased velocity is the result of aortic valvular stenosis, then the left ventricular outflow tract will have a normal velocity.

Doppler recordings of flow velocities across the aortic valve are best obtained from the apical, suprasternal, and high right parasternal locations. With pulsed Doppler echocardiography, the sample volume is placed in the outflow tract proximal to the aortic valve and then gradually moved across the valve into the ascending aorta. This technique allows the examiner to record the peak velocity in the left ventricular outflow tract and to determine the precise level at which the increased flow velocity occurred. With valvular aortic stenosis, a dramatic increase in peak velocity usually occurs as the sample volume is moved into the ascending aorta.[6] In practice, Doppler recordings are made from multiple echocardiographic windows to find the highest value for the peak velocity of the aortic jet. In children, either continuous-wave or high pulse repetition

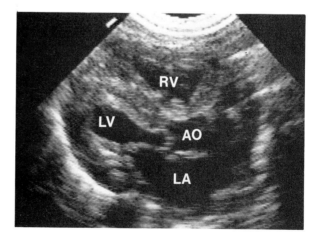

FIG 9–33.
Parasternal long-axis view from an infant with critical aortic valvular stenosis. The aortic valve annulus is small and the valve leaflets are thickened and domed. A clear systolic opening cannot be visualized. The left ventricular (LV) cavity is small and smooth-walled. The LV is markedly hypertrophied; the echo-bright areas throughout the endocardium represent endocardial fibroelastosis. AO = aorta; LA = left atrium; RV = right ventricle.

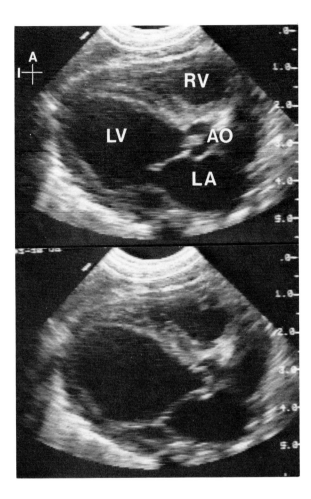

FIG 9–34.
Parasternal long-axis views in diastole (*top*) and systole (*bottom*) from a newborn with critical aortic valvular stenosis. In this patient as well, the aortic valve leaflets are thickened and domed and a clear systolic opening cannot be seen. The left ventricle (LV) is markedly dilated and has a diminished shortening fraction. A = anterior; I = inferior; LA = left atrium; RV = right ventricle.

frequency Doppler can be used to record the high-velocity jet, and the findings are nearly identical regardless of which Doppler technology is used (Figs 9–35 to 9–37).

The location of the poststenotic dilatation may provide an important clue about which echocardiographic window is the best to use. For example, a marked enlargement of the right lateral border of the ascending aorta suggests that the best alignment with the jet would be obtained from the high right parasternal window. For the high right parasternal Doppler examination, the patient is placed in a steep right lateral decubitus position. The transducer is positioned in the second or third right intercostal space as close to the sternal border as possible, and the ultrasound beam is aimed toward the cardiac apex. The absence of poststenotic dilatation suggests that the suprasternal notch or apical windows should be used. For the suprasternal notch examination, the patient lies with his or her neck hyperextended. The transducer is placed in the supraster-

nal notch and angled anteriorly and somewhat rightward. The aortic stenosis jet is usually recorded at the same anterior level as the flow in the superior vena cava.

Once the highest value for the peak velocity is found and a clear recording of the entire Doppler envelope throughout systole is made, several different indicators of the severity of the stenosis can be calculated. The techniques for calculating these indexes are discussed in detail in Chapter 4.

Peak instantaneous pressure gradient.—Using the simplified Bernoulli equation, the peak instantaneous pressure gradient across the stenotic aortic valve can be estimated from Doppler recordings of the peak velocity of the aortic jet.[6, 39–48] Figure 9–36 was recorded from the ascending aorta of a 10-year-old male with a bicuspid aortic valve. The continuous-wave Doppler recording obtained from the right parasternal region shows a peak velocity of 4 m/sec. This predicts a peak instantaneous pressure gradient of 4×4^2 or 64 mm Hg across the aortic valve. If the peak velocity proximal to the valve is greater than 1.0 m/sec, the expanded Bernoulli equation should be used to minimize errors in predicting the peak gradient (see Chapter 4). The peak velocity proximal to the valve can be recorded with the pulsed Doppler instrument or, in some cases, can be measured from the continuous-wave Doppler recording of the aortic stenotic jet.

In children with aortic valvular stenosis, the peak-to-peak pressure gradient measured at cardiac catheterization is often used to determine the severity of the stenosis and the need for intervention. Currently, the most widely used noninvasive technique for estimating the severity of aortic

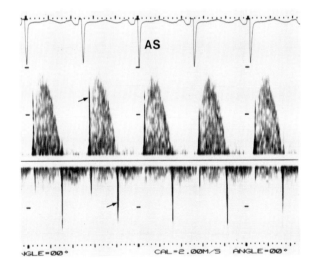

FIG 9–35.
Continuous-wave Doppler recording from the suprasternal notch of a patient with aortic stenosis (AS). A high-velocity jet is seen in systole directed toward the transducer (above the baseline). The peak velocity of the jet is approximately 3.8 m/sec. *Arrows* indicate signals arising from the valve leaflets as they open and close and pass through the area of the Doppler ultrasound beam.

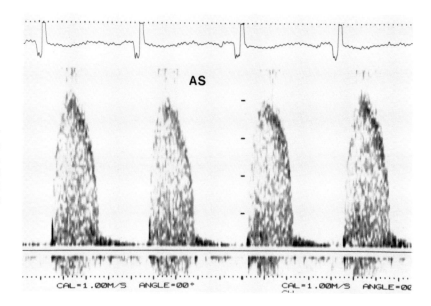

FIG 9–36.
Continuous-wave Doppler recording from the right parasternal region of a child with aortic stenosis (AS). A high-velocity jet is seen in systole above the baseline (flow toward the transducer). The peak velocity of the jet is 4 m/sec, which predicts a peak instantaneous pressure gradient of 64 mm Hg across the aortic valve.

stenosis is measurement of the peak instantaneous pressure gradient with Doppler echocardiography. In some children, the Doppler-derived peak instantaneous pressure gradient correlates well with the catheterization-measured peak-to-peak pressure gradient;[39–41] however, the correlation between the two measurements is not nearly as close as it is in the case of valvular pulmonary stenosis. In other children, especially those with mild-to-moderate degrees of obstruction, the Doppler-derived peak instantaneous pressure gradient does not correlate well with the catheterization-measured peak-to-peak pressure gradient,[42–44] and differences between the two pressure gradients can be as high as 30 mm Hg (the Doppler peak gradient is almost always higher). The reasons for this discrepancy are discussed in detail in Chapter 4. When simultaneous Doppler and cardiac catheterization studies are performed, the Doppler-predicted peak instantaneous pressure gradient correlates closely with that measured at cardiac catheterization.[44, 48] However, the peak instantaneous pressure gradient is not routinely measured at cardiac catheterization as an indicator of the need for intervention; therefore, the clinician has no suitable reference standard to which the Doppler peak instantaneous pressure gradient can be compared.

Another limitation of the use of the peak gradient to predict the severity of aortic stenosis is that this pressure gradient is affected by the amount of transvalvular flow. Therefore, in children with critical aortic stenosis, left ventricular dysfunction, and low cardiac output, a low peak velocity may be present in the ascending aorta, even in the presence of severe stenosis. Conversely, a high peak velocity can be detected in the ascending aorta in children with mild aortic stenosis and increased flow across the valve (i.e., associated aortic insufficiency).

The Doppler peak instantaneous pressure gradient can be used to assess the adequacy of surgical valvotomy or balloon angioplasty. Some investigators have reported poorer correlations between the Doppler peak gradient and the catheterization gradient in the first 48 hours after balloon valvuloplasty, presumably because of the physiologic instability that occurs during this time period.[49] Beyond 48 hours, the correlations improve considerably. In the postoperative patient, aortic insufficiency may be significant enough to increase the flow velocities proximal to the valve, in which case an expanded Bernoulli equation should be used to predict the peak gradient.

Mean pressure gradient.—The Doppler mean gradient is another noninvasive estimate of the severity of aortic stenosis which has proven useful in the evaluation of adult patients with aortic stenosis.[43–47, 49] The Doppler-predicted mean pressure gradient is directly comparable to the mean pressure gradient measured at cardiac catheterization;[45–47] in pediatric patients, however, little information is available relating either the Doppler or the catheterization mean pressure gradient to the severity of stenosis and the need for intervention. The mean gradient across the aortic valve can be calculated using the techniques outlined in Chapter 4 and illustrated in Figure 9–38. In a group of children with aortic valve stenosis, we found that all children with a Doppler mean gradient >27 mm Hg had a catheterization peak-to-peak pressure gradient of ≥75 mm Hg and therefore required intervention.[50] All children with a Doppler mean gradient < 17 mm Hg had a catheterization peak-to-peak pressure gradient <50 mm Hg and did not require intervention. Children with Doppler mean gradients ≥17 and ≤27 mm Hg comprised an intermediate group, with peak-to-peak pressure gradients ≥50 and <75 mm Hg. In this group, Doppler mean gradient alone was not sufficient information to predict which child would need intervention; however, the presence of symptoms or an abnormal exercise test provided the additional information necessary for an accurate noninvasive assessment of the severity of the aortic stenosis (Fig 9–39).

In children with aortic stenosis, we found that a Doppler mean gradient >27 mm Hg or ≥17 and ≤27 mm Hg in the presence of symptoms or an abnormal exercise treadmill test predicted the need for intervention with 92% sensitivity and 82% specificity (Fig 9–40).

The Doppler mean gradient provides an additional important noninvasive measurement of the severity of aortic valve stenosis in pediatric patients. The Doppler mean pressure gradient has several advantages over the Doppler peak instantaneous pressure gradient as a noninvasive indicator of the hemodynamic severity of the obstruction. First, the Doppler mean gradient is directly comparable to the catheterization mean pressure gradient. No such catheterization reference standard exists for the Doppler peak instantaneous pressure gradient. Second, the Doppler mean

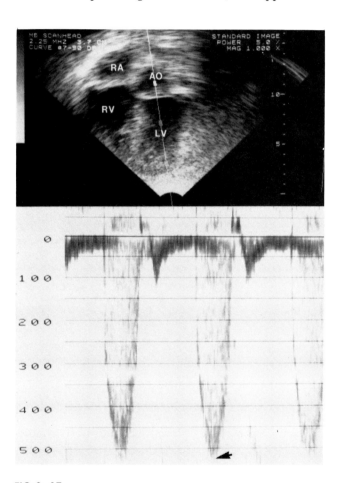

FIG 9–37.
Pulsed Doppler recording of the ascending aorta (AO) from the apical four-chamber view of a child with severe aortic valve stenosis. The freeze-frame image, *top*, shows the location of the sample volume during the Doppler recording. The Doppler tracing, *bottom*, shows a high-velocity jet in systole below the baseline, indicating flow away from the transducer across the aortic valve. The peak velocity of the jet (*arrow*) is 5.5 m/sec, which predicts a peak pressure gradient of 120 mm Hg across the aortic valve. LV = left ventricle; RA = right atrium; RV = right ventricle. (From Snider AR: *Clin Perinatol* 1988; 15:537. Used by permission.)

gradient is the average of all the instantaneous gradients throughout systole and is therefore not so dependent on a clear recording of the peak velocity. Doppler peak instantaneous pressure gradient is solely dependent on an accurate recording of the peak systolic velocity and is more sensitive to small measurement errors. Last, the mean transvalvular pressure gradient is the basis for calculation of valve area using the Gorlin equation. Thus, for a normal stroke volume and heart rate, the Doppler mean pressure gradient has a more direct relationship to aortic valve area than the Doppler peak instantaneous pressure gradient.

Aortic valve area.—Both the Doppler mean and peak pressure gradients are dependent on transvalvular flow and are not as reliable as the aortic valve area in indicating the severity of the aortic stenosis. Aortic valve area can be calculated from the Doppler examination using either the Gorlin equation or the continuity equation as outlined in Chapter 4. In children with isolated aortic valve stenosis, excellent correlation has been found between the Doppler and the catheterization techniques using the Gorlin formula.[51] Several recent studies have shown excellent correlation between aortic valve area calculated by Doppler using the continuity equation and that calculated at cardiac catheterization in adult patients.[47, 52–56] Similar studies to validate the accuracy of the continuity equation in small children with aortic stenosis have not yet been performed. Noninvasive estimate of aortic valve area may prove to be an excellent technique for assessing the severity of aortic stenosis in children; however, a prospective study of a large number of patients is necessary to validate the use of this Doppler technique in children and to establish the significance of a given Doppler-computed valve area in regard to prognosis and treatment.

Systolic time intervals.—Another indicator of the severity of the aortic stenosis is the time to the peak velocity. In aortic stenosis, the time from aortic valve opening to the peak velocity of the jet is delayed (Fig 9–41).[6, 39, 41] Hatle and co-workers found that the ratio of the time to peak velocity of the jet [acceleration time (AT)] divided by the left ventricular ejection time (LVET) was useful in assessing the severity of the obstruction.[39] In normal patients, the AT/LVET ratio was less than 0.30. For AT/LVET ratio greater than 0.30, the pressure gradient was greater than 50 mm Hg. With a ratio of 0.55 or more, obstruction severe enough to indicate surgical intervention is usually present. When using this ratio to assess the severity of the aortic stenosis, it is necessary to be aware that severe mitral regurgitation or left ventricular failure can prolong the ratio by shortening the left ventricular ejection time. Similarly, associated aortic regurgitation can shorten the AT/LVET ratio by increasing the left ventricular ejection time.

Color-flow Doppler examination.—Color-flow Doppler examination of the aortic valve can be performed from parasternal, apical, subcostal, or suprasternal notch locations. A high-velocity, mosaic jet can be seen on the ve-

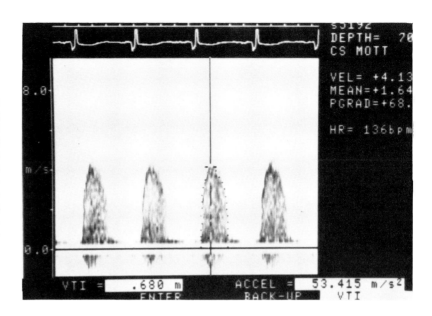

FIG 9–38.
Doppler spectral tracing illustrating the technique used to obtain the mean pressure gradient. Using a digitizing system and an on-line computer, the outer margin of the Doppler spectral recording is traced throughout systole. The computer measures the peak velocity and calculates the instantaneous peak pressure gradient every two to three milliseconds. The mean gradient is obtained by averaging all the peak instantaneous gradients throughout systole. The mean gradient is not obtained by substituting the mean velocity in the Bernoulli equation.

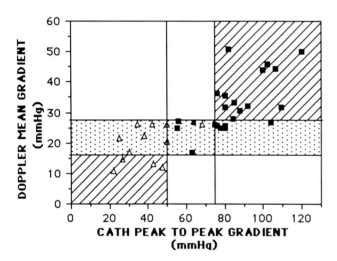

FIG 9–39.
Graphic comparison of the Doppler-derived mean pressure gradient and the peak-to-peak pressure gradient measured at catheterization in 36 children with aortic valve stenosis. All children with a Doppler mean gradient >27 mm Hg (represented in the box with diagonal lines at the upper right corner of the graph) had a catheterization peak-to-peak pressure gradient of ≥75 mm Hg and required intervention. All children with a Doppler mean gradient <17 mm Hg (represented in the box with diagonal lines at the lower left corner) had a catheterization peak-to-peak gradient <50 mm Hg and did not require intervention. Children with Doppler mean gradients ≥17 and ≤27 mm Hg comprised an intermediate group with peak-to-peak pressure gradients ≥50 and <75 mm Hg. In this group (represented by the dotted area on the graph), Doppler mean gradient alone was not sufficient information to predict which child would need intervention.

locity/variance map in systole (Plate 33). Just proximal to the valve, there is usually a small area of color reversal that represents aliasing caused by acceleration of flow proximal to the stenotic valve. The proximal flow acceleration occurs because of a decrease in flow area before the valve (i.e., as a result of muscle hypertrophy).[12] The spatial display of the jet on the color Doppler examination can be used to align the pulsed or continuous-wave Doppler beam and the jet flow.

Subvalvular Aortic Stenosis

Subvalvular aortic stenosis accounts for 10% to 20% of all forms of left ventricular outflow obstruction. Three types of subvalvular aortic stenosis have been described. In the discrete membranous type, a thin fibrous diaphragm encircles the left ventricular outflow tract. The membrane can be located a few millimeters below the aortic valve and, in this location, has attachments to the base of the anterior mitral valve leaflet and to the ventricular septum just below the right aortic cusp. Alternatively, the membrane can be located 2 to 3 cm below the aortic valve and, in this location, usually has connections onto the anterior mitral valve leaflet. A second type of subvalvular aortic stenosis is a thicker, fibromuscular obstruction that forms a collarlike obstruction around the left ventricular outflow tract a few centimeters below the aortic valve. In the third and most severe form, a fibromuscular obstruction narrows the left ventricular outflow tract for several centimeters, thus forming a tunnel subaortic stenosis.[57, 58]

M-Mode Echocardiographic Features
On the M-mode echocardiographic examination of pa-

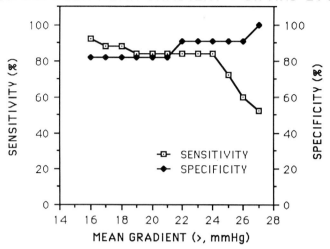

SENSITIVITY AND SPECIFICITY FOR DOPPLER MEAN GRADIENT + SX AND ETT

FIG 9–40.
Graph of the sensitivity and specificity for predicting the need for intervention when the criteria for intervention is a Doppler mean gradient of >27 mm Hg or ≥17 and ≤27 mm Hg in the presence of symptoms or an abnormal exercise treadmill test (ETT). Note that a Doppler gradient >27 mm Hg or ≥17 and ≤27 mm Hg in the presence of symptoms or an abnormal ETT predicted the need for intervention with 92% sensitivity and 82% specificity.

tients with subvalvular aortic stenosis, there are several characteristic findings. These include early systolic closure of the aortic valve, coarse systolic aortic flutter, and a diminished mitral-to-septal distance in the left ventricular outflow tract (Fig 9–42).[59, 60] The early systolic closure is caused by a jet stream and is explained by the Venturi principle. Because the obstruction is high in the left ventricular outflow tract rather than low in the body of the left ventricle, the jet formed by the subaortic stenosis passes through the aortic valve in early systole. As the jet passes through the flexible aortic valve cusps, the low-pressure area bordering the jet allows the cusps to move back toward each other (partial closure).

In patients with severe obstruction caused by subvalvular aortic stenosis, the M-mode echocardiogram shows severe concentric left ventricular hypertrophy. As with other forms of ventricular obstruction, the left ventricular posterior wall thickness does not correlate closely with the catheterization pressure gradient. In patients with tunnel subaortic stenosis, systolic anterior motion of the mitral valve is frequently present.

Two-Dimensional Echocardiographic Features

Subvalvular aortic stenosis is best visualized in the parasternal and apical views. The discrete fibrous membrane is seen as a thin linear echo in the left ventricular outflow tract (Fig 9–43).[32, 61] These thin membranes may be difficult to image in the parasternal-long axis view, where they are aligned parallel with the beam and in the direction

of the lateral resolution of the equipment. Often, in the parasternal long-axis view, only a small portion of the membrane adjacent to the ventricular septum can be seen. In the apical views, the subaortic membrane is aligned perpendicular to the beam and in the direction of the axial resolution of the equipment. As a result, subaortic membranes are usually well visualized in the apical views. When the subaortic membrane is located just millimeters away from the aortic valve, it can be difficult to distinguish echoes that arise from the membrane from those arising from the aortic fibrous annulus. A careful examination of this region, performed by tilting the transducer anteriorly and posteriorly and reviewing the information in slow motion, will usually differentiate these two conditions.

With a discrete subaortic membrane, the jet through the stenosis often damages the aortic valve. On the two-dimensional echocardiogram, the valve leaflets often appear thickened and Doppler examination may show evidence of aortic insufficiency. With subaortic stenosis, there is no poststenotic dilatation of the ascending aorta.

Discrete subaortic membrane may occur as an isolated defect or in association with other abnormalities. For example, subaortic membrane is frequently associated with a ventricular septal defect or ventricular septal aneurysm

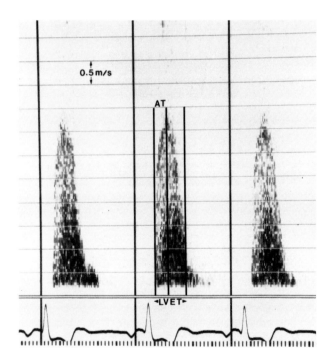

FIG 9–41.
Continuous-wave Doppler recording from a patient with aortic stenosis demonstrating the method used to measure the acceleration time (AT) and the left ventricular ejection time (LVET). The AT is measured from the onset of flow to the peak velocity of the jet. The left ventricular ejection time is measured from the onset of flow to the cessation of flow across the aortic valve. The ratio of AT/LVET in normal patients is less than 0.3. For ratios greater than 0.3, the pressure gradient across the aortic valve is >50 mm Hg.

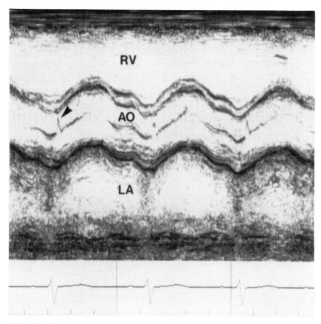

FIG 9–42.
M-mode echocardiogram from the aorta (AO) of a child with sub-valvular aortic stenosis. There is early systolic closure (*arrow*) of the AO valve caused by a jet stream and explained by the Venturi principle. The jet formed by the subaortic stenosis passes through the aortic valve in early systole. As the jet passes through the flexible aortic valve cusps, the low-pressure area bordering the jet allows the cusps to move back toward each other (partial closure). LA = left atrium; RV = right ventricle.

and double-chambered right ventricle. Also, subaortic membrane may occur with multiple left-heart obstructive lesions (supravalvular mitral ring, parachute mitral valve deformity, bicuspid aortic valve, and coarctation of the aorta), a condition known as Shone complex.[62]

The fibromuscular collar is a thick muscular ring that forms lower in the left ventricular outflow tract than most discrete membranes. This muscular obstruction can easily be seen in parasternal, apical, and subcostal views (Fig 9–44) as a thick, fibrous shelf projecting into the outflow tract.[61, 63] In tunnel subaortic stenosis, an extensive length of the left ventricular outflow tract is narrowed (Fig 9–45). The left ventricular walls are usually thicker and the cavity is more compromised. Unlike hypertrophic cardiomyopathy, the muscular obstruction in tunnel subaortic stenosis usually produces concentric left ventricular hypertrophy.[63]

Fibromuscular forms of subaortic stenosis are frequently associated with other cardiac defects such as ventricular septal defect, multiple left heart obstructions (i.e., Shone complex), and other left-to-right shunts. The ventricular septal defect can be located above or below the fibromuscular obstruction. One common association is supracristal ventricular septal defect, fibromuscular subaortic stenosis, and severe aortic coarctation with tubular hypoplasia of the transverse arch (Fig 9–45).

Doppler Echocardiographic Features

The peak pressure gradient across the discrete subaortic membrane can be calculated from the simplified Bernoulli equation and a Doppler recording of the peak velocity of the systolic jet (Fig 9–46). In some cases, the membrane is far enough away from the aortic valve to allow placement of the sample volume of the pulsed or high pulse repetition frequency Doppler instrument between the membrane and the aortic valve. In other cases, the membrane is so close to the aortic valve that sampling of the ascending aorta is necessary to record the subaortic stenosis jet. The peak velocity of the jet can be recorded from apical or suprasternal notch windows.

When there are multiple restrictive orifices in series (i.e., fibromuscular collar and bicuspid aortic valve), the Doppler peak gradient may overestimate the catheteriza-

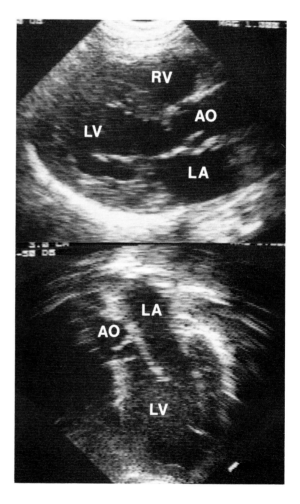

FIG 9–43.
Parasternal (*top*) and apical (*bottom*) long-axis views from a patient with subvalvular aortic stenosis caused by a discrete fibrous membrane in the left ventricular (LV) outflow tract just beneath the aortic (AO) valve. LA = left atrium; RV = right ventricle.

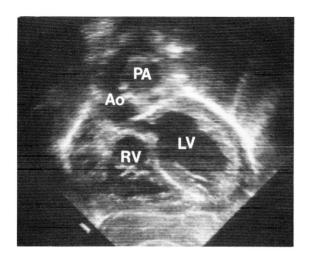

FIG 9–44.
Subcostal coronal view of the left ventricle (LV) from a child with subvalvular aortic stenosis caused by a fibromuscular collar, which appears as a thick muscular ring just below the aortic (AO) valve. Note the marked concentric LV hypertrophy. PA = pulmonary artery; RV = right ventricle.

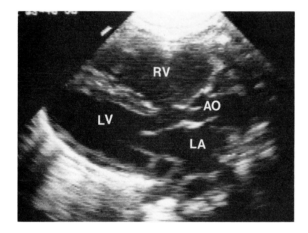

FIG 9–45.
Parasternal long-axis view from a patient with a large outlet (supracristal) ventricular septal defect and long tunnel subvalvular aortic stenosis. The entire left ventricular (LV) outflow tract is narrow. In other echocardiographic views, this patient was found to have a persistent left superior vena cava draining to the coronary sinus, a severe aortic coarctation, and tubular hypoplasia of the transverse aortic arch. AO = aorta; LA = left atrium; RV = right ventricle.

In a child in whom a large ventricular septal defect is located proximal to the subaortic stenosis, the left-to-right shunt through the ventricular septal defect can decompress the left ventricle. Thus, a minimal left ventricular outflow tract gradient may be found, even in the presence of severe subaortic stenosis. When the ventricular septal defect is closed, the full extent of the stenosis is revealed.[57, 64] In cases such as these, the severity of the subaortic stenosis can usually be predicted preoperatively from the two-dimensional echocardiogram (e.g., the amount of left ventricular hypertrophy, the size of the outflow tract).

Doppler color-flow mapping is a useful technique for

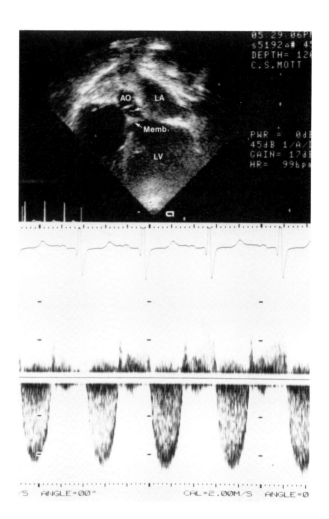

FIG 9–46.
Simultaneous imaging and continuous-wave Doppler examination of the left ventricular (LV) outflow tract of a patient with a subvalvular membrane (MEMB). The two-dimensional echocardiogram, *top*, shows the position of the continous-wave beam at the time of the Doppler tracing, *bottom*. The arrow indicates the focal zone of the continuous-wave beam and not a sample volume. The Doppler tracing shows a high-velocity jet in systole below the baseline, indicating flow away from the transducer. The peak velocity of the jet is 4.5 m/sec, indicating a peak pressure gradient across the subaortic membrane of 81 mm Hg. AO = aorta; LA = left atrium.

tion-measured peak-to-peak gradient.[14–16] The reasons for this discrepancy are discussed in detail in this chapter in the section on valvular pulmonary stenosis. In cases of very severe tunnel subaortic stenosis and a long narrow orifice in the left ventricular outflow tract, the Doppler-predicted peak gradient may underestimate the catheterization gradient because of failure to take into account the pressure drop caused by viscous friction along the flow path.

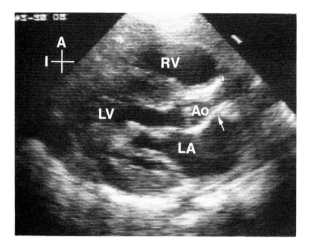

FIG 9–47.
Parasternal long-axis view from a patient with supravalvular aortic stenosis and an hourglass deformity (*arrow*) of the ascending aorta (Ao). There is an internal stricture above the Ao sinuses involving some length of the Ao and accompanied by an external narrowing of the Ao in the region of the stricture. In addition, there is marked concentric hypertrophy of the left ventricle (LV). The Ao valve leaflets are thickened and myxomatous. A = anterior; I = inferior; LA = left atrium; RV = right ventricle.

confirming the presence of obstruction proximal to the aortic valve. On the color-flow Doppler examination, a mosaic, high-velocity jet is seen in systole in the left ventricular outflow tract beneath the aortic valve (Plate 34). Disturbed flow usually persists into the ascending aorta in systole. In diastole, aortic insufficiency is often present.

Supravalvular Aortic Stenosis

Three specific anatomic types of supravalvular aortic stenosis have been described.[1] The membranous type consists of a simple fibrous diaphragm just above the aortic sinuses of Valsalva, with minimal to no narrowing of the external aorta. In the second type, there is an internal stricture above the aortic sinuses involving some length of the aorta and accompanied by an external narrowing of the aorta in the region of the stricture. The external narrowing gives the aorta the appearance of an hourglass deformity. In the third type of supravalvular aortic stenosis, a severely narrowed and hypoplastic segment of the ascending aorta is present from immediately above the sinuses of Valsalva to the origin of the innominate artery. Blood flow to the arch vessels and descending aorta is usually by way of a patent ductus arteriosus.

Two-Dimensional Echocardiographic Features

Supravalvular aortic stenosis can best be imaged from the parasternal and apical long-axis views, the subcostal views of the left ventricular outflow tract, or the suprasternal long- and short-axis views. In the parasternal and apical long-axis views in the normal heart, the aortic diameter increases at the level of the sinuses of Valsalva and

then decreases at the superior border of the aortic sinuses. The diameter of the ascending aorta above the aortic sinus, however, is the same as the diameter of the aortic valve annulus in the normal heart. In supravalvular aortic stenosis with an hourglass deformity, the diameter of the ascending aorta is considerably smaller than that of the aortic annulus (Fig 9–47). In supravalvular aortic stenosis with tubular hypoplasia, the narrowing at the top of the aortic sinuses is severe and extends all the way to the origin of the innominate artery (Fig 9–48). The innominate, left carotid, and left subclavian arteries are not hypoplastic, and the transverse and descending aorta are of normal size. In supravalvular aortic stenosis with a fibrous diaphragm (Fig 9–49), the external ascending aortic diameter is normal; however, an echo-bright membrane is seen stretching across the superior margin of the sinuses of Valsalva.[65, 66]

With severe supravalvular aortic stenosis, the aortic valve and coronary arteries are exposed to much higher pressures than usual. As a result, the aortic valve often appears thickened and myxomatous on the two-dimensional echocardiogram. In some cases, the valve prolapses in diastole into the left ventricular outflow tract. In addition, the main coronary arteries are extremely dilated. With severe stenosis, concentric left ventricular hypertrophy occurs.

In children with supravalvular aortic stenosis, the intimal hyperplasia that contributes to formation of the fibrous diaphragm may extend across the orifice of the coronary artery (especially the left coronary artery) and cause coronary ostial stenosis. In severe cases, myocardial ischemia and even infarction can occur as a result of coronary ostial stenosis. Thus, the ostia of the coronary arteries should be carefully examined in the parasternal short-axis view for evidence of a membrane covering the ostium or for evidence of ostial narrowing with poststenotic dila-

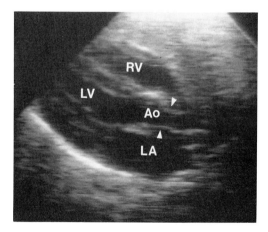

FIG 9–48.
Parasternal long-axis view from an infant with supravalvular aortic stenosis and tubular hypoplasia (*arrow*) of the ascending aorta (Ao). Narrowing begins at tht top of the Ao sinuses and extends to the origin of the innominate artery. LA = left atrium; LV = left ventricle; RV = right ventricle.

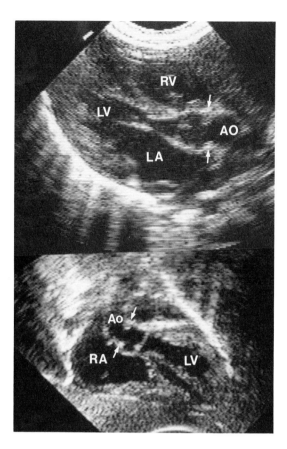

FIG 9–49.
Parasternal long-axis (*top*) and subcostal coronal (*bottom*) views from a child with supravalvular aortic stenosis with a discrete fibrous diaphragm (*arrow*) in the ascending aorta (AO). The echo-bright membrane is seen stretching across the margin of the sinuses of Valsalva; the external Ao diameter, however, is normal. LA = left atrium; LV = left ventricle; RA = right atrium; RV = right ventricle.

tation of the coronary artery. In addition, intimal hyperplasia in the aorta distal to the obstruction can frequently be seen in the suprasternal notch views (Fig 9–50).

Supravalvular aortic stenosis frequently occurs with mental retardation and characteristic elfin facies (Williams syndrome).[67] In this setting, association with peripheral pulmonary arterial stenosis is common.[68, 69] Other frequently associated lesions include coarctation of the aorta and stenosis of the brachiocephalic vessels.[69] In many cases, the position of the supravalvular aortic stenosis causes a jet that is preferentially directed toward the innominate artery. When this occurs, a dilated innominate artery can be seen in the suprasternal views.

Doppler Echocardiographic Features

Doppler echocardiography can be used to estimate the peak instantaneous pressure gradient across the area of supravalvular aortic stenosis. In discrete membranous supravalvular stenosis, the Doppler peak gradient correlates fairly well with the catheterization peak-to-peak gradient.

In other forms of supravalvular aortic stenosis, Doppler peak gradient may under- or overestimate the catheterization peak-to-peak gradient for the reasons outlined in the section on pulmonary valvular stenosis. For example, if multiple levels of obstruction are present, the Doppler peak gradient will overestimate the catheterization gradient. If a long, narrow segment of stenosis is present, the Doppler peak gradient may underestimate the catheterization gradient because of failure to take into account the pressure drop caused by viscous friction along the flow path. With tubular hypoplasia of the ascending aorta, Doppler examination of the descending aorta shows evidence of a right-to-left shunt through a patent ductus arteriosus.

The jet flow through the area of supravalvular stenosis is often directed toward the innominate artery; consequently, the highest value of the peak velocity is often obtained by aligning the Doppler beam parallel with the innominate artery in the suprasternal views. The spatial display of the jet on the color-flow Doppler examination is also useful for obtaining a minimal intercept angle between the jet flow and Doppler ultrasound beam.

The nonimaging continuous-wave Doppler probe should be used with caution in patients with supravalvular aortic stenosis. These children often have multiple areas of arterial stenosis, any of which could produce a high-velocity, systolic jet oriented in the same direction as the jet flow across the supravalvular aortic stenosis. For example, with a nonimaging continuous-wave Doppler transducer positioned in the suprasternal notch, it would be extremely difficult to distinguish the jet originating from a stenotic left carotid artery or left upper lobe pulmonary artery from the jet across the supravalvular obstruction. Even with the use of a simultaneous imaging and continuous-wave Doppler transducer, it may be difficult to separate the jets that arise from all the different areas of arterial stenosis.

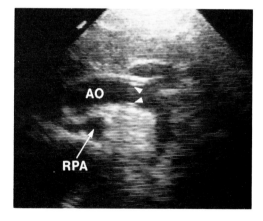

FIG 9–50.
Suprasternal long-axis view from a child with supravalvular aortic stenosis. There is marked intimal hyperplasia (*arrows*) throughout the aortic (AO) arch. RPA = right pulmonary artery.

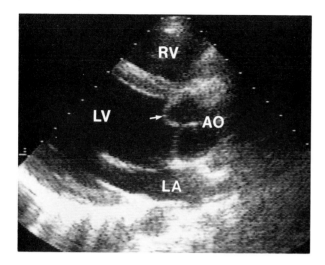

FIG 9–51.
Parasternal long-axis view from a patient with aortic (AO) valvular insufficiency following spontaneous closure of a membranous ventricular septal defect and prolapse (arrow) of the right coronary cusp of the AO valve. The prolapsed cusp is seen bowing into the left ventricle (LV) in diastole. The LV is markedly dilated. LA = left atrium; RV = right ventricle.

Aortic Insufficiency

In pediatric patients, aortic insufficiency frequently occurs in association with several congenital heart defects. These defects include aortic cusp prolapsed into a ventricular septal defect (Fig 9–51), bicuspid aortic valve (Fig 9–52), aortico-left ventricular tunnel, sinus of Valsalva aneurysm, Marfan syndrome or other connective tissue disorders, and conditions with a large, dilated aorta that overrides the ventricular septum (i.e., tetralogy of Fallot, persistent truncus arteriosus). In only two of these defects (bicuspid aortic valve and aortico-left ventricular tunnel) does aortic insufficiency occur as the sole initial symptom. The anatomic features of aortico-left ventricular tunnel will be reviewed later in this chapter. In the remainder of this section, the echocardiographic features of aortic insufficiency will be discussed.

M-Mode and Two-Dimensional Echocardiographic Features

Aortic insufficiency causes an increased filling of the left ventricle in diastole (an increased preload) and therefore leads to an increased left ventricular end-diastolic dimension. The left ventricular response to an increased diastolic filling is an increase in shortening fraction. As long as ventricular function is good, the left ventricle can eject the normal stroke volume plus the regurgitant volume, so that left ventricular end-systolic dimension remains normal. If the left ventricle begins to fail and can no longer eject the extra regurgitant volume, the left ventricular end-systolic dimension begins to increase. Thus, an increasing left ventricular end-systolic dimension is a serious sign of an inability of the left ventricle to handle

the increased volume load. M-mode echocardiographic studies in adult patients with aortic insufficiency suggest that, in order to prevent irreversible myocardial damage, surgical intervention should occur before the left ventricular end-systolic dimension reaches a value of 5.5 cm.[70] A comparable value has not been determined for pediatric patients, primarily because their left ventricular dimensions are changing with body growth. In our patients with aortic insufficiency, we plot serial measurements of the left ventricular end-diastolic and end-systolic dimensions on the graphs for normal values of these dimensions at different body surface areas. If the left ventricular end-systolic dimension is within normal limits and follows the same percentile line with increasing body surface area, we do not usually recommend surgical intervention, even if the left ventricular end-diastolic dimension is very abnormal. If the left ventricular end-systolic dimension begins

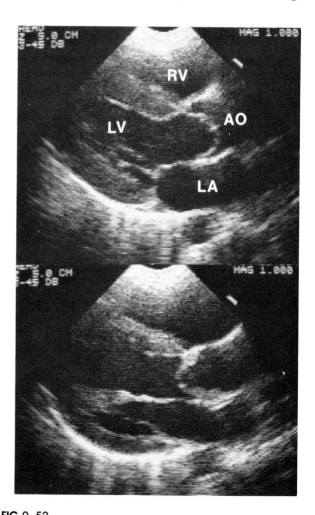

FIG 9–52.
Parasternal long-axis views in systole (above) and diastole (below) from a child with a bicuspid aortic valve and severe aortic insufficiency. In systole, the aortic (AO) valve is stenotic and domed. In diastole, the AO valve prolapses into the left ventricular (LV) outflow tract, creating the appearance of a reverse dome. LA = left atrium; RV = right ventricle.

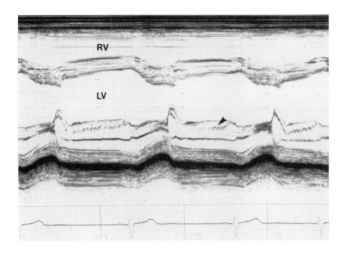

FIG 9–53.
M-mode echocardiogram of the left ventricle (LV) from a patient with severe aortic regurgitation. There is coarse, diastolic fluttering of the anterior mitral valve leaflet (*arrow*), caused by the aortic regurgitation jet hitting the anterior mitral valve leaflet in diastole. RV = right ventricle.

to increase above the percentile line along which it had previously tracked, then we would consider that patient at risk of developing irreversible myocardial damage if surgical intervention is not performed.

If the aortic insufficiency jet is directed posteriorly and strikes the mitral valve leaflets, coarse diastolic fluttering and diminished diastolic excursion of the mitral valve leaflets can be seen on the M-mode echocardiogram (Fig 9–53). If left ventricular compliance is decreased, the left atrium may be dilated as well.

On the two-dimensional echocardiogram, the dilated left ventricle can be visualized. In addition, the regurgitant orifice can often be seen in diastole in the short-axis views of the aortic valve (Fig 9–54). The diastolic runoff of blood from the aorta to the left ventricle causes a lowered aortic diastolic pressure, widened aortic pulse pressure, and bounding pulsations of the descending aorta that can be seen in the subcostal views of the descending aorta or suprasternal views of the aortic arch.

Doppler Echocardiographic Features

In patients with aortic insufficiency, the Doppler examination from the cardiac apex shows normal forward flow in systole below the baseline (away from the transducer) and reverse flow in diastole above the baseline (toward the transducer) (Fig 9–55). Regurgitant flow signals begin immediately at the time of aortic valve closure and continue throughout diastole. The peak velocity of the regurgitant jet is usually high in early diastole and remains high throughout diastole because of the large pressure difference that exists throughout diastole between the aorta and the left ventricle. When using Doppler ultrasound from the cardiac apex to detect an aortic insufficiency jet, care must be taken not to mistake Doppler signals from the mitral valve inflow for a regurgitant aortic jet. The position

of the sample volume, the timing of the Doppler flow signals (aortic insufficiency starts before mitral valve opening), and the peak velocity of the flow signals can help distinguish aortic insufficiency from mitral valve inflow.

In addition, in patients with aortic insufficiency, the Doppler examination from the suprasternal notch view usually shows a reverse flow signal in the ascending or descending aorta in diastole, indicating a runoff of blood from the aorta to the left ventricle (Plate 35).

The Doppler technique for detection of aortic insufficiency is very sensitive, and minor amounts of aortic insufficiency can be detected even when no diastolic murmur is heard. Nevertheless, physiologic amounts of aortic insufficiency have not been found on the Doppler examination of normal children.[24]

Techniques for quantification of the severity of aortic insufficiency are discussed in detail in Chapter 4 and will only be mentioned in this section.

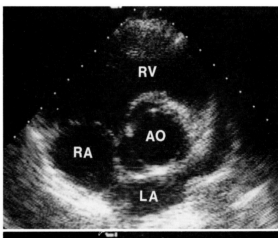
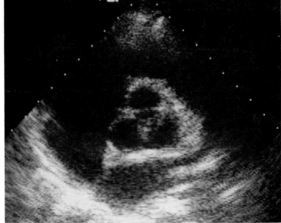

FIG 9–54.
Parasternal short-axis views in systole (*top*) and diastole (*bottom*) from a patient with aortic valve stenosis and aortic insufficiency. In diastole, when the aortic valve should be fully closed, a triangular regurgitant orifice can be seen. AO = aorta; LA = left atrium; RA = right atrium; RV = right ventricle.

FIG 9-55.
Pulse Doppler recording from a patient with aortic insufficiency. The freeze-frame image of the apical five-chamber view, *right*, shows the position of the sample volume (*arrow*) in the left ventricular (LV) outflow tract just below the aortic (Ao) valve when the Doppler tracing was recorded. The Doppler spectral tracing, *left*, shows normal forward flow away from the transducer and below the baseline in systole. In diastole, there is a high-velocity jet (*black arrow*) above the baseline, indicating regurgitant flow through the Ao valve and toward the transducer. LA = left atrium; RA = right atrium; RV = right ventricle.

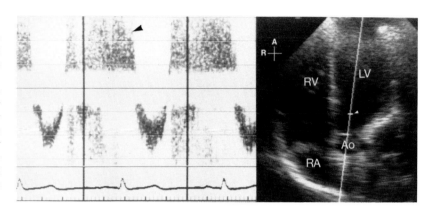

The continuous-wave Doppler recording can be used to assess the severity of the aortic insufficiency. In this technique, a clear recording of the outer envelope of the insufficiency jet throughout diastole is required (Fig 9-56). The continuous-wave Doppler measurements that have been used to estimate the severity of the insufficiency include (1) the deceleration slope, (2) velocity half-time, and (3) the pressure half-time.[71-73] Pulsed Doppler echocardiography has also been used to assess the severity of aortic insufficiency. The pulsed Doppler methods include (1) measurement of regurgitant fraction, (2) mapping of the extension of the jet into the left ventricle, and (3) measurement of the retrograde diastolic flow area in the descending thoracic or abdominal aorta.[74-77] The color-flow Doppler examination provides a spatial display of the aortic insufficiency jet, which is useful for alignment of the jet flow and the continuous-wave Doppler beam (Plate 36). Measurements of the jet dimensions on the color-flow Doppler have been used to assess the severity of the aortic insufficiency; however, this technique has serious limitations which are discussed in Chapter 4.[78, 79]

Aortico-Left Ventricular Tunnel

Aortico-left ventricular tunnel is one of the few congenital defects that presents with severe aortic insufficiency at birth. The tunnel forms an abnormal communication between the aorta and the left ventricle. The aortic end of the tunnel is usually located in the anterior aortic wall above the level of the right coronary artery. The ventricular end of the tunnel opens into the left ventricle just below the right and left aortic cusps. The extracardiac vessel-like segment of the tunnel lies between the aorta and pulmonary artery, while an intracardiac segment passes through the conus septum, thus connecting the aortic lumen to the left ventricle while bypassing the normal aortic valve. Aneurysmal dilatation of either segment of the tunnel occurs frequently.[1]

As the tunnel passes through the conus septum, it lies behind the right ventricular infundibulum and often causes the posterior wall of the infundibulum to bulge into the

right ventricular cavity. In many patients, this distortion of the right ventricular infundibulum is most likely responsible for development of right ventricular outflow obstruction (subvalvular and valvular). In some cases, the

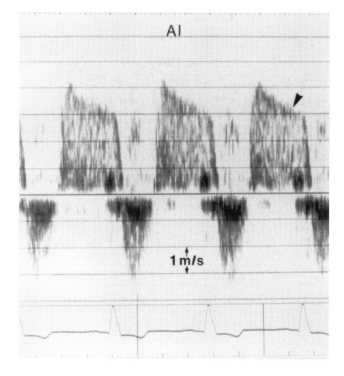

FIG 9-56.
A continuous-wave Doppler recording obtained from the cardiac apex of a patient with aortic insufficiency (AI). This tracing demonstrates the clear recording of the outer envelope of the insufficiency jet throughout diastole that is required to obtain quantitative information from the continuous-wave Doppler examination. The *arrow* indicates peak velocity at end-diastole at the onset of the QRS signal. This velocity is used to calculate the pressure gradient between the aorta and left ventricle at end-diastole and thus estimate left ventricular end-diastolic pressure (see Chapter 4).

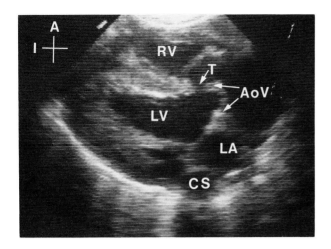

FIG 9–57.
Parasternal long-axis view from a newborn infant with an aortico-left ventricular tunnel (T). In this view, there are two passageways for blood to exit from the left ventricle (LV). The posterior passageway leads from the LV through a normally positioned aortic valve (AoV) to the ascending aorta. The anterior passageway leads from the LV through the ventricular septum and terminates in the ascending aorta above the right coronary artery. This represents the tunnel. A = anterior; CS = coronary sinus; I = inferior; LA = left atrium; RV = right ventricle.

aortic valve is congenitally thickened and stenotic and may be bicuspid.[80, 81]

Aortico-left ventricular tunnel can be distinguished anatomically from ruptured sinus of Valsalva aneurysm because the abnormal communication in the tunnel deformity opens into the aorta above the coronary arteries. In a ruptured sinus of Valsalva aneurysm, the aortic end of the communication is situated below the coronary arteries.

On the two-dimensional echocardiographic examination of newborn infants with an aortico-left ventricular tunnel, the right ventricular anterior wall, the septum, and the left ventricular posterior wall are markedly thickened, and the left ventricular end-diastolic dimension and shortening fraction are increased, suggesting a left ventricular volume overload. In the parasternal and apical long-axis views and the suprasternal views (Fig 9–57), there are two passageways for blood to exit from the left ventricle. The posterior passageway leads from the left ventricle through a normally positioned aortic valve to the ascending aorta. The anterior passageway leads from the left ventricle, through the ventricular septum, and terminates in the ascending aorta above the right coronary artery. At first glance, the left ventricular end of the tunnel may resemble a large subaortic ventricular septal defect; however, closer inspection shows that the left ventricle communicates with the aorta rather than the right ventricle through this opening. Usually, the ascending aorta above the aortic valve and the extracardiac portion of the tunnel are aneurysmally dilated. In these views, the annulus of the aortic valve may be somewhat narrowed and the aortic leaflets may be thickened and stenotic.[82]

In the parasternal short-axis view at the level of the aortic valve, a cross-section of the tunnel can be seen anterior and slightly rightward of the cross-section of the aortic valve (Fig 9–58). In cross-section, these two structures resemble a figure-of-eight. In this view, the encroachment of the tunnel on the right ventricular outflow tract can be seen. As the plane of sound is titled superiorly above the level of the aortic valve, the right coronary artery can be seen. Above the plane of the right coronary artery, the anterior and posterior passageways become confluent. This is the level at which the tunnel enters the ascending aorta. To distinguish aortico-left ventricular tunnel from ruptured sinus of Valsalva aneurysm, it is important to determine the spatial relationship between the aortic end of the communication and the right coronary artery. The parasternal long- and short-axis views are particularly useful for obtaining this information.

As the transducer is tilted more anteriorly in the apical and subcostal four-chamber views, the tunnel is seen protruding anteriorly into the right ventricular outflow tract (Fig 9–59).

Pulsed and color-flow Doppler examinations show evidence of severe aortic insufficiency through the tunnel into the left ventricle. Descending aorta Doppler examination usually shows significant retrograde flow in diastole.

As long as the tunnel remains open and provides another egress of blood from the left ventricle, Doppler examination of the aortic valve will not be a useful technique for assessing the severity of aortic stenosis. In this situation, the examiner will need to rely on the two-dimensional appearance of the valve (i.e., leaflet mobility, annulus size) to assess the severity of the obstruction.

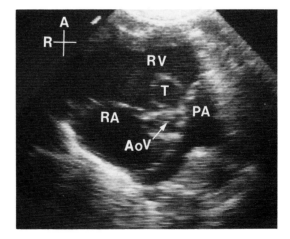

FIG 9–58.
Parasternal short-axis view at the base of the heart from the same infant as in Figure 9–57. In this view, the tunnel (T) is seen in cross-section anterior to the aortic valve (AoV). Together, these two structures resemble a figure-of-eight. A = anterior; PA = pulmonary artery; R = right; RA = right atrium; RV = right ventricle.

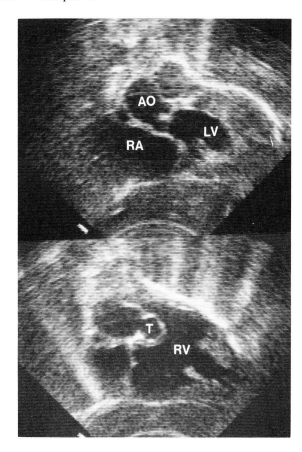

FIG 9–59.
Subcostal coronal views from an infant with an aortico-left ventricular tunnel (T). In the *top frame,* the plane of sound passes through the left ventricle (LV), the normal posterior aortic valve, and the ascending aorta (AO). The *bottom frame* was obtained by tilting the transducer anteriorly. In this view, the plane of sound passes through the right ventricle (RV) and the tunnel, which protrudes anteriorly into the right ventricular outflow tract. RA = right atrium.

Sinus of Valsalva Aneurysm

The symptoms of sinus of Valsalva aneurysm may develop early in life or as late as the fifth or sixth decade. The orifice of the aneurysm is just above the aortic valve fibrous annulus, arising close to the floor of the sinus of Valsalva. Any aortic cusp may be involved or two or three cusps may be involved. Most commonly, the right aortic cusp is the site of the aneurysm, while the posterior aortic cusp is the second most common site. The left aortic cusp is rarely involved. The expansion of the aneurysm is usually in the direction of the least resistance; hence, the most common site of expansion is into the right heart chambers. The aneurysm may simply expand into a chamber, or it can rupture and develop communications with that chamber. Thus, rupture of a sinus of Valsalva aneurysm into a right heart chamber results in a left-to-right shunt, while rupture of a sinus of Valsalva aneurysm into the left ventricle results in aortic insufficiency.[1]

Sinus of Valsalva aneurysms can be congenital or can occur as a complication of Marfan syndrome or endocarditis. Unruptured sinus of Valsalva aneurysm may cause right ventricular outflow obstruction, tricuspid regurgitation, coronary occlusion, or obstruction of the right pulmonary artery branch or descending aorta.[83, 84] On the two-dimensional echocardiogram, the enlarged sinus of Valsalva can be seen on the parasternal views (Fig 9–60). By tilting the transducer in various directions, the sinus of Valsalva aneurysm can usually be imaged to its farthest extension.[83–85] Pulsed and color-flow Doppler techniques can be used to detect rupture of the aneurysm into a cardiac chamber.[86] If rupture has occurred into the right atrium, right ventricle, pulmonary artery, or left atrium, a continuous, high-velocity jet will be seen in the receiving chamber. If rupture has occurred into the left ventricle, a high velocity diastolic jet will be detected in that chamber. In

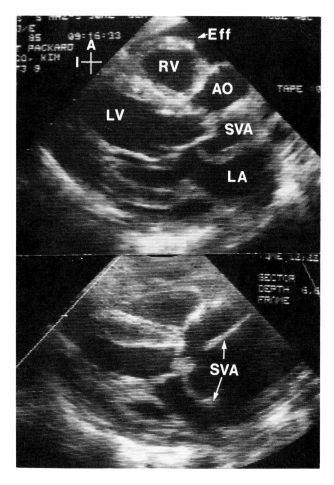

FIG 9–60.
Parasternal long-axis views from a patient with a sinus of Valsalva aneurysm (SVA) that developed as a complication of bacterial endocarditis of the aortic valve. In this view, the SVA is seen protruding posteriorly. AO = aorta; Eff = effusion; LA = left atrium; LV = left ventricle; RV = right ventricle.

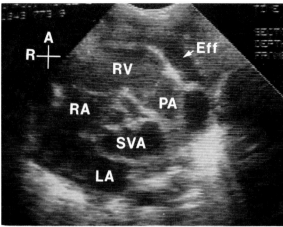

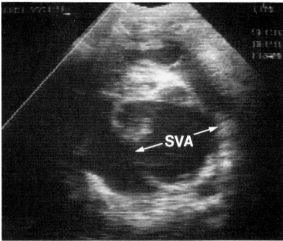

FIG 9–61.
Parasternal short-axis views at the base of the heart from the same patient as in Figure 9–60. The sinus of Valsalva aneurysm (SVA) can be seen protruding to the left and posteriorly. The SVA has encroached considerably on the main and right pulmonary artery (PA) branches. Eff = effusion; RV = right ventricle; RA = right atrium.

addition to direct imaging of the aneurysm, the two-dimensional and Doppler echocardiogram can be used to detect complications of the aneurysm (Fig 9–61).[84]

REFERENCES

1. Goor DA, Lillehei CW: *Congenital Malformations of the Heart.* New York, Grune and Stratton, 1975.
2. Heger JJ, Weyman AE: A review of M-mode and cross-sectional echocardiographic findings of the pulmonary valve. *J Clin Ultrasound* 1979; 7:98–107.
3. Weyman AE, Hurwitz RA, Girod DA, et al: Cross-sectional echocardiographic visualization of the stenotic pulmonary valve. *Circulation* 1977; 56:769–774.
4. Trowitzsch E, Colan SD, Sanders SP: Two-dimensional echocardiographic evaluation of right ventricular size and function in newborns with severe right ventricular outflow tract obstruction. *J Am Coll Cardiol* 1985; 6:388–393.
5. Weyman AE, Dillon JC, Feigenbaum H, et al: Echocardiographic pattern of pulmonary valve motion in valvular pulmonary stenosis. *Am J Cardiol* 1974; 34:644–649.
6. Hatle L, Angelsen B: *Doppler Ultrasound in Cardiology,* ed 2, Philadelphia, Lea and Febiger, 1985, pp 97–293.
7. Lima CO, Sahn DJ, Valdes-Cruz LM, et al: Noninvasive prediction of transvalvular pressure gradient in patients with pulmonary stenosis by quantitative two-dimensional echocardiographic Doppler studies. *Circulation* 1983; 67:866–871.
8. Johnson GL, Kwan OL, Handshoe S, et al: Accuracy of combined two-dimensional echocardiography and continuous wave Doppler recordings in the estimation of pressure gradient in right ventricular outlet obstruction. *J Am Coll Cardiol* 1984; 3:1013–1018.
9. Frantz EG, Silverman NH: Doppler ultrasound evaluation of valvar pulmonary stenosis from multiple transducer positions in children requiring pulmonary valvuloplasty. *Am J Cardiol* 1988; 61:844–849.
10. Stevenson JG, Kawabori I: Noninvasive determination of pressure gradients in children: Two methods employing pulsed Doppler echocardiography. *J Am Coll Cardiol* 1984; 3:179–192.
11. Snider AR, Stevenson JG, French JW, et al: Comparison of high pulse repetition frequency and continuous wave Doppler echocardiography for velocity measurement and gradient prediction in children with valvular and congenital heart disease. *J Am Coll Cardiol* 1986; 7:873–879.
12. Sahn DJ, Chung KJ, Tamura T, et al: Factors affecting jet visualization by Doppler color flow mapping echo: In vitro studies. *Circulation* 1986; 74(suppl 2):271.
13. Kveselis DA, Rocchini AP, Snider AR, et al: Results of balloon valvuloplasty in the treatment of congenital valvar pulmonary stenosis in children. *Am J Cardiol* 1985; 56:527–532.
14. Yoganathan A, Valdes-Cruz L, Schmidt-Dohna J, et al: Continuous wave Doppler velocities and gradients across fixed tunnel stenoses in an in vitro flow model. *Circulation* 1987; 76:657–666.
15. Houston AB, Simpson IA, Sheldon CD, et al: Doppler ultrasound in the estimation of the severity of pulmonary infundibular stenosis in infants and children. *Br Heart J* 1986; 55:381–384.
16. Simpson IA, Valdes-Cruz LM, Yoganathan AP, et al: Spatial velocity distribution and acceleration in serial subvalve tunnel and valvular obstructions: An in vitro study using Doppler color flow mapping. *J Am Coll Cardiol* 1989; 13:241–248.
17. Rowland TW, Rosenthal A, Castenada AR: Double chambered right ventricle: Experience with 17 cases. *Am Heart J* 1975; 89:445–462.
18. Matina D, Van Doesburg NH, Fouron J-C, et al: Subxiphoid two-dimensional echocardiographic diagnosis of double-chambered right ventricle. *Circulation* 1983; 67:885–888.
19. Baumstark A, Fellows KE, Rosenthal A: Combined double chambered right ventricle and discrete subaortic stenosis. *Circulation* 1978; 57:299–303.

20. Hastreiter AR, Joorabchi B, Pujatti G, et al: Cardiovascular lesions associated with congenital rubella. *J Pediatr* 1967; 71:59–66.

21. Roberts N, Moes CAF: Supravalvular pulmonary stenosis. *J Pediatr* 1973; 82:838–844.

22. Snider AR, Enderlein ME, Teitel DF, et al: Two-dimensional echocardiographic determination of aortic and pulmonary artery sizes from infancy to adulthood in normal subjects. *Am J Cardiol* 1984; 53:218–224.

23. Kostucki W, Vandenbossche J-L, Friart A, et al: Pulsed Doppler regurgitant flow patterns of normal valves. *Am J Cardiol* 1986; 58:309–313.

24. Yoshida K, Yoshikawa J, Shakudo M, et al: Color Doppler evaluation of valvular regurgitation in normal subjects. *Circulation* 1988; 78:840–847.

25. Patel AK, Rowe GG, Dhanani SP, et al: Pulsed Doppler echocardiography in diagnosis of pulmonary regurgitation: Its value and limitations. *Am J Cardiol* 1982; 49:1801–1805.

26. Waggoner AD, Quinones MA, Young JB, et al: Pulsed Doppler echocardiographic detection of right-side valve regurgitation. *Am J Cardiol* 1981; 47:279–286.

27. Nanda NC, Gramiak R, Manning J, et al: Echocardiographic recognition of the congenital bicuspid aortic valve. *Circulation* 1974; 49:870–875.

28. Fowles RE, Martin RP, Abrams JM, et al: Two-dimensional echocardiographic features of bicuspid aortic valve. *Chest* 1979; 75:434–440.

29. Radford DJ, Bloom KR, Izukawa T, et al: Echocardiographic assessment of bicuspid aortic valves: Angiographic and pathological correlates. *Circulation* 1976; 53:80–85.

30. Fernicola DJ, Mann JM, Roberts WC: Congenitally quadricuspid aortic valve: Analysis of six necropsy patients. *Am J Cardiol* 1989; 63:136–138.

31. Coeurderoy A, Biron Y, Laurent M, et al: Quadricuspid aortique congenitale. *Arch Mal Coeur* 1986; 79:745–748.

32. Williams DE, Sahn DJ, Friedman WF: Cross-sectional echocardiographic localization of sites of left ventricular outflow tract obstruction. *Am J Cardiol* 1976; 37:250–255.

33. Weyman AE, Feigenbaum H, Hurwitz RA, et al: Cross-sectional echocardiographic assessment of the severity of aortic stenosis in children. *Circulation* 1977; 55:773–778.

34. Huhta JC, Glasow P, Murphy DJ, et al: Surgery without catheterization for congenital heart defects: Management of 100 patients. *J Am Coll Cardiol* 1987; 9:823–829.

35. Krabill KA, Ring S, Foker JE, et al: Echocardiographic v. cardiac catheterization diagnosis of infants with congenital heart disease requiring cardiac surgery. *Am J Cardiol* 1987; 60:351–354.

36. Huhta JC, Latson LA, Gutgesell HP, et al: Echocardiography in the diagnosis and management of symptomatic aortic valve stenosis in infants. *Circulation* 1984; 70:438–444.

37. Huhta JC, Carpenter RJ Jr, Moise KJ Jr, et al: Prenatal diagnosis and postnatal management of critical aortic stenosis. *Circulation* 1987; 75:573–576.

38. Latson LA, Cheatham JP, Gutgesell HP: Relation of the echocardiographic estimate of left ventricular size to mortality in infants with severe left ventricular outflow obstruction. *Am J Cardiol* 1981; 48:887–891.

39. Hatle L, Angelsen BA, Tromsdal A: Non-invasive assessment of aortic stenosis by Doppler ultrasound. *Br Heart J* 1980; 43:284–292.

40. Young JB, Quinones MA, Waggoner AD, et al: Diagnosis and quantification of aortic stenosis with pulsed Doppler echocardiography. *Am J Cardiol* 1980; 45:937–944.

41. Oliveira LC, Sahn DJ, Valdes-Cruz LM, et al: Prediction of the severity of left ventricular outflow tract obstruction by quantitative two-dimensional echocardiographic Doppler studies. *Circulation* 1983; 68:348–354.

42. Berger M, Berdoff RL, Gallerstein PE, et al: Evaluation of aortic stenosis by continuous wave Doppler ultrasound. *J Am Coll Cardiol* 1984; 3:150–156.

43. Smith MD, Dawson PL, Elion JL, et al: Correlation of continuous wave Doppler velocities with cardiac catheterization gradient: An experimental model of aortic stenosis. *J Am Coll Cardiol* 1985; 6:1306–1314.

44. Currie PJ, Hagler DJ, Seward JB, et al: Instantaneous pressure gradient: A simultaneous Doppler and dual catheter correlative study. *J Am Coll Cardiol* 1986; 7:800–806.

45. Agatston AS, Chengot M, Rao A, et al: Doppler diagnosis of valvular aortic stenosis in patients over 60 years of age. *Am J Cardiol* 1985; 56:106–109.

46. Yeager M, Yock PG, Popp RL: Comparison of Doppler-derived pressure gradient to that determined at cardiac catheterization in adults with aortic valve stenosis: Implications for management. *Am J Cardiol* 1986; 57:644–648.

47. Oh JK, Taliercio CP, Holmes DR Jr, et al: Prediction of the severity of aortic stenosis by Doppler aortic valve area determination: Prospective Doppler-catheterization correlation in 100 patients. *J Am Coll Cardiol* 1988; 11:1227–1234.

48. Currie PJ, Seward JB, Reeder GS, et al: Continuous-wave Doppler echocardiographic assessment of severity of calcific aortic stenosis: A simultaneous Doppler-catheter correlative study in 100 adult patients. *Circulation* 1985; 71:1162–1169.

49. Nishimura RA, Holmes DR Jr, Reeder GS, et al: Doppler evaluation of results of percutaneous aortic balloon valvuloplasty in calcific aortic stenosis. *Circulation* 1988; 78:791–799.

50. Bengur AR, Snider AR, Serwer GA, et al: Doppler mean gradient in children with aortic stenosis. *Circulation* 1988; 78(suppl 2):395.

51. Kosturakis D, Allen HD, Goldberg SJ, et al: Noninvasive quantification of stenotic semilunar valve areas by Doppler echocardiography. *J Am Coll Cardiol* 1984; 3:1256–1262.

52. Otto CM, Pearlman AS, Comess KA, et al: Determination of the stenotic aortic valve area in adults using Doppler echocardiography. *J Am Coll Cardiol* 1986; 7:509–517.

53. Fan P-H, Kapur KK, Nanda NC: Color-guided Doppler echocardiographic assessment of aortic valve stenosis. *J Am Coll Cardiol* 1988; 12:441–449.

54. Skjaerpe T, Hegrenaes L, Hatle L: Noninvasive estimation of valve area in patients with aortic stenosis

by Doppler ultrasound and two-dimensional echocardiography. *Circulation* 1985; 72:810–818.

55. Zoghbi WA, Farmer KL, Soto JG, et al: Accurate noninvasive quantification of stenotic aortic valve area by Doppler echocardiography. *Circulation* 1986; 73:452–459.

56. Richards KL, Cannon SR, Miller JF, et al: Calculation of aortic valve area by Doppler echocardiography: A direct application of the continuity equation. *Circulation* 1986; 73:964 969.

57. Newfeld EA, Muster AJ, Paul MH, et al: Discrete subvalvular aortic stenosis in childhood. Study of 51 patients. *Am J Cardiol* 1976; 38:53–61.

58. Reis RL, Peterson LM, Mason DT, et al: Congenital fixed subvalvular aortic stenosis. An anatomical classification and correlations with operative results. *Circulation* 1971; 43(suppl 1):1–18.

59. Ten Cate FJ, Van Dorp WG, Hugenholtz PG, et al: Fixed subaortic stenosis, value of echocardiography for diagnosis and differentiation between various types. *Br Heart J* 1979; 41:159–166.

60. Krueger SK, French JW, Forker AD, et al: Echocardiography in discrete subaortic stenosis. *Circulation* 1979; 59:506–513.

61. Weyman AE, Feigenbaum H, Hurwitz RA, et al: Cross-sectional echocardiography in evaluating patients with discrete subaortic stenosis. *Am J Cardiol* 1976; 37:358–365.

62. Shone JD, Sellers RD, Anderson RL, et al: The developmental complex of parachute mitral valve, supravalvular ring of the left atrium, subaortic stenosis, and coarctation of aorta. *Am J Cardiol* 1963; 11:714–718.

63. Maron BJ, Redwood DR, Roberts WC, et al: Tunnel subaortic stenosis: Left ventricular outflow tract obstruction produced by fibromuscular narrowing. *Circulation* 1976; 54:404–416.

64. Fisher DJ, Snider AR, Silverman NH, et al: Ventricular septal defect with silent discrete subaortic stenosis. *Pediatr Cardiol* 1982; 2:265–269.

65. Weyman AE, Caldwell RL, Hurwitz RA, et al: Cross-sectional echocardiographic characterization of aortic obstruction. 1. Supravalvular aortic stenosis and aortic hypoplasia. *Circulation* 1978; 57:491–497.

66. Vogt J, Rupprath G, Grimm T, et al: Qualitative and quantitative evaluation of supravalvar aortic stenosis by cross-sectional echocardiography. A report of 80 patients. *Pediatr Cardiol* 1982; 3:13–17.

67. Williams JCP, Barratt-Boyes BG, Lowe JB: Supravalvular aortic stenosis. *Circulation* 1961; 24:1311–1318.

68. Beuren AJ, Schulze C, Eberle P, et al: The syndrome of supravalvular aortic stenosis, peripheral pulmonary stenosis, mental retardation, and similar facial appearance. *Am J Cardiol* 1964; 13:471–483.

69. Johnson LW, Fishman RA, Schneider B, et al: Familial supravalvular aortic stenosis. Report of a large family and review of the literature. *Chest* 1976; 70:494–500.

70. Bonow RO, Henry WL, Ebstein SE: Echocardiographic changes in asymptomatic patients with aortic regurgitation (AR): Observations on the optimum time to operate. *Circulation* 1978; 58:23.

71. Labovitz AJ, Ferrara RP, Kern MJ, et al: Quantitative evaluation of aortic insufficiency by continuous

wave Doppler echocardiography. *J Am Coll Cardiol* 1986; 8:1341–1347.

72. Beyer RW, Ramirez M, Josephson MA, et al: Correlation of continuous-wave Doppler assessment of chronic aortic regurgitation with hemodynamics and angiography. *Am J Cardiol* 1987; 60:852–856.

73. Grayburn PA, Handshoe R, Smith MD, et al: Quantitative assessment of the hemodynamic consequences of aortic regurgitation by means of continuous wave Doppler recordings. *J Am Coll Cardiol* 1987; 10:135–141.

74. Goldberg SJ, Allen HD: Quantitative assessment by Doppler echocardiography of pulmonary or aortic regurgitation. *Am J Cardiol* 1985; 56:131–135.

75. Rokey R, Sterling LL, Zoghbi WA, et al: Determination of regurgitant fraction by pulsed Doppler two-dimensional echocardiography. *J Am Coll Cardiol* 1986; 7:1273–1278.

76. Ciobanu M, Abbasi AS, Allen M, et al: Pulsed Doppler echocardiography in the diagnosis and estimation of severity of aortic insufficinecy. *Am J Cardiol* 1982; 49:339–343.

77. Takenaka K, Dabestani A, Gardin JM, et al: A simple Doppler echocardiographic method for estimating severity of aortic regurgitation. *Am J Cardiol* 1986; 57:1340–1343.

78. Perry GJ, Helmcke F, Nanda NC, et al: Evaluation of aortic insufficiency by Doppler color flow mapping. *J Am Coll Cardiol* 1987; 9:952–959.

79. Switzer DF, Yoganathan AP, Nanda NC, et al: Calibration of color Doppler flow mapping during extreme hemodynamic conditions in vitro: A foundation for a reliable quantitative grading system for aortic incompetence. *Circulation* 1987; 75:837–846.

80. Levy MJ, Lillehei CW, Anderson RC, et al: Aortico-left ventricular tunnel. *Circulation* 1963; 27:841–853.

81. Perez-Martinez V, Quero M, Castro C, et al: Aortico-left ventricular tunnel. A clinical and pathologic review of this uncommon entity. *Am Heart J* 1973; 85:237–245.

82. Turley K, Silverman NH, Teitel D, et al: Repair of aortico-left ventricular tunnel in the neonate: Surgical, anatomic, and echocardiographic considerations. *Circulation* 1982; 65:1015–1020.

83. Engel PJ, Held JS, Van der Bel-Kahn J, et al: Echocardiographic diagnosis of congenital sinus of Valsalva aneurysm with dissection of the interventricular septum. *Circulation* 1981; 63:705–711.

84. Shaffer EM, Snider AR, Beekman RH, et al: Sinus of Valsalva aneurysm complicating bacterial endocarditis in an infant: Diagnosis with two-dimensional and Doppler echocardiography. *J Am Coll Cardiol* 1987; 9:588–591.

85. Terdjman M, Bourdarias J-P, Farcot J-C, et al: Aneurysms of sinus of Valsalva: Two-dimensional echocardiographic diagnosis and recognition of rupture into the right heart cavities. *J Am Coll Cardiol* 1984; 3:1227–1235.

86. Yokoi K, Kambe T, Ichimiya S, et al: Ruptured aneurysm of the right sinus of Valsalva: Two pulsed Doppler echocardiographic studies. *J Clin Ultrasound* 1981; 9:505–510.

10

Abnormal Vascular Connections and Structures

PATENT DUCTUS ARTERIOSUS

Patent ductus arteriosus is a common cardiac abnormality that can occur as an isolated defect or in association with various congenital cardiac defects. The medical and surgical management of an infant with a patent ductus arteriosus requires knowledge of the direction and magnitude of the ductal shunt. In most instances, two-dimensional echocardiography can accurately define the presence and morphologic characteristics of the patent ductus arteriosus; however, the hemodynamic characteristics of the patent ductus arteriosus cannot usually be defined with two-dimensional echocardiography alone. Doppler echocardiography provides a method for diagnosing the direction and magnitude of ductal shunts, for assessing the relative pulmonary and systemic vascular resistances, and for estimating pulmonary artery systolic, mean, and diastolic pressures.

Direct Visualization of the Patent Ductus Arteriosus

The patent ductus arteriosus can be imaged directly from left parasternal, high left parasternal, and suprasternal locations. In the parasternal short-axis view at the base of the heart, the patent ductus arteriosus can be seen arising from the main pulmonary artery between the right and left pulmonary artery branches and connecting to the descending thoracic aorta (Fig 10–1).[1] To optimize visualization of the patent ductus arteriosus in the parasternal short-axis view, the transducer should be angled leftward and superiorly toward the pulmonary artery bifurcation. In addition, with a slight clockwise rotation of the transducer back toward the parasternal long-axis view, a longer length of the descending thoracic aorta and usually the entire length of the patent ductus arteriosus can be visualized (Fig 10–2). The patent ductus arteriosus is imaged in the direction of the lateral resolution of the equipment in this view. Thus, even with the use of a high-frequency trans-

ducer, such as a 7.5 MHz probe, a ductus lumen of 1 mm or less cannot usually be visualized directly by two-dimensional echocardiography.

In the suprasternal long-axis view, the patent ductus arteriosus can be seen connecting the descending aorta (just past the left subclavian artery) and the main pulmonary artery.[2] Figure 10–3 is a suprasternal long-axis view from a patient with pulmonary atresia and a long, narrow patent ductus arteriosus. Note the reverse angle of the patent ductus arteriosus and the absence of aortic isthmus narrowing caused by severe right ventricular outflow tract obstruction *in utero* with altered fetal flow patterns.

In most cases of isolated patent ductus arteriosus, the ductus cannot be imaged in the suprasternal long-axis view without tilting the plane of sound toward the left pulmonary artery. In this projection, the patent ductus arteriosus is seen between the origin of the left pulmonary artery and the descending aorta. In patients without a patent ductus arteriosus, it is important not to mistakenly diagnose the area where the left pulmonary artery crosses over the descending aorta as a patent ductus arteriosus.

Figure 10–4 is a high left parasternal view of a patent ductus arteriosus. This view is obtained by sliding the transducer down from the suprasternal notch toward the left parasternal position.[3] The plane of sound is oriented in the same direction as a suprasternal long-axis view through the left pulmonary artery.

Several factors contribute to the limits on our ability to visualize the patent ductus arteriosus directly with two-dimensional echocardiography. First, the patent ductus arteriosus is nearly always imaged in the direction of the lateral resolution of the equipment. Although it is possible to image a wide, short patent ductus arteriosus in a larger patient, it may be extremely difficult to visualize the patent ductus arteriosus with certainty in a premature infant. An ultrasound system with excellent lateral resolution and a high-frequency imaging transducer is necessary. Second, the patent ductus arteriosus may be long and tortuous and

264

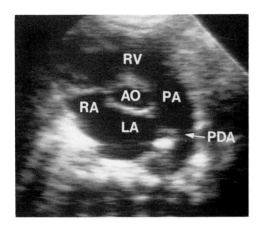

FIG 10–1.
Parasternal short-axis view at the base of the heart from a newborn infant with a large patent ductus arteriosus (PDA) connecting the pulmonary artery (PA) to the descending aorta. AO = aorta; LA = left atrium; RA = right atrium; RV = right ventricle.

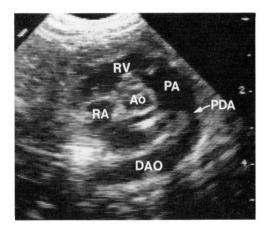

FIG 10–2.
Parasternal short-axis view from an infant with a large patent ductus arteriosus (PDA). The transducer has been rotated slightly to image a longer length of the descending aorta (DAO). The PDA is seen connecting the main pulmonary artery (PA) and the DAO. Ao = aorta; LA = left atrium; RA = right atrium; RV = right ventricle.

curve into and out of the imaging plane, thus making visualization of the entire patent ductus arteriosus extremely difficult, even with optimal instrumentation.

Cardiac Chamber Dimensions

As the pulmonary vascular resistance decreases after birth, the left-to-right shunting of blood through the patent ductus arteriosus increases, leading to increased pulmonary blood flow, increased pulmonary venous return, and consequently, left atrial and left ventricular volume overload. In a premature infant with a compliant left atrium, the left atrial/aortic root ratio measured from the M-mode echocardiogram is useful for the indirect assessment of the

size of the ductal shunt.[4–8] With a significant shunt, the left atrial/aortic root ratio is greater than 1.3. In some instances, however, the left atrial/aortic ratio can be very misleading. For example, the left atrium can be enlarged in a superior-inferior direction or a right-left direction and the ratio (which relies on an anterior-posterior measurement of the left atrial dimension) can still be normal. Conversely, abnormally increased left atrial/aortic root ratios can be created by unusual transducer positions or by car-

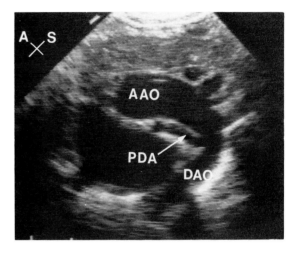

FIG 10–3.
Suprasternal long-axis view from an infant with tricuspid and pulmonary atresia. A long, narrow patent ductus arteriosus (PDA) is present. The reverse angle of the PDA and the lack of isthmus narrowing in the aortic arch suggest altered fetal flows *in utero* as a result of severe right ventricular outflow obstruction. A = anterior; AAO = ascending aorta; DAO = descending aorta; S = superior.

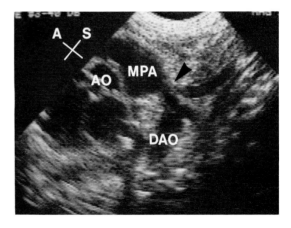

FIG 10–4.
High left parasternal view from an infant with a patent ductus arteriosus *(arrow)*. The patent ductus arteriosus is seen connecting the main pulmonary artery (MPA) to the descending aorta (DAO). This view, which is obtained with the transducer positioned between the suprasternal notch and the standard parasternal region, is particularly useful for imaging the patent ductus arteriosus. A = anterior; AO = aorta; S = superior.

diac rotation. Because of the ability to image the left atrium in several planes, a more accurate estimate of left atrial size can be obtained with two-dimensional echocardiography.

On the two-dimensional echocardiogram of an infant with a large patent ductus arteriosus, the left atrium is considerably larger than the right atrium or aortic root; and the atrial septum bows prominently toward the right, indicating left atrial dilatation. The parasternal long-axis view and the apical and subcostal four-chamber views are particularly useful for visualizing the enlarged left atrium. In addition, the left ventricular diastolic dimension is increased because of increased preload. In most cases, stroke volume is increased so that the left ventricle appears hypercontractile and has a normal end-systolic dimension. Left ventricular dilatation is easily detected in the parasternal long- and short-axis views and the apical and subcostal four-chamber views. Because of the large runoff of blood in diastole from the descending aorta to the main pulmonary artery through the patent ductus arteriosus, the aortic pulse pressure is widened and the descending aorta pulsations in the subcostal views are increased.

Doppler Echocardiographic Features of Patent Ductus Arteriosus

Doppler Examination of the Main Pulmonary Artery

Doppler echocardiography has been used to detect turbulent blood flow across the patent ductus arteriosus. This technique is especially useful for confirming the presence of a small, tortuous patent ductus arteriosus that cannot be visualized directly on the two-dimensional echocardiogram. In children with a patent ductus arteriosus, blood flows from the aorta into the main pulmonary artery throughout systole and diastole as long as systemic vascular resistance exceeds pulmonary vascular resistance. Several different flow patterns can be seen on the Doppler examination of the main pulmonary artery from the parasternal window. If the Doppler sample volume is positioned in the distal main pulmonary artery near the origin of the left pulmonary artery, continuous disturbed flow directed toward the transducer can be seen.[9–11] These signals represent the shunt flow through the patent ductus arteriosus throughout systole and diastole. If pulmonary artery pressure is normal, the velocity of the flow signals will be high. With elevated pulmonary artery pressure, the velocity of the flow signals will be diminished. If the sample volume is placed in the main pulmonary artery adjacent to the pulmonary valve and away from the orifice of the ductus arteriosus (Fig 10–5), the systolic portion of the left-to-right shunt may be directed away from the region of the sample volume. Instead, signals from the forward flow through the pulmonary valve predominate and are located below the baseline. Signals from the diastolic portion of the left-to-right shunt can still be seen above the baseline when the pulmonary valve closes. With the sample volume positioned in the midportion of the main pulmonary artery, it is even possible to record diastolic flow

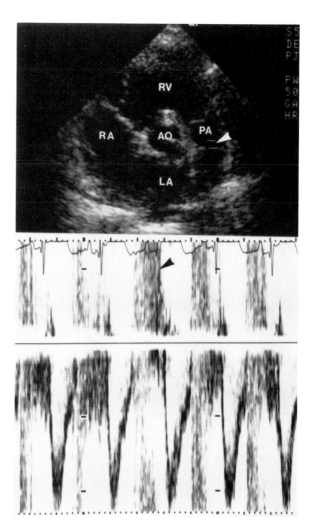

FIG 10–5.
Doppler recording from the pulmonary artery (PA) of an infant with a patent ductus arteriosus. The freeze-frame image of the parasternal short-axis view (top) shows the position of the sample volume (arrow) at the time of the Doppler recording. The Doppler tracing on the bottom shows forward flow in systole below the baseline and therefore away from the transducer. This represents the normal flow from the right ventricle (RV) to the PA in systole. In diastole, high-velocity, disturbed flow (arrow), seen above and below the baseline, represents the left-to-right shunt in diastole through the patent ductus arteriosus. AO = aorta; LA = left atrium; RA = right atrium.

signals below the baseline. Presumably, these signals arise as the jet flow from the patent ductus arteriosus strikes the closed pulmonary valve in diastole and swirls back on itself, giving rise to Doppler signals directed away from the transducer.[12]

Direct Doppler Examination of the Patent Ductus Arteriosus

Following the initial descriptions of the main pulmonary artery Doppler findings in patients with a patent ductus arteriosus, several investigators reported the results of direct interrogation of the ductus arteriosus with pulsed

TABLE 10–1.

Flow Patterns Detectable by Direct Doppler Examination of the PDA*

1. Isolated L → R PDA shunt: Continuous positive flow with a peak velocity in late systole
2. Isolated R → L PDA shunt: Continuous negative flow with a peak velocity in early systole
3. Bidirectional PDA shunt and severe PAH: R → L shunt in systole and L → R shunt in late systole extending to late diastole

*L = left; PDA = patent ductus arteriosus; PAH = pulmonary artery hypertension; and R = right.

and continuous-wave Doppler.[13–15] Direct Doppler interrogation of the ductus arteriosus has many advantages over pulmonary artery Doppler interrogation. First, a small patent ductus arteriosus shunt can be missed by sampling only in the pulmonary artery. Second, direct ductus examination has the advantage of being able to differentiate a patent ductus arteriosus from other defects that cause disturbed diastolic flow in the pulmonary artery (i.e., aortopulmonary window, anomalous origin of a coronary artery from the pulmonary artery, bronchial collateral vessels, etc.). Third, Doppler sampling in the main pulmonary artery does not permit detection of a right-to-left ductus shunt.

Several different flow patterns can be observed when the ductus arteriosus is sampled directly using pulsed or continuous-wave Doppler (Table 10–1). Patients with an isolated left-to-right ductal shunt and no other cardiac abnormalities have a continuous positive flow with a peak velocity in late systole. Figure 10–6 was taken from a newborn infant with a left-to-right ductus shunt. Note the continuous flow toward the transducer with a peak velocity in late systole. Peak systolic pressure gradients across the patent ductus arteriosus can be calculated by substituting the peak velocity in late systole in the simplified Bernoulli equation. Doppler gradients have correlated closely with catheterization measurements of the peak instantaneous gradient between the aorta and pulmonary artery in systole.[15] If the blood pressure is measured at the time of the Doppler examination, the pulmonary artery systolic pressure can be calculated as the systolic blood pressure minus the Doppler peak gradient.

Patients with an isolated right-to-left ductal shunt (as may occur in infants with aortic arch interruption and severe pulmonary hypertension) have a continuous negative flow away from the transducer with a peak velocity in early systole.[13, 14]

Bidirectional ductal shunting is detectable in infants with a patent ductus arteriosus and very severe pulmonary artery hypertension.[13, 14, 16] In these cases, the right-to-left shunt occurs as a negative deflection in systole, and the left-to-right shunt occurs as a positive deflection beginning in late systole and extending into late diastole (Fig 10–7). Patients with no oxygen saturation differences above and below the patent ductus arteriosus have a right-to-left shunt that peaks in early systole, while patients with oxygen saturation differences of 5% to 30% above and below the patent ductus arteriosus have a right-to-left shunt that peaks in mid- to late systole. When diagnosing a right-to-left ductal shunt (especially when using continuous-wave Doppler), care must be taken not to confuse normal systolic flow in the adjacent left pulmonary artery with a right-to-left ductal shunt (Fig 10–8).

In patients with bidirectional ductal shunting and pulmonary artery hypertension who develop high pulmonary vascular resistance, the right-to-left shunt begins in diastole, abbreviates the left-to-right diastolic shunt, and extends into early systole as a high-velocity reverse flow. The left-to-right shunt (if present) occurs in late systole to early diastole (Figs 10–9 and 10–10).

In assessing peak velocity of the patent ductus arterio-

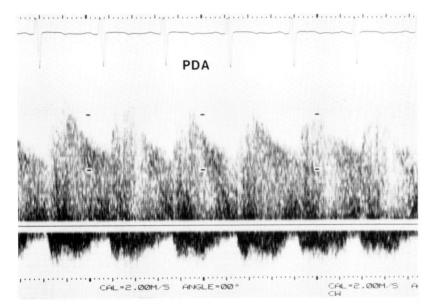

PDA

CAL=2.00M/S ANGLE=00° CAL=2.00M/S A
CW

FIG 10–6.
Continuous-wave Doppler tracing from the parasternal location of an infant with a patent ductus arteriosus (PDA). A high-velocity continuous flow is seen above the baseline, indicating flow toward the transducer from the descending aorta through the PDA to the pulmonary artery. The peak velocity is reached in late systole and is approximately 4.2 m/sec. This flow pattern is characteristic of a PDA with an isolated left-to-right shunt.

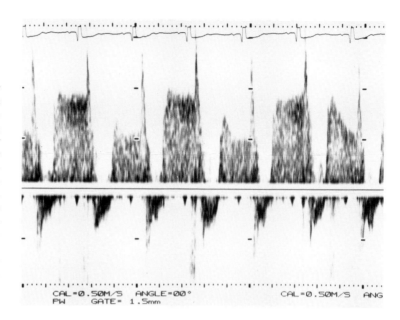

FIG 10–7.
Pulsed Doppler tracing from an infant with pulmonary artery hypertension and a patent ductus arteriosus. This tracing shows evidence of bidirectional shunting through the patent ductus arteriosus. The negative deflection in systole below the baseline arises from the right-to-left shunt through the patent ductus arteriosus from the pulmonary artery to the descending aorta (away from the transducer). The positive deflection, beginning in late systole and extending into late diastole, arises from the left-to-right shunt through the patent ductus arteriosus from the descending aorta to the pulmonary artery (toward the transducer). In this case, the peak velocity of the right-to-left shunt (below the baseline) occurs in mid-to-late systole, indicating that the oxygen saturation difference above and below the patent ductus arteriosus is 5% to 30%.

sus flow with pulsed Doppler, it is necessary to be aware that maximal velocities of the left-to-right shunt are recorded with the sample volume on the pulmonary end of the ductus arteriosus and maximal velocities of the right-to-left shunt are recorded on the aortic end of the ductus arteriosus.

Doppler Examination of the Descending Aorta

With a large patent ductus arteriosus and low pulmonary artery diastolic pressures, blood flows from the aorta into the pulmonary artery in diastole. Evidence of a diastolic runoff or "steal" of blood from the aorta can be seen on the Doppler examination of the aorta. If the Doppler sample volume is positioned in the descending aorta below the ductus arteriosus in the suprasternal notch view (Fig 10–11), forward flow signals are seen in systole below the baseline. In diastole, flow signals are seen above the baseline indicating flow up the descending aorta toward the ductus arteriosus and main pulmonary artery.[17] The retrograde diastolic flow signals are usually M-shaped, with peaks at early diastole and after atrial contraction. If the Doppler sample volume is positioned in the descending aorta above the ductus arteriosus, the diastolic runoff signals will be below the baseline, indicating flow away from the transducer toward the ductus arteriosus. Serwer and colleagues showed a good correlation between clinical estimates of shunt size and the ratio of the retrograde flow area to the forward flow area.[17] Reverse diastolic flow has also been recorded on Doppler tracings from the brachial

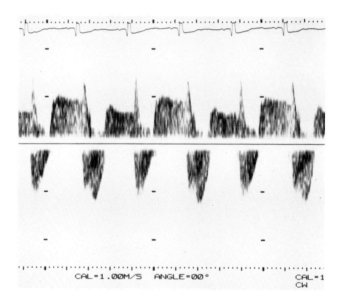

FIG 10–8.
Continuous-wave Doppler tracing from the same infant as in Figure 10–7. With continuous-wave Doppler, it is possible to record flow signals from both the patent ductus arteriosus and the adjacent left pulmonary artery. Care must be taken not to confuse systolic flow from the left pulmonary artery (below the baseline and peaking early) with the systolic right to left shunt through the patent ductus arteriosus. The flow in the left pulmonary artery begins at the onset of systole and peaks early. The right-to-left shunt begins later in systole and peaks in mid-to-late systole.

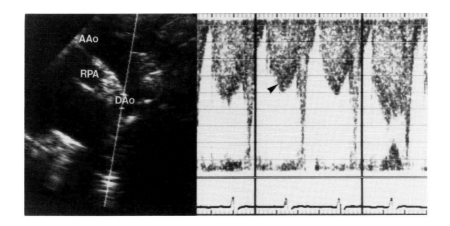

FIG 10-9.
Doppler spectral recording of the descending aorta from the suprasternal long-axis view of an infant with trisomy 18, ventricular septal defect, patent ductus arteriosus, and severe pulmonary vascular obstructive disease. The freeze-frame image, *left,* shows the position of the sample volume in the descending aorta (DAo) at the time of the Doppler recording. The Doppler spectral tracing, *right,* shows evidence of forward flow in systole down the descending aorta. In diastole, there are Doppler flow signals below the baseline *(arrow),* indicating a right-to-left shunt from the ductus arteriosus to the DAo. These flow patterns are characteristic of patients with bidirectional ductal shunting and pulmonary artery hypertension who develop high pulmonary vascular resistance. In these cases, the right-to-left shunt begins in diastole, abbreviates the left-to-right shunt, and extends into early systole as a high-velocity reverse flow. The left-to-right shunt (if present) occurs in late systole to early diastole. AAo = ascending aorta; RPA = right pulmonary artery. (From Snider AR: Doppler echocardiography in congenital heart disease, in Berger M (ed): *Doppler Echocardiography in Heart Disease.* New York, Marcel Dekker, 1987, p 294. Used by permission.)

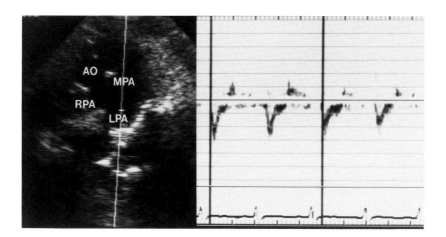

FIG 10-10.
Doppler recording of the main pulmonary artery (MPA) from the parasternal short-axis view of the same patient as in Figure 10-9. The freeze-frame image *(left)* shows the position of the Doppler sample volume in the MPA toward the origin of the ductus arteriosus at the time of the Doppler recording. The Doppler spectral tracing *(right)* shows evidence of pulmonary artery hypertension and no evidence of a left-to-right shunt through the ductus arteriosus. AO = aorta; LPA = left pulmonary artery; RPA = right pulmonary artery. (From Snider AR: Doppler echocardiography in congenital heart disease, in Berger M (ed): *Doppler Echocardiography in Heart Disease.* New York, Marcel Dekker, 1987, p 293. Used by permission.)

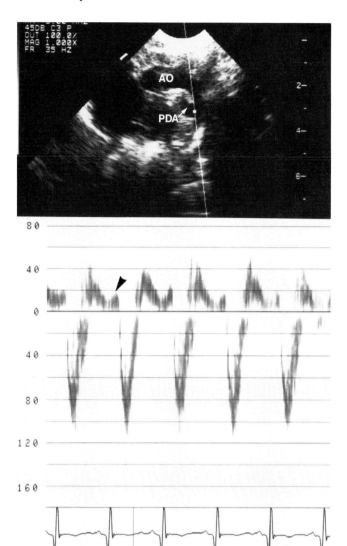

FIG 10–11.
Doppler spectral recording *(bottom)* from the descending aorta of a patient with a large patent ductus arteriosus (PDA). The freeze-frame image *(top)* shows the position of the sample volume at the origin of the PDA at the time of the Doppler recording. The Doppler tracing shows forward flow signals in systole below the baseline, indicating flow down the descending aorta away from the transducer. In diastole, flow signals are seen above the baseline *(arrow)*, indicating flow up the descending aorta toward the PDA and main pulmonary artery. The retrograde diastolic flow signals are M-shaped, with peaks in early diastole and following atrial contraction. Diastolic runoff indicates a sizeable left-to-right shunt through a PDA. AO = aorta.

arteries,[11] femoral arteries,[18] subclavian arteries, carotid arteries, and cerebral arteries[19, 20] of infants with a large ductus shunt (Fig 10–12). The amount of reverse flow in these arteries is useful for assessing the shunt size, as a large left-to-right ductus shunt is required to cause diastolic runoff from peripheral arteries. There is some speculation that

the diastolic steal of blood from the descending aorta and cerebral arteries of preterm infants with a patent ductus arteriosus predisposes these infants to complications such as necrotizing enterocolitis and intraventricular hemorrhage. After surgical ligation of the patent ductus arteriosus, descending aorta and cerebral artery Doppler flow patterns in these infants return to normal (Fig 10–13).

The finding of retrograde flow of blood in the descending aorta is not specific for a patent ductus arteriosus. This Doppler pattern can be found in any defect in which a diastolic runoff of blood from the aorta occurs.[21]

Color-Flow Doppler Examination of the Patent Ductus Arteriosus

Doppler color-flow mapping has improved the ease and speed with which it is possible to visualize the patent ductus arteriosus.[22, 23] With color-flow Doppler, flow can be detected in the patent ductus arteriosus that is too small to be imaged clearly on the two-dimensional echocardiogram. With the color Doppler display of the ductus jet, it is possible to obtain better alignment of the pulsed or continous-wave Doppler beam with the jet flow and thus improve the estimation of pulmonary artery pressures. One limitation of two-dimensional color flow mapping is that it may lack the temporal resolution to identify clearly the exact timing of bidirectional shunts in patients with fast heart rates.

Plate 37 is a parasternal short axis-view from an infant with a left-to-right ductus shunt and low pulmonary artery pressure. The color-flow signals clearly outline the small patent ductus arteriosus, which was difficult to visualize directly with two-dimensional echocardiography alone. The high-velocity jet flow through the patent ductus arteriosus is displayed as a mosaic flow area layered along the left lateral border of the main pulmonary artery. The mosaic of colors is caused by aliasing (color reversal) and the presence of disturbed flow (variance mapping) (Plate 38). Plate 39 is a parasternal short-axis view from an infant with a patent ductus arteriosus and severe pulmonary artery hypertension. In this patient, the low peak velocity of the ductus jet did not exceed the Nyquist limit of the color Doppler system; hence, the ductus jet appears as a pure red flow area (flow directed toward the transducer).

In infants with a large left-to-right shunt through a patent ductus arteriosus, color-flow mapping of the descending aorta often shows evidence of diastolic retrograde flow. Diastolic retrograde flow appears as a red flow area (flow toward the transducer) in the lower thoracic aorta in diastole.

Doppler Quantitation of the Magnitude of the Ductal Shunt

Using the techniques outlined in Chapter 4, the pulmonary blood flow, systemic blood flow, and pulmonary-to-systemic flow ratio can be calculated from the two-dimensional and Doppler echocardiographic examinations in children with a patent ductus arteriosus. Because the left-to-right shunt is downstream from the main pulmonary

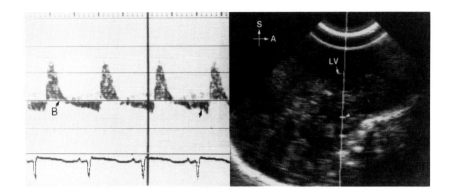

FIG 10-12.

Doppler spectral tracing *(left)* from a basal cerebral artery of an infant with a large patent ductus arteriosus and retrograde diastolic flow. The freeze-frame image of the sagittal view of the brain *(right)* shows the position of the sample volume *(white arrow)* when the spectral tracing was recorded. The spectral tracing shows Doppler signals *(black arrow)* in mid- to late diastole below the baseline *(B)*, indicating retrograde diastolic flow. A = anterior; LV = lateral ventricle; S = superior. (From Martin CG, Snider AR, Katz SM, et al: Abnormal cerebral blood flow patterns in preterm infants with a large patent ductus arteriosus. *J Pediatr* 1982; 101:590. Used by permission.)

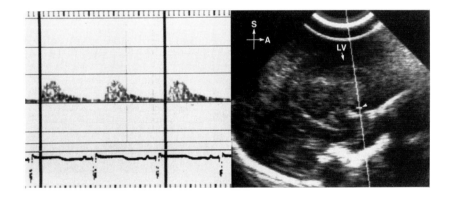

FIG 10-13.

Doppler spectral tracing *(left)* from a basal cerebral artery of the same infant as in Figure 10-12 after ligation of the patent ductus arteriosus. Now, flow in the cerebral artery is normal (i.e., forward flow is present throughout systole and diastole, resulting in Doppler signals displayed above the baseline). A = anterior; LV = lateral ventricle; S = superior. (From Snider AR, Howard EA: The evaluation of cerebral artery flow patterns with Doppler ultrasonography, in Berman W Jr (ed): *Pulsed Doppler Ultrasound in Clinical Pediatrics.* New York, Futura Publishing, 1983, p 109. Used by permission.)

artery, sampling of flow velocities in the right ventricular outflow tract or at the pulmonary valve provides the Doppler information necessary to calculate systemic blood flow (not pulmonary blood flow). Similarly, sampling of flow velocities at the aortic valve provides the Doppler information necessary to calculate pulmonary blood flow (not systemic blood flow).

Using the Doppler technique, close correlations have been found between Doppler and catheterization estimates of pulmonary-to-systemic flow ratio in infants with a patent ductus arteriosus.[24]

ARTERIOVENOUS FISTULA

Coronary Arteriovenous Fistula

Congenital coronary artery fistula is a rare defect reported to occur in 1 in 50,000 patients with congenital heart disease and 1 in 500 patients undergoing coronary arteriography.[25] In the presence of a significant shunt, the physical examination may be nearly identical to that of a patient with a patent ductus arteriosus except for subtle differences in the location of the murmur.[26] Visualization of coronary arteries by two-dimensional echocardiography,

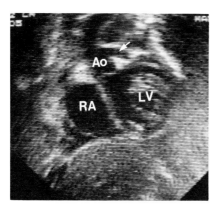

FIG 10–14.
Subcostal view of the left ventricular (LV) outflow tract from a patient with a coronary artery fistula. A massively dilated left coronary artery *(arrow)* can be seen arising from the aorta (Ao). This finding is highly suggestive of the presence of a coronary arteriovenous fistula. RA = right atrium.

together with additional information obtained from the Doppler examination, provides an excellent technique for the noninvasive diagnosis of coronary artery fistula.

Most commonly, coronary artery fistulas originate from the right coronary artery[27] but may arise from the left coronary artery, both coronary arteries, or an anomalous single coronary artery.[28] The low-pressure chambers are the usual drainage sites. In one review of 58 patients with coronary fistulas,[28] the right ventricle and pulmonary artery were the most common drainage sites. In another review of 101 patients with coronary fistulas,[29] the most common drainage site was the pulmonary artery. In both of these series, a left circumflex coronary artery to right ventricle fistula was exceedingly rare, occurring in only 4 of the total 159 patients from both series.

The two-dimensional echocardiographic diagnosis of a coronary artery fistula requires a high index of suspicion and should be considered in any child with a continuous murmur. This diagnosis should be suspected when two-dimensional imaging of the main coronary arteries in the parasternal short-axis view shows one coronary artery to be massively dilated while the other coronary artery is of normal size.[30, 31] Usually, the dilatation is uniform, involves the entire main coronary artery, and extends into the involved branches. Multiple two-dimensional echocardiographic planes should be used to follow the dilated coronary artery throughout the course of the fistula to its site of entry (Fig 10–14 and 10–15).[32–36] The site of entry of the fistula into a cardiac chamber or vessel cannot always be visualized directly with two-dimensional echocardiography; however, the site of entry can usually be located with the help of contrast or Doppler echocardiography. If flow through the fistula is very large, the chamber or vessel that receives the fistula can be dilated.

Some suggested views for visualization of portions of the coronary arteries are:

1. Left main coronary artery-parasternal short-axis view at the base of the heart, apical four-chamber view aiming anteriorly toward the aortic root, subcostal four-chamber view of the left ventricular outflow tract.

2. Bifurcation of the left main coronary artery-parasternal short-axis view at the base of the heart with clockwise transducer rotation, parasternal long-axis view of the right ventricular outflow tract.

3. Left anterior descending coronary artery-parasternal short-axis view, parasternal long-axis view of the right ventricular outflow tract (Fig 10–16).

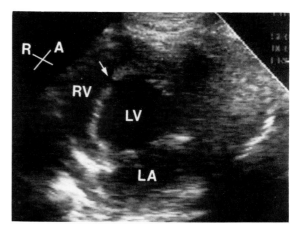

FIG 10–15.
Foreshortened apical view showing an area of echocardiographic dropout *(arrow)* in the apical portion of the ventricular septum. This area represents the site of entry of a coronary artery fistula from the left circumflex coronary artery through the ventricular septum to the right ventricle (RV). A = anterior; LA = left atrium; LV = left ventricle; R = right. (From Barton CW, Snider AR, Rosenthal A: Two-dimensional and Doppler echocardiographic features of left circumflex coronary artery to right ventricle fistula: Case report and literature review. *Pediatr Cardiol* 1986; 7:168. Used by permission.)

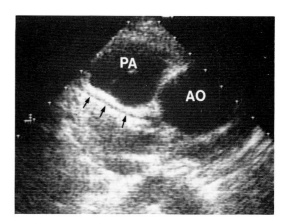

FIG 10–16.
Visualization of the left anterior descending coronary artery *(arrows)* from the parasternal long-axis view of the right ventricular outflow tract. AO = aorta; PA = pulmonary artery.

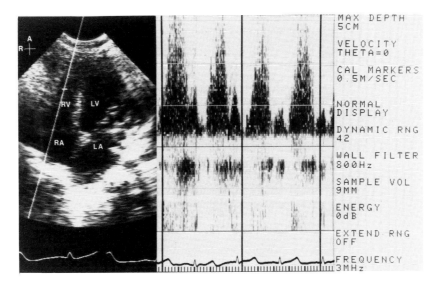

FIG 10–17.
Doppler spectral tracing recorded from the right ventricle (RV). The two-dimensional apical four-chamber view *(left)* shows the Doppler cursor line positioned in the RV. The sample volume is placed opposite the site of entry of a left circumflex coronary artery fistula into the RV. The Doppler spectral tracing *(right)* shows disturbed flow above the baseline, beginning in mid-systole and extending into early diastole. A = apex; LA = left atrium; LV = left ventricle; R = right; RA = right atrium. (From Barton CW, Snider AR, Rosenthal A: Two-dimensional and Doppler echocardiographic features of left circumflex coronary artery to right ventricle fistula: Case report and literature review. *Pediatr Cardiol* 1986; 7:168. Used by permission.)

4. Circumflex coronary artery-parasternal short-axis view, apical and subcostal four-chamber views tilting the transducer anteriorly to the ascending aorta and posteriorly to the posterior atrioventricular groove.

5. Right coronary artery-parasternal short-axis view, apical and subcostal four-chamber views tilting the transducer anteriorly to the aortic root and posteriorly to the posterior atrioventricular groove.

6. Posterior descending coronary artery-apical and subcostal four-chamber views tilting the transducer posteriorly to image the posterior surface of the heart.

When the site of entry of the fistula cannot be visualized directly, Doppler echocardiography can be used to detect disturbed flow at the site of entry of the fistula.[37–44] Initially, pulsed Doppler echocardiography was used to detect continuous disturbed flow at the site of entry of the fistula; however, this technique required a time-consuming, methodical search of multiple cardiac chambers and vessels with the small sample volume. In some instances where the fistula was small, disturbed flow at the entry site could not be found with pulsed Doppler. The introduction of color-flow mapping techniques improved the screening capabilities of Doppler echocardiography for locating the site of entry of the fistula. With the color-flow mapping technique, large spatial areas of the cardiac chambers and vessels can be interrogated at one time. The site of entry of the fistula is diagnosed by pulsed or color-flow Doppler by detecting continuous, disturbed flow that enters a cardiac chamber or vessel (Fig 10–17 and Plate 40).

With a large flow through the coronary artery fistula, pulsed Doppler examination of the ascending or descending aorta shows evidence of diastolic flow reversal caused by runoff of blood from the aorta into the fistula (Fig 10–18).[42, 44]

Using injections into the left heart at the time of cardiac catheterization, two-dimensional contrast echocardiography can be used to image the fistula and its site or sites of entry into the heart.[30, 43]

Pulmonary Arteriovenous Fistula

In the pediatric age range, pulmonary arteriovenous fistula is a rare malformation that requires a high index of suspicion for a successful echocardiographic diagnosis. In cases where a large flow occurs through the fistula, the pulmonary artery branches may be dilated and tortuous and increased flow velocities may be present on Doppler examination of the pulmonary veins.

The diagnosis can be confirmed with peripheral venous contrast echocardiography (see Chapter 3). Following a contrast injection, contrast echoes are seen filling the right atrium and right ventricle. Several cardiac cycles later, contrast echoes appear in the left atrium and left ventricle. The contrast material reaches the left heart by flowing through the arteriovenous fistula, thus avoiding filtration in the pulmonary capillary bed. The timing of the appearance of the contrast echoes in the left atrium allows differentiation of a pulmonary fistula from a right-to-left atrial shunt. In the right-to-left shunt, contrast echoes opacify the right atrium and then the left atrium on the same or subsequent cardiac cycle. In pulmonary fistula, contrast echoes opacify the right atrium and then the left atrium several cardiac cycles later (usually two or three beats later).

Cerebral Arteriovenous Fistula

Cerebral arteriovenous malformation enlarging the vein of Galen is rare.[45–49] This defect is the result of a direct arterial fistula or an adjacent arteriovenous malformation that increases flow through the vein of Galen and deep venous system, causing aneurysmal dilatation.[50] Newborn infants with this disorder often develop symptoms of congestive heart failure and cyanosis. Infants with severe congestive heart failure caused by an intracranial arteriovenous malformation are critically ill and prompt diagnosis is essential. Two-dimensional ultrasonography of the heart and brain provides a rapid, efficient method for the detection of intracranial arteriovenous malformation.

Indirect Evidence of a Cerebral Arteriovenous Fistula

Besides the complex adjustments that occur on conversion to extrauterine circulation, the newborn infant with a large intracranial arteriovenous malformation has an additional circulatory burden. Shortly after birth, when the pulmonary vascular resistances are still elevated, the decrease in the total systemic vascular resistance caused by

the presence of a large arteriovenous malformation promotes right-to-left ductal shunting. The large venous return to the right atrium from the arteriovenous fistula augments right-to-left atrial shunting. In the presence of a large right-to-left ductal shunt, the pulmonary blood flow and left atrial volume are decreased, and further right-to-left atrial shunting occurs because the flap valve of the foramen ovale remains open.[51] This persistence of fetal circulatory pathways can be detected by contrast, Doppler, or color-flow Doppler echocardiographic techniques.

In addition, increased blood flow to the low-resistance fistula leads to dilatation of the ascending aorta and carotid arteries, which can be detected by two-dimensional suprasternal notch echocardiography. For example, from the suprasternal long-axis view, the ascending aorta, innominate artery, and both carotid arteries are very enlarged and tortuous. The left subclavian artery and descending aorta are usually of normal caliber. Increased systemic venous return from the arteriovenous fistula leads to superior vena caval, right atrial, and right ventricular dilatation, also detectable by two-dimensional echocardiography. In the suprasternal short-axis view (Fig 10–19), the superior vena cava and innominate veins are markedly dilated. Usually, the superior vena cava diameter exceeds that of the adjacent transverse aorta. Right atrial, right ventricular, and pulmonary artery enlargement can be seen in the parasternal short-axis and apical and subcostal four-chamber views.[51]

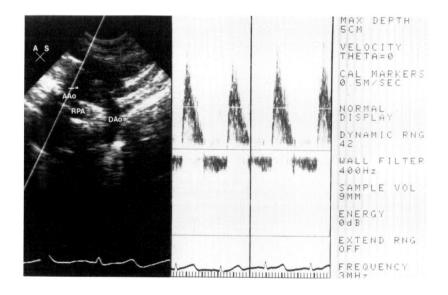

FIG 10–18.

Doppler spectral tracing recorded from the ascending aorta (AAO) of the same patient as in Figure 10–17. At *left* is the two-dimensional suprasternal long-axis view of the aortic arch. The Doppler cursor line is positioned in the AAo. The sample volume is indicated by the *arrow*. At *right* is the Doppler spectral tracing, showing normal laminar flow above the baseline in the AAo during systole. There is retrograde flow below the baseline in diastole, caused by a runoff

of blood through the fistula. A = anterior; DAo = descending aorta; RPA = right pulmonary artery; S = superior. (From Barton CW, Snider AR, Rosenthal A: Two-dimensional and Doppler echocardiographic features of left circumflex coronary artery to right ventricle fistula: Case report and literature review. *Pediatr Cardiol* 1986; 7:169. Used by permission.)

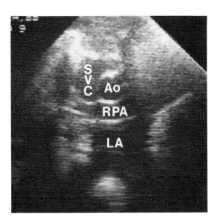

FIG 10–19.
Suprasternal short-axis view from an infant with a cerebral arteriovenous fistula. Increased systemic venous return from the arteriovenous fistula causes marked superior vena caval (SVC) dilatation. Ao = aorta; LA = left atrium; RPA = right pulmonary artery.

The presence of the cerebral arteriovenous malformation causes the systemic vascular resistance to be quite low. As a result, pulsed Doppler examination of the ascending aorta and carotid arteries shows evidence of low-velocity, antegrade diastolic flow. Pulsed Doppler examination of the descending aorta distal to the left subclavian artery shows evidence of retrograde diastolic flow from the descending aorta to the fistula.

Direct Visualization of the Cerebral Arteriovenous Malformation

For direct visualization of the cerebral arteriovenous malformation, the transducer is positioned in the anterior fontanel and tilted from anterior to posterior in a coronal body plane and from right to left in a sagittal body plane (Figs 10–20 and 10–21). A transverse view of the defect can be obtained by applying the transducer to the temporal bone in a horizontal plane. In all three views, the cerebral arteriovenous malformation appears as a large, fluid-filled (echolucent) structure within the brain. In some cases, the afferent and efferent vessels connecting to the malformation can be seen.[50–52]

A Doppler or contrast echocardiogram can be used to distinguish the vein of Galen aneurysm from other causes of an echolucent structure in the brain (i.e., cyst, enlarged ventricle, etc.). Pulsed or color-flow Doppler examination of the cerebral arteriovenous malformation shows evidence of continuous, disturbed flow in the malformation, thus confirming its vascular nature.[50, 52] With contrast echocardiography, the persistence of fetal circulatory patterns allows microcavitations from a peripheral venous contrast injection to pass from right to left at atrial level, travel in the ascending aorta to the carotid arteries, and opacify the arteriovenous malformation (see Figs 10–20 and 10–21). Other echolucent structures in the brain are nonvascular and do not opacify with contrast echoes. Microcavitations in the fistula bypass filtration by the systemic capillary bed and reappear rapidly in the superior vena cava. Superior

vena caval recirculation can be readily detected by two-dimensional suprasternal notch echocardiography.[51]

Because infants with congestive heart failure and cyanosis caused by an arteriovenous malformation are usually critically ill, rapid diagnosis is essential. We found that two-dimensional ultrasonography allows accurate, rapid detection of the intracranial arteriovenous malformation but does not provide the detailed anatomic delineation of the feeding vessels necessary before surgery. If the diagnosis can be made by ultrasonography without cardiac catheterization, both the additional stress of catheterization and use of contrast agents at catheterization can

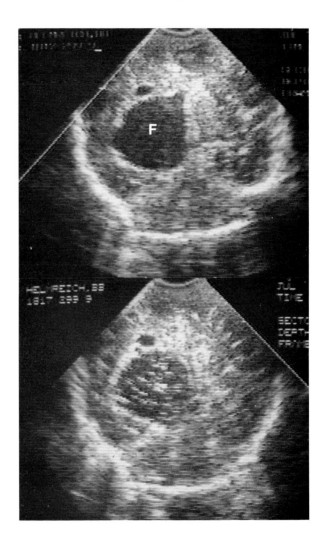

FIG 10–20.
Coronal plane through the brain of an infant with a large cerebral arteriovenous fistula (F). The fistula appears as an echo-free space in the midportion of the brain. Following injection of a contrast agent into a peripheral arm vein *(bottom)*, contrast echoes are seen filling the fistula. These contrast microbubbles pass from right to left at atrial level, travel in the ascending aorta to the carotid arteries, and opacify the fistula. The appearance of contrast echoes in the fistula proves that the echolucent structure is not a nonvascular cystic malformation.

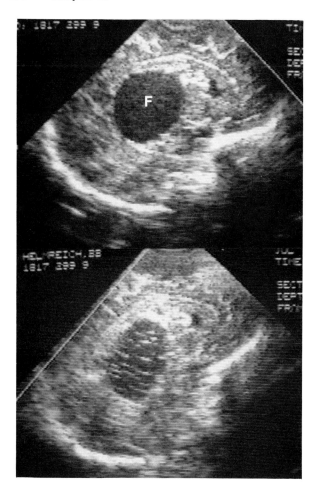

FIG 10–21.
Sagittal view of the brain from the same infant as in Figure 10–20. The fistula (F) is again seen in the midportion of the brain. Following a peripheral venous contrast injection *(bottom)*, contrast echoes are seen in the fistula.

be avoided. Once the diagnosis is made by two-dimensional ultrasonography, the use of contrast agents can be reserved for more detailed anatomic studies, such as selective cerebral arteriograms in several views or computerized tomography with contrast in several planes before surgery.[51]

ABNORMALITIES OF SYSTEMIC VENOUS RETURN

Persistent Left Superior Vena Cava

Persistent left superior vena cava is a common anomaly that occurs in 0.5% of the general population and 3% to 10% of children with congenital heart disease.[53, 54] There are four varieties of persistent left superior vena cava. In more than 90% of cases, the persistent left superior vena cava drains to the right atrium by way of the coronary sinus. In the second type, the persistent left superior vena cava drains to the coronary sinus and a defect exists in the wall between the left atrium and coronary sinus. In the third

form, the persistent left superior vena cava opens into the roof of the left atrium. In the fourth variety, the persistent left superior vena cava drains to the pulmonary vein.[55]

Persistent Left Superior Vena Cava Draining to the Coronary Sinus

Persistent left superior vena cava draining to the coronary sinus can be found as an isolated anomaly or in association with congenital heart disease (especially secundum atrial septal defect, tetralogy of Fallot, and tricuspid atresia). The finding of an enlarged coronary sinus on the two-dimensional echocardiogram should first alert the echocardiographer to the possibility that a persistent left superior vena cava connecting to the coronary sinus is present. The coronary sinus can be enlarged in three circumstances: (1) defects in which there is anomalous venous drainage to the coronary sinus (i.e., persistent left superior vena cava, total anomalous pulmonary venous return to the coronary sinus); (2) defects in which right atrial pressure is high, leading to passive congestion of flow in the coronary sinus (i.e., tricuspid atresia), and (3) defects with increased left main coronary artery blood flow and increased coronary sinus return (i.e., severe left ventricular hypertrophy caused by systemic hypertension). The coronary sinus that is enlarged because of anomalous drainage is more markedly dilated than the coronary sinus that is enlarged because of the latter two conditions.

The enlarged coronary sinus can be seen in cross-section in the parasternal long-axis view as a circular structure lying just superior to the posterior mitral valve leaflet in the atrioventricular groove (Fig 10–22).[56, 57] In the normal patient, the circular coronary sinus is small and barely visible in this view. In patients with a persistent left su-

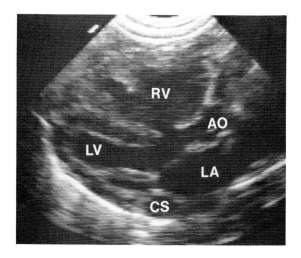

FIG 10–22.
Parasternal long-axis view from a patient with a large ventricular septal defect and a persistent left superior vena cava draining to the coronary sinus (CS). In the long-axis view, the CS is imaged in cross-section as it courses from left to right in the atrioventricular groove just above the mitral valve. AO = aorta; LA = left atrium; LV = left ventricle; RV = right ventricle.

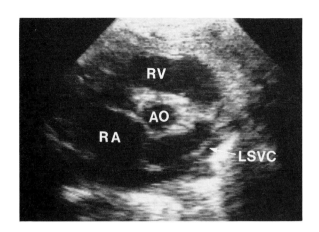

FIG 10–23.
Parasternal short-axis view demonstrating a persistent left superior vena cava (LSVC) draining to the coronary sinus. The coronary sinus and LSVC are seen in longitudinal section in the atrioventricular groove. AO = aorta; RA = right atrium; RV = right ventricle.

perior vena cava to the coronary sinus, the enlarged coronary sinus is extremely visible in this plane. The enlarged coronary sinus lies in the atrioventricular groove, within or anterior to the posterior pericardial echo. This feature helps distinguish the enlarged coronary sinus from the pulmonary veins or descending thoracic aorta, both of which lie posterior to the pericardial echo.

The enlarged coronary sinus can be seen in the parasternal short-axis view at the level of the anterior mitral valve leaflet and just below the standard short-axis plane through the aorta.[56] In this view, the enlarged coronary sinus appears as a crescent-shaped structure posterior to the left ventricle and continuous with the right atrium (Fig 10–23). This appearance occurs because the coronary sinus is sectioned longitudinally as it encircles the heart in the atrioventricular groove. Care should be taken not to mistake the enlarged coronary sinus in this view for a posterior pericardial effusion. Pericardial effusions are not continuous with the right atrium and are usually seen inferior to the level of the anterior mitral valve leaflet.

In the apical and subcostal four-chamber views, the enlarged coronary sinus appears as an oval-shaped structure along the lateral border of the left atrium (Fig 10–24). With posterior angulation of the transducer in the four-chamber views, the enlarged coronary sinus can be seen along its entire length to its ostium in the right atrium (Fig 10–25). In this angled four-chamber view, care must be taken not to mistake the ostium of the coronary sinus for a primum atrial septal defect. The coronary sinus ostium is seen in a plane posterior to the atrioventricular valves, while the primum atrial septum is seen in the plane of the atrioventricular valves.

The persistent left superior vena cava can be imaged directly from the suprasternal views. If the transducer is tilted leftward from the standard suprasternal long-axis view, the left superior vena cava can be seen descending in front and to the left of the aortic arch and pulmonary

hilum toward the atrioventricular groove (Fig 10–26). In some cases, the left superior vena cava and the entire coronary sinus can be imaged from this projection. With slight leftward rotation of the transducer in the suprasternal short-axis view, the left superior vena cava can be seen descending to the left of the transverse aorta. The suprasternal short-axis view is also especially useful for determining if a right superior vena cava is present and, if so, whether the two superior venae cavae communicate by way of a bridging vein. Often, if two superior venae cavae are present and of equal size, the communciating vein is absent or poorly developed. In these cases, no communicating or

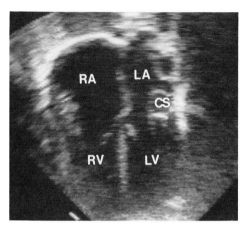

FIG 10–24.
Apical four-chamber view from a patient with a persistent left superior vena cava draining to the coronary sinus (CS), seen situated along the left lateral wall of the left atrium (LA). LV = left ventricle; RA = right atrium; RV = right ventricle.

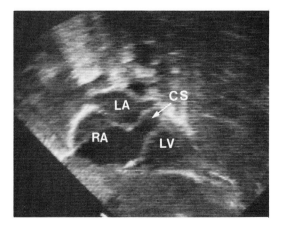

FIG 10–25.
Subcostal four-chamber view with the plane of sound tilted posteriorly to image the coronary sinus (CS). The CS is enlarged because a persistent left superior vena cava is present. LA = left atrium; LV = left ventricle; RA = right atrium.

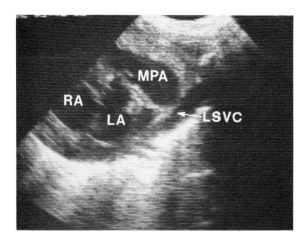

FIG 10–26.
Suprasternal long-axis view, with the plane of sound tilted to the left, in a patient with persistent left superior vena cava (LSVC) draining to the coronary sinus. In this view, the LSVC drains to the left and in front of the aortic arch and pulmonary hilum as it courses toward the atrioventricular groove. The entire coronary sinus and its drainage into the right atrium (RA) can also be seen. LA = left atrium; MPA = main pulmonary artery.

innominate vein is seen in cross-section anterior to the innominate artery and superior to the aortic arch in the suprasternal long-axis view. Also, no venous structure is seen in the suprasternal short-axis view superior to the transverse aorta. When attempting to visualize the communicating vein with suprasternal notch echocardiography, care must be taken to use a transducer with excellent near-field resolution and not to obliterate the vein by pushing down on the transducer in the suprasternal notch. Often, the right superior vena cava is absent or too small to be visualized in the suprasternal short-axis view (Fig 10–27). In these cases, the innominate vein is well developed and the systemic veins appear to be the mirror image of normal in the suprasternal short-axis view. The right innominate vein courses from right to left above the aortic arch to join the left innominate vein along the left side of the aortic arch.

The persistent left superior vena cava can also be imaged in the parasternal short-axis view at the base of the heart (see Fig 10–23). With the transducer tilted superiorly toward the pulmonary artery bifurcation, the left superior vena cava is seen coursing anterior to the main pulmonary artery toward the atrioventricular sulcus.

Pulsed and color-flow Doppler can be used to confirm the diagnosis of a persistent left superior vena cava. If the structure in question is a left superior vena cava, a venous flow pattern (low-velocity, biphasic flow) with flow directed toward the heart (away from the transducer in the suprasternal views) can be recorded. If Doppler examination reveals a venous flow pattern with flow directed away from the heart, the abnormal structure does not represent a persistent left superior vena cava. Vessels that resemble a persistent left superior vena cava but have venous flow

directed away from the heart on Doppler examination occur primarily in two situations. First, infants with total anomalous pulmonary venous return through the left vertical vein to the innominate vein to the right superior vena cava have a left vertical vein that resembles a left superior vena cava. This structure connects the pulmonary venous confluence to the innominate vein and ultimately the right superior vena cava and, on Doppler examination, has a venous flow pattern with flow directed away from the heart. Second, some infants with mitral atresia and intact atrial septum have a levoatrial cardinal vein that resembles a left superior vena cava and connects the left atrium to the innominate vein and right superior vena cava. In these children as well, Doppler examination of the levoatrial cardinal vein shows venous flow directed away from the heart.

If for some reason the left superior vena cava cannot be imaged directly (i.e., inadequate suprasternal views) and the patient has an enlarged coronary sinus, the presence of a left superior vena cava draining to the coronary sinus can be confirmed by left arm vein contrast injections. Following a left arm vein injection, contrast echoes are seen first in the coronary sinus and, subsequently, in the right atrium and right ventricle (see Figure 3–51).

Persistent Left Superior Vena Cava Draining to the Coronary Sinus With a Defect in the Wall of the Coronary Sinus

Patients with a persistent left superior vena cava draining to the coronary sinus and a defect in the wall between the left atrium and coronary sinus have the same two-dimensional echocardiographic features as patients with-

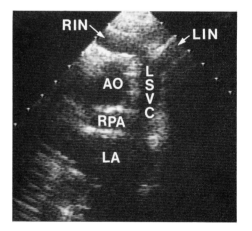

FIG 10–27.
Suprasternal short-axis view from a patient with a persistent left superior vena cava (LSVC) draining to the coronary sinus and absent right superior vena cava. The course of the innominate veins is a mirror image of normal. The right innominate vein (RIN) courses from right to left above the aortic arch (AO) to join the left innominate vein (LIN) along the left side of the aortic arch. From there, the LSVC descends on the left of the AO toward the coronary sinus. LA = left atrium; RPA = right pulmonary artery.

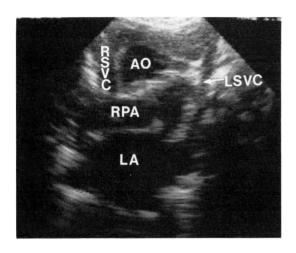

FIG 10–28.
Suprasternal short-axis view from a patient with a persistent left superior vena cava (LSVC) draining to the left atrium (LA). The LSVC descends alongside the aorta (AO) and terminates in the roof of the LA between the left upper pulmonary vein and the left atrial appendage. RPA = right pulmonary artery; RSVC = right superior vena cava.

out a defect in the wall of the coronary sinus. If a high index of suspicion exists for the presence of this defect, it may be possible to image directly the defect in the wall of the coronary sinus. Depending on the relative pressures in the two atria, either right-to-left or left-to-right shunting can occur across the defect in the wall between the left atrium and coronary sinus. Pulsed and color-flow Doppler may be useful for detecting these abnormal shunts. Also, contrast echocardiography may show contrast echoes filling the coronary sinus and left atrium nearly simultaneously.

Persistent Left Superior Vena Cava Draining to the Left Atrium

In this defect, the persistent left superior vena cava descends in front of the aorta and terminates in the roof of the left atrium between the left upper pulmonary vein and the left atrial appendage. The connection of the left superior vena cava to the left atrium can be seen in suprasternal and subcostal views (Figs 10–28 and 10–29). This type of defect is invariably associated with other congenital cardiac defects (i.e., atrial septal defects, atrioventricular septal defects, patent ductus arteriosus, tetralogy of Fallot, dextrocardia, etc.).

Persistent Left Superior Vena Cava Draining to the Left Pulmonary Vein

In this defect, the left superior vena cava drains to the origin of the left pulmonary veins rather than directly to the left atrium. This defect can be diagnosed if the connection to the pulmonary veins occurs near their communication with the left atrium. If the connection to the pulmonary veins occurs farther out in the hilum of the left

lung, direct visualization of the defect may be obscured by the surrounding lung tissue.

Interrupted Inferior Vena Cava

Portions of the normal right-sided inferior vena cava may be absent or may have anomalous connections. A large variety of inferior vena cava anomalies have been reported. This section will review the echocardiographic features of the most common inferior vena cava defect — interruption of a segment of the inferior vena cava.

Azygous Continuation of the Inferior Vena Cava

In azygous continuation of the inferior vena cava, the intrathoracic segment of the inferior vena cava connecting the hepatic veins and abdominal portion of the inferior vena cava to the right atrium is absent. Instead, the hepatic veins drain separately or by way of a common hepatic vein directly to the right atrium. The abdominal portion of the inferior vena cava is present, enters the right chest, and continues as the azygous vein which connects posteriorly to the right superior vena cava.

On the subcostal sagittal view in the abdomen, the hepatic veins are seen entering the right atrium and no continuity can be seen from the hepatic veins to an abdominal inferior vena cava (Fig 10–30).[58] The subcostal cross-sectional views of the lower abdomen show a large vessel posterior and to the right of the spine. This vessel represents the abdominal portion of the right inferior vena cava. This vessel enters the right chest as the azygous vein, which can often be seen in the subcostal sagittal view (Fig 10–31).

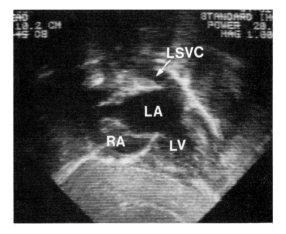

FIG 10–29.
Subcostal four-chamber view from the same patient as in Figure 10–28. The persistent left superior vena cava (LSVC) can be seen draining to the roof of the left atrium (LA). LV = left ventricle; RA = right atrium.

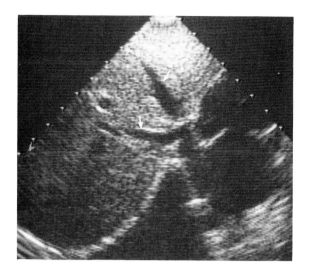

FIG 10–30.
Subcostal sagittal view in the abdomen from a patient with interrupted inferior vena cava. The hepatic veins *(arrows)* are seen entering the right atrium; no continuity can be seen from the hepatic veins to an abdominal inferior vena cava.

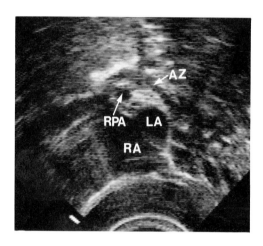

FIG 10–31.
Subcostal sagittal view from a patient with interrupted inferior vena cava and azygous (AZ) continuation of the inferior vena cava. A very large AZ vein can be seen entering the posterior side of the superior vena cava. LA = left atrium; RA = right atrium; RPA = right pulmonary artery.

Hemiazygous Continuation of the Inferior Vena Cava

In this defect, the abdominal portion of the right inferior vena cava is absent, but the intrathoracic segment connecting the hepatic veins to the right atrium is present. Blood from the lower body returns to the heart by way of a left-sided inferior vena cava which can drain directly to the left atrium, to the left superior vena cava, or to the coronary sinus.

As in the previous defect, subcostal sagittal views in the abdomen show the hepatic veins draining to the right atrium with no continuity to a right-sided abdominal inferior vena cava. The subcostal short-axis view of the lower abdomen shows the posterior and leftward lower inferior vena cava (Fig 10–32). In the subcostal sagittal views, this vessel is located slightly to the left of the descending aorta in the abdomen (Fig 10–33). By tilting the transducer cra-

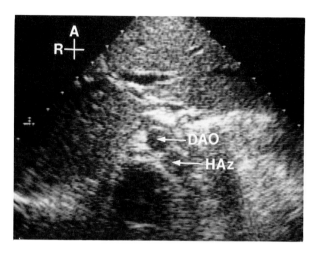

FIG 10–32.
Subcostal short-axis view of the lower abdomen in a patient with interrupted inferior vena cava and hemiazygous (HAz) continuation of lower body venous drainage to a left superior vena cava. In the cross-section of the lower abdomen, the descending aorta (DAO) is seen to the left of the spine. Posterior and leftward of the DAO, the HAZ vein is seen. The posterior location is a clue that this vessel is a HAz vein. A = anterior; R = right.

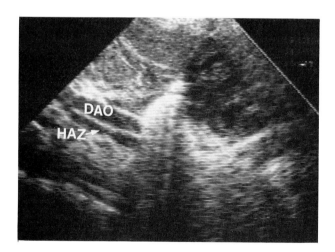

FIG 10–33.
Subcostal sagittal view in the abdomen from a patient with an interrupted inferior vena cava and hemiazygous (HAz) continuation to the coronary sinus. The HAz vein in the abdomen is to the left of the descending aorta (DAO).

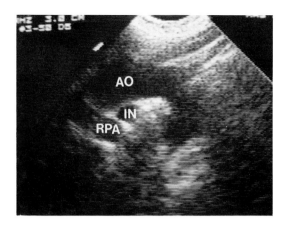

FIG 10–34.
Suprasternal long-axis view from a patient with anomalous course of the left innominate vein (IN) underneath the aortic arch (AO). The IN vein is seen superior to the right pulmonary artery (RPA).

nially, this vessel can be traced to its entry in the left chest. In rare instances, the left-sided inferior vena cava crosses the midline at the level of the diaphragm and continues in the right chest as the azygous vein.[55]

Anomalous Course of the Innominate Vein

Anomalous course of the left innominate vein beneath the aortic arch is a rare defect which is encountered infrequently and usually as an incidental finding at the time of postmortem examination. Suprasternal notch echocardiography provides a technique for direct visualization of the size, connections, and course of the left innominate vein.

In the suprasternal long-axis view, the left innominate vein is seen in cross-section under the aortic arch superior to the right pulmonary artery (Fig 10–34). In the suprasternal short-axis view, the left innominate vein is seen in longitudinal section below the transverse aorta and above the right pulmonary artery (Fig 10–35). By tilting the transducer toward the patient's left side, the innominate vein can be imaged coursing toward the left arm. By tilting the transducer toward the patient's right side, the innominate vein can be followed to its insertion in the lowermost portion of the superior vena cava. Doppler examination of the innominate vein shows a venous flow pattern directed away from the transducer.[59]

We have seen this defect frequently in the setting of a right aortic arch or an outlet ventricular septal defect and severe pulmonary stenosis (i.e., tetralogy of Fallot).

Anomalous course of the left innominate vein has not been reported to cause cardiac symptoms. The importance of recognizing this defect is to prevent mistakenly identifying the innominate vein as another cardiac structure. Because the innominate vein in this defect is located beneath the aortic arch, it is most likely to be mistakenly identified as the right pulmonary artery. Hence, the potential exists for the echocardiographer to measure the

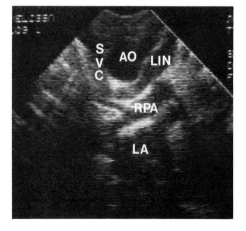

FIG 10–35.
Suprasternal short-axis view from a patient with anomalous drainage of the left innominate vein (LIN) underneath the aortic arch (AO). The LIN can be seen under the AO and superior to the right pulmonary artery (RPA). The LIN drains to the lowermost portion of the superior vena cava (SVC). LA = left atrium.

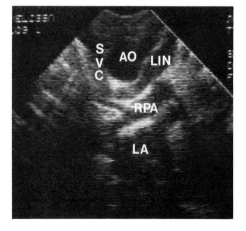

wrong vessel and to report an erroneous right pulmonary artery size; an even more serious potential exists for the cardiac surgeon to identify the wrong vessel as the right pulmonary artery. For example, when performing a Blalock-Taussig shunt procedure, the surgeon might look under the aortic arch for the right pulmonary artery, see the anomalous vessel carrying desaturated blood beneath the arch, and mistake it for the right pulmonary artery. The two-dimensional echocardiographic diagnosis of anomalous course of the left innominate vein can be made only if the suprasternal views are routinely included as a part of the echocardiographic examination and the echocardiographer is aware of the existence of the anomaly.[59]

ABNORMALITIES OF PULMONARY VENOUS RETURN

Anomalous pulmonary venous return is a group of abnormalities in which one or more pulmonary veins drain into the systemic venous return. There are innumerable variations in this group of anomalies; in this section, however, we will review the echocardiographic features of the most common types of anomalous pulmonary venous return found in patients with situs solitus. The pulmonary venous anomalies associated with situs ambiguus will be discussed in Chapter 14. For the sake of clarity, partial anomalous pulmonary venous return will be used to describe conditions in which one or two pulmonary veins drain abnormally; total anomalous pulmonary venous return will refer to conditions in which all four pulmonary veins drain abnormally.

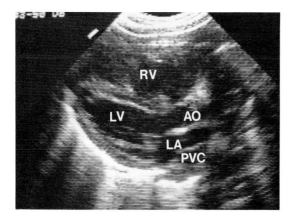

FIG 10–36.
Parasternal long-axis view from an infant with total anomalous pulmonary venous return to the coronary sinus. The pulmonary veins join to form a pulmonary venous confluence (PVC) that lies posterior and separated from the left atrium (LA). AO = aorta; LV = left ventricle; RV = right ventricle.

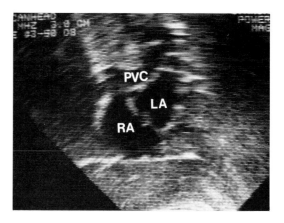

FIG 10–37.
Subcostal four-chamber view from an infant with the supracardiac form of total anomalous pulmonary venous return. The four individual pulmonary veins can be seen joining to form a pulmonary venous confluence (PVC), which lies superior to the left atrium (LA). RA = right atrium.

Total Anomalous Pulmonary Venous Return

Total anomalous pulmonary venous return is a condition in which the pulmonary veins join to form a confluence that drains back to the right atrium rather than the left atrium. Infants with total anomalous pulmonary venous return are usually cyanotic and in severe respiratory distress, and this defect can be difficult to differentiate clinically from persistent pulmonary artery hypertension or pulmonary disease in the newborn. The M-mode and two-dimensional echocardiograms in all three conditions show four normally positioned cardiac valves and chambers, two normally positioned great arteries, and right heart dominance. On the two-dimensional echocardiogram, total anomalous pulmonary venous return can be diagnosed by identifying the pulmonary venous confluence that lies posterior to and separated from the left atrium (Fig 10–36).[60–65] Usually, the individual pulmonary veins can be seen connecting to the pulmonary venous confluence (Fig 10–37) and the pulmonary venous confluence can be followed to the final site of drainage into the systemic venous return.[63]

In the intracardiac form of total anomalous pulmonary venous return (i.e., drainage to the coronary sinus or directly to the right atrium), the pulmonary venous confluence is directly posterior to the left atrium and, thus, is well visualized in the parasternal, apical, and subcostal views (see Fig 10–36).[56] In the supracardiac form of total anomalous pulmonary venous return (i.e., drainage to the superior vena cava directly or by way of a left vertical vein), the pulmonary venous confluence is usually superior to the left atrium and, thus, is best visualized in the suprasternal short-axis and subcostal sagittal views (Fig 10–38).[2, 66] In infracardiac total anomalous pulmonary venous return (i.e., to the hepatic portal system or the hepatic veins), the pulmonary veins usually converge like the

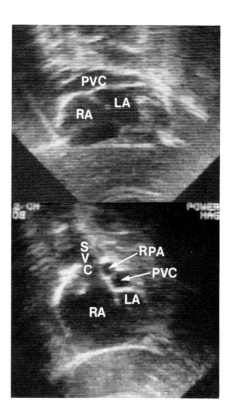

FIG 10–38.
Subcostal four-chamber (top) and sagittal (bottom) views from an infant with total anomalous pulmonary venous return to the left vertical vein to the innominate vein to the right superior vena cava (SVC). In the subcostal four-chamber view, the pulmonary venous confluence (PVC) can be seen superior to the left atrium (LA). In the subcostal sagittal view, the PVC is situated superior to the LA and inferior to the right pulmonary artery (RPA). A very dilated SVC can be seen. RA = right atrium.

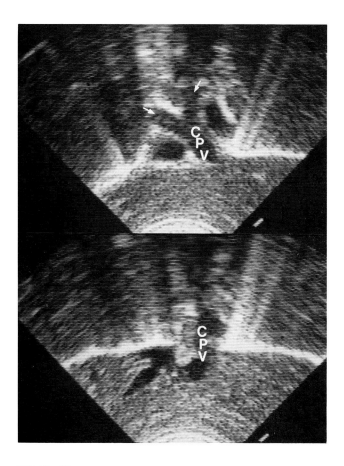

FIG 10–39.
Subcostal coronal views from the abdomen of an infant with infracardiac total anomalous pulmonary venous return. The *top frame* was obtained by tilting the transducer posterior to the left atrium to visualize the pulmonary veins *(arrows)*. The *bottom frame* was obtained by tilting the plane of sound even more posteriorly to follow the venous drainage below the diaphragm. In this instance, the pulmonary veins converged like the branches of a tree just above the diaphragm. A pulmonary venous confluence did not exist as a distinct separate chamber. Instead, a common pulmonary vein (CPV) drained through the diaphragm and inserted into the left hepatic vein.

branches of a tree just above the diaphragm (Fig 10–39); therefore, the pulmonary venous confluence is often small and inferior to the left atrium or may not exist as a distinct, separate chamber. In infracardiac total anomalous pulmonary venous return, the pulmonary venous confluence is usually best visualized from apical four-chamber or subcostal views.[64, 67]

Because of its size, shape, and posterior location, the pulmonary venous confluence can sometimes be difficult to image directly. Also, because of the technical limitations associated with examining small infants with respiratory distress, it can be difficult to visualize with certainty the wall separating the true left atrium from the common pulmonary venous chamber. Thus, imaging of the pulmonary veins behind the left atrium does not prove that these veins drain to the left atrium. They may, in fact, be separated

from the left atrium by the anterior wall of the pulmonary venous confluence. Without the use of high-frequency transducers and the ability to focus the beam in the far field, the wall of the pulmonary venous confluence might not be visualized (Fig 10–40).

Usually, the pulmonary venous confluence can be followed to the final site of drainage in the right atrium. In total anomalous pulmonary venous return to the coronary sinus, the pulmonary venous confluence can be seen connecting to an enlarged coronary sinus in the parasternal long- and short-axis views (Figs 10–41 and 10–42). Evidence of an enlarged coronary sinus can also be seen in other echocardiographic planes.[56, 63] In total anomalous pulmonary venous return to the superior vena cava by way of the left vertical vein and innominate vein, the entire anomalous supracardiac connection can be seen in the suprasternal short-axis view (Fig 10–43). In this view, the anomalous pulmonary venous connection resembles a large vascular collar surrounding the transverse aorta. In the suprasternal long-axis view (Fig 10–44), the markedly dilated innominate vein can be seen in cross-section anterior to the innominate artery.[2, 63, 66] In some infants, the entire anomalous connection can be seen from the subcostal four-chamber view of the left ventricular outflow tract. In infracardiac or infradiaphragmatic total anomalous pulmonary venous return, a common pulmonary vein exits the pulmonary venous confluence, passes through the diaphragm (usually anterior to the aorta), and drains into a systemic vein in the abdomen. Some common sites of drainage include the hepatic portal system and the left hepatic vein. In the subcostal sagittal view in the abdomen, the common pulmonary vein is usually imaged in a plane to the left of the inferior vena cava. This vessel is usually seen anterior to the descending aorta and can be traced back through the diaphragm to its origin from the pul-

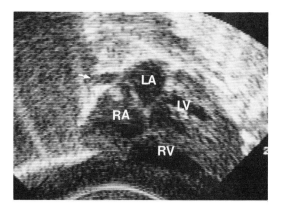

FIG 10–40.
Subcostal four-chamber view from an infant with total anomalous pulmonary venous return. The right upper pulmonary vein is imaged behind the left atrium (LA). Imaging of the pulmonary vein adjacent to the left atrium does not prove that it drains to the left atrium. In this case, the pulmonary veins drained to a confluence and the wall separating the pulmonary veins from the LA was difficult to image. LV = left ventricle; RA = right atrium; RV = right ventricle.

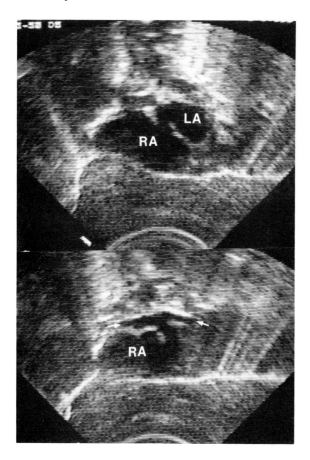

FIG 10–41.
Subcostal four-chamber views from an infant with total anomalous pulmonary venous return to the coronary sinus. In the *top frame,* the plane of sound has been positioned to image the left atrium (LA) and right atrium (RA). No pulmonary veins can be seen draining to the LA, and the RA is very dilated. A secundum atrial septal defect is present. In the *bottom frame,* the plane of sound has been tilted posteriorly to visualize the pulmonary veins *(arrows).* The pulmonary veins drain by way of an enlarged coronary sinus to the RA.

monary venous confluence (Fig 10–45). Often, three large vessels (the inferior vena cava, descending aorta, and common pulmonary vein) are seen in cross-section in the subcostal short-axis view.[64, 67]

In infants with total anomalous pulmonary venous return, pulsed and/or color-flow Doppler examination can be very useful for confirming the presence of pulmonary venous flow in any anomalous structure believed to be the common pulmonary vein on the two-dimensional echocardiogram.[67, 68] For example, Figure 10–46 is a subcostal sagittal view of the descending aorta of an infant with total anomalous pulmonary venous return to the hepatic-portal system. A vascular structure thought to represent the common pulmonary vein was imaged anterior to the descending aorta. The Doppler examination of this structure shows a venous flow pattern with the direction of flow toward the transducer. Therefore, the vascular structure cannot represent a systemic vein in the abdomen because systemic

venous flow would be directed toward the heart and away from the transducer in this view. Anomalous pulmonary venous drainage below the diaphragm gives rise to flow signals directed away from the heart and toward the transducer. Likewise, Doppler examination of the left vertical vein shows venous flow signals directed away from the heart (Fig 10–47), while systemic veins in the thorax would have flow directed toward the heart. Thus, the Doppler examination is very useful for confirming that the unusual structure seen on the two-dimensional echocardiogram is indeed the common pulmonary vein and not some other anomalous systemic vein (in which flow would be directed toward the heart) (Plate 41).

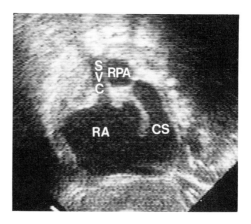

FIG 10–42.
Subcostal sagittal view from the same patient as in Figure 10–41. The pulmonary veins drain by a very enlarged coronary sinus (CS) to the right atrium (RA). RPA = right pulmonary artery; SVC = superior vena cava.

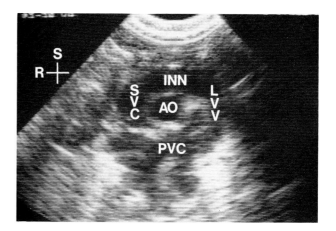

FIG 10–43.
Suprasternal short-axis view from an infant with total anomalous pulmonary venous return to the left vertical vein (LVV) to the innominate vein (INN) to the right superior vena cava (SVC). The pulmonary venous confluence (PVC) can be seen underneath the aortic (AO) arch. R = right; S = superior.

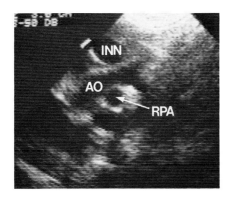

FIG 10–44.
Suprasternal long-axis view from an infant with total anomalous pulmonary venous return to the left vertical vein to the innominate (INN) vein to the superior vena cava. In this view, a markedly dilated INN vein can be seen superior to the aortic (AO) arch. Few diseases cause this degree of dilatation of the INN vein. RPA = right pulmonary artery.

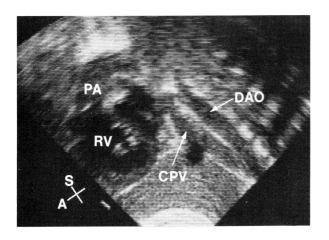

FIG 10–45.
Subcostal sagittal view from a patient with infracardiac total anomalous pulmonary venous return. The pulmonary veins drain by a common pulmonary vein (CPV) that passes through the diaphragm anterior to the descending aorta (DAO). A = anterior; PA = pulmonary artery; RV = right ventricle; S = superior.

In infants with total anomalous pulmonary venous return, Doppler echocardiography provides additional useful information. For example, children with this defect have obligatory right-to-left atrial shunting which can be detected by pulsed or color-flow Doppler. In addition, the Doppler examination often shows evidence of a patent ductus arteriosus that shunts predominately right to left because of elevated pulmonary vascular resistances. Finally, Doppler echocardiography can be used to detect obstruction to pulmonary venous flow (Fig 10–48 and Plate 42).[68] In supracardiac total anomalous pulmonary venous return, the left vertical vein can become obstructed as it ascends

between the left pulmonary artery and the left mainstem bronchus. Sampling of flow velocities in the left vertical vein superior to the left pulmonary artery shows high-velocity (>2 m/sec), continuous disturbed flow signals when significant obstruction is present. In supracardiac total anomalous pulmonary venous return, obstruction occurs less frequently at the junction of the innominate vein and superior vena cava and at the junction of the superior vena cava and right atrium. The entire anomalous vascular channel should be interrogated with Doppler echocardiography to exclude obstruction to pulmonary venous return. In in-

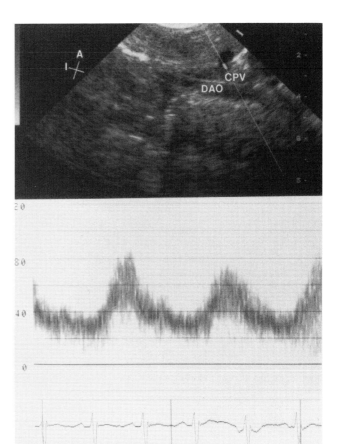

FIG 10–46.
Pulsed Doppler recording from the common pulmonary vein (CPV) of an infant with total anomalous pulmonary venous return below the diaphragm. The freeze-frame image, *top,* shows the location of the sample volume in the CPV at the time of the Doppler recording. The Doppler tracing, *bottom,* shows a venous pattern of flow signals above the baseline throughout systole and diastole. This indicates forward flow down the CPV away from the heart and toward the transducer which was located in the abdomen. Note the high peak velocities of the venous flow signals, suggesting obstruction to forward flow in the CPV. A = anterior; DAO = descending aorta; I = inferior. (From Snider AR: Two-dimensional and Doppler echocardiographic evaluation of heart disease in the neonate and fetus. *Clin in Perinatol* 1988; 15:553. Used by permission.)

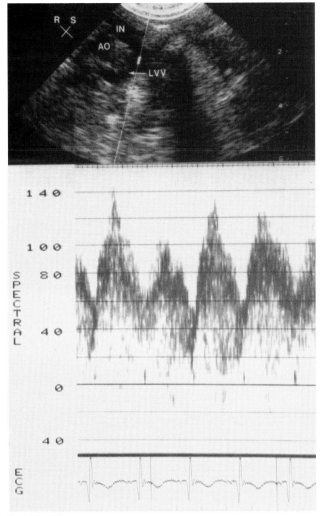

FIG 10–47.
Doppler spectral recording *(bottom)* from the left vertical vein (LVV) of a patient with a supracardiac form of total anomalous pulmonary venous return. The freeze-frame image *(top)* shows the position of the sample volume in the LVV at the time of the Doppler tracing. The Doppler recording shows continuous forward flow above the baseline and toward the transducer throughout systole and diastole. This flow signal indicates that the direction of flow in the LVV is toward the transducer and away from the heart. This type of flow signal distinguishes a persistent left superior vena cava that is draining to the heart from total anomalous pulmonary venous return and an LVV draining away from the heart. AO = aorta; IN = innominate vein; R = right; S = superior.

tracardiac total anomalous pulmonary venous return, obstruction is uncommon. Doppler echocardiographic examination is difficult in this defect because of the absence of a long common pulmonary vein to interrogate and the difficulty in aligning the Doppler beam with flow in the pulmonary venous confluence. In infracardiac total anomalous pulmonary venous return, the entire common pulmonary vein should be examined with Doppler echocardiography for evidence of obstruction. Obstruction in this defect often occurs where the common pulmonary vein passes through the diaphragm or where this vein connects

to the systemic vein in the abdomen.

On the M-mode and two-dimensional echocardiogram, children with total anomalous pulmonary venous return usually have right atrial, right ventricular, and main pulmonary artery enlargement. The right ventricle is hypertrophic and there is echocardiographic evidence of pulmonary artery hypertension. Ventricular septal motion is usually flat or frankly paradoxical. The left atrium and left ventricle are normal or slightly decreased in size.

Rarely, "mixed" forms of total anomalous pulmonary venous return occur in which the pulmonary veins drain

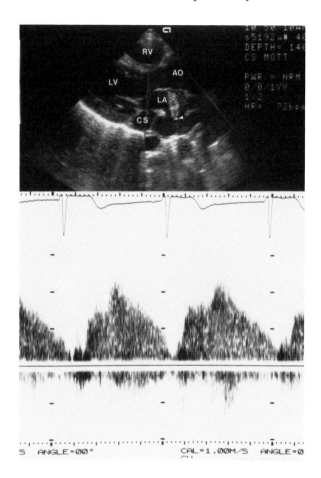

FIG 10–48.
Doppler spectral recording from a patient who has had repair of total anomalous pulmonary venous return above the diaphragm. Following repair, this patient developed pulmonary venous obstruction involving the right upper and right lower pulmonary veins. The parasternal long-axis view *(top)* was obtained from a Doppler color-flow mapping examination. The jet from the obstructed pulmonary vein is shown in shades of gray. The jet was used to align the continuous-wave Doppler beam *(arrow)* parallel with the jet flow through the obstructed pulmonary vein. The Doppler tracing *(bottom)* shows a nearly continuous flow throughout systole and diastole with a very high peak velocity (greater than 2 m/sec). This flow signal indicates pulmonary venous obstruction. Because this patient also has interrupted inferior vena cava with hemiazygous drainage to the coronary sinus (CS), the CS is very enlarged. AO = aorta; LA = left atrium; LV = left ventricle; RV = right ventricle.

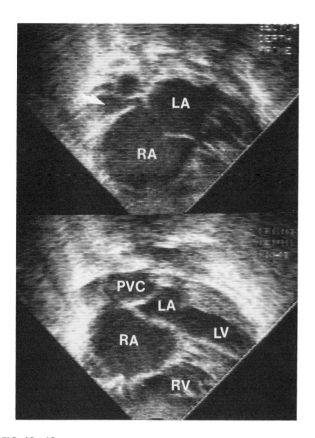

FIG 10–49.
Apical four-chamber views from a patient with a mixed form of anomalous pulmonary venous drainage. In the *top frame*, the plane of sound has been tilted far posteriorly. The right upper pulmonary vein *(arrow)* is seen draining to the right atrium (RA). In the *bottom frame*, the plane of sound has been tilted more anteriorly. The remaining three pulmonary veins are seen draining to a pulmonary venous confluence (PVC) which is separate from the left atrium (LA). LV = left ventricle; RV = right ventricle.

to two separate systemic venous sites. In any child with total anomalous pulmonary venous return, attempts should be made using multiple two-dimensional echocardiographic views and Doppler color-flow mapping to visualize the connection of all four pulmonary veins to the confluence. If only two pulmonary veins can be seen draining to the pulmonary venous confluence, one should be suspicious that a "mixed" form of the disease is present (Fig 10–49).

Partial Anomalous Pulmonary Venous Return

Partial anomalous pulmonary venous return is a defect in which one or two pulmonary veins drain anomalously to the systemic venous return. This condition is frequently associated with atrial septal defects (of any type) and persistent left superior vena cava. Although any pulmonary vein or combination of pulmonary veins can drain anomalously to any systemic venous site, anomalous drainage of the right pulmonary veins is more common. The echo-

cardiographic detection of partial anomalous pulmonary venous return requires a high index of suspicion that this defect is present and a thorough attempt to visualize the connections of all four pulmonary veins on the two-dimensional echocardiogram. The use of color-flow mapping has greatly enhanced the ability to locate all the pulmonary veins.

One very common form of partial anomalous pulmonary venous return is anomalous drainage of the right upper pulmonary vein to the right side of the atrial septum or to the base of the superior vena cava in patients with sinus venosus atrial septal defect (Fig 10–50). As mentioned above, however, partial anomalous pulmonary venous return can occur with any type of atrial septal defect (Fig 10–51).

If only one pulmonary vein drains to the right atrium, the M-mode and two-dimensional echocardiogram shows no evidence of right atrial or right ventricular volume overload from the anomalous pulmonary venous drainage. If two pulmonary veins drain anomalously, mild right heart dilatation may be present.

AORTIC ARCH ANOMALIES

Anomalies of the aortic arch may appear either in isolation or in conjunction with other intracardiac defects. This section will examine aortic arch anomalies as if they occur in isolation, with the awareness that intracardiac defects often coexist. The three general classes of abnormalities to be discussed are (1) abnormal formation of the aortic arch typified by mirror image right aortic arches, vascular rings, and cervical aortic arches; (2) coarctation of the aorta and, in its most severe form, interruption of the aortic arch; and (3) aortic aneurysms.

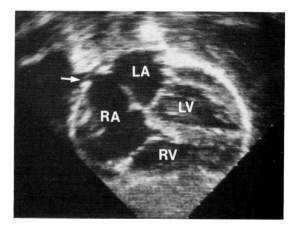

FIG 10–50.
Subcostal four-chamber view from a patient with a sinus venosus atrial septal defect and anomalous drainage of the right upper pulmonary vein *(arrow)* to the right atrium (RA). LA = left atrium; LV = left ventricle; RV = right ventricle.

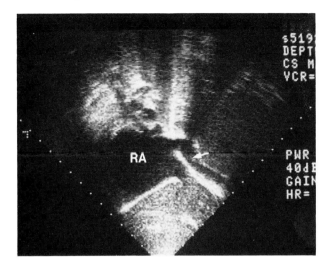

FIG 10–51.
Subcostal sagittal view from a patient with anomalous drainage of the right lower pulmonary vein *(arrow)* to the right atrium (RA) and a secundum atrial septal defect. The right lower pulmonary vein enters the posterior wall of the right atrium just superior to the orifice of the inferior vena cava.

Abnormal Formation of the Aortic Arch

The aortic arch is imaged predominantly from the suprasternal notch approach.[2, 3] The parasternal long-axis view shows the proximal portion of the ascending aorta and a cross-section of descending aorta as it passes posterior to the left atrium; nevertheless, it gives little information about the morphology of the arch itself. The parasternal short-axis view also images only the proximal aorta. Subcostal and apical views may permit imaging of more of the aortic arch, particularly in neonates,[2] but these views usually allow imaging of the arch only to the origin of the first arch vessel. In some patients the entire aortic arch can be imaged from the subcostal views, which may be helpful. In many patients, however, none of these views provides the anatomic information needed to make a definite diagnosis.

From the suprasternal notch, the aortic arch is well imaged with the scan plane passing through its long axis (suprasternal long-axis view) or at an angle perpendicular to the axis of the aortic arch, showing it in cross-section (suprasternal short-axis)[69] as described in Chapter 3. In the patient with a normal left aortic arch, the ascending aorta, transverse aorta, and descending aorta are all seen with the origins of three arch vessels. Beneath the aortic arch is the right pulmonary artery seen in cross-section.

Mirror-image Right Aortic Arch

From an isolated suprasternal long-axis view it is not possible to distinguish between a left aortic arch and a mirror-image right aortic arch. To make this distinction, the scan plane should first be adjusted to best image the aortic arch. From this position, the scan plane can be tilted either to the left or the right to look for the tracheal air

column and tracheal rings.[70] If the scan plane is tilted left to image the tracheal air column, a right aortic arch is present (Fig 10–52). If the scan plane is tilted to the right to find the tracheal air column, a left aortic arch is present. It must be emphasized that this distinction is made by the examiner. A videotape review of the images is not diagnostic. In our practice, an annotation is placed on the recorded image to denote the presence of a right aortic arch.

Turning the transducer 90 degrees permits imaging of the arch in a coronal view—suprasternal short axis view. In the normal situation the ascending aorta is imaged in cross-section, below which is seen the right pulmonary artery traversing from left to right (see Chapter 3). As the scan plane is moved from caudad to cephalad, the ascending aorta is followed superiorly and the first arch ves-

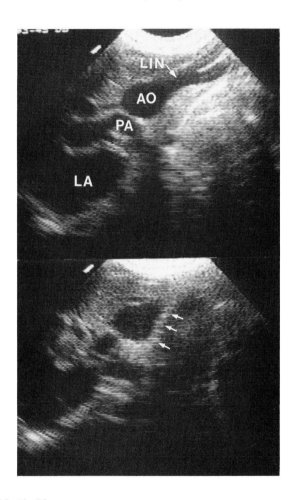

FIG 10–52.
Suprasternal short-axis views from a patient with a right aortic arch. In the *top frame*, the first branch off the aorta (AO) is the left innominate artery (LIN). The bifurcation of the LIN into left common carotid and left subclavian arteries can be seen. When the first branch off the AO is to the left, one should be highly suspicious that a right aortic arch is present. In the *bottom frame*, the plane of sound has been tilted slightly posteriorly and the AO can be seen to the right of the tracheal rings *(arrows)*. This proves the existence of a right aortic arch. LA = left atrium; PA = pulmonary artery.

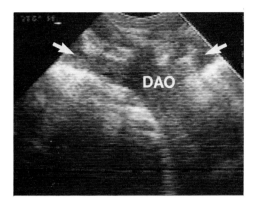

FIG 10–53.
Suprasternal short-axis view with the plane of sound tilted far posteriorly to visualize the descending aorta in a patient with a vascular ring. In this patient, the aorta arched to the right. Following that, the aortic arch was retroesophageal and the descending aorta (DAO) descended to the left in the thorax and abdomen. *Arrows* indicate second and third branches off the arch.

sel is seen to originate.[69, 71] This vessel is important, as it allows confirmation of the diagnosis of a right aortic arch. When a normal left aortic arch is present, this vessel is the right innominate artery which runs rightward and bifurcates into the right carotid and right subclavian arteries. If this first vessel goes leftward, a mirror image right aortic arch is present (see Figure 10–52). If the first vessel is not seen to bifurcate, a vascular anomaly, such as anomalous right subclavian artery with a left aortic arch or a more complex vascular ring with a right aortic arch, may be present. Movement of the scan plane in a more cephalad and posterior position produces an image of the descending aorta along its long axis, but in a plane orthogonal to that obtained in the standard suprasternal long-axis view. This is helpful for determining if the descending aorta crosses from side to side within the thoracic cage or remains on the same side of the spine.

Finally, examination of the abdomen in cross section allows visualization of the descending aorta below the diaphragm to ascertain on which side of the spine it now lies.[71] This permits a complete description of the course of the aorta from the thoracic to the abdominal region.

Vascular Rings

The echocardiographic examination should begin with the suprasternal long-axis view to determine the side of the aortic arch. In the presence of a left aortic arch, an anomalous right subclavian artery is the only vascular ring anomaly that can exist. Definitive diagnosis of a left aortic arch with an anomalous right subclavian artery is made by the discovery of a non-bifurcating first arch vessel in the suprasternal short-axis view.

If a right aortic arch is found, a careful search must be made for a left arch that can be followed to the descending aorta[72, 73] (Fig 10–53). The left arch is usually small or atretic. A left carotid or innominate artery must not be mistaken

for a patent left arch. Doppler flow studies — particularly color Doppler mapping — can aid in this distinction by documenting flow to the descending aorta.[74] As the transverse portion of the right aortic arch turns posteriorly, it will cross behind the trachea and be lost from the echocardiographic view until it emerges from behind the trachea.

The suprasternal short-axis view is next employed to evaluate the origin of the first arch vessel. In the presence of a right aortic arch and a non-bifurcating first arch vessel, this vessel must be a left carotid artery with the left subclavian artery arising anomalously from the descending aorta. Moving posteriorly to image the descending aorta, the left subclavian artery may be seen to arise, coursing leftward.

Careful attention must also be paid to the descending aorta in the region of the ductus arteriosus. In many vascular rings, the presence of the ductus arteriosus is an important element often comprising the left side of the ring. Even when the ductus arteriosus is not patent, it may be an important factor in the symptomatology associated with a vascular ring. Often the ductus arteriosus is seen to originate from a diverticulum off the descending aorta. Even in the presence of only a ductal ligament, the presence of this diverticulum provides important information about the makeup of the vascular ring itself. In summary, the questions to be answered are:

1. Are there bilateral patent arches, or only a right arch?
2. What is the nature of the first arch vessel?
3. Is a patent ductus arteriosus or ductus diverticulum present?

Cervical Aortic Arch

Cervical aortic arches present as pulsatile neck masses and may be identified from the suprasternal long-axis view.[75–78] They course farther cephalad than the normal aortic arch, extending past the suprasternal notch into the neck, and may be either left- or right-sided arches.[76] A true cervical aortic arch must be distinguished from a high thoracic aortic arch that does not extend into the neck. Although this lesion is easily seen from the suprasternal long-axis view, it requires moving the transducer onto the neck over the pulsatile mass to accurately describe the most cephalic extension of the arch.

Other anomalies of the aortic arch, such as buckling of the innominate artery, must also be sought.[79] In this lesion, the innominate artery is elongated, turning back on itself before bifurcating, and must not be mistaken for a non-bifurcating vessel.

Coarctation of the Aorta

Coarctation of the aorta is also best imaged from the suprasternal notch. Certain intracardiac findings suggest the possibility that a coarctation of the aorta may exist before the arch is imaged. Left ventricular outflow obstructive lesions, significant right ventricular hypertrophy without obvious explanation, and absence of pulsations of the descending aorta as imaged from the abdomen all suggest the possibility of a coarctation. The echocardiographic examination using the suprasternal long-axis view provides an image of the entire arch, with the area of coarctation seen near the origin of the left subclavian artery[2, 80] (Figs 10–54 and 10–55). When imaging a coarctation, one must be absolutely certain that the entire aortic arch is imaged, particularly in the region of the origin of the left subclavian artery. Inadequate imaging of this area may often lead to an inappropriate diagnosis. Subcostal views (Fig 10–56) and a high left parasternal view (Fig 10–57) may also be helpful. The coarctation may either be a long-segment narrowing or, more commonly, a short segment obstruction caused by a posterior aortic shelf. In the region of the duc-

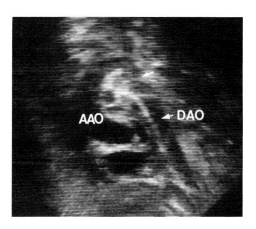

FIG 10–56.
Subcostal long-axis view from an infant with a severe coarctation of the aorta *(arrow)*. A posterior ledge is seen, which is typical of an aortic coarctation. AAO = ascending aorta; DAO = descending aorta.

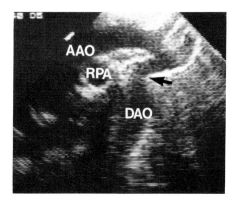

FIG 10–54.
Suprasternal long-axis view from a child with a severe coarctation *(arrow)* of the descending aorta (DAO). There is a prominent posterior ledge in the area of the coarctation. AAO = ascending aorta; RPA = right pulmonary artery.

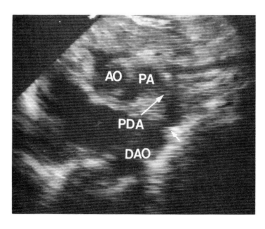

FIG 10–57.
High left parasternal view from an infant with a severe coarctation of the aorta *(arrow)* and a patent ductus arteriosus (PDA). The PDA connects the main pulmonary artery (MPA) to the descending aorta (DAO) in the area of the coarctation. A prominent ledge *(arrow)* is seen opposite the insertion of the PDA. AO = ascending aorta.

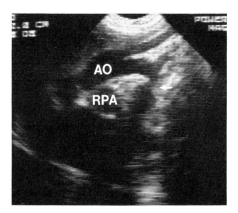

FIG 10–55.
Suprasternal long-axis view from an infant with severe coarctation of the aorta *(arrow)*. Note the marked post-stenotic dilatation of the descending aorta distal to the coarctation. AO = aorta; RPA = right pulmonary artery.

tus arteriosus, an anterior shelf may normally exist just proximal to the aortic origin of the ductus. It is important not to mistake this for a coarctation shelf. In addition, the size of the transverse arch must also be noted as it invariably is somewhat small, particularly in the newborn with severe coarctation (Fig 10–58). The distance from the origin of the left subclavian artery to the coarctation must also be noted.

Doppler flow velocity evaluation of the coarctation is extremely important (Fig 10–59 and Plate 43). Our practice is to begin with color-flow imaging of the descending aorta, looking for turbulent jets in the region suspected of possessing a coarctation. Once such jets are imaged, the continuous-wave Doppler beam is directed into this area for flow velocity recording. Doppler echocardiography of

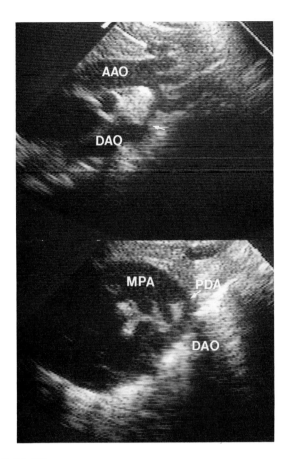

FIG 10–58.
Suprasternal long-axis views from a newborn infant with a severe coarctation of the aorta and a patent ductus arteriosus (PDA). The *top frame* is a standard suprasternal long-axis view through the entire aortic arch. Proximal to the coarctation, the entire aortic isthmus is elongated and hypoplastic. In the *bottom frame,* the plane of sound has been tilted to the left. In this view, the arch formed by the connection of the main pulmonary artery (MPA) and the PDA to the descending aorta (DAO) is seen. AAO = ascending aorta.

coarctation flow shows a high-velocity jet with antegrade flow extending throughout diastole.[81, 82] The magnitude of the peak flow velocity is indicative of the coarctation gradient present (see Fig 10–59). However, when proximal aortic blood flow velocity is high as a result of obstruction, correction for this is necessary before the coarctation gradient can be calculated. The expanded Bernoulli equation described in Chapter 3 must be used. If the proximal velocity is normal, such a correction is not necessary. Using careful imaging techniques and confirmation of the characteristic Doppler flow pattern of coarctations, the diagnosis of coarctation may be made with a high degree of sensitivity and specificity.[80] When a patent ductus arteriosus is present, no gradient may be measured across a coarctation and a normal Doppler flow velocity pattern can be misleading. In this situation, careful imaging alone must be employed to make the correct diagnosis.

The most severe form of coarctation is total interrup-

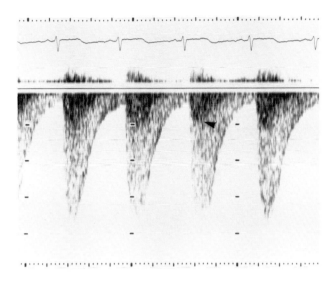

FIG 10–59.
Continuous-wave Doppler examination obtained from the suprasternal notch of a child with a coarctation of the aorta. Flow signals are seen in systole continuing throughout diastole below the baseline, indicating flow away from the transducer. These flow signals arise from blood flow down the descending aorta. The peak velocity of the flow is 3.6 m/sec. Superimposed on the high-velocity flow signals through the coarctation are low-velocity signals *(arrows)* from the descending aorta proximal to the coarctation. These flow signals have a peak velocity of 1 m/sec, which is normal. Because the velocity proximal to the coarctation is normal, the peak gradient across the coarctation can be calculated simply as 4×3.6^2 or 52 mm Hg.

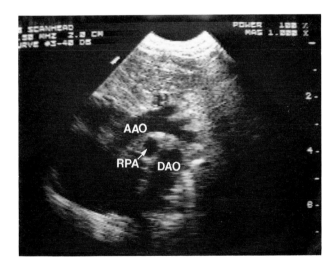

FIG 10–60.
Suprasternal long-axis view from an infant with an interruption of the aortic arch beyond the origin of the left subclavian artery (type A). The vessels to the head and neck arose from the ascending aorta (AAO). DAO = descending aorta; RPA = right pulmonary artery.

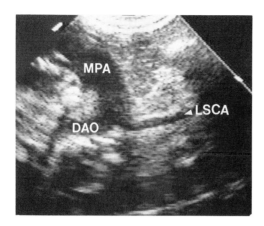

FIG 10–61.
Suprasternal long-axis view with the plane of sound tilted toward the left in a patient with an interruption of the aortic arch between the left common carotid and left subclavian arteries (type B). In this view, the arch formed by the connection of the main pulmonary artery (MPA) to the patent ductus arteriosus to the descending aorta (DAO) is seen. The left subclavian artery (LSCA) can be seen arising from the DAO just opposite the patent ductus arteriosus. This view is particularly useful for identifying which head vessels, if any, arise from the DAO in patients with interruption of the aortic arch.

tion of the aortic arch (Figs 10–60 to 10–62). Such an interruption may be only a short segment, or it may be a long segment with a marked distance between the proximal and distal segments of the aorta. This is also imaged from the suprasternal long-axis approach, showing a relatively small ascending aorta giving rise to at least one arch vessel and a much larger descending aorta with the ductus arteriosus at its proximal end.[83] The arch vessels may originate from either the proximal or distal segments. The most common situation is for the innominate and left carotid arteries to originate from the proximal segment and for the left subclavian artery to arise from the distal segment (Fig 10–61). The interruption may also be between the right carotid artery and the left carotid artery (Fig 10–62) or distal to the left subclavian artery.[84] Caution again should be exercised that the ductus arteriosus connecting the main pulmonary artery to the descending aorta is not mistaken for the true aortic arch (Fig 10–62). This distinction is based upon seeing no arch vessels arise from the main pulmonary artery-ductus arteriosus-descending aorta arch. With adequate patency of the ductus arteriosus, the descending aorta may be normally pulsatile, and one must rely on accurate imaging from the suprasternal notch to define the true ascending aorta. Color-flow mapping may show total absence of high-velocity jets in the descending aorta, provided the ductus arteriosus is adequately patent. Some restriction of the ductus arteriosus may result in high-velocity jets in the descending aorta that can mimic the appearance of coarctation. Adequate imaging is mandatory to distinguish between these two entities.

From a surgical standpoint, total characterization of the interrupted aortic arch with accurate description of the

vessels originating from the proximal and distal segments, together with the degree of separation of the proximal and distal segments, is of paramount importance.

Aneurysms

Aneurysms of the proximal aorta are usually easily recognized from the parasternal long-axis view, the parasternal short-axis view, and the suprasternal long-axis

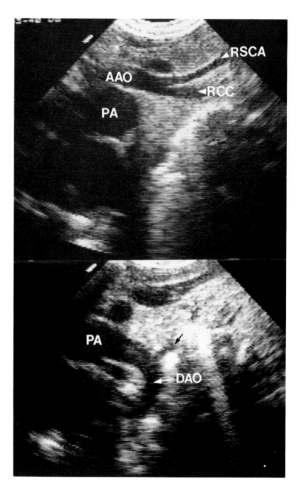

FIG 10–62.
Suprasternal long-axis views from an infant with *d*-transposition of the great arteries, tricuspid atresia, and interruption of the aortic arch. In this infant, the interruption in the aortic arch occurred between the right common carotid (RCC) and left common carotid arteries (type C). This form of interrupted arch is particularly common in children with complex malformations such as tricuspid atresia. In the *top frame*, the right subclavian artery (RSCA) and RCC can be seen arising from the ascending aorta (AAO). The *bottom frame* was obtained by tilting the plane of sound to the left. In this view, the arch formed by the connection of the main pulmonary artery (PA) to the patent ductus arteriosus to the descending aorta (DAO) can be seen. The left common carotid artery *(arrow)* can be seen arising from the DAO. The left subclavian artery was visualized in a slightly different plane.

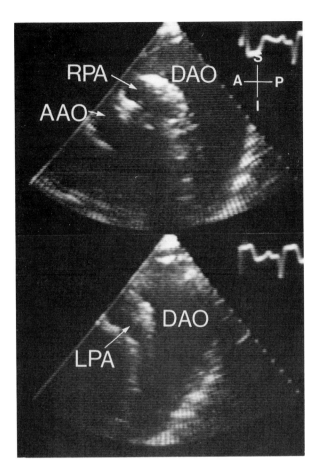

FIG 10–63.
Suprasternal long-axis views from an adolescent with Marfan syndrome and aneurysmal dilatation of the descending aorta (DAO). A = anterior; AAO = ascending aorta; I = inferior; LPA = left pulmonary artery; P = posterior; RPA = right pulmonary artery; S = superior.

view.[85] Marked dilatation of the aortic root, particularly in connective tissue diseases such as Marfan syndrome, is quite evident. Careful measurement of aortic root size is mandatory for serial studies to allow assessment of disease progression. The aortic valve must also be examined, particularly with Doppler echocardiography, to determine if insufficiency exists.

Aneurysms may also occur in the descending aorta (Fig 10–63), particularly at the site of a previous coarctation repair. Such aneurysms may occur either after surgical repair or balloon angioplasty. The aortic arch must be imaged not only in the suprasternal long-axis view but also in the suprasternal coronal plane to allow imaging of lateral wall aneurysms. When a patient has had a subclavian flap angioplasty for repair of coarctation, the incidence of bulges at the site of repair increases. These bulges must be distinguished from true aneurysms by careful measurement of their size and comparison to published normal data.[86–88] Careful note of the aortic diameter must be made to allow for assessment of progression on serial studies. Doppler

color-flow mapping may show some swirling within the aneurysms, or the flow may be quite laminar. Again, imaging is of prime importance for detection of such aneurysms.

When a dissecting aneurysm is suspected, both the false lumen and the communication between the true and false lumen must be identified.[86, 89] Echocardiographic examination from several projections — parasternal long-axis, parasternal short-axis, and suprasternal long-axis — must be employed. The intimal flap that forms at the entrance to the false lumen may show an undulating motion that may extend along the inner portion of the dissected wall. Color-flow Doppler mapping can also show flow into and out of the false lumen.[90] The absence of such flow should not rule out a dissecting aneurysm, as clot may fill a large portion of the false lumen. Complications of the dissecting aneurysm such as aortic regurgitation, rupture into a cardiac chamber or the pericardial space, and obstruction of the arch vessels must also be sought.

PULMONARY ARTERY ANOMALIES

This section will discuss abnormal formation of the pulmonary arteries, manifest by abnormal origin of one or both pulmonary arteries. The three major defects to be discussed are (1) pulmonary sling or origin of the left pulmonary artery from the right pulmonary artery, (2) origin of the right pulmonary artery from the ascending aorta, and (3) complete absence of the right pulmonary artery.

Pulmonary Sling

Pulmonary sling or abnormal origin of the left pulmonary artery from the right pulmonary artery occurs when the left pulmonary artery originates from the proximal right pulmonary artery rather than the main pulmonary artery and then courses posterior before turning leftward to pass posterior to the trachea. This encircles the trachea with the main pulmonary artery anterior, the left pulmonary artery to the right and posterior, and the ductus arteriosus or ductal ligament on the left. The esophagus is not affected by this defect, as the left pulmonary artery passes anterior to the esophagus, thus separating it from the trachea. Infants generally present early in life with significant respiratory distress that improves rapidly with intubation.

Echocardiographically, the diagnosis should first be suspected from the parasternal short-axis view.[91] In this view, the normal origin of the left pulmonary artery is absent. The main pulmonary artery continues in a smooth course into the right pulmonary artery. Once the right pulmonary artery turns rightward, the origin of the left pulmonary artery is seen. Only the proximal segment of the left pulmonary artery is seen, as it turns behind the trachea and cannot be seen. It is necessary to distinguish a true pulmonary sling from delayed origin of the left pulmonary artery. Slight rotation of the heart within the thorax can mimic abnormal insertion of the left pulmonary artery. If the left pulmonary artery can be followed from its origin to the hilum of the lung, a sling is not present.

The subcostal coronal view provides an excellent view of the main pulmonary artery as it arises from the right ventricle, coursing slightly superior and then posterior to give rise, in the normal patient, to the right and left pulmonary artery branches. In the presence of a pulmonary sling, the main pulmonary artery can be seen coursing in the usual direction and then turning rightward, smoothly merging into the right pulmonary artery with no left pulmonary artery evident. Once the main pulmonary artery has turned rightward to lie in a left-to-right orientation, the left pulmonary artery can be seen to arise, coursing posteriorly. The posterior course is usually short, as it then disappears from the echocardiographic view because it passes behind the trachea. If the tracheal air column can be visualized, the origin of the left pulmonary artery is seen to be rightward of the trachea, diagnostic for anomalous origin of the left pulmonary artery.

Turning to the subcostal sagittal view, the initial proximal portion of the left pulmonary artery can again be seen as it courses slightly superiorly, then turns directly posterior following its origin from the right pulmonary artery. Its origin is more clearly rightward, being seen superior to the right atrium rather than the left atrium, as is the usual situation.[91] Sweeping the scan plane leftward may then show the left pulmonary artery in cross-section as it emerges from behind the trachea to lie anterior to the esophagus and the descending aorta. In this view it is important not to misinterpret a patent ductus arteriosus arising from the main pulmonary artery as the left pulmonary artery. Although the position of the patent ductus arteriosus may simulate a left pulmonary artery, its course can be identified, going from the main pulmonary artery into the descending aorta.

Abnormalities of the Right Pulmonary Artery

The right pulmonary artery may either arise anomalously from the ascending aorta or be completely absent, with the right lung supplied by bronchial collateral vessels. In either of these entities the left pulmonary artery may be normal if no other cardiac defects are present. Origin of the right pulmonary artery from the ascending aorta hemodynamically mimics truncus arteriosus, yet anatomically it is quite different, with separate aortic and pulmonary valves and usually no conotruncal or septal defects. From the subcostal coronal view, the main pulmonary artery is seen to arise in the normal manner and continue into a normal left pulmonary artery. The distal right pulmonary artery is seen superior to the left atrium but does not continue back to the main pulmonary artery.[92] Instead, it courses slightly anterior to join the lateral wall of the ascending aorta. From the suprasternal long-axis view the right pulmonary artery is no longer seen beneath the aortic arch. Doppler flow studies show continuous flow in the right pulmonary artery, with retrograde diastolic flow in

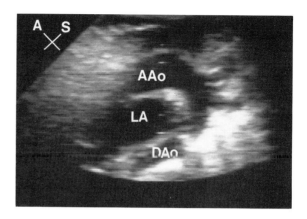

FIG 10–64.
Suprasternal long-axis view from an infant with truncus arteriosus and absent right pulmonary artery. In the suprasternal long-axis view, there is no evidence of a right pulmonary artery underneath the aortic arch. In this patient, the right lung was supplied by bronchial collateral vessels arising from the descending aorta (DAO). A = anterior; AAo = ascending aorta; LA = left atrium; S = superior.

the aorta. Even though there may be no associated anomalies, there is usually pulmonary hypertension in the left pulmonary artery and right ventricle, with Doppler findings of that condition present.

Complete absence of the right pulmonary artery presents with no right pulmonary artery seen in the suprasternal views (Fig 10–64). Differentiation of this lesion from the origin of the right pulmonary artery from the ascending aorta depends upon seeing no vessel beneath the aortic arch or to the right of the aorta superior to the left atrium.

CORONARY ARTERY ANOMALIES

This section will focus on abnormalities of the coronary arteries of both a congenital and acquired nature other than arteriovenous fistulae, which were discussed above. Coronary artery stenosis and coronary artery atheromatous disease will not be covered, with discussion emphasizing entities more common in the younger patient. The lesions to be discussed are anomalous origin of the left coronary artery from the pulmonary artery and coronary artery aneurysms. As coronary vessels are small even in their dilated state, meticulous imaging with high-frequency transducers is necessary to accurately describe anomalies that may be present.

Anomalous Origin of the Left Coronary Artery From the Pulmonary Artery

In this situation the left coronary artery arises anomalously from the pulmonary artery, usually arising from the posterior margin of the pulmonary artery. This condition results in a steal of blood away from the myocardium, with retrograde flow through the left coronary artery system into the pulmonary artery with resultant myocardial ischemia and ventricular dysfunction mimicking that seen in congestive cardiomyopathy.

Echocardiographically, this condition should be suspected when a dilated, poorly functioning ventricle is present.[93] Segmental left ventricular dysfunction may exist, but more commonly, patients have global hypokinesis evident in the parasternal long-axis view, with wall motion patterns and ventricular volumes indistinguishable from those of patients with congestive cardiomyopathies.[94] In the parasternal short-axis view, dilatation of the origin of the right coronary artery is seen.[95] Normal coronary diameters range from 2 mm in infants to 5 mm in older children and adults.[96, 97] Moreover, the more longstanding the disease process, the more dilated the right coronary artery will be. Careful imaging of the left aortic root must be performed to see if the left coronary artery ostium is present. Even when the left coronary artery arises from the pulmonary artery, it still runs posterior to the pulmonary trunk in its normal position, although there is no direct communication with the aorta. The examiner must be careful not to mistake artifactual target dropout caused by lateral resolution problems for a left coronary ostium.[95] In addition, the transverse pericardial sinus that lies to the left and posterior of the aorta must not be mistaken for the proximal left coronary artery.[95] If there is question about the origin of the left coronary artery, the examiner should next image the pulmonary artery from the high left parasternal projection, with the scan plane imaging the pulmonary artery in an anterior-posterior direction. The insertion of the left coronary artery into the posterior wall of the pulmonary artery can be seen in this view. In addition, color-flow mapping from this projection will show flow from the coronary artery into the main pulmonary artery (Plate 44).[98] However, the degree of such shunt flow depends upon the degree of collateralization that has developed between the right and left coronary system and the pulmonary artery pressure. In the newborn, flow may be low and much more difficult to detect than in the older patient. Care must be taken to avoid confusion with flow from a patent ductus arteriosus. Diastolic ductal flow usually is along the superior left border of the pulmonary artery, whereas diastolic flow from an anomalous left coronary artery usually is along the posterior left border of the pulmonary artery.[99] The aortic root should next be imaged from the subcostal coronal projection. In this view the prominent right coronary artery is again seen, with no identifiable origin of the left coronary artery from the left coronary sinus of the aortic root. Again, the left coronary artery may be seen lying within the atrioventricular groove, although it cannot be traced to the aortic root. In summary to make this diagnosis, no one view should be used in isolation. Because of the small size of the vessels involved, multiple views are necessary, together with Doppler techniques, to establish this diagnosis.

Coronary Artery Aneurysms

Coronary artery aneurysms are usually associated with Kawasaki disease, but may be a consequence of other disease processes. Aneurysms may be present anywhere along the coronary artery system, but in general, only proximal aneurysms are imaged by echocardiography.[96, 100] When a patient suspected of having coronary artery aneurysms is being examined, careful imaging of the coronary arteries from their origin at the aortic root as far distally as it is possible to image must be performed. The examination should begin by imaging the coronary arteries from the parasternal short-axis view, carefully measuring the size of the coronary arteries at their origin. In general, in the presence of coronary artery aneurysms, the origins are dilated, although this is not a consistent finding in all patients. To image the left coronary artery, the transducer is rotated slightly clockwise and inferior from the standard parasternal short-axis view to image the left coronary artery as it passes through the left atrioventricular groove (Fig 10–65). It can usually be imaged to its bifurcation into the circumflex and anterior descending branches. Aneurysms may again be noted anywhere along the length; their diameter as well as their shape, which may be either saccular or fusiform, should be noted.

From the parasternal short-axis view imaging the tricuspid valve and pulmonary valve, the transducer may be tilted slightly cephalad to image the atrioventricular groove anterior to the tricuspid valve in which the right coronary artery lies (Figs 10–66 and 10–67). Patients with increased myocardial fat allow better imaging of the right coronary artery because of the differing densities of the vessel walls and the adjacent fat. Clots that form within coronary aneurysms may also be seen (Fig 10–68).

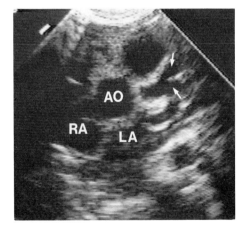

FIG 10–65.
Parasternal short-axis view from a patient with Kawasaki disease and multiple aneurysms in the left main, circumflex, and left anterior descending coronary arteries *(arrows)*. AO = aorta; LA = left atrium; RA = right atrium.

The coronary arteries can also be imaged well from the subcostal coronal and apical four-chamber view, scanning superiorly from the inlet region of the heart to image the aortic root (Fig 10–69). Slight clockwise rotation of the scan plane may be needed to image the left and right atrioventricular grooves in which the coronary vessels lie. Again, high-frequency transducers are needed to accurately define the size of the coronary vessels. In any view, coronary vessels should normally be less than 3 mm in diameter. A diameter greater than published normal values for the patient's age should raise the question of aneurysm formation.

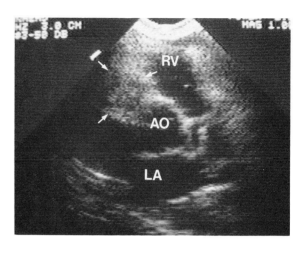

FIG 10–68.
Parasternal short-axis view from a patient with Kawasaki disease and multiple coronary artery aneurysms. Aneurysmal dilatation of the left main coronary artery is present. An enormous aneurysm filled with thrombus is seen in the right coronary artery (arrows). AO = aorta; LA = left atrium; RV = right ventricle.

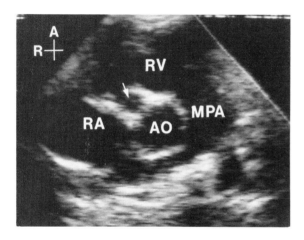

FIG 10–66.
Parasternal short-axis view from a patient with Kawasaki disease and a large circular aneurysm (arrow) of the right main coronary artery. A = anterior; AO = aorta; MPA = main pulmonary artery; R = right; RA = right atrium; RV = right ventricle.

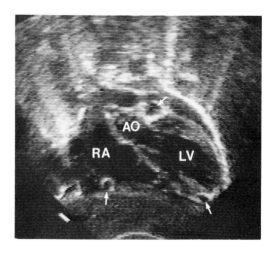

FIG 10–69.
Subcostal view of the left ventricular (LV) outflow tract from a patient with Kawasaki disease and multiple aneurysms (arrows) of the proximal and distal coronary arteries. Aneurysms are seen in the left circumflex coronary artery, at the distal end of the left anterior descending coronary artery, and in the right coronary artery. AO = aorta; RA = right atrium.

REFERENCES

1. Sahn DJ, Allen HD: Real-time cross-sectional echocardiographic imaging and measurement of the patent ductus arteriosus in infants and children. *Circulation* 1978; 58:343–354.
2. Snider AR, Silverman NH: Suprasternal notch echocardiography: A two-dimensional technique for evaluating congenital heart disease. *Circulation* 1981; 63:165–173.

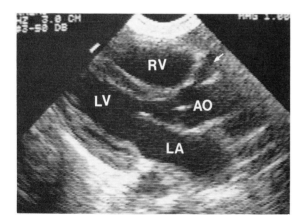

FIG 10–67.
Parasternal long-axis view from a patient with Kawasaki disease and a long aneurysmal dilatation (arrow) of the right main coronary artery. AO = aorta; LA = left atrium; LV = left ventricle; RV = right ventricle.

3. Huhta JC, Gutgesell HP, Latson LA, et al: Two-dimensional echocardiographc assessment of the aorta in infants and children with congenital heart disease. *Circulation* 1984; 70:417–424.

4. Silverman NH, Lewis AB, Heyman MA, et al: Echocardiographic assessment of ductus arteriosus shunt in premature infants. *Circulation* 1974; 50:821–825.

5. Baylen B, Meyer RA, Korfhagen J, et al: Left ventricular performance in the critically ill premature infant with patent ductus arteriosus and pulmonary disease. *Circulation* 1977; 55:182–188.

6. Goldberg SJ, Allen HD, Sahn DJ: Echocardiographic detection and management of patent ductus arteriosus and neonates with respiratory distress syndrome: A two-and-one-half year prospective study. *J Clin Ultrasound* 1977; 5:161–169.

7. Laird WP, Fixler DE: Echocardiography of premature infants with pulmonary disease: A noninvasive method for detecting large ductal left-to-right shunts. *Radiology* 1977; 122:455–457.

8. Halliday HL, Hirata T, Brady JP: Echocardiographic findings of large patent ductus arteriosus in the very low birthweight infant before and after treatment with indomethacin. *Arch Dis Child* 1979; 54:744–749.

9. Gentile R, Stevenson G, Dooley T, et al: Pulsed Doppler echocardiographic determination of time of ductal closure in normal newborn infants. *J Pediatr* 1981; 98:443–448.

10. Stevenson JG, Kawabori I, Guntheroth WG: Pulsed Doppler echocardiographic diagnosis of patent ductus arteriosus: Sensitivity, specificity, limitations, and technical features. *Cathet Cardiovasc Diagn* 1980; 6:255–263.

11. Feldtman RW, Andrassy RJ, Alexander JA, et al: Doppler ultrasonic flow detection as an adjunct in the diagnosis of patent ductus arteriosus in premature infants. *J Thorac Cardiovasc Surg* 1976; 72:288–290.

12. Daniels O, Hopman JCW, Stelinga GBA, et al: Doppler flow characteristics in the main pulmonary artery and LA/Ao ratio before and after ductal closure in healthy newborns. *Pediatr Cardiol* 1982; 3:99–104.

13. Cloez JL, Isaaz K, Pernot C: Pulsed Doppler flow characteristics of ductus arteriosus in infants with associated congenital anomalies of the heart or great arteries. *Am J Cardiol* 1986; 57:845–851.

14. Hiraishi S, Horiguchi Y, Misawa H, et al: Noninvasive Doppler echocardiographic evaluation of shunt flow dynamics of the ductus arteriosus. *Circulation* 1987; 75:1146–1153.

15. Musewe NN, Smallhorn JF, Benson LN, et al: Validation of Doppler-derived pulmonary arterial pressure in patients with ductus arteriosus under different hemodynamic states. *Circulation* 1987; 76:1081–1091.

16. Stevenson JG, Kawabori I, Guntheroth WG: Noninvasive detection of pulmonary hypertension in patent ductus arteriosus by pulsed Doppler echocardiography. *Circulation* 1979; 60:355–359.

17. Serwer GA, Armstrong BE, Anderson PAW: Noninvasive detection of retrograde descending aortic flow in infants using continuous wave Doppler ultrasonography. *J Pediatr* 1980; 97:394–400.

18. Alverson DC, Eldridge M, Aldrich M, et al: Effect of patent ductus arteriosus on lower extremity blood flow velocity patterns in preterm infants. *Am J Perinatol* 1984; 1:216–221.

19. Perlman J, Hill A, Volpe J: The effect of patent ductus arteriosus on flow velocity in the anterior cerebral arteries: Ductal steal in the premature newborn infant. *J Pediatr* 1981; 99:767–771.

20. Martin CG, Snider AR, Katz SM, et al: Abnormal cerebral blood flow patterns in preterm infants with a large patent ductus arteriosus. *J Pediatr* 1982; 101:587–593.

21. Snider AR: Doppler echocardiography in congenital heart disease, in Berger M (ed): *Doppler Echocardiography in Heart Disease*. New York, Marcel Dekker, Inc., 1987, pp 199–331.

22. Swensson RE, Valdes-Cruz LM, Sahn DJ, et al: Real-time Doppler color flow mapping for detection of patent ductus arteriosus. *Pediatr Cardiol* 1986; 8:1105–1112.

23. Liao P-K, Su W-J, Hung J-S: Doppler echocardiographic flow characteristics of isolated patent ductus arteriosus: Better delineation by Doppler color flow mapping. *J Am Coll Cardiol* 1988; 12:1285–1291.

24. Barron JV, Sahn DJ, Valdes-Cruz, LM, et al: Clinical utility of two-dimensional Doppler echocardiographic techniques for estimating pulmonary to systemic blood flow ratios in children with left-to-right shunting atrial septal defect, ventricular septal defect or patent ductus arteriosus. *J Am Coll Cardiol* 1984; 3:169–178.

25. Wenger NK: Rare causes of coronary artery disease, in Hurst JW (ed): *The Heart*. New York, McGraw-Hill, 1978, pp 1348–1349.

26. Ellis AJ, Schattenberg TT, Feldt RH, et al: Congenital coronary artery fistula: Surgical considerations and results of operation. *Mayo Clin Proc* 1972; 47:567–571.

27. Oldham HN Jr, Ebert PA, Young WA, et al: Surgical management of congenital coronary artery fistula. *Ann Thorac Surg* 1971; 12:503–513.

28. Urrutia-S CO, Falaschi G, Ott DA, et al: Surgical management of 56 patients with congenital coronary artery fistulas. *Ann Thorac Surg* 1983; 35:300–307.

29. Hobbs RE, Millit HD, Raghavan PV, et al: Coronary artery fistulae: A 10 year review. *Cleveland Clinic Q* 1982; 49:191–197.

30. Reeder GS, Tajik AJ, Smith HC: Visualization of coronary artery fistula by two-dimensional echocardiography. *Mayo Clin Proc* 1980; 55:185–189.

31. Yoshikawa J, Katao H, Yanagihara K, et al: Non-invasive visualization of the dilated main coronary arteries in coronary artery fistulas by cross-sectional echocardiography. *Circulation* 1982; 64:600–603.

32. Weyman AE, Feigenbaum H, Dillon JC, et al: Non-invasive visualization of the left main coronary artery by cross-sectional echocardiography. *Circulation* 1976; 54:169–174.

33. Ogawa S, Chen CC, Hubbard FE, et al: A new approach to visualize the left main coronary artery using apical cross-sectional echocardiography. *Am J Cardiol* 1980; 45:301–304.

34. Rodgers DM, Wolf NM, Barrett MJ, et al: Two-di-

mensional echocardiographic features of coronary arteriovenous fistula. *Am Heart J* 1982; 104:872–874.

35. Kronzon I, Winer HE, Cohen M: Non-invasive diagnosis of left coronary arteriovenous fistula communicating with the right ventricle. *Am J Cardiol* 1982; 49:1811–1813.

36. Satomi G, Endo M, Takao A, et al: A case of right coronary artery to left ventricle fistula: Two dimensional echocardiographic study. *Pediatr Cardiol* 1983; 4:229–232.

37. Pickoff AS, Wolff GS, Bennett VL, et al: Pulsed Doppler echocardiographic detection of coronary artery to right ventricle fistula. *Pediatr Cardiol* 1982; 2:145–149.

38. Agatson AS, Chapman E, Hildner FJ, et al: Diagnosis of a right coronary artery-right atrial fistula using two-dimensional and Doppler echocardiography. *Am J Cardiol* 1984; 54:238–239.

39. Chen CC, Hwang B, Hsuing MC, et al: Recognition of coronary arterial fistula by Doppler 2-dimensional echocardiography. *Am J Cardiol* 1984; 53:392–394.

40. Miyatake K, Okamoto M, Kinoshita N, et al: Doppler echocardiographic features of coronary arteriovenous fistula. *Br Heart J* 1984; 51:508–518.

41. Griffiths SP, Ellis K, Hordof AJ, et al: Spontaneous complete closure of a congenital coronary artery fistula. *J Am Coll Cardiol* 1983; 2:1169–1173.

42. Friedman DM, Rutkowski M: Coronary artery fistula: A pulsed Doppler/two-dimensional echocardiographic study. *Am J Cardiol* 1985; 55:1652–1655.

43. Cooper MJ, Bernstein D, Silverman NH: Recognition of left coronary artery fistula to the left and right ventricles by contrast echocardiography. *J Am Coll Cardiol* 1985; 6:923–926.

44. Barton CW, Snider AR, Rosenthal A: Two-dimensional and Doppler echocardiographic features of left circumflex coronary artery to right ventricle fistula: Case report and literature review. *Pediatr Cardiol* 1986; 7:167–170.

45. Glatt BS, Rowe RD: Cerebral arteriovenous fistula associated with congestive heart failure in the newborn. *Pediatrics* 1960; 26:596–603.

46. Gold AP, Ransohoff J, Carter S: Vein of Galen malformation. *Acta Neurol Scand* 1964; 40(suppl 2):31.

47. Sunderland CO, Morgan CL, Lees HM: Cerebral arteriovenous fistula producing temporary heart failure in a newborn infant. *Clin Pediatr* 1971; 10:309–311.

48. Holden AM, Fyler DC, Shillito J, et al: Congestive heart failure from intracranial arteriovenous fistula in infancy. *Pediatrics* 1972; 49:30–39.

49. Watson DG, Smith RR, Brann AW: Arteriovenous malformations of the vein of Galen. *Am J Dis Child* 1976; 130:520–525.

50. Hirsch JH, Cyr D, Eberhardt H, et al: Ultrasonographic diagnosis of an aneurysm of the vein of Galen in utero by duplex scanning. *J Ultrasound Med* 1983; 2:231–233.

51. Snider AR, Soifer SJ, Silverman NH: Detection of intracranial arteriovenous fistula by two-dimensional ultrasonography. *Circulation* 1981; 63:1179–1185.

52. Sivakoff M, Nouri S: Diagnosis of vein of Galen arteriovenous malformation by two-dimensional ultrasound and pulsed Doppler method. *Pediatrics* 1982; 69:84–88.

53. Cha EM, Khoury GH: Persistent left superior vena cava. *Radiology* 1972; 103:375–381.

54. Winter FS: Persistent left superior vena cava. Survey of world literature and report of thirty additional cases. *Angiology* 1954; 5:90–132.

55. Goor DA, Lillehei CW: *Congenital Malformations of the Heart.* New York, Grune and Stratton, 1975, pp 380–413.

56. Snider AR, Ports TA, Silverman NH: Venous anomalies of the coronary sinus: Detection by M-mode, two-dimensional, and contrast echocardiography. *Circulation* 1979; 60:721–727.

57. Cohen BE, Winer HE, Kronzon I: Echocardiographic findings in patients with left superior vena cava and dilated coronary sinus. *Am J Cardiol* 1979; 44:158–161.

58. Huhta JC, Smallhorn JF, Macartney FJ, et al: Cross-sectional echocardiographic diagnosis of systemic venous return. *Br Heart J* 1982; 48:388–403.

59. Shaffer EW, Snider AR, Peters J, et al: Echocardiographic detection of anomalous course of the left innominate vein. *Int J Cardiac Imaging* 1985; 1:167–169.

60. Paquet M, Gutgesell H: Echocardiographic features of total anomalous pulmonary venous connection. *Circulation* 1975; 52:599–605.

61. Orsmond GS, Ruttenberg HS, Bessinger FB, et al: Echocardiographic features of total anomalous pulmonary venous connection to the coronary sinus. *Am J Cardiol* 1978; 41:597–601.

62. Aziz KU, Paul MH, Bharati S, et al: Echocardiographic features of total anomalous pulmonary venous drainage into the coronary sinus. *Am J Cardiol* 1978; 42:108–113.

63. Sahn DJ, Allen HD, Lange LW, et al: Cross-sectional echocardiographic diagnosis of the sites of total anomalous pulmonary venous drainage. *Circulation* 1979; 60:1317–1325.

64. Snider AR, Silverman NH, Turley K, et al: Evaluation of infradiaphragmatic total anomalous pulmonary venous connection with two-dimensional echocardiography. *Circulation* 1982; 66:1129–1132.

65. Smallhorn JF, Sutherland GR, Tommasini G, et al: Assessment of total anomalous pulmonary venous connection by two-dimensional echocardiography. *Br Heart J* 1981; 46:613–623.

66. Sahn DJ, Goldberg SJ, Allen HD, et al: Cross-sectional echocardiographic imaging of supracardiac total anomalous pulmonary venous drainage to a vertical vein in a patient with Holt-Oram syndrome. *Chest* 1981; 79:113–115.

67. Cooper MJ, Teitel DF, Silverman NH, et al: Study of the infradiaphragmatic total anomalous pulmonary venous connection with cross-sectional and pulsed Doppler echocardiography. *Circulation* 1984; 70:412–416.

68. Smallhorn JF, Freedom RM: Pulsed Doppler echocardiography in the preoperative evaluation of total anomalous pulmonary venous connection. *J Am Coll Cardiol* 1986; 8:1413–1420.

69. Shrivastava S, Berry JM, Einzig S, et al: Parasternal cross-sectional echocardiographic determination of aortic arch situs: A new approach. *Am J Cardiol* 1985; 55:1236–1238.

70. Kveselis DA, Snider AR, Dick M II, et al: Echocardiographic diagnosis of right aortic arch with a retroesophageal segment and left descending aorta. *Am J Cardiol* 1986; 57:1198–1199.

71. Celano V, Pieroni DR, Gingell RL, et al: Two-dimensional echocardiographic recognition of the right aortic arch. *Am J Cardiol* 1983; 51:1507–1512.

72. Enderlein MA, Silverman NH, Stanger P, et al: Usefulness of suprasternal notch echocardiography for diagnosis of double aortic arch. *Am J Cardiol* 1986; 57:359–361.

73. Sahn DJ, Valdes-Cruz LM, Ovitt TW, et al: Two dimensional echocardiography and intravenous digital video subtraction angiography for diagnosis and evaluation of double aortic arch. *Am J Cardiol* 1982; 50:342–346.

74. Kan MN, Nanda NC, Stopa AR: Diagnosis of double aortic arch by cross sectional echocardiography with Doppler colour flow mapping. *Br Heart J* 1987; 58:284–286.

75. D'Cruz IA, Stanley A, Vitullo D, et al: Noninvasive diagnosis of right cervical aortic arch. *Chest* 1983; 83:820–822.

76. Morris T, Ruttley M: Left cervical aortic arch associated with aortic aneurysm. *Br Heart J* 1978; 40:87–90.

77. Kronzon I, Mehta SS, Zelefsky M: Cervical aorta presenting as superior mediastinal mass: Diagnosis by echography. *Br J Radiol* 1974; 47:900–902.

78. Mullins CE, Gillette PC, McNamara DG: The complex of cervical aortic arch. *Pediatrics* 1973; 51:210–215.

79. Brand A, Branski D, Kerem E, et al: Usefulness of echocardiography and radionuclide ventriculography for diagnosing buckling of the innominate artery in children. *Am J Cardiol* 1986; 57:492–493.

80. Nihoyannopoulos P, Karas S, Sapsford RN, et al: Accuracy of two-dimensional echocardiography in the diagnosis of aortic arch obstruction. *J Am Coll Cardiol* 1987; 10:1072–1077.

81. Sanders SP, MacPherson D, Yeager SB: Temporal flow velocity profile in the descending aorta in coarctation. *J Am Coll Cardiol* 1986; 7:603–609.

82. Shaddy RE, Snider AR, Silverman NH, et al: Pulsed Doppler findings in patients with coarctation of the aorta. *Circulation* 1986; 73:82–88.

83. Riggs TW, Berry TE, Aziz KU, et al: Two-dimensional echocardiographc features of interruption of the aortic arch. *Am J Cardiol* 1982; 50:1385–1390.

84. Smallhorn JF, Anderson RH, Macartney FJ: Cross-sectional echocardiographc recognition of interruption of aortic arch between left carotid and subclavian arteries. *Br Heart J* 1982; 48:229–235.

85. Mathew T, Nanda NC: Two-dimensional and Doppler echocardiographic evaluation of aortic aneurysm and dissection. *Am J Cardiol* 1984; 54:379–385.

86. Come PC: Improved cross-sectional echocardiographic technique for visualization of the retrocardiac descending aorta in its long axis. *Am J Cardiol* 1983; 51:1029–1032.

87. Iliceto S, Antonelli G, Biasco G, et al: Two-dimensional echocardiographc evaluation of aneurysms of the descending thoracic aorta. *Circulation* 1982; 66:1045–1049.

88. Mintz GS, Kotler MN, Segal BL, et al: Two dimensional echocardiographic recognition of the descending thoracic aorta. *Am J Cardiol* 1979; 44:232–238.

89. Diehl JT, Kaiser LR, Howard RJ, et al: Two-dimensional echocardiography for diagnosing acute ascending aortic dissection. *Can J Surg* 1985; 28:345–347.

90. Iliceto S, Nanda NC, Rizzon P, et al: Color Doppler evaluation of aortic dissection. *Circulation* 1987; 75:748–755.

91. Yeager SB, Chin AJ, Sanders SP: Two-dimensional echocardiographic diagnosis of pulmonary artery sling in infancy. *J Am Coll Cardiol* 1986; 7:625–629.

92. Lo RN, Mok CK, Leung MP, et al: Cross-sectional and pulsed Doppler echocardiographic features of anomalous origin of right pulmonary artery from the ascending aorta. *Am J Cardiol* 1987; 60:921–924.

93. Shapiro J, Boxer R, Krongrad E: Echocardiography in infants with anomalous origin of the left coronary artery. *Pediatr Cardiol* 1979; 1:23–28.

94. Rein AJJT, Colan SD, Parness IA, et al: Regional and global left ventricular function in infants with anomalous origin of the left coronary artery from the pulmonary trunk: Preoperative and postoperative assessment. *Circulation* 1987; 75:115–123.

95. Schmidt KG, Cooper MJ, Silverman NH, et al: Pulmonary artery origin of the left coronary artery: Diagnosis by two-dimensional echocardiography, pulsed Doppler ultrasound, and color flow mapping. *J Am Coll Cardiol* 1988; 11:396–402.

96. Arjunan K, Daniels SR, Meyer RA, et al: Coronary artery caliber in normal children and patients with Kawasaki disease but without aneurysms: An echocardiographic and angiographic study. *J Am Coll Cardiol* 1986; 8:1119–1124.

97. Vered Z, Katz M, Rath S, et al: Two-dimensional echocardiographc analysis of proximal left main coronary artery in humans. *Am Heart J* 1986; 112:972–976.

98. Swensson RE, Murillo-Olivas A, Elias W, et al: Noninvasive Doppler color flow mapping for detection of anomalous origin of the left coronary artery from the pulmonary artery and evaluation of surgical repair. *J Am Coll Cardiol* 1988; 11:659–661.

99. Fyfe DA, Sade RM, Gillette PC, et al: Pre- and postoperative Doppler echocardiographic evaluation of anomalous left coronary artery arising from the pulmonary artery. *J Ultrasound Med* 1987; 6:101–103.

100. Ching KJ, Fulton DR, Lapp R, et al: One-year follow-up of cardiac and coronary artery disease in infants and children with Kawasaki disease. *Am Heart J* 1988; 115:1263–1267.

11

Abnormalities Within the Cardiac Chambers

This chapter will discuss lesions that are identified within the cardiac chambers but are acquired rather than a result of abnormal cardiogenesis. The origin of these lesions may be external to the heart, such as metastatic tumors or foreign bodies, or intrinsic to the heart, such as primary myocardial tumors, thrombi, or vegetations. We will examine five major classifications of such lesions: (1) neoplasms, both primary and metastatic, (2) thrombi, (3) vegetations, (4) foreign bodies, and (5) ventricular aneurysms. The diagnostic characteristics of each and where they are most likely to be found will be presented.

CARDIAC NEOPLASMS

Primary Cardiac Tumors

This section discusses specific myocardial tumors that may be encountered and compares the echocardiographic findings in each. It should be recognized that such lesions may be seen in multiple views or may only be evident in a single view and that all views must be closely examined for the presence of these abnormalities. No one view is more likely to show a specific lesion than any other, but when a lesion is found, it should be inspected in multiple views so that the examiner can more fully appreciate the location, size, and characteristics of the lesion. In addition, when one lesion is found, the entire heart must be carefully inspected to make certain that multiple lesions are not present. Many primary myocardial tumors may be multiple, and the presence or absence of such multiple lesions has clinical importance.

Myxomas

Myxomas may be found in any of the cardiac chambers, although they are seen more commonly in the left atrium and left ventricle.[1-4] Left atrial myxomas generally are attached to the lower atrial septum by a stalk that permits the main mass of the tumor to move within the atrial cavity (Figs 11–1 and 11–2). The myxoma often prolapses into or through the mitral valve orifice during ventricular diastole and may obstruct the mitral valve.[1] The point of attachment can be anywhere along the atrial septum or the mitral valve. It is rare to find a myxoma attached to an atrial free wall. A wide base of attachment rather than a stalk should raise the possibility that the tumor is not a myxoma. The main tissue mass is usually somewhat globular and lobulated. Whenever these tumors are present, careful M-mode and Doppler interrogation of the mitral valve must be performed to exclude the possibility of significant mitral obstruction or insufficiency as a consequence of the tumor mass (Fig 11–3).

Right atrial myxomas have also been described and are similar in appearance to left atrial myxomas.[5,6] They are also attached by stalks, again usually to the atrial septum, but can be on the atrial free wall. Multiple tumors have also been described.[5]

Left ventricular myxomas are also seen and are more common in the younger patient. Particular attention must be directed to the left ventricle in examining the patient after a previous left atrial myxoma has been removed because seeding of the ventricular cavity at the time of tumor removal may occur. Tumors characteristically appear as lobulated lesions attached by a stalk to the ventricular endocardium, most commonly either at the ventricular apex or along the interventricular septum. The apical four-chamber view is usually the most useful (Fig 11–4) although it does not permit careful examination of the outlet septum and left ventricular outflow tract where many such tumors may occur. Again, these tumors are highly mobile within the left ventricular cavity, and the presence of a

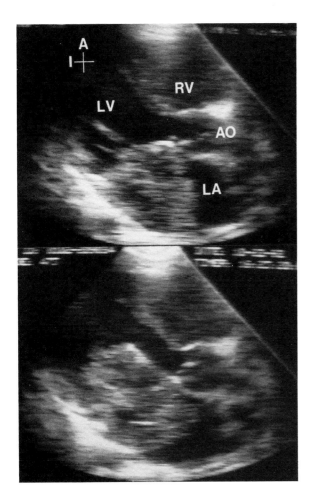

FIG 11–1.
Parasternal long-axis views in systole *(above)* and diastole *(below)* from a patient with a large myxoma filling the left atrium (LA). The myxoma has a globular appearance and is heterogeneous, containing echolucent and echo-bright areas. In diastole, the tumor prolapses through and occludes the mitral valve. A = anterior; I = inferior; AO = aorta; LV = left ventricle; RV = right ventricle.

large area of connection between the tumor mass and the myocardium rather than a stalk should suggest that the tumor is not a myxoma.

Right ventricular myxomas also occur but are the least common.[7, 8] They may be attached either to the anterior free wall or to the outflow tract and may prolapse into the pulmonary artery during systole.[9] Again, the highly mobile nature of this tumor, together with the narrow stalk attachment, should suggest the diagnosis of myxoma.

From a clinical standpoint, the information needed is the location of the tumor attachment, the size of the lesion, the number of lesions present, and the hemodynamic consequences of the lesion. Such tumors must be differentiated from mobile thrombi, although in some instances this differentiation may be difficult. Thrombi, as will be discussed below, are usually not as mobile as a myxoma and in general have a broader point of attachment. Thrombi also tend to be irregular rather than globular in shape. Attempts at

tissue characterization using echocardiography have been made, but by and large these have proved difficult.[10]

Rhabdomyomas

Cardiac rhabdomyomas are the most common cardiac tumor to occur in infants and children. These tumors are highly associated with tuberous sclerosis and are found in 30% to 50% of patients examined with tuberous sclerosis.[11] These lesions range in size from very tiny to quite large and are often multiple. Their echocardiographic appearance tends to be that of a homogeneous, echo-bright lesion.[12] They have a propensity for the ventricles and are found predominantly in the left ventricular papillary muscles and along both sides of the ventricular septum (Figs 11–5 to 11–7). They may, however, also be found along

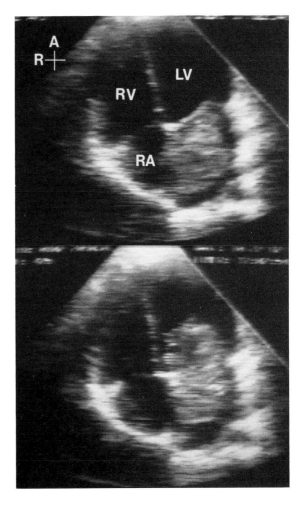

FIG 11–2.
Apical four-chamber views in systole *(above)* and diastole *(below)* from the same patient as in Figure 11–1. The myxoma is seen filling the left atrium and prolapsing through the mitral valve in diastole. The myxoma is attached to the left atrial side of the atrial septum. A = anterior; LV = left ventricle; R = right; RA = right atrium; RV = right ventricle.

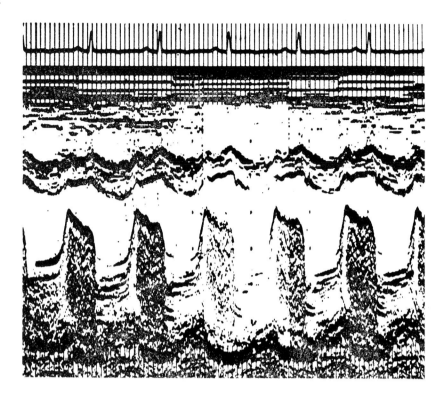

FIG 11–3.
M-mode echocardiogram from a patient with a left atrial myxoma. The echoes arising from the myxoma fill the space behind the anterior mitral valve leaflet in diastole. Between the anterior mitral valve leaflet and the tumor echoes is a clear space, which indicates that the tumor passes into the mitral valve after the leaflet opens. This leading edge is characteristic of echoes that arise from a myxoma.

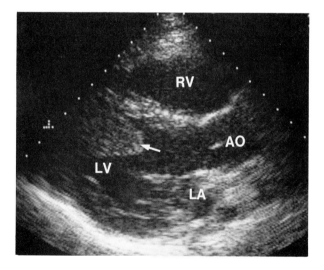

FIG 11–4.
Echocardiogram from an adolescent male who had removal of a left atrial myxoma one year before this study. On the one-year follow-up examination, another myxoma *(arrow)* was found in the apical portion of the left ventricle (LV). LA = left atrium.

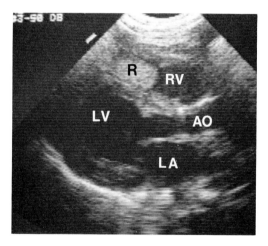

FIG 11–5.
Parasternal long-axis view from a patient with tuberous sclerosis and a large rhabdomyoma (R) filling the apical portion of the right ventricle (RV). AO = aorta; LA = left atrium; LV = left ventricle.

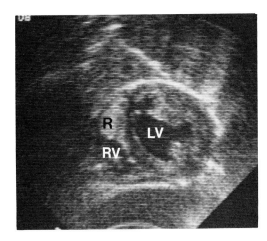

FIG 11–6.
Subcostal view of the ventricles from a patient with tuberous sclerosis and multiple rhabdomyoma. A rhabdomyoma (R) is seen in the apical portion of the right ventricle (RV) and in the papillary muscle of the left ventricle (LV).

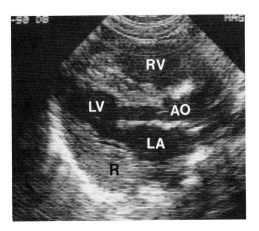

FIG 11–7.
Parasternal long-axis view from an infant with a large rhabdomyoma (R) on the left ventricular (LV) posterior wall. This tumor involved the mitral valve and its chordae. AO = aorta; LA = left atrium; RV = right ventricle.

the atrial septum in either the right or the left atrium (Fig 11–8). They usually are intramyocardial with limited extension into the cavity. They are usually not free-floating within the cavity and do not have a propensity for systemic or pulmonary embolization. Large lesions may become obstructive to either ventricular outflow tracts (Figs 11–9 and 11–10). Doppler examination can be quite helpful in this situation. In any child with suspected or proven tuberous sclerosis, careful examination of the heart is indicated. In fact, cardiac rhabdomyomas may be the first clue that a patient has tuberous sclerosis, and such lesions have even been identified within the fetal heart (Fig 11–11).[13] In gen-

eral, cardiac rhabdomyomas appear as echo-bright areas in the cardiac muscle, but care must be exercised to differentiate such lesions from normal reflections of the ventricular trabeculae. Careful adjustment of the gain controls of the echocardiographic instrument is necessary to avoid false-positive diagnoses.

Close follow-up of these patients is recommended. These lesions may increase in size to become obstructive, particularly in the left and right ventricular outflow tracts, or they may regress. We have seen lesions totally disappear over time and be of no clinical significance. In addition, lesions found at the crux of the heart in the inlet must also be carefully followed, as they can lead to interference with the cardiac conduction system and creation of heart block.

Other Primary Tumors

Other tumors that may arise primarily within the heart are rhabdomyosarcomas and lesions of the pericardium,

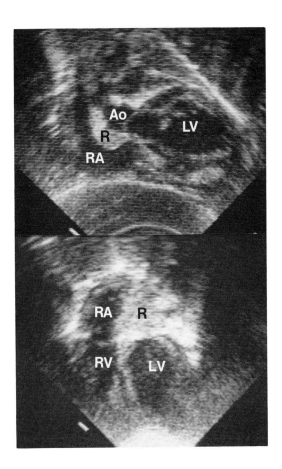

FIG 11–8.
Subcostal four-chamber view of the left ventricular (LV) outflow tract *(top)* and apical four-chamber view *(bottom)* from an infant with a large rhabdomyoma (R). This rhabdomyoma extended along the posterior left atrial wall, as seen in the apical four-chamber view. It then extended up through the atrial septum to the area of the ascending aorta and superior vena cava, as seen in the subcostal view. Ao = aorta; RA = right atrium; RV = right ventricle.

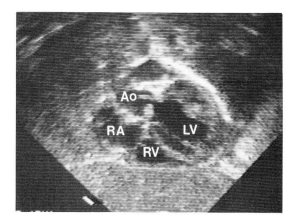

FIG 11–9.
Subcostal view of the left ventricular (LV) outflow tract from a patient with a rhabdomyoma protruding into the LV just beneath the aortic valve leaflets. This rhabdomyoma caused a considerable pressure gradient across the LV outflow tract in systole. Ao = aorta; RA = right atrium; RV = right ventricle.

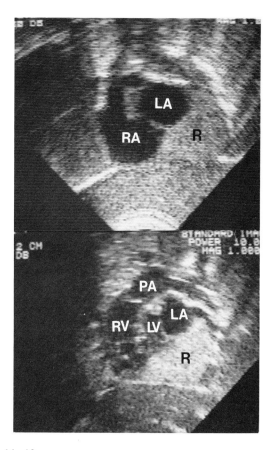

FIG 11–10.
Subcostal four-chamber *(top)* and sagittal *(bottom)* views from an infant with a large posterior rhabdomyoma (R). The rhabdomyoma filled the pericardial sac and was attached to the posterior surfaces of both ventricles. LA = left atrium; PA = pulmonary artery; RA = right atrium; RV = right ventricle.

particularly pericardial cysts and mesotheliomas.[14–16] Such tumors may arise anywhere within the heart and have even been reported to arise as a primary lesion within the pulmonary trunk.[14] Intracardiac tumors of this nature generally are more sessile than myxomas and are more irregular than cardiac rhabdomyomas. They may invade the entire thickness of the ventricular wall and result in significant myocardial dysfunction. Differentiation from a thrombus may be difficult, but when extension of the tumor mass into the myocardial tissue is seen, thrombus is excluded.

Pericardial lesions are again rare but can present significant clinical problems, particularly because of restriction to cardiac filling. Asymmetric echo-free spaces attached to the pericardium should raise the possibility of such lesions. Lesions extrinsic to the heart may be eliminated, as they do not move with the cardiac motion, whereas pericardial lesions do. Such lesions may be cystic, with a single, large, fluid-filled area or multiple fluid-filled areas with septa. Tumors such as mesotheliomas, even though they arise in the pericardium, may invade cardiac musculature and be visualized within the free wall or septal structures. Additional pericardial fluid may also be present.

Careful localization of the lesion must be performed. Multiple views, particularly a combination of parasternal views together with subcostal or apical four-chamber views, are needed to permit a three-dimensional reconstruction. It is also important to note whether these lesions extend superiorly to involve the great vessels or remain localized to the cardiac chambers. Pericardial cysts are typically located at the right costophrenic angle or left costophrenic angle and generally do not involve the base of the heart and the great vessels, whereas malignant mesotheliomas

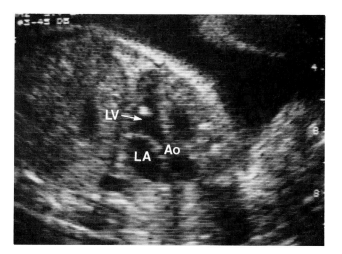

FIG 11–11.
Echocardiogram from a fetus found to have a rhabdomyoma *in utero*. The rhabdomyoma appears as an echo-bright spot in the area of the left ventricular (LV) papillary muscles. Ao = aorta; LA = left atrium.

classically are seen extending from the cardiac apex to the base and often will involve the great vessels.[16]

Primary malignant lesions of the heart can result in rupture of the cardiac structures with resultant hemopericardium and the potential for tamponade.[17] This can also result in clot formation within the pericardium, which can be confused with an extracardiac mass. Whenever pericardial effusion is present in the context of a primary myocardial neoplasm, careful inspection of all cardiac walls for potential rupture is indicated.

Metastatic Cardiac Lesions

Numerous tumors can invade the heart, although such involvement is rare.[18–24] Most metastatic tumors do not invade the intravascular space but are confined to the pericardial space or invasion of the myocardial walls. However, when such chamber involvement occurs, it can be difficult to distinguish between primary and metastatic lesions. One useful criterion is the presence of tumor in cardiac structures usually not affected by primary tumors. Such structures are the cardiac veins, particularly the inferior and superior vena cava, and the pulmonary veins. Any tumor seen extending into the inferior vena cava should be suspected of being metastatic. Wilm's tumor, hepatomas, and some rhabdomyosarcomas can involve the great veins. The subcostal long-axis view is particularly helpful in defining the caudal extension of the tumor. In addition, any tumor involving a pulmonary vein should again be suspected of arising as a metastatic rather than a primary lesion, especially when no clear point of attachment is seen.[18, 19] Atrial myxomas tend to be more nonhomogeneous and lobulated, to change shape during the cardiac cycle, and to show a clear point of attachment to the cardiac chamber walls. Metastatic lesions do not show these features.

Lymphomas predominantly invade the pericardium and are the most common form of metastatic involvement, particularly in children.[23] This results in pericardial thickening with effusions and extrinsic masses compressing the ventricle. In general, extrinsic compression produces only mild hemodynamic consequences in terms of obstructive lesions, although significant restriction to normal cardiac filling may occur. Detection of cardiac metastases obviously has important therapeutic and prognostic implications and, therefore, echocardiography is advised in any situation where the potential for cardiac metastasis exists.

Extrinsic Tumors Compressing the Heart

Compression of cardiac structures by tumors extrinsic to the heart can occur; however, hemodynamically significant compression is rare. Some of the more common tumors that can compress the heart are thoracic lymphomas, neuroblastomas, and thymomas (Fig 11–12). Several echocardiographic features are helpful for distinguishing a normal, large thymus from a thymoma. The normal thymus gives rise to homogeneous echoes and does not distort or

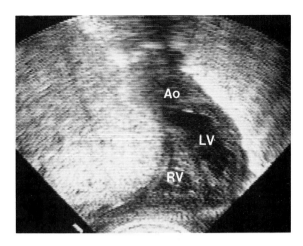

FIG 11–12.
Subcostal four-chamber view from a patient with a large mediastinal mass compressing the right ventricular (RV) chamber. Ao = aorta; LV = left ventricle.

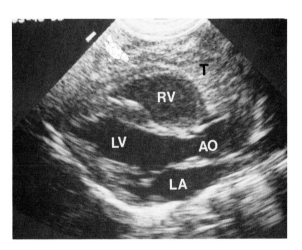

FIG 11–13.
Parasternal long-axis view from a normal infant demonstrating the appearance of a normal thymus (T) around the heart. AO = aorta; LA = left atrium; LV = left ventricle; RV = right ventricle.

compress any cardiac structures (Figs 11–13 and 11–14). Thymic tumors are usually nonhomogeneous, containing echo-bright and echolucent (fluid-filled) areas (Fig 11–15). These tumors usually compress and distort the right ventricular outflow tract, the main pulmonary artery, the aortic arch, and/or the arch vessels.

BACTERIAL ENDOCARDITIS

With higher-resolution imaging, visualization of intracardiac vegetations now is possible in many instances. There are vegetations that still may not be large enough to be imaged, and echocardiographic examination without

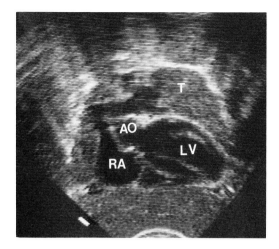

FIG 11–14.
Subcostal four-chamber view of the left ventricular (LV) outflow tract from a normal infant with a large thymus (T). The thymus has the consistency of liver tissue and does not compress the heart. AO = aorta; RA = right atrium.

visualization of vegetations does not rule out the presence of endocarditis. In any patient suspected of having endocarditis, however, careful examination should be performed to look for vegetations and to assess the potential hemodynamic consequences of the endocarditis. When vegetations are detected, the prognostic significance of the vegetations is still debatable. In a large series from Buda and coworkers,[25] 50 patients with culture-proven endocarditis were reported in whom 42% were found to have vegetations by two-dimensional echocardiography. A major complication occurred in 86% of those patients with identifiable vegetations, compared to only 62% of those without visualized vegetations. In addition, the mortality rate was increased in those patients in whom vegetations were seen. The authors, therefore, felt that visualization of a vegetation defined a high-risk group of patients with infective endocarditis. However, a subsequent study by Lutes and coworkers[26] did not find patients with vegetations to be at any higher risk of developing a major complication but did find that patients with identifiable vegetations required surgical intervention more often.

In children, differing results have also been reported. In one series, echocardiographic abnormalities were identified in only 36%, but the presence of such lesions was unrelated to the causative organism or to the need for early operation.[27] In another series, however, 82% of children studied with endocarditis had lesions identified.[28] A high percentage of patients with echocardiographic lesions had a major complication of their disease. Such lesions also resolved slowly after appropriate therapy over many months. It is debatable if the presence of lesions is at all indicative of ultimate clinical outcome. Nevertheless, the presence of such lesions clearly points to the potential for hemodynamic involvement and rapid deterioration, particularly with left-sided lesions. Echocardiography is,

therefore, an important tool for serial assessment of patients as they undergo therapy.

Echocardiographic features of infective endocarditis generally consist of initial thickening of the valve leaflets followed by the appearance of irregularly shaped lesions attached to either the valve leaflet tissue or chordal tissue (Figs 11–16 to 11–20). Lesions can be present anywhere along the valve apparatus, from well-localized lesions at

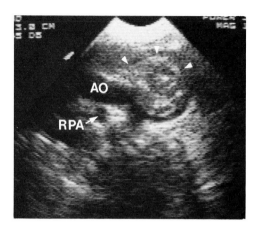

FIG 11–15.
Suprasternal long-axis view from an infant with a thymic tumor. The thymic tumor is the circular area seen above the aortic arch which is distorting the vessels to the head and neck. Unlike the normal thymus, thymic tumors are heterogeneous, containing echolucent and echo-bright areas. They also compress adjacent cardiac structures. AO = aorta; RPA = right pulmonary artery.

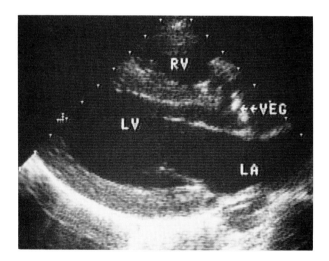

FIG 11–16.
Parasternal long-axis view from a patient with a large ventricular septal defect, pulmonary vascular obstructive disease, and subacute bacterial endocarditis. Large vegetations (VEG) were attached to the tricuspid valve chordae. These vegetations prolapse through the ventricular septal defect into the left ventricular (LV) outflow tract in diastole. LA = left atrium; RV = right ventricle.

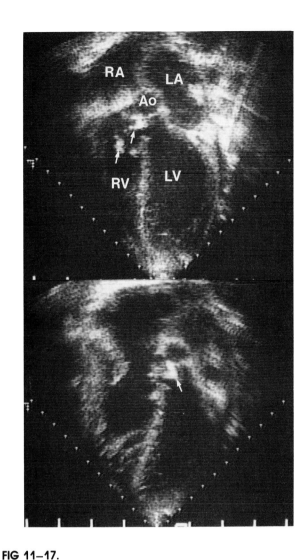

FIG 11–17.
Apical four-chamber views from the same patient as in Figure 11–16. As diastole proceeds, the vegetation *(arrows, top)* can be seen prolapsing through the ventricular septal defect into the left ventricular (LV) outflow tract *(arrow, bottom)*. Ao = aorta; LA = left atrium; RA = right atrium; RV = right ventricle.

the base of the valve attachments to the fibrous annulus, to the edges of the free leaflets, and extending down to the chordal attachments. Any valve may be involved, with the aortic and mitral valves being involved most often.[25] Right-sided structures may also be involved but less commonly.[29, 30] This is probably related to less turbulence present across right-sided valves. Lesions tend to be downstream from turbulent flow and, therefore, in atrioventricular valve regurgitation, tend to be on the atrial side of the valve, whereas in semilunar valve involvement they tend to be on the great vessel side of the valve. In ventricular septal defects, lesions occur on the right ventricular side of the defect and can often extend for great distances through the right ventricular cavity; in some cases, they can even extend through the pulmonary valve.[29] Measurement of vegetation size can be difficult because of the irregular contour

of the lesions. Assessment in several views is mandatory to fully appreciate the overall three-dimensional size of the lesion.

Although different types of organisms produce lesions with different characteristics, it is certainly not possible to diagnose the causative organism based solely upon the echocardiographic findings. However, group D streptococ-

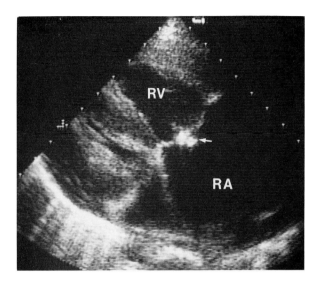

FIG 11–18.
Parasternal long-axis view through the right ventricular (RV) inflow tract of the same patient as in Figure 11–16. A prominent vegetation *(arrow)* is seen attached to the right atrial (RA) side of the tricuspid valve.

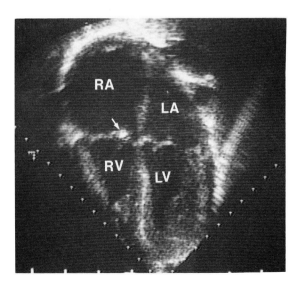

FIG 11–19.
Apical four-chamber view from the same patient as in Figure 11–16. From the apical four-chamber view, the vegetation *(arrow)* is again seen attached to the right atrial (RA) side of the tricuspid valve. LA = left atrium; LV = left ventricle; RV = right ventricle.

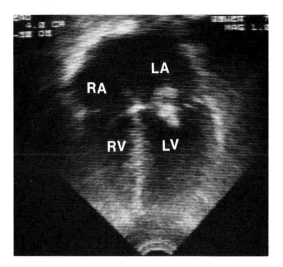

FIG 11–20.
Apical four-chamber view from a patient with bacterial endocarditis and an enormous vegetation attached to the mitral valve. LA = left atrium; LV = left ventricle; RA = right atrium; RV = right ventricle.

cal lesions and gram-negative lesions tend to produce long filamentous strands; fungal lesions and staphylococcal lesions, on the other hand, tend to produce globular masses. Staphylococcal lesions can even mimic the appearance of a left atrial myxoma when attached to the mitral valve on the atrial side.[31] However, the lack of a stalk attachment to the atrial septum should suggest that the examiner is not dealing with an atrial myxoma but rather a vegetation or other neoplasm, as discussed above. This distinction is further complicated by the realization that atrial myxomas also may become infected secondarily; therefore, an atrial myxoma with positive blood cultures can exist. The echocardiographic appearance of the lesion should at least suggest one diagnosis rather than the other.[32]

The aortic root itself is also a target for bacterial lesions. Aortic root abscess and aneurysm formation in the sinuses of Valsalva have been reported (Fig 11–21).[33, 34]

Finally, the hemodynamic consequences of all lesions must be carefully assessed. Doppler flow gradients across all valves and evidence of valvular regurgitation must be carefully sought. In addition, the presence of new regurgitant jets in the absence of true vegetations but in the clinical situation of endocarditis is strong evidence for infective endocarditis. Color-flow imaging of all valves is mandatory to detect small regurgitant jets and also to point out when multiple jets occur, again implying more involvement of the affected valve.

Serial studies are useful for tracking the course of the patient's disease. However, vegetations require a fair time to regress and, therefore, a patient should not be considered necessarily a therapeutic failure if the lesion remains. That it is slowly resolving in size is the important issue, together with the patient's clinical status. Sudden disappearance of a lesion should raise the question of embolization, and

careful evaluation of the patient for the site of embolization must be undertaken. As on initial study, serial assessment of vegetation size must be done in multiple views to assess the size accurately. In addition, it is necessary to be highly cognizant of the effects of different gain settings upon apparent lesion size. As higher gain settings are employed, there is an apparent increase in the lesion size.

In summary, to be visualized, vegetations must be greater than 1 mm in size. These lesions place the patient at an increased risk for embolic events and are slow to resolve. Even after adequate treatment, resolution of the lesions can take several months, and the acute disappearance of a lesion must raise the question of embolization. Long, filamentous lesions are usually associated with group D streptococcal or gram-negative organisms, while large, globular lesions are usually associated with either fungal or staphylococcal organisms. In general, lesions occur on the low-pressure side of the jet (i.e., on the great vessel side of the semilunar valves, the right ventricular side of a ventricular septal defect, or the atrial side of an atrioventricular valve). Careful examination of all valves must be performed from many different views to exclude vegetations. When one lesion is found, all aspects of that structure must be examined, and Doppler interrogation of the involved structure is mandatory to assess the degree of hemodynamic impairment. Serial assessment is usually indicated, particularly to assess the ongoing changes in the hemodynamic status.

FOREIGN BODIES

The most common foreign body encountered is the intravascular catheter, either placed in the heart by design

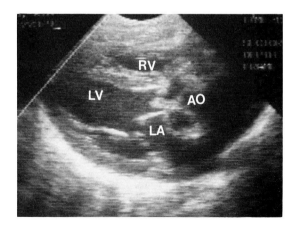

FIG 11–21.
Parasternal long-axis view from a newborn infant with aortic valve stenosis who developed bacterial endocarditis of the aortic valve. The infection extended into the aortic root and caused the development of a sinus of Valsalva aneurysm. The aneurysmal dilatation involves the posterior coronary cusp. The aortic valve leaflet is thickened and prolapsing into the left ventricle (LV). AO = aorta; LA = left atrium; RV = right ventricle.

or having migrated to the heart from a more distal site. The purpose of the echocardiographic examination is to define the location of the catheter and any hemodynamic effects it may be creating (i.e., valvular insufficiency) and to ascertain if any thrombi or vegetation have formed on the catheter. Thrombus and vegetation formation are discussed in detail elsewhere.

Catheters are constructed of material with acoustic density different from that of muscle and blood; therefore, sound velocity through the catheter wall is altered so that the width of the catheter, as measured from the ultrasound image, differs from the actual diameter. This tends to make the walls appear thicker than they are, although the lumen of the catheter is still easily seen in most cases. In addition, the entire length of the catheter does not lie within the same two-dimensional plane and tends to come in and out of the plane, with only portions of the catheter visible at any one time. It is therefore necessary to make minor alterations from the standard echocardiographic planes to image the catheter along its entire length and to follow it to its tip. Finally, locating the tip of the catheter can be very difficult. For these reasons, it is possible to determine where the body of the catheter is located but often difficult to tell with certainty where the tip is located.

Umbilical venous catheters are easily visualized entering the heart from the inferior vena cava. In general, their tips should be positioned at approximately the right atrial-inferior vena caval junction; often, however, they have been advanced further into the heart, either crossing the atrial septum to lie in the left atrium or crossing the tricuspid valve to lie in the right ventricle. It is important that the catheter tip be localized as precisely as possible. A large catheter placed within the heart (i.e., for extracorporeal membrane oxygenation) should also have its tip just within the right atrium (Fig 11–22). Because the tips of these catheters are somewhat larger, it is easier to clearly ascertain their exact location. Particularly with larger catheters but also with small umbilical catheters, perforation of the cardiac walls does occur. From imaging alone, it can be difficult to determine if the tip has simply been pushed up against the wall or completely through it. The presence of a pericardial effusion clearly points to perforation but is not absolutely diagnostic. Contrast echocardiography can be very helpful in this situation. Saline is injected into the catheter in question and microcavitations that appear in the pericardial space clearly document perforation (see Chapter 3).

Endocardial pacing catheters raise specific questions. The appearance of these catheters is different from fluid-filled catheters as there is no central echo-free space. By design, they lie next to the endocardial surface so that it is difficult to diagnose perforation of the cardiac wall. Again, the presence of a pericardial effusion suggests perforation but definitive diagnosis of this can be quite difficult and usually requires detection of an acute change in pacing parameters.

Of equal importance are the hemodynamic consequences of an in-dwelling catheter on atrioventricular valve

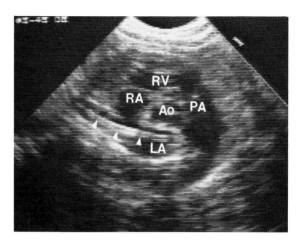

FIG 11–22.
Parasternal short-axis view from a newborn infant in whom an umbilical venous catheter *(arrows)* has been passed inadvertently across the foramen ovale into the left atrium. Ao = aorta; LA = left atrium; RA = right atrium; RV = right ventricle; PA = pulmonary artery.

function specifically. Careful Doppler assessment of the atrioventricular valve, particularly with color mapping in the region where the catheter crosses the valve, is extremely important.

ANEURYSM OF THE LEFT VENTRICLE

Left ventricular aneurysms can be acquired as a consequence of myocardial infarction, cardiovascular surgery, trauma, or endocarditis, or they can be congenital. The majority of acquired aneurysms are located at the left ventricular apex but can involve any region of the left ventricle.[35–37] Congenital aneurysms can occur at either the base of the heart with a large dilated area posterior to the left atrium[38, 39] or at the apex, being either a true aneurysm or a diverticulum.[40]

An aneurysm can be defined as an abnormal bulge or outpouching in the left ventricular contour that occurs during both systole and diastole. The area of the aneurysm itself may be akinetic or dyskinetic, with paradoxical motion during the cardiac cycle. In the setting of myocardial disease, dyskinetic segments can be precursors of areas of aneurysm formation. The examiner must be cautious to differentiate between a true aneurysm and more global hypokinesis by demonstrating a clear difference between the motion of the walls of the aneurysm and the surrounding myocardium.

Once an area of an aneurysm or potential aneurysm is identified, careful delineation of all boundaries of this area is necessary. Imaging must be performed in a minimum of two views to delineate fully the boundaries of the aneurysm (Figs 11–23 and 11–24). Ideally, three orthogonal planes should be used.

Left ventricular aneurysms have a variable influence upon left ventricular function. Usual indexes of function

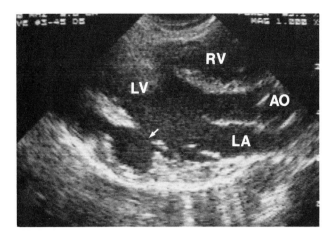

FIG 11–23.
Parasternal long-axis view from an adolescent male with a large pseudoaneurysm *(arrow)* of the left ventricular posterior wall. In the area of the aneurysm, there is a disruption in the left ventricular (LV) myocardium. AO = aorta; LV = left ventricle; RV = right ventricle.

measured with M-mode techniques are of no value or only limited value, as the area contributing to the measurement may not be affected. Various indexes for quantitation of function in the presence of an aneurysm have been proposed.[41] Calculation of ejection fraction from two-dimensional echocardiography is helpful, as is regional ejection fraction calculation. Qualitative description of segment motion, whether hyperkinetic, akinetic, or dyskinetic, should also be performed. Finally, careful attention should be directed toward identification of any thrombi associated with the aneurysm itself, as will be discussed below.

For aneurysms involving the basilar area of the heart near the mitral valve annulus, the neck or entrance of the aneurysm is often small, and phasic flow can often be demonstrated into and out of this area by color-flow mapping. In some instances, the aneurysm can serve as a reservoir, with hemodynamic effects upon the left ventricle similar to that of mitral regurgitation. In addition, aneurysms associated with the mitral valve ring may produce mitral regurgitation by distorting the annulus. Contrast studies have also been used to demonstrate flow patterns into and out of submitral aneurysms,[42] although color-flow Doppler mapping may make this unnecessary.

Distinction must also be made between a true aneurysm and a pseudoaneurysm, defined as an acquired blood-filled space external to the cardiac chambers but communicating with the left ventricle through a hole in the ventricular wall.[43, 44] Echocardiographically, the pseudoaneurysm is recognized by the sharp discontinuity of the endocardial image at the site of communication with the left ventricular cavity and the presence of a narrow orifice leading to the relatively larger diameter aneurysm. The body of the pseudoaneurysm is often in a different plane from that of the communication with the left ventricular cavity; therefore, multiple views are necessary to delineate fully the size and location of the pseudoaneurysm as well

as the site of communication with the left ventricle. The majority tend to be located posterior to the left ventricle, and the apical four-chamber view and subcostal views tend to be the most useful. Doppler color-flow mapping can be useful for delineation of phasic flow into and out of the pseudoaneurysm, more clearly defining the communication site.[45]

Aneurysms of other chambers do occur, but with less frequency. Left atrial aneurysms[46] can arise from the atrial appendage or posterior free wall. They are best imaged from the subcostal view or apical four-chamber view and are recognized by their well-defined connection with the left atrium, their position within the posterior pericardial space, and their phasic flow.

Finally, aneurysms of other structures occur, but also with less frequency. Aneurysms of the right ventricle usually occur in patients after cardiovascular surgery (see Chapter 13). Aneurysms following endocarditis of the right ventricle and aortic root have been reported.[47, 48] Aneurysms of the mitral valve leaflets also occur with the leaflet extending back into the left atrial cavity and, in some cases, becoming adherent to the left atrial wall.[49]

INTRACAVITARY THROMBI

Although intravascular thrombi are uncommon in a patient with a normal heart, specific situations increase the risk for thrombus formation. These include dilated cardiomyopathy, ventricular aneurysm, dilated atria (especially when either atrial fibrillation or flutter is present), the presence of intravascular catheters, myocardial infarction, prosthetic valves, recently placed intracardiac patches, and certain hypercoagulable states. Using definite echo-

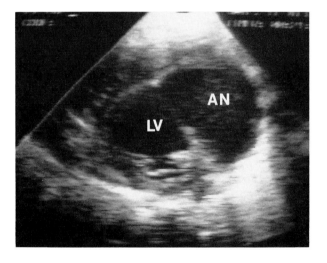

FIG 11–24.
Parasternal short-axis view from a patient with an aneurysm (AN) of the left ventricle (LV). A wide neck connects the aneurysm to the LV.

cardiographic criteria, the sensitivity for thrombus detection has been estimated to be as high as 95%, with a specificity of 86%. Echocardiographic criteria for thrombus diagnosis include:

1. An echogenic mass present within a cardiac chamber contiguous with the endocardium in at least one area.
2. The mass visible in at least two different views.
3. Usually, the thrombus attached to the chamber wall along a broad area.

In addition, thrombi tend to have bright, relatively smooth borders and a homogeneous appearance. Specific areas more likely to harbor thrombi include the ventricular apex, the atrial appendages, and intravascular catheters.

All echocardiographic views may be helpful, depending on the location of the thrombus. When a question of intraventricular thrombi arises, careful attention must be paid to the apical four-chamber view, as it images the apex best. The apex is the most common site for ventricular thrombus formation, particularly in the presence of a dilated cardiomyopathy. It is important not to foreshorten the view and, as a result, not fully image the apex. The sagittal subcostal view permits imaging of both the right ventricular and left ventricular apex from an orthogonal view to further define the apical regions of both ventricles.

Atrial thrombi are best imaged from those views that permit imaging of the atrial appendages. The subcostal sagittal view permits imaging of the right atrial appendage, while the subcostal coronal and, to a lesser degree, the apical four-chamber view permit imaging of the left atrial appendage. Although most atrial thrombi are relatively fixed in position, some may be highly mobile and may mimic a left atrial myxoma. Differentiation can be difficult and should rest on the location of the mass and the manner of its attachment to the atrial wall. The edges of a myxoma may be smoother than a thrombus, but this is not always the case. Thrombi can form in other low flow areas of the atria such as on the downstream side of the eustachian valve (Figs 11–25 to 11–27).

Thrombi may be present at birth, especially in infants whose mothers have clotting disorders such an anti-thrombin III deficiency. We have seen one infant with fatal thrombosis of the aortic arch and one infant with thrombus formation in the pulmonary artery whose mothers had antithrombin III deficiency (Figs 11–28 and 11–29).

Thrombi associated with prosthetic valves may be recognized by the presence of multiple strong irregular echoes associated with the valve. Care must be taken to not confuse the normal enhanced echogenicity of the prosthetic valve with the presence of thrombi. Imaging of the valve in multiple views is useful in making this distinction. In addition, the leaflets of the valve may show diminished or jerky motion when a thrombus is present. Doppler examination will show increased velocity of flow with an increased mean gradient across the valve. Secondary signs of valve obstruction, such as dilatation of the proximal chamber, are also likely to be present.

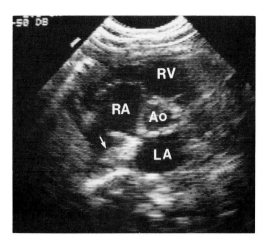

FIG 11–25.
Parasternal short-axis view from a 6-week-old infant with a thrombus *(arrow)* extending up the inferior vena cava, along the eustachian valve, and to the atrial septum. Ao = aorta; LA = left atrium; RA = right atrium; RV = right ventricle.

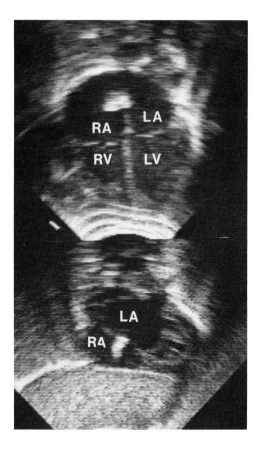

FIG 11–26.
Apical *(top)* and subcostal *(bottom)* four-chamber views from the same patient as in Figure 11–25. The attachment of the thrombus to the atrial septum in the region of the fossa ovalis is clearly seen. LA = left atrium; LV = left ventricle; RA = right atrium; RV = right ventricle.

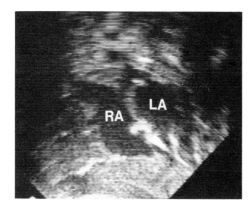

FIG 11–27.
Subcostal sagittal view from the same patient as in Figure 11–25. The thrombus is seen extending from the inferior vena cava along the eustachian valve to the area of the fossa ovalis. LA = left atrium; RA = right atrium.

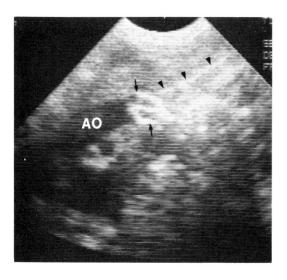

FIG 11–28.
Suprasternal long-axis view of the aortic (AO) arch of an infant born with a large thrombus filling the transverse aorta and extending into the head and neck vessels (arrows).

Finally, thrombi associated with intravascular catheters may occur wherever a catheter has been placed (Fig 11–30). Most commonly, these thrombi occur in the right atrium or right ventricle associated with a right atrial catheter placed for chronic intravenous administration of medication or nutrition or a transvenous pacing catheter. Nevertheless, in neonates, thrombi have been associated with umbilical artery catheters placed in the descending aorta. Such thrombi may persist or be detected after catheter removal. When the catheter is still present, care must again be exercised to distinguish between the normal echogenicity of the catheter and a thrombus. Catheter echoes are, in general, parallel lines that are smooth. The presence

of irregular echoes associated with a catheter or the presence of additional echoes extending off the walls of the catheter must raise the possibility of thrombus formation.

Distinction between thrombus and tumor remains difficult and may not be possible in all cases. Helpful distinguishing factors are:

1. The underlying cardiovascular disease, e.g., thrombi are likely to be present with dilated cardiomyopathy.
2. The presence of intravascular foreign material.
3. The manner of attachment of the mass in question to the underlying myocardium (a small area of attachment is more likely with a tumor).

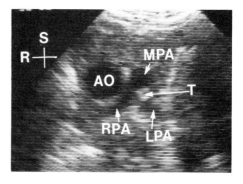

FIG 11–29.
High parasternal view from a newborn infant whose mother had an anti-thrombin III deficiency. At birth, this infant was noted to have a large circular thrombus (T) located in the main pulmonary artery (MPA) near the pulmonary artery bifurcation. AO = aorta; LPA = left pulmonary artery; R = right; RPA = right pulmonary artery; S = superior.

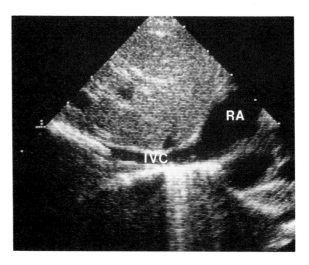

FIG 11–30.
Subcostal sagittal view of the inferior vena cava (IVC) and its junction with the right atrium (RA) in a patient with a large thrombus filling the IVC. The thrombus is the caste of a previous catheter that had been left in the IVC. Note that this thrombus caste actually has an echolucent area representing the previous catheter lumen.

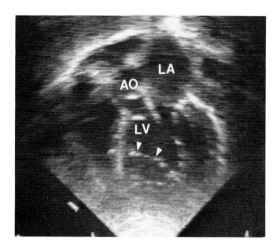

FIG 11–31.
Apical five-chamber view from a patient with a subaortic membrane and a false tendon *(arrows)* traversing the apical portion of the left ventricle (LV). This is a normal finding. AO = aorta; LA = left atrium.

FALSE TENDONS

Within the ventricular cavity, false tendons as well as chordae from the atrioventricular valves may be seen. In the left ventricle, chordae from the mitral valve do not insert on the ventricular septum normally. Yet, fibromuscular bands connecting the septum and free wall as well as the papillary muscles and the septum can be seen. It becomes important to distinguish false tendons from abnormal chordal attachments as well as other pathologic structures. It has been estimated that false tendons can be seen in 50% of children, occurring in both normal and abnormal hearts.[50]

False tendons are best imaged from either the apical four-chamber view or the subcostal coronal view (Fig 11–31). They usually traverse the left ventricular minor axis from the septum to the free wall but can extend into the outflow tract. They are usually thin structures and never attach to the mitral apparatus. When present in the outflow tract, they must be differentiated from a subaortic membrane that may attach to the mitral apparatus.

REFERENCES

1. Panidis IP, Mintz GS, McAllister M: Hemodynamic consequences of left atrial myxomas as assessed by Doppler ultrasound. *Am Heart J* 1986; 111:927–931.
2. Barold SS, Hicks GL, Nanda NC, et al: Mitral valve myxoma diagnosed by two-dimensional echocardiography. *Am J Cardiol* 1987; 59:182–183.
3. Gosse P, Herpin D, Roudaut R, et al: Myxoma of the mitral valve diagnosed by echocardiography. *Am Heart J* 1986; 111:803–805.
4. Abramowitz R, Majdan JF, Plzak LF, et al: Two-dimensional echocardiographic diagnosis of separate myxomas of both the left atrium and left ventricle. *Am J Cardiol* 1984; 53:379–380.
5. Gladden JR, Dreiling RJ, Gollub SB, et al: Two-dimensional echocardiographic features of multiple right atrial myxomas. *Am J Cardiol* 1983; 52:1364–1365.
6. Goli VD, Thadani U, Thomas SR, et al: Doppler echocardiographic profiles in obstructive right and left atrial myxomas. *J Am Coll Cardiol* 1987; 9:701–703.
7. Chia BL, Lim CH, Sheares JH, et al: Echocardiographic findings in right ventricular myxoma. *Am J Cardiol* 1986; 58:663–664.
8. Viswanathan B, Luber JM Jr, Bell-Thomson J: Right ventricular myxoma. *Ann Thorac Surg* 1985; 39:280–281.
9. Nanda NC, Barold SS, Gramiak R, et al: Echocardiographic features of right ventricular outflow tumor prolapsing into the pulmonary artery. *Am J Cardiol* 1977; 40:272–276.
10. Green SE, Joynt LF, Fitzgerald PJ, et al: In vivo ultrasonic tissue characterization of human intracardiac masses. *Am J Cardiol* 1983; 51:231–236.
11. Bass JL, Breningstall GN, Swaiman KF: Echocardiographic incidence of cardiac rhabdomyoma in tuberous sclerosis. *Am J Cardiol* 1985; 55:1379–1382.
12. Fischer DR, Beerman LB, Park SC, et al: Diagnosis of intracardiac rhabdomyoma by two-dimensional echocardiography. *Am J Cardiol* 1984; 53:978–979.
13. Gresser CD, Shime J, Rakowski H, et al: Fetal cardiac tumor: A prenatal echocardiographic marker for tuberous sclerosis. *Am J Obstet Gynecol* 1987; 156:689–690.
14. Wright EC, Wellons HA, Martin RP: Primary pulmonary artery sarcoma diagnosed noninvasively by two-dimensional echocardiography. *Circulation* 1983; 67:459–462.
15. Hynes JK, Tajik AJ, Osborn MJ, et al: Two-dimensional echocardiographic diagnosis of pericardial cyst. *Mayo Clin Proc* 1983; 58:60–63.
16. Agatston AS, Robinson MJ, Trigo L, et al: Echocardiographic findings in primary pericardial mesothelioma. *Am Heart J* 1986; 111:986–988.
17. Armstrong WF, Buck JD, Hoffman R, et al: Cardiac involvement by lymphoma: detection and follow-up by two-dimensional echocardiography. *Am Heart J* 1986; 112:627–631.
18. Lutas EM, Stelzer P: Echocardiographic demonstration of right atrial rupture in a patient with right-sided cardiac tumor. *Chest* 1983; 83:921–922.
19. Cohen DE, Mora C, Keefe DL: Echocardiographic findings of metastatic chondrosarcoma involving the left atrium. *Am Heart J* 1986; 111:993–996.
20. Mich RJ, Gillam LD, Weyman AE: Osteogenic sarcomas mimicking left atrial myxomas: Clinical and two-dimensional echocardiographic features. *J Am Coll Cardiol* 1985; 6:1422–1427.
21. Kutalek SP, Panidis IP, Kotler MN, et al: Metastatic tumors of the heart detected by two-dimensional echocardiography. *Am Heart J* 1985; 109:343–349.
22. Chia BL, Choo MH, Tan L, et al: Two-dimensional echocardiographic abnormalities of right atrial metastatic tumors in hepatoma. *Chest* 1985; 87:399–401.
23. Grenadier E, Lima CO, Barron JV, et al: Two-dimen-

sional echocardiography for evaluation of metastatic cardiac tumors in pediatric patients. *Am Heart J* 1984; 107:122–126.

24. Johnson MH, Soulen RL: Echocardiography of cardiac metastases. *Am J Roentgen* 1983; 141:677–681.

25. Buda AJ, Zotz RJ, LeMire MS, et al: Prognostic significance of vegetations detected by two-dimensional echocardiography in infective endocarditis. *Am J Cardiol* 1986; 58:649–650.

26. Lutas EM, Roberts RB, Devereux RB, et al: Relation between the presence of echocardiographic vegetations and the complication rate in infective endocarditis. *Am Heart J* 1986; 112:107–113.

27. Bricker JT, Latson LA, Huhta JC, et al: Echocardiographic evaluation of infective endocarditis in children. *Am J Cardiol* 1985; 55:1433–1435.

28. Kavey RE, Frank DM, Byrum CJ, et al: Two-dimensional echocardiographic assessment of infective endocarditis in children. *Am J Dis Child* 1983; 13:851–856.

29. Agathangelou NE, dos Santos LA, Lewis BS: Real-time 2-dimensional echocardiographic imaging of right-sided cardiac vegetations in ventricular septal defect. *Am J Cardiol* 1983; 52:420–421.

30. Robbins MJ, Frater RW, Soeiro R, et al: Influence of vegetation size on clinical outcome of right-sided infective endocarditis. *Am J Med* 1986; 80:165–171.

31. Zee-Cheng CS, Gibbs HR, Johnson KP, et al: Giant vegetation due to Staphylococcus aureus endocarditis imulating left atrial myxoma. *Am Heart J* 1986; 111:414–417.

32. Quinn TJ, Codini MA, Harris AA: Infected cardiac myxoma. *Am J Cardiol* 1984; 53:381–382.

33. Saner HE, Asinger RW, Homans DC, et al: Two-dimensional echocardiographic identification of complicated aortic root endocarditis: Implications for surgery. *J Am Coll Cardiol* 1987; 10:859–868.

34. Shaffer EM, Snider AR, Beekman RH, et al: Sinus of Valsalva aneurysm complicating bacterial endocarditis in an infant. Diagnosis with two-dimensional and Doppler echocardiography. *J Am Coll Cardiol* 1987; 9:588–591.

35. Baur HR, Daniel JA, Nelson RR: Detection of left ventricular aneurysm on two dimensional echocardiography. *Am J Cardiol* 1982; 50:191–196.

36. Weyman AE, Peskoe SM, Williams ES, et al: Detection of left ventricular aneurysms by cross-sectional echocardiography. *Circulation* 1976; 54:936–944.

37. Visser CA, Kan G, Meltzer RS, et al: Incidence, timing and prognostic value of left ventricular aneurysm formation after myocardial infarction: A prospective. *Am J Cardiol* 1986; 57:729–732.

38. Shaddy R, Silverman NH, Stanger P, et al: Two-dimensional echocardiographic recognition and repair of subvalvular mitral aneurysm of the left ventricle in an infant. *J Am Coll Cardiol* 1985; 5:765–769.

39. Davis MD, Caspi A, Lewis BS, et al: Two-dimensional echocardiographic features of submitral left ventricular aneurysm. *Am Heart J* 1982; 103:289–290.

40. Hamaoka K, Onaka M, Tanaka T, et al: Congenital ventricular aneurysm and diverticulum in children. *Pediatr Cardiol* 1987; 8:169–175.

41. Ryan T, Petrovic O, Armstrong WF, et al: Quantitative two-dimensional echocardiographic assessment of patients undergoing left ventricular aneurysmectomy. *Am Heart J* 1986; 111:714–720.

42. Shah VK, Vaidya KA, Daruwala DF, et al: Submitral aneurysm diagnosed by left ventricular contrast echocardiography. *Am Heart J* 1988; 115:682–684.

43. Saner HE, Asinger RW, Daniel JA, et al: Two-dimensional echocardiographic identification of left ventricular pseudoaneurysm. *Am Heart J* 1986; 112:977–985.

44. Gatewood RP Jr, Nanda NC: Differentiation of left ventricular pseudoaneurysm from true aneurysm with two-dimensional echocardiography. *Am J Cardiol* 1980; 46:869–878.

45. Roelandt JR, Sutherland GR, Yoshida K, et al: Improved diagnosis and characterization of left ventricular pseudoaneurysm by Doppler color flow imaging. *J Am Coll Cardiol* 1988; 12:807–811.

46. Foale RA, Gibson TC, Guyer DE, et al: Congenital aneurysms of the left atrium: Recognition by cross-sectional echocardiography. *Circulation* 1982; 66:1065–1069.

47. Garty B, Berant M, Weinhouse E, et al: False aneurysm of the right ventricle due to endocarditis in a child. *Pediatr Cardiol* 1987; 8:275–277.

48. Sapsford RN, Fitchett DH, Tarin D, et al: Aneurysm of left ventricle secondary to bacterial endocarditis. *J Thorac Cardiovasc Surg* 1979; 78:79–86.

49. Lewis BS, Colsen PR, Rosenfeld T, et al: An unusual case of mitral valve aneurysm: Two dimensional echocardiographic and cineangiocardiographic features. *Am J Cardiol* 1982; 49:1293–1296.

50. Brenner JI, Baker K, Ringel RE, et al: Echocardiographic evidence of left ventricular bands in infants and children. *J Am Coll Cardiol* 1984; 3:1515–1520.

Cardiomyopathies

The term cardiomyopathy refers to a variety of myocardial abnormalities. Although most cases of cardiomyopathy are not congenital, this chapter is included because cardiomyopathies are a frequently encountered problem in the care of children with cardiac disorders.

From an etiologic point of view, cardiomyopathies can be classified as primary or secondary cardiomyopathies (Table 12–1). Primary cardiomyopathies have no associated cardiovascular or systemic disease to account for the myocardial abnormalities; secondary cardiomyopathies occur because of an associated disease. Cardiomyopathies can be further classified according to their anatomic and functional features into congestive, hypertrophic or obstructive, and restrictive types.[1] [3]

With echocardiography, the anatomic and functional nature of the cardiomyopathy can be defined; however, it is usually not possible to determine the cause or the precise histologic type of cardiomyopathy from the echocardiogram. Many of the echocardiographic findings provide the clinician with information that is invaluable in the search for the exact etiology and appropriate management of the cardiomyopathy.[2]

CONGESTIVE CARDIOMYOPATHY

M-Mode Echocardiographic Features

The presence of a dilated, poorly contractile left ventricle makes congestive cardiomyopathy easy to recognize by M-mode and two-dimensional echocardiography. On the M-mode echocardiogram, the left ventricular end-diastolic and end-systolic dimensions are usually well above the normal limits for body surface area (Fig 12–1). Usually, the left atrium is also enlarged. On the M-mode echocardiogram at the level of the anterior mitral valve leaflet, marked E point-septal separation is found, and E point-septal separation normalized for end-diastolic dimension is markedly increased, well above the values found in chil-

dren with left ventricular volume overload (see Chapter 4 for details of how to calculate these indexes).[4]

The left ventricular shortening fraction is markedly depressed—values as low as 8% to 10% are not uncommon. Likewise, the heart rate-corrected mean velocity of circumferential fiber shortening is extremely low, and evaluation of the wall stress-fiber shortening relationship shows that this index is low because of depressed contractility rather than high afterload (see Chapter 4).[4, 5]

Digitized M-mode tracings of the left ventricular cavity and posterior wall show that the peak rate of shortening of the left ventricle and the peak rate of thickening of the left ventricular posterior wall are markedly depressed.[6, 7]

All of these M-mode echocardiographic measurements provide a valuable technique for the serial assessment of systolic function in the child with a congestive cardiomyopathy.

Two-Dimensional Echocardiographic Features

In congestive cardiomyopathy, marked left ventricular enlargement and poor contractility create a dramatic and easily recognized two-dimensional echocardiographic image (Fig 12–2). The enlarged left atrium and left ventricle can be visualized in the parasternal long- and short-axis, apical, and subcostal four-chamber views (Figs 12–3 and 12–4). In real time, a global hypokinesia of all the left ventricular walls is present, and the ejection fraction calculated from two-dimensional volume analysis is extremely low.

The low flow velocities in the left heart chambers create an increased risk for thrombus formation in patients with congestive cardiomyopathy. A freshly formed thrombus can be extremely difficult to detect on the two-dimensional echocardiogram; therefore, the left atrium and left ventricle should be carefully searched in each view, using multiple transducer angulations and various instrument gain settings. Special attention should be directed toward

TABLE 12–1.

Classification of Cardiomyopathies*

Primary cardiomyopathies
  Congestive
    Endocardial fibroelastosis of infancy
    Idiopathic type
  Restrictive
    Hypertrophic type with ventricular hypertrophy and small cavities
    Endomyocardial fibrosis
  Obstructive or hypertrophic type
    Idiopathic hypertrophic subaortic stenosis
Secondary cardiomyopathies
  Infective
    Virus
    Diphtheritic
  Metabolic
    Carnitine deficiency
    Glycogenosis type II (Pompe's disease)
  Neurologic or muscular disease
    Friedreich's ataxia
    Muscular dystrophy (Duchenne's)
  Collagen disease
    Systemic lupus erythematosis

*From Harris LC, Nghiem QX: Cardiomyopathies in infants and children. *Prog Cardiovasc Dis* 1972; 15:255–287. Used by permission.

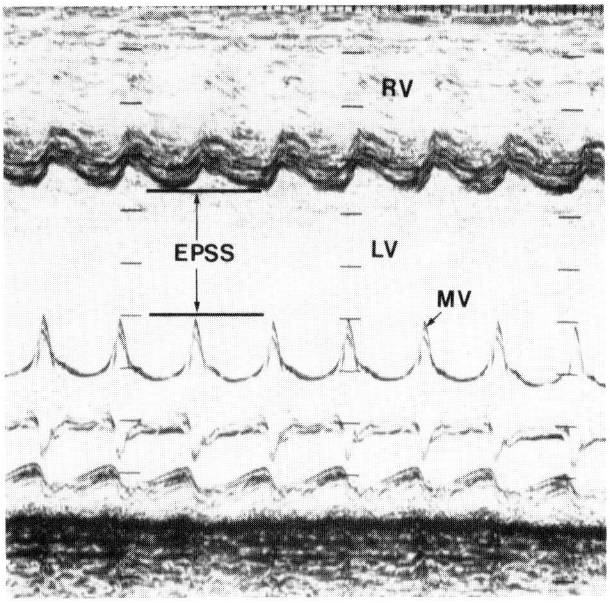

imaging the left atrial appendage and cardiac apex—two areas that are difficult to examine in congestive cardiomyopathy patients and that are frequent sites for thrombus formation (Fig 12–4). Because the left ventricle is so enlarged in congestive cardiomyopathy, the left ventricular apex is rotated posteriorly and inferiorly and is difficult to image because of the adjacent lung tissue. To clearly image this portion of the left ventricle, the patient can be placed in a steep left lateral decubitus position. When the patient is in this position, a cutout area in the mattress can facilitate placement of the transducer over the cardiac apex. Similarly, in patients with a dilated left atrium, the left

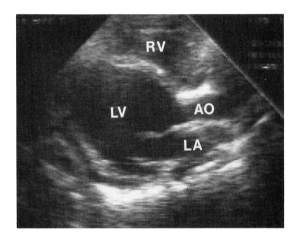

FIG 12–2.
Parasternal long-axis view from a child with congestive cardiomyopathy. The left ventricle (LV) is markedly dilated and globular. AO = aorta; LA = left atrium; RV = right ventricle.

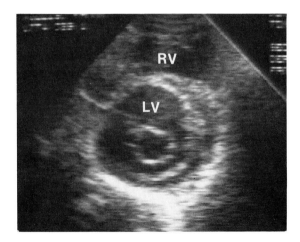

FIG 12–3.
Parasternal short-axis view at the level of the mitral valve from the same patient as in Figure 12–2. The left ventricle (LV) is markedly dilated and there is marked separation between the anterior mitral valve leaflet and the ventricular septum. RV = right ventricle.

FIG 12–1.
M-mode echocardiogram of the left ventricle (LV) from a patient with congestive cardiomyopathy. The LV end-diastolic and end-systolic dimensions are markedly increased. In addition, there is a wide separation between the maximum excursion of the mitral valve (MV) and the most posterior excursion of the ventricular septum. This distance is called the E point-septal separation (EPSS). In this patient, EPSS measured 2.5 cm, which is well above the 95th percentile. RV = right ventricle.

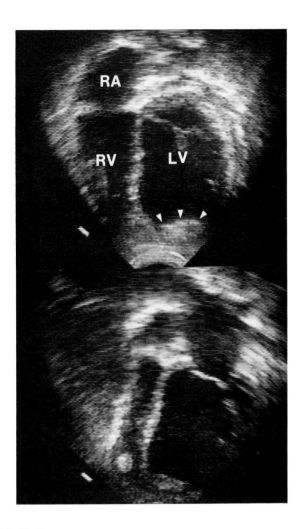

FIG 12–4.
Apical four-chamber views from a patient with congestive cardiomyopathy. The *top frame* was taken with the transducer oriented far posteriorly to image the posterior portion of the left ventricular (LV) apex. A thrombus *(arrows)* is seen in the dilated and noncontractile portion of the LV apex. In the *bottom frame,* the transducer has been rotated slightly rightward and anteriorly to examine the right ventricular (RV) apex. A dense, circular thrombus is seen in the apex of the RV. RA = right atrium.

atrial appendage is often obscured by the adjacent lung tissue. The left atrial appendage can usually be visualized in the parasternal short-axis view at the base of the heart by having the patient lie in a steep left lateral decubitus position and hold his or her breath out at end-expiration. Alternatively, the left atrial appendage can be visualized in some patients in the subcostal four-chamber view through the left ventricle.

In infants with endocardial fibroelastosis, the left ventricle can be dilated or contracted. Usually, the left ventricle is dilated and the endocardium is thick, pearly-white, stiff, and rubbery. These fibroelastotic changes usually involve the left ventricle and left atrium but can also involve the endocardial surface of the right ventricle. The right atrium is rarely involved. Endocardial fibroelastotic changes

may be spread diffusely throughout the affected chambers or may have a patchy distribution. On the two-dimensional echocardiogram, endocardial fibroelastosis can be seen as an area of echogenicity along the endocardial surface. Endocardial fibroelastosis with a patchy distribution is easier to detect on the two-dimensional echocardiogram than that with a diffuse distribution. In the patchy distribution, the lesions stand out as echo-bright areas surrounded by normal endocardium. When the entire endocardium is involved, it is more difficult to determine if the endocardial echoes are too bright.

In children with echocardiographic findings that suggest congestive cardiomyopathy, it is important that anomalous origin of the left main coronary artery from the pulmonary artery be excluded as a cause of depressed myocardial contractility. To exclude this surgically treatable abnormality, a clear demonstration of the left main coronary artery arising normally from the aorta should be obtained in the parasternal short-axis view.

Doppler Echocardiographic Features

In patients with congestive cardiomyopathy, several indexes measured from the ascending aorta Doppler tracing are useful for assessment of left ventricular systolic function. These indexes include aortic peak velocity, peak and mean acceleration rates, acceleration time, deceleration rates, and deceleration time (see Chapter 4).

In patients with dilated cardiomyopathy, peak aortic velocity is markedly decreased compared to that of normal subjects (cardiomyopathy patients = 47 cm/sec, range 35 to 62 cm/sec and normal subjects = 92 cm/sec, range 72 to 120 cm/sec). The aortic velocity time integral is also very decreased in cardiomyopathy patients (6.7 cm, range 3.5 to 9.1; normal subjects = 15.7 cm, range 12.6 to 22.5). Aortic acceleration time is shorter in cardiomyopathy patients (73 msec, range 55 to 98 msec) compared to normals (98 msec, range 83 to 118 msec); however, there is considerable overlap in the values for this time interval between the two patient groups. Mean aortic acceleration is significantly reduced in cardiomyopathy patients (659 cm/sec^2, range 389 to 921 cm/sec^2) compared to normals (955 cm/sec^2, range 735 to 1,318 cm/sec^2), but again, there is overlap in this data between the two groups. Deceleration time and mean deceleration rate are lower in cardiomyopathy patients but are less useful indexes for assessing systolic function.[8]

Left ventricular diastolic filling abnormalities have also been detected in patients with congestive cardiomyopathy on the mitral valve Doppler examination. Cardiomyopathy patients with no significant mitral regurgitation have a reduced peak E velocity and increased A/E velocity ratio compared to normal subjects. Cardiomyopathy patients with mitral regurgitation have normal peak E and A velocities and normal A/E velocity ratio but a shortened deceleration half-time. Thus, filling abnormalities are frequently present on the mitral valve Doppler examination of cardiomyopathy patients but can be masked by high filling pressures (i.e., significant mitral regurgitation).[9]

In children with congestive cardiomyopathy, left atrial and left ventricular enlargement can lead to dilatation of the aortic and mitral valve fibrous rings and, consequently, insufficiency of these two valves. Sometimes, aortic and mitral regurgitation is caused not by valve dilatation but by involvement of the valve leaflets in the myopathic process (i.e., endocardial fibroelastosis can involve the valve surfaces, chordae, and papillary muscles). Pulsed and color-flow Doppler techniques are particularly useful for the detection and quantitation of aortic and mitral insufficiency.

HYPERTROPHIC CARDIOMYOPATHY

Hypertrophic cardiomyopathy is a primary disorder of heart muscle characterized by symmetric or asymmetric hypertrophy of the left and/or right ventricle. In pediatric patients, the most common form of hypertrophic cardiomyopathy is classic idiopathic hypertrophic subaortic stenosis with asymmetric septal hypertrophy and marked septal cardiac muscle cell disorganization.[10] This disease process includes abnormalities of systolic and diastolic function. In systole, an intraventricular pressure gradient may be present or absent. When present, the gradient may be persistent at rest, spontaneously variable (labile), or provocable (latent). In diastole, abnormalities of ventricular relaxation and passive chamber stiffness are present. Usually, patients with more extensive hypertrophy exhibit more severe abnormalities of systolic and diastolic function.[11]

M-Mode Echocardiographic Features

The three hallmarks of hypertrophic cardiomyopathy are asymmetric septal hypertrophy, septal disorganization, and systolic anterior motion of the anterior mitral leaflet. None of these findings is pathognomonic of hypertrophic cardiomyopathy; however, because they are uncommonly found in children with other cardiac disorders, these three findings are each highly specific for hypertrophic cardiomyopathy. In the diagnosis of hypertrophic cardiomyopathy, the specificity of asymmetric septal hypertrophy, marked septal disorganization, and systolic anterior motion of the mitral valve is 90%, 93%, and 97% respectively.[12] Two of these findings (asymmetric septal hypertrophy and systolic anterior motion of the mitral valve) are easily detected with M-mode echocardiography.

In patients with hypertrophic cardiomyopathy, the M-mode echocardiogram shows marked hypertrophy of the left ventricle, usually with much more striking involvement of the ventricular system (Fig 12–5). The ratio of the ventricular septal thickness to the left ventricular posterior wall thickness in diastole greatly exceeds 1.3, the upper limit of normal. Left ventricular end-diastolic dimension is usually normal; however, left ventricular end-systolic dimension is decreased, and shortening fraction is usually normal or supranormal.[13]

The subaortic obstruction in hypertrophic cardiomy-

opathy is caused by abnormal apposition in systole between the anterior mitral valve leaflet and the ventricular septum (Fig 12–5). It is believed that rapid early nonobstructed systolic ejection, through an outflow tract narrowed by subaortic septal hypertrophy, draws the anterior mitral leaflet toward the septum by Venturi forces. The subsequent mitral leaflet-septal contact, caused by the high-velocity systolic ejection jet passing close to the mitral leaflets, results not only in subaortic obstruction but also in concomitant mitral regurgitation.[11] Several studies have shown direct correlations between pressure gradient and the time of onset and duration of the mitral leaflet-septal contact. Large gradients are associated with mitral leaflet-septal contact that begins early in systole and is prolonged. Thus, when mitral leaflet-septal contact first develops in early systole, the majority of the left ventricular stroke volume encounters the obstruction, the pressure gradient is high, and left ventricular ejection time is prolonged. When the mitral leaflet-septal contact develops in mid-systole, a large percentage of left ventricular emptying has occurred before the subaortic obstruction has developed; therefore, the pressure gradient is low and the ejection time is normal or slightly prolonged. Systolic anterior motion

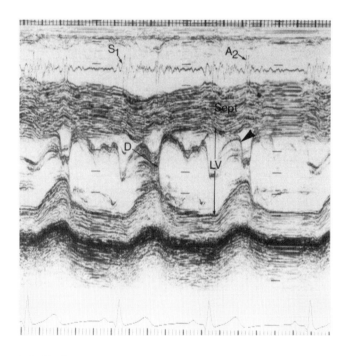

FIG 12–5.
M-mode echocardiogram from the left ventricle (LV) of a patient with idiopathic hypertrophic subaortic stenosis. There is marked asymmetric thickening of the ventricular septum. The ratio of septal to LV posterior wall thickness is greater than 1.3. In addition, systolic anterior motion of the mitral valve is seen *(arrow)*. These findings are highly specific for idiopathic hypertrophic subaortic stenosis. A_2 = aortic closing component of the second heart sound; D = mitral leaflet separation in the beginning of diastole; S_1 = the first heart sound on the phonocardiogram.

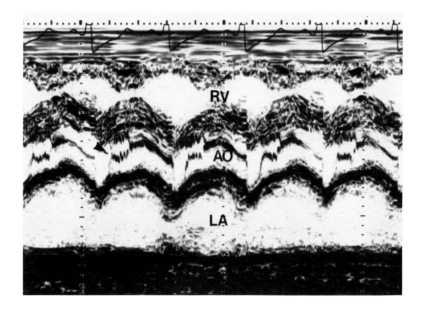

FIG 12–6.
M-mode echocardiogram through the aorta (AO) of a patient with idiopathic hypertrophic subaortic stenosis. Midsystolic closure of the aortic valve leaflets is seen *(black arrow)*. This finding is highly suggestive of idiopathic hypertrophic subaortic stenosis. In midsys- tole, a high-velocity jet, surrounded by low pressure areas, passes through the aortic valve. The low-pressure areas allow the flexible aortic valve leaflets to drift partially closed. LA = left atrium; RV = right ventricle.

without septal contact causes no subaortic obstruction and either no gradient or a small impulse gradient of 10 mm Hg or less.[14]

On the M-mode echocardiogram in patients with hypertrophic cardiomyopathy, mid-systolic closure of the aortic valve leaflets is commonly found (Fig 12–6). The mechanism for midsystolic closure of the aortic valve in hypertrophic cardiomyopathy is the same as for early systolic closure of the aortic valve in discrete membranous subaortic stenosis (see Chapter 9). In midsystole, a high-velocity jet surrounded by low pressure areas passes through the aortic valve. The low pressure areas allow the flexible aortic valve leaflets to drift partially closed. In hypertrophic cardiomyopathy, the obstruction is located farther from the aortic valve than it is in subaortic membrane; hence, the jet reaches the valve later in systole.

In patients with hypertrophic cardiomyopathy, diastolic filling abnormalities can be detected on the digitized M-mode echocardiogram (see Chapter 4 for details of the technique). The isovolumic relaxation period is considerably longer in patients with hypertrophic cardiomyopathy compared to normal subjects, and the peak filling rate of the left ventricle is reduced. Furthermore, the percentage of the total change in left ventricular diastolic dimension that occurs in the rapid filling period is decreased.[15–17] All of these findings suggest an impairment in left ventricular early relaxation properties.

Two-Dimensional Echocardiographic Features

In patients with hypertrophic cardiomyopathy, two-dimensional echocardiography provides a more complete picture of the full extent and distribution of myocardial involvement.[18, 19] On the two-dimensional echocardiogram, the entire left ventricle is usually very hypertrophic but the ventricular septum is involved to a far greater degree. Hypertrophy of the ventricular septum is usually greatest in the midportion (muscular septum), and the membranous and outlet septum are usually not involved. Thus, in longitudinal sections, the ventricular septum has a cigar shape (Fig 12–7). The thickness of the septum and left ventricular posterior wall can best be evaluated in the parasternal long- and short-axis views and the apical and subcostal four-chamber views (Figs 12–8 and 12–9).

Although the classic form of idiopathic hypertrophic subaortic stenosis involves primarily the septum and left ventricular posterior wall, any or all ventricular walls can be involved. For example, the left ventricular posterior wall can be thicker than any other cardiac wall, or the hypertrophy can be limited to the left ventricular apex.[20, 21] In infants with hypertrophic cardiomyopathy, the right ventricle is frequently involved.[22] There is usually severe concentric hypertrophy of the right ventricle, and hypertrophy of the muscle bands of the crista supraventricularis can lead to severe right ventricular outflow obstruction.

Systolic anterior motion of the anterior mitral leaflet can also be observed on the two-dimensional echocardiogram in the parasternal long-axis view (Fig 12–10). Usually, the two-dimensional echocardiogram must be viewed in slow motion to detect systolic anterior motion of the mitral valve, especially if the patient has a rapid heart rate. In the parasternal long-axis view, an echo-bright area is

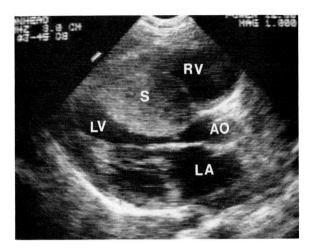

FIG 12–7.
Parasternal long-axis view from a patient with idiopathic hypertrophic subaortic stenosis. There is marked asymmetric hypertrophy of the ventricular septum (S). The septum is far greater in thickness than the left ventricular (LV) posterior wall. AO = aorta; LA = left atrium; RV = right ventricle.

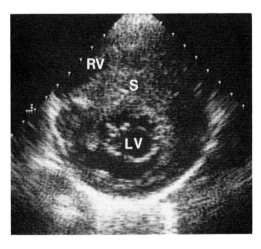

FIG 12–8.
Parasternal short-axis view from a patient with severe idiopathic hypertrophic subaortic stenosis. The ventricular septum (S) is far thicker than the left ventricular (LV) posterior wall. RV = right ventricle.

often seen in the left ventricular outflow tract where the mitral leaflet contacts the septum. The bright echoes in this area arise from a fibrotic, plaquelike lesion that occurs because of injury to the septal endocardium by the mitral leaflet. In addition, mitral valve prolapse is frequently present; mitral regurgitation is invariably present. With severe mitral regurgitation, left atrial dimensions may be increased.

Most children with hypertrophic cardiomyopathy have a normal left ventricular end-diastolic volume and a small left ventricular end-systolic volume on the two-dimen-

sional echocardiogram. The ejection fraction is markedly elevated and obliteration of the apical portion of the left ventricular cavity in systole is common.

Doppler Echocardiographic Features

Systolic Flow Abnormalities

In patients with hypertrophic cardiomyopathy, pulsed Doppler mapping of the left ventricular outflow velocities

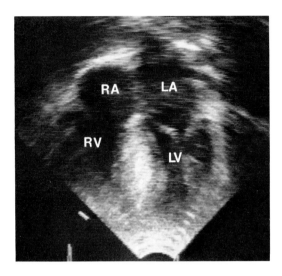

FIG 12–9.
Apical four-chamber view from a patient with idiopathic hypertrophic subaortic stenosis. The ventricular septum is markedly thickened and echo-bright. Note the small size of the left ventricular (LV) chamber. LA = left atrium; RA = right atrium; RV = right ventricle.

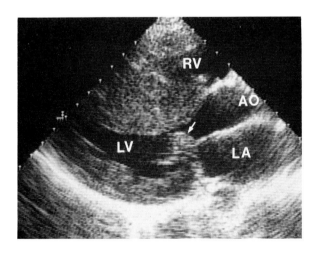

FIG 12–10.
Parasternal long-axis view from a patient with idiopathic hypertrophic subaortic stenosis. There is marked thickening of the ventricular septum. In addition, systolic anterior motion of the mitral valve (arrow) can be seen in this frame. AO = aorta; LA = left atrium; LV = left ventricle; RV = right ventricle.

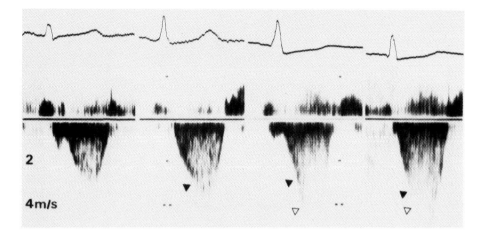

FIG 12–11.
Four examples of left ventricular outflow tract jets recorded by continuous-wave Doppler ultrasound in patients with hypertrophic cardiomyopathy. The increasing slope as the jet accelerates toward the peak velocities *(black arrow)* is typical for left ventricular outflow signals in patients with hypertrophic cardiomyopathy. There is usually a decrease in the amplitude of the signal at the peak velocity

(white arrow). This dagger shape is very typical of the left ventricular outflow jet in hypertrophic cardiomyopathy. (From Yock PG, Hatle L, Popp RL: Patterns and timing of Doppler-detected intracavitary and aortic flow in hypertrophic cardiomyopathy. *J Am Coll Cardiol* 1986; 8:1049. Used by permission.)

has shown a consistent pattern of flow acceleration in the left ventricle.[23, 24] Four different flow patterns can be observed at four different anatomic regions of the left ventricle as the sample volume is moved from the apex toward the aortic valve. At the base of the papillary muscles, maximal velocities range from about 0.4 to 1.7 m/sec, and there is a sharp peak in velocity occurring at end-systole. In patients with severe apical hypertrophy, the peak velocity in this region can be higher. Farther up, at the level of the papillary muscle tips, the velocities are somewhat higher and exhibit a rounded, earlier peak. This is the level at which flow begins to accelerate, probably because septal hypertrophy narrows the left ventricular outflow tract area somewhat. Farther upstream at the level of the chordae and mitral leaflet tips, the left ventricular outflow tract jet begins. Here, there is a definite increase in velocity. A short distance beyond this level (in the fourth anatomic area), the highest jet velocities are recorded; however, the high velocity jet extends for only 1 to 2 cm upstream. Higher in the left ventricular outflow tract and across the aortic valve, velocities are lower.[24]

Maximum left ventricular outflow velocities can be recorded with continuous-wave Doppler examination from the cardiac apex. In hypertrophic cardiomyopathy, the outflow jet is best recorded with the Doppler beam aimed midway between the mitral inflow and aortic outflow. The outflow jet is not directed toward the aortic leaflets but rather posterior and lateral to the aortic valve. In the majority of cases, the outflow jet shows a gradual increase in velocity in the first portion of systole (Fig 12–11). Following a shoulder or inflection point on the curve in early systole, the slope of the velocity curve increases rapidly as the jet approaches maximum velocity. The inflection point represents the onset of obstruction and occurs immediately before mitral leaflet-septal contact. The peak velocities occur when the left ventricular outflow tract is narrowed to its smallest area during mitral leaflet-septal contact.[24–26] Thus, the left ventricular outflow velocities have a characteristic timing and shape that resembles a dagger.[25] In addition, a decrease in the amplitude or intensity of the Doppler outflow tract signal occurs just before the peak velocity is reached. In some patients, the decrease in amplitude makes clear recording of the peak velocity impossible. The decreased amplitude occurs because a decreased number of targets or red blood cells are moving at these high velocities. This suggests a decreased flow during this part of ejection. Thus, left ventricular outflow Doppler signals suggest a high-velocity, low volume flow jet in mid-to-late systole.[24–26]

Simultaneous M-mode and continuous-wave Doppler echocardiographic studies have shown that the flow velocity is already increased in the left ventricular outflow tract (to a mean of 1.5 m/sec) at the onset of systolic anterior motion on the M-mode recording. The abrupt increase in velocity at the shoulder point occurs when the mitral leaflets begin to encroach on the septum, narrowing the outflow tract; the highest outflow velocities occur at the time of maximum anterior displacement of the mitral valve.[24] In addition, color-flow mapping studies show the highest-velocity, mosaic jet to be localized in the area of mitral leaflet-septal contact. The peak gradient calculated from continuous-wave Doppler recording of this jet corresponds exactly with peak instantaneous pressure gradient measured by transducers mounted on needles and placed intraoperatively on either side of the subaortic obstruction.[25]

Because of the shape of the left ventricular outflow tract, aortic flow velocities are best recorded from a suprasternal notch transducer position. At the level of the aortic valve, the Doppler recording shows an early peak compared to normal subjects. The early peak velocity is followed by a sudden deceleration of aortic flow in early systole (Fig 12–12). Peak velocities at the aortic valve are markedly less than those in the left ventricular outflow jet. In the ascending aorta, velocity profiles are extremely variable, depending on the position of the sample volume; however, in all cases, peak aortic velocity occurs well before peak left ventricular outflow tract velocity. Aortic valve midsystolic closure occurs at the time of peak left ventricular outflow tract velocity.[23, 24]

These characteristic features of the aortic Doppler recordings suggest that flow in the left ventricular outflow tract diminishes in mid-to-late systole, even in the presence of high outflow velocities. The aortic velocities peak earlier than the left ventricular outflow tract velocities, so that while the left ventricular outflow jet velocities are still increasing, aortic velocities and flow area are decreasing, the latter indicated by partial closure of the aortic leaflets.[24]

As stated earlier, the aortic velocity profile is extremely variable, depending on the sample volume position in the ascending aorta. These different velocity profiles (i.e., bifid tracing, tracings with negative late systolic velocities, etc.) are probably caused by the entry of a narrow aortic jet into the wider, fixed-diameter ascending aorta flow area and the formation of eddies. It is likely that the early deceleration of flow and resultant eddy formation in the ascending aorta contribute to midsystolic closure of the aortic valve leaflets.[24]

In patients with hypertrophic cardiomyopathy, mitral regurgitation invariably accompanies an obstructive pressure gradient and the degree of regurgitation is directly related to the severity of the obstruction.[11] The systolic velocities of mitral regurgitation can be recorded with continuous-wave Doppler ultrasound from the cardiac apex and with color-flow mapping techniques from the parasternal and apical windows. The onset of the regurgitation is coincident with the first heart sound and, thus, occurs well before the onset of the left ventricular outflow jet. The jets of mitral regurgitation and left ventricular outflow tract obstruction are both high-velocity, systolic jets, directed away from the transducer in the apical view and separated by only a small distance. Nevertheless, these jets can easily be distinguished by the following important features: (1) the left ventricular outflow tract jet has a slow upstroke and terminal acceleration to a late peak velocity; (2) the mitral regurgitation jet has a higher peak velocity than the left ventricular outflow jet (greater left ventricular-left atrial pressure gradient compared to the left ventricular-aortic gradient); (3) the onset of the mitral regurgitation jet is much earlier, beginning at the time of mitral closure; and (4) pulsed and color-flow mapping techniques show the spatial location of the jet and thereby help distinguish the two jets.[24]

Diastolic Flow Abnormalities

Diastolic dysfunction in hypertrophic cardiomyopathy is mainly related to impaired relaxation and decreased chamber compliance. Examination of the mitral inflow Doppler tracing may provide evidence of diastolic filling abnormalities (see Chapter 4).[27] In patients with hypertrophic cardiomyopathy and no significant mitral regurgitation, peak E velocity is decreased, deceleration of early diastolic flow is reduced, and E/A ratio is decreased.[28–31]

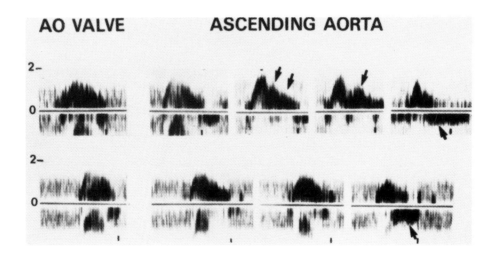

FIG 12–12.
Examples of Doppler tracings from the ascending aorta (AO) from two patients with hypertrophic cardiomyopathy. The contour of the velocity traces changes dramatically with changes in the position of the sample volume in the ascending AO. The diastolic closures and reverse flows *(arrows)* noted in the ascending AO are probably a result of eddy currents in the great vessel. (From Yock PG, Hatle L, Popp RL: Patterns and timing of Doppler-detected intracavitary and aortic flow in hypertrophic cardiomyopathy. *J Am Coll Cardiol* 1986; 8:1056. Used by permission.)

The presence of significant mitral regurgitation tends to increase left ventricular filling pressure and normalize the mitral valve Doppler filling indexes. Thus, patients with hypertrophic cardiomyopathy and significant mitral regurgitation have normal peak E and A velocities, normal deceleration rate of early diastolic flow, and normal E/A ratio.[29,31] In a group of children with nonobstructive hypertrophic cardiomyopathy and no significant mitral regurgitation, we found a prolonged isovolumic relaxation time, decreased peak E velocity, and decreased percentage of the total Doppler area in the first 33% of diastole.[32] These findings suggest that early relaxation is impaired in patients with hypertrophic cardiomyopathy, even when there is no resting gradient.

Another diastolic flow abnormality frequently found in patients with hypertrophic cardiomyopathy is aortic insufficiency. Approximately one-third of patients with hypertrophic cardiomyopathy have aortic insufficiency that can be detected by Doppler echocardiographic techniques.[33] It is believed that aortic insufficiency is the result of damage to the valve cusps by the high-velocity jet in the left ventricular outflow tract.

Genetic Transmission

In most cases, hypertrophic cardiomyopathy has an autosomal dominant pattern of inheritance with near complete penetration of the gene expression.[1–3] Thus, 50% of the children of an affected parent can be expected to have the disease. For this reason, if we discover a child with idiopathic hypertrophic subaortic stenosis, we recommend that the child's family members undergo a complete echocardiographic evaluation. When screening the young siblings of a child with hypertrophic cardiomyopathy, it is important to note that the echocardiographic features of the disease may not become apparent until adolescence or early adulthood. Therefore, when young siblings of an affected child have a normal echocardiogram, we recommend repeating the examination in early adulthood.

RESTRICTIVE CARDIOMYOPATHY

Restrictive cardiomyopathy is an extremely rare disease in childhood. The contracted form of endocardial fibroelastosis can be considered as a restrictive cardiomyopathy in which the fibrotic endocardium offers the restriction to ventricular filling. The few cases of restrictive cardiomyopathy that we have seen in pediatric patients have been of undetermined etiology.

M-Mode and Two-Dimensional Echocardiographic Features

Restrictive cardiomyopathy is a disease characterized by diminished myocardial compliance, with large increases in early diastolic ventricular pressures for small changes in volume and an abrupt, premature cessation of filling in the first one-third of diastole.[34,35] The presence of the disease is suggested on the two-dimensional echocardiogram by the finding of very enlarged atria in the presence of normal-sized ventricles with variable systolic function.[34]

M-mode and two-dimensional echocardiography in patients with restrictive cardiomyopathy show normal left and right ventricular end-diastolic dimensions. Left ventricular shortening fraction is usually normal or low. On the M-mode echocardiogram, an abrupt increase in left ventricular dimension is seen in early diastole (abrupt posterior motion of the left ventricular posterior wall and anterior motion of the septum) followed by no further increase in chamber dimension (flat posterior wall and septal motion) throughout the remainder of diastole.[35–37] On the two-dimensional echocardiogram, this abrupt cessation of early diastolic filling creates the appearance of a jerky, spasmodic wall motion in real-time.

The most striking two-dimensional echocardiographic feature of restrictive cardiomyopathy is the enormous biatrial enlargement seen in the apical and subcostal four-chamber views (Figs 12–13 and 12–14). Very few, if any, diseases in pediatric patients cause this degree of biatrial enlargement in the presence of normal-sized ventricular chambers.

Doppler Echocardiographic Features

Doppler Findings in Restrictive Cardiomyopathy

Patients with restrictive cardiomyopathy exhibit abnormalities of the mitral and tricuspid inflow Doppler and of systemic venous flow.[34] On the mitral valve Doppler examination, the peak E velocity and the percentage of the total Doppler area occurring under the E wave (see Chapter 4) are normal; however, the peak A velocity and the percentage of the total Doppler area occurring under the A wave are decreased (Fig 12–15). As a result, the E/A velocity and area ratios are increased. Mitral deceleration time is shortened (<150 msec) and shortens even further during inspiration. In normal subjects, mitral deceleration time does not shorten with inspiration. Left ventricular isovolumic relaxation time is also shortened compared to normal subjects. Similar findings are present on the tricuspid valve Doppler of patients with restrictive cardiomyopathy. The tricuspid peak A velocity and A area fraction are decreased; the E/A velocity and area ratios are increased, and deceleration time is shortened (<150 msec). Further shortening of deceleration time occurs with inspiration.[34]

The shortened mitral and tricuspid deceleration time, a striking Doppler finding in patients with restrictive cardiomyopathy, is caused by a more rapid equalization of atrial and early ventricular diastolic pressures. This rapid equalization probably occurs because of the large, abnormal rapid filling waves caused by decreased ventricular compliance. The further shortening of the tricuspid valve deceleration time with inspiration probably occurs because of an inability of the right ventricle to accept an increase

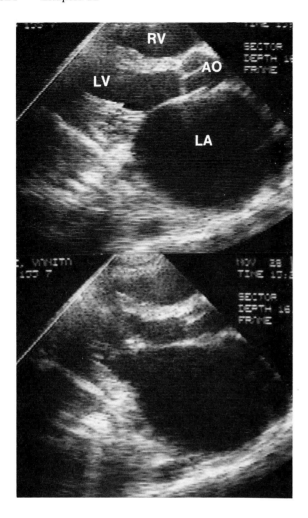

FIG 12-13.
Parasternal long-axis views in systole *(above)* and diastole *(below)* from a patient with restrictive cardiomyopathy. There is marked enlargement of the left atrium (LA), with a near normal-sized left ventricle (LV). These findings are highly suggestive of diminished myocardial compliance with an abrupt premature cessation of filling in early diastole. Note that there is very little change in LV dimension from systole to diastole. AO = aorta; RV = right ventricle.

in venous return without an abrupt pressure increase and an even earlier atrial-ventricular pressure equalization. Because left ventricular volume does not increase with inspiration, the shortening of the mitral valve deceleration time (and increase in left ventricular rapid filling wave) with inspiration is probably caused by a further decrease in left ventricular compliance as a result of displacement of the septum into the left ventricle.[34]

Mid-diastolic mitral and tricuspid regurgitation is seen in a high percentage of patients with restrictive cardiomyopathy (Fig 12-16). In some patients, ventricular diastolic pressure exceeds atrial pressure at the peak of the rapid filling wave. The pressure reversal results in a flow reversal (mid-diastolic regurgitation).[34]

Abnormal systemic venous flow velocity patterns are

seen in all patients with restrictive cardiomyopathy. In the systemic veins of normal subjects, forward flow occurs during systole and diastole, with the systolic flow being the dominant flow. With atrial contraction, small flow reversals occur which decrease or disappear during inspiration. In restrictive cardiomyopathy patients, forward flow during systole is diminished or absent, and most of the forward flow occurs during diastole (Fig 12-17). In addition, these patients have abnormally large or prolonged flow reversals during atrial contraction or systole which increase with inspiration. These venous flow patterns reflect decreased right ventricular compliance with an inability to accept an increase in venous return without an abnormal pressure increase and flow reversal.[34]

Some patients with restrictive cardiomyopathy have Doppler evidence of forward diastolic flow in the main pulmonary artery in inspiration. This occurs because, at the peak of the rapid filling wave, right ventricular diastolic pressure exceeds pulmonary artery diastolic pressure.[34]

It is not at all uncommon to detect insufficiency of any or all of the cardiac valves in patients with restrictive cardiomyopathy.

Differentiation of Constrictive Pericarditis and Restrictive Cardiomyopathy

Several M-mode and Doppler echocardiographic findings are useful in distinguishing patients with restrictive cardiomyopathy from those with constrictive pericarditis.[37, 38] On the M-mode echocardiogram, patients with constrictive pericarditis have a larger increase in left ventricular

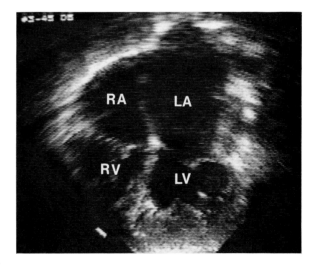

FIG 12-14.
Apical four-chamber view from the same patient as in Figure 12-13. From the apical view, the right atrium (RA) and the left atrium (LA) are both seen to be markedly enlarged. The right ventricle (RV) and the left ventricle (LV) are normal in size. The apical portion of the LV is markedly hypertrophic. The findings of severe biatrial enlargement in the presence of near normal-sized ventricular chambers is highly suggestive of restrictive cardiomyopathy.

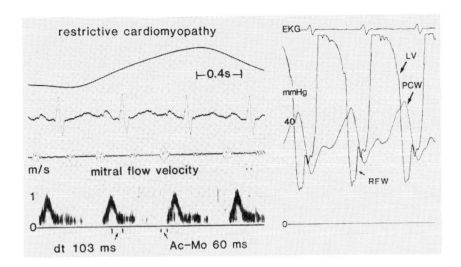

FIG 12–15.
Mitral valve Doppler recording from a patient with restrictive disease. The left ventricular (LV) and pulmonary capillary wedge (PCW) pressure tracings are also included. The Doppler tracing shows a markedly shortened mitral deceleration time (dt), minimal flow with atrial contraction, and an increased left ventricular rapid filling wave (RFW) and end diastolic pressure. These findings are highly suggestive of restrictive disease. Ac-Mo = time interval between the aortic closing component of the second heart sound and the mitral opening on the Doppler tracing. (From Appleton CP, Hatle LK, Popp RL: *J Am Coll Cardiol* 1988; 11:760. Used by permission.)

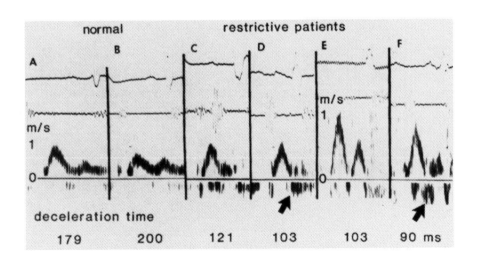

FIG 12–16.
Mitral Doppler recordings from two normal patients *(panels A and B)* and four patients with restrictive disease *(panels C to F).* The velocity of early diastolic filling is as large or larger in the patients with restrictive disease as it is in the normal subjects. Patients with restrictive disease also have a markedly shortened deceleration time. Low velocity *(panel C)* and reversal of flow *(panel D)* are seen with atrial contraction. In *panels E and F,* the peak velocity with atrial contraction is normal, but in *panel F,* there is mid-diastolic reversal of flow, representing diastolic mitral regurgitation. These findings are commonly present in patients with restrictive disease. (From Appleton CP, Hatle LK, Popp RL: Demonstration of restrictive ventricular physiology by Doppler echocardiography. *J Am Coll Cardiol* 1988; 11:762. Used by permission.)

diastolic dimension from inspiration to expiration than patients with restrictive cardiomyopathy (5.4 ± 1.5 mm vs. 1.8 ± 1.0 mm, respectively).[38]

On the mitral valve Doppler examination, patients with constrictive pericarditis have a much more pronounced lengthening of isovolumic relaxation time and a more pronounced decrease in peak E velocity from expiration to inspiration compared to normal subjects and patients with restrictive cardiomyopathy. In restrictive cardiomyopathy, respiratory variation in these variables is much less than 15%, while respiratory variation in these variables is greater than 25% in constrictive pericarditis.[38]

On the tricuspid valve Doppler, the increase in peak E and peak A velocity from expiration to inspiration is far greater in patients with constrictive pericarditis compared to normal subjects or patients with restrictive cardiomyopathy. The respiratory variation in tricuspid flow velocities shows more variability; and overlap of the data between patient groups makes the tricuspid Doppler findings less sensitive as a diagnostic indicator of constrictive disease.[38]

In addition, patients with constrictive pericarditis and restrictive cardiomyopathy have a shortening of mitral and tricuspid deceleration time compared to normal subjects. However, unlike patients with restrictive cardiomyopathy, patients with constrictive disease do not have a further shortening of deceleration time with inspiration. Also, in contrast to findings in restrictive cardiomyopathy, patients with constrictive pericarditis seldom have diastolic atrioventricular valve regurgitation, and mitral and tricuspid peak A velocities are normal.[38]

The greater respiratory changes in transvalvular flow velocities in constrictive pericarditis is probably caused by the fixed total cardiac volume imposed by the rigid pericardial sac. Since the cardiac volume is fixed in constrictive pericarditis, an increased filling of the right heart will impede filling of the left heart (by displacement of the ventricular septum). However, blood can flow from the atria to the ventricles with atrial contraction because chamber compliance in early diastole is normal and this flow does not increase total cardiac volume. In restrictive cardiomyopathy, impedance to ventricular filling increases throughout diastole so that the proportion of filling with atrial contraction is reduced. With inspiration and an increase in systemic venous return, a larger and more abrupt right ventricular rapid filling wave occurs. This leads to a premature cessation of filling in early diastole and in inspiratory shortening of the tricuspid deceleration time. Because of the lack of pericardial constraint and the presence of a less compliant septum, right ventricular filling alterations have less effect on left ventricular filling in restrictive cardiomyopathy.[38]

SECONDARY CARDIOMYOPATHIES

Cardiomyopathy in Infants of Diabetic Mothers

Nearly one-half of infants born to diabetic mothers will have a hypertrophic cardiomyopathy indistinguishable on echocardiographic examination from idiopathic hypertrophic subaortic stenosis. Hypertrophy usually involves both ventricles, and the ventricular septum is disproportionately thickened (Fig 12–18).[39, 40] Subaortic and/or subpulmonic pressure gradients may be present; however, the disease is often accompanied by persistent pulmonary hy-

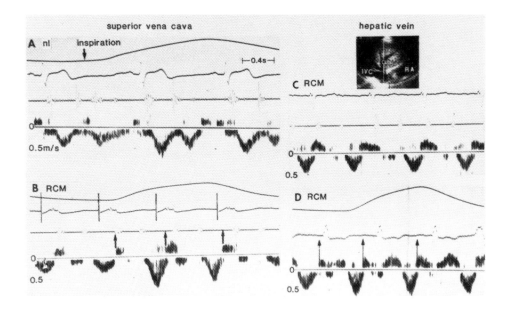

FIG 12–17.
Superior vena cava *(left)* and hepatic vein *(right)* flow recordings from a normal (nl) subject *(panel A)* and three patients with restrictive cardiomyopathy (RCM) *(panels B to D)*. In the normal patient, *panel A,* superior vena caval flow is biphasic with the highest velocities occurring during systole. Small flow reversals occur with atrial contraction and do not increase with inspiration. In the RCM patient in *panel B,* the superior vena caval flow shows a diastolic forward flow followed by presystolic flow reversals that become larger and begin earlier with inspiration *(arrows).* In *panel C,* hepatic vein flow from a patient with RCM and atrial fibrillation is shown. There is only forward flow during diastole followed by diastolic reversal of flow. *Panel D* is a hepatic vein tracing from a patient with RCM, sinus rhythm, and moderately severe tricuspid regurgitation. Forward flow occurs during diastole followed by presystolic flow reversals that increase and begin earlier in diastole with inspiration. IVC = inferior vena cava; RA = right atrium. (From Appleton CP, Hatle LK, Popp RL: Demonstration of restrictive ventricular physiology by Doppler echocardiography. *J Am Coll Cardiol* 1988; 11:763. Used by permission.)

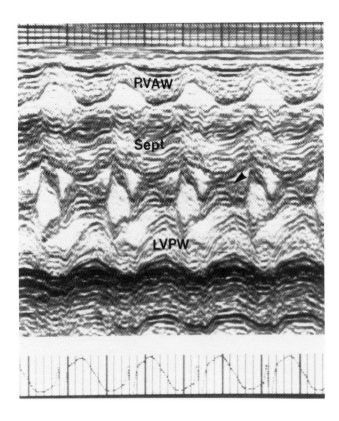

FIG 12–18.

M-mode echocardiogram of the left ventricle from a newborn infant born to a diabetic mother. The M-mode echocardiogram closely resembles that of the patient in Figure 12–5 with idiopathic hypertrophic subaortic stenosis. There is marked asymmetric thickening of the ventricular septum (Sept). In addition, there is systolic anterior motion of the mitral valve *(arrow)*. LVPW = left ventricular posterior wall; RVAW = right ventricular anterior wall.

pertension rather than right ventricular outflow obstruction.[2] The hypertrophy generally regresses in the first six to eight months of life, and this factor, plus the history of diabetes in the mother, helps differentiate the disease from other types of hypertrophic cardiomyopathy.

Type II Glycogen Storage Disease

Infants with glycogen storage disease type II or Pompe's disease often have a hypertrophic cardiomyopathy. This disease is characterized by massive hypertrophy of the left ventricle and sometimes the right ventricle (Figs 12–19 to 12–21). Hypertrophy is usually concentric, and the ventricular cavity dimensions are normal to enlarged. Unlike idiopathic hypertrophic subaortic stenosis, left ventricular shortening fraction is usually markedly decreased. This diagnosis should be considered in any infant who is "floppy," who has congestive heart failure, and who has severe cardiac hypertrophy on the echocardiogram.[1, 2]

Friedreich's Ataxia

Cardiac involvement is the most frequent cause of death in Friedreich's ataxia, and it is estimated that 80% to 90% of patients with this disease have echocardiographic abnormalities.[41] Concentric left ventricular hypertrophy is

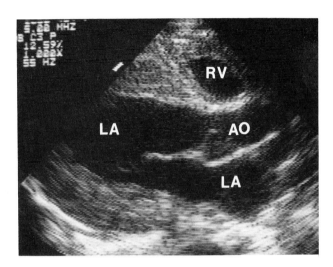

FIG 12–19.

Parasternal long-axis view from an infant with Pompe's disease and cardiac involvement. There is marked concentric hypertrophy of the left ventricle (LV). In addition, the LV is markedly dilated and had a markedly diminished shortening fraction. AO = aorta; LA = left atrium; RV = right ventricle.

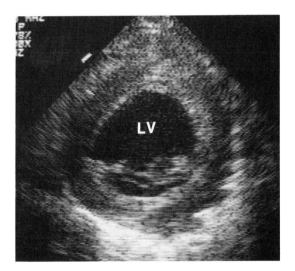

FIG 12–20.

Parasternal short-axis view through the left ventricle (LV) of the same patient as in Figure 12–19. The LV is concentrically hypertrophied and markedly dilated.

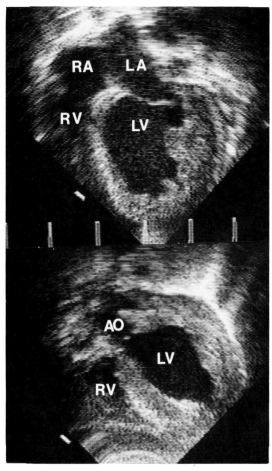

FIG 12–21.
Apical four-chamber *(top)* and long axis *(bottom)* views from the same patient as in Figure 12–19. The left ventricular (LV) myocardium is echo-bright and concentrically hypertrophied. The LV is markedly dilated. AO = aorta; LA = left atrium; RA = right atrium; RV = right ventricle.

found in two-thirds of the patients with cardiac involvement. In these patients, the papillary muscles are thickened and echodense, the left ventricular cavity dimensions are normal, and the shortening fraction is normal.

Approximately 8% to 9% of patients have asymmetric septal hypertrophy, and another 8% to 9% have a dilated cardiomyopathy with increased left ventricular cavity dimensions and decreased shortening fraction.[41] Thus, a wide spectrum of cardiac abnormalities are present in Friedreich's ataxia.

Systemic Carnitine Deficiency

Thirty percent of patients with systemic carnitine deficiency and 20% of patients with plasma carnitine deficiency have a congestive cardiomyopathy characterized by left ventricular dilatation, left atrial dilatation, and decreased left ventricular shortening fraction.[42, 43] After treatment with *l*-carnitine, most patients show dramatic

improvement in cardiac size and function on the echocardiogram. Thus, because this disease represents the only form of congestive cardiomyopathy that can be reversed with medical therapy, measurement of carnitine levels is warranted in all patients that present with echocardiographic features of idiopathic congestive cardiomyopathy.

REFERENCES

1. Harris LC, Nghiem QX: Cardiomyopathies in infants and children. *Prog Cardiovasc Dis* 1972; 15:255–287.
2. Meyer RA: Cardiomyopathy in the young. *J Am Soc Echo* 1988; 1:88–93.
3. Goodwin JF: Prospects and predictions for the cardiomyopathies. *Circulation* 1974; 50:210–219.
4. Engle SJ, DiSessa TG, Perloff JK, et al: Mitral valve E point to ventricular septal separation in infants and children. *Am J Cardiol* 1983; 52:1084–1087.
5. Colan SD, Borow KM, Neumann A: Left ventricular end-systolic wall stress-velocity of fiber shortening relation: A load-independent index of myocardial contractility. *J Am Coll Cardiol* 1984; 4:715–724.
6. Kugler JD, Gutgesell HP, Nihill MR: Instantaneous rates of left ventricular wall motion in infants and children. Computer-assisted determinations from single-cycle echocardiograms. *Pediatr Cardiol* 1979; 1:15–21.
7. Gibson DG, Brown D: Measurement of instantaneous left ventricular dimension and filling rate in man, using echocardiography. *Br Heart J* 1973; 35:1141–1149.
8. Gardin JM, Iseri LT, Elkayam U, et al: Evaluation of dilated cardiomyopathy by pulsed Doppler echocardiography. *Am Heart J* 1983; 106:1057–1065.
9. Takenaka K, Dabestani A, Gardin JM, et al: Pulsed Doppler echocardiographic study of left ventricular filling in dilated cardiomyopathy. *Am J Cardiol* 1986; 58:143–147.
10. Maron BJ, Roberts WC: Quantitative analysis of cardiac muscle cell disorganization in the ventricular septum of patients with hypertrophic cardiomyopathy. *Circulation* 1979; 59:689–706.
11. Wigle ED: Hypertrophic cardiomyopathy: A 1987 viewpoint. *Circulation* 1987; 75:311–322.
12. Maron BJ, Epstein SE: Hypertrophic cardiomyopathy. Recent observations regarding the specificity of three hallmarks of the disease: Asymmetric septal hypertrophy, septal disorganization and systolic anterior motion of the anterior mitral leaflet. *Am J Cardiol* 1980; 45:141–154.
13. Gotsman MS, Lewis BS: Left ventricular volumes and compliance in hypertrophic cardiomyopathy. *Chest* 1974; 66:498–505.
14. Pollick C, Rakowski H, Wigle ED: Muscular subaortic stenosis: The quantitative relationship between systolic anterior motion and the pressure gradient. *Circulation* 1984; 69:43–49.
15. Hanrath P, Mathey DG, Siegert R, et al: Left ventricular relaxation and filling pattern in different forms of ventricular hypertrophy. An echocardiographic study. *Am J Cardiol* 1980; 45:15–23.

16. Hanrath P, Mathey DG, Kremer P, et al: Effect of verapamil on left ventricular isovolumic relaxation time and regional left ventricular filling in hypertrophic cardiomyopathy. *Am J Cardiol* 1980; 45:1258–1264.

17. Hanrath P, Schluter M, Kremer P, et al: The assessment of left ventricular function in hypertrophic cardiomyopathy by echocardiography. *Eur Heart J* 1983; 4(suppl F):39–46.

18. Tajik AJ, Giuliani ER: Echocardiographic observations in idiopathic hypertrophic subaortic stenosis. *Mayo Clin Proc* 1974; 49:89–95.

19. Martin RP, Rakowski H, French J, et al: Idiopathic hypertrophic subaortic stenosis viewed by wide-angle, phased-array echocardiography. *Circulation* 1979; 59:1206–1217.

20. Panidis IP, Nestico P, Hakki AH, et al: Systolic and diastolic left ventricular performance at rest and during exercise in apical hypertrophic cardiomyopathy. *Am J Cardiol* 1986; 57:356–358.

21. Rovelli EG, Parenti F, Devizzi S: Apical hypertrophic cardiomyopathy of "Japanese type" in a western European person. *Am J Cardiol* 1986; 57:358–359.

22. Barr PA, Celermajer JM, Bowdler JD, et al: Idiopathic hypertrophic obstructive cardiomyopathy causing severe right ventricular outflow tract obstruction in infancy. *Br Heart J* 1973; 35:1109–1115.

23. Hatle L, Angelsen B: *Doppler Ultrasound in Cardiology*, ed 2. Philadelphia, Lea and Febiger, 1985, pp 97–293.

24. Yock PG, Hatle L, Popp RL: Patterns and timing of Doppler-detected intracavitary and aortic flow in hypertrophic cardiomyopathy. *J Am Coll Cardiol* 1986; 8:1047–1058.

25. Stewart WJ, Schiavone WA, Salcedo EE, et al: Intraoperative Doppler echocardiography in hypertrophic cardiomyopathy: Correlations with the obstructive gradient. *J Am Coll Cardiol* 1987; 10:327–335.

26. Sasson Z, Yock PG, Hatle LK, et al: Doppler echocardiographic determination of the pressure gradient in hypertrophic cardiomyopathy. *J Am Coll Cardiol* 1988; 11:752–756.

27. Appleton CP, Hatle LK, Popp RL: Relation of transmitral flow velocity patterns to left ventricular diastolic function: New insights from a combined hemodynamic and Doppler echocardiographic study. *J Am Coll Cardiol* 1988; 12:426–440.

28. Kitabatake A, Inoue M, Asao M, et al: Transmitral blood flow reflecting diastolic behavior of the left ventricle in health and disease: A study by pulsed Doppler technique. *Jpn Circ J* 1982; 46:92–102.

29. Takenaka K, Dabestani A, Gardin J, et al: Left ventricular filling in hypertrophic cardiomyopathy: A pulsed Doppler echocardiographic study. *J Am Coll Cardiol* 1986; 7:1263–1271.

30. Maron BJ, Spirito P, Green KJ, et al: Noninvasive assessment of left ventricular diastolic function by pulsed Doppler echocardiography in patients with hypertrophic cardiomyopathy. *J Am Coll Cardiol* 1987; 10:733–742.

31. Bryg RJ, Pearson AC, Williams GA, et al: Left ventricular systolic and diastolic flow abnormalities determined by Doppler echocardiography in obstructive hypertrophic cardiomyopathy. *Am J Cardiol* 1987; 59:925–931.

32. Gidding SS, Snider AR, Rocchini AP, et al: Left ventricular diastolic filling in children with hypertrophic cardiomyopathy: Assessment with pulsed Doppler echocardiography. *J Am Coll Cardiol* 1986; 8:310–316.

33. Theard MA, Bhatia SJS, Plappert T, et al: Doppler echocardiographic study of the frequency and severity of aortic regurgitation in hypertrophic cardiomyopathy. *Am J Cardiol* 1987; 60:1143–1147.

34. Appleton CP, Hatle LK, Popp RL: Demonstration of restrictive ventricular physiology by Doppler echocardiography. *J Am Coll Cardiol* 1988; 11:757–768.

35. Chew CYC, Ziady GM, Raphael MJ, et al: Primary restrictive cardiomyopathy: Nontropical endomyocardial fibrosis and hypereosinophilic heart disease. *Br Heart J* 1977; 39:399–413.

36. Mehta AV, Ferrer PL, Pickoff AS, et al: M-mode echocardiographic findings in children with idiopathic restrictive cardiomyopathy. *Pediatr Cardiol* 1984; 5:273–279.

37. Janos GG, Arjunan K, Meyer RA, et al: Differentiation of constrictive pericarditis and restrictive cardiomyopathy using digitized echocardiography. *J Am Coll Cardiol* 1983; 1:541–549.

38. Hatle LK, Appleton CP, Popp RL: Differentiation of constrictive pericarditis and restrictive cardiomyopathy by Doppler echocardiography. *Circulation* 1989; 79:357–370.

39. Gutgesell HP, Speer ME, Rosenberg HS: Characterization of the cardiomyopathy in infants of diabetic mothers. *Circulation* 1980; 61:441–450.

40. Mace S, Hirschfeld SS, Riggs T, et al: Echocardiographic abnormalities in infants of diabetic mothers. *J Pediatr* 1979; 95:1013–1019.

41. Alboliras ET, Shub C, Gomez MR, et al: Spectrum of cardiac involvement in Friedreich's ataxia: Clinical, electrocardiographic and echocardiographic observations. *Am J Cardiol* 1986; 58:518–524.

42. Tripp ME, Katcher ML, Peters HA, et al: Systemic carnitine deficiency presenting as familial endocardial fibroelastosis. *N Engl J Med* 1981; 305:385–390.

43. Winter SC, Szabo-Aczel S, Curry CJR, et al: Plasma carnitine deficiency: Clinical observations in 51 pediatric patients. *Am J Dis Child* 1987; 141:660–665.

13

Echocardiographic Evaluation of the Postoperative Patient

SYSTEMIC ARTERY TO PULMONARY ARTERY SHUNTS

In children with decreased pulmonary blood flow or right ventricular-pulmonary artery discontinuity, surgical systemic artery to pulmonary artery shunts are often created in an attempt to provide a controlled source of pulmonary blood flow. Many surgical shunts are difficult to image directly on the two-dimensional echocardiogram because they are interposed between the aorta and a pulmonary artery branch. For example, the Waterston shunt between the ascending aorta and right pulmonary artery is often hidden from view by the overlying ascending aorta, and the Potts shunt between the descending aorta and left pulmonary artery is often hidden from view by the overlying left pulmonary artery branch. The central or front shunt between the ascending aorta and main pulmonary artery is hidden by the overlying bony sternum. On the other hand, the Blalock-Taussig shunt between the subclavian artery and a branch pulmonary artery is located some distance away from the aorta and main pulmonary artery and has considerably more length than other shunts. For these reasons, direct visualization of Blalock-Taussig shunts is far easier than for other shunts.

The majority of shunts that can be visualized directly on the two-dimensional echocardiogram are usually imaged in the suprasternal views. For example, the right Blalock-Taussig shunt can be seen in the suprasternal short-axis view (Fig 13–1). In this view, the right subclavian artery or a prosthetic tube courses from the base of the right innominate artery to the top of the right pulmonary artery just proximal to the origin of the right upper lobe branch. In some patients, it may be possible to image constrictions in the shunt (usually at the pulmonary artery end) or distortion of the right pulmonary artery created by the shunt. The left Blalock-Taussig shunt can usually be imaged in the suprasternal long-axis view with the transducer tilted toward the left pulmonary artery branch (Fig 13–2). It may

not be possible to image the entire length of the left Blalock-Taussig shunt in one plane; therefore, the transducer should be angled in multiple positions to image the shunt all the way from its origin to its insertion.

When a surgical shunt cannot be imaged directly on the two-dimensional echocardiogram with certainty, color-flow Doppler techniques are very helpful for localizing the shunt (Plate 45). On the color Doppler, flow in the shunt is displayed as a high-velocity, mosaic flow that is continuous throughout systole and diastole (Plate 46). Thus, the disturbed flow pattern outlines the area of the shunt and continues into the pulmonary artery. The color flow Doppler examination is extremely useful for (1) localizing a shunt that cannot be visualized directly, (2) determining if the shunt is patent, and (3) optimizing alignment of the pulsed and continuous-wave Doppler beam with flow in the shunt.

Pulsed and continuous-wave Doppler examination of the child with a surgical shunt can provide useful information about the size of the shunt and the pulmonary artery pressure.[1, 2] With high pulse repetition frequency or continuous-wave Doppler, the high velocities through the shunt can be displayed unambiguously (Fig 13–3). If flow is sampled at the insertion of the shunt into the pulmonary artery, the Doppler examination shows a continuous, high-velocity jet directed toward the pulmonary artery. In the pulmonary artery itself, Doppler examination shows evidence of continuous disturbed flow. From the Doppler examination of the shunt, the peak pressure gradient between the aorta and the pulmonary artery can be calculated in systole and diastole from the simplified Bernoulli equation. For this calculation, the peak velocities of the shunt in systole and diastole are substituted in the equation: pressure gradient = $4 \times$ peak velocity^2. If the arm blood pressure is recorded at the time of the Doppler examination, the pulmonary artery systolic and diastolic pressure can be calculated as: arm blood pressure in systole or diastole minus peak pressure gradient in systole or diastole. With

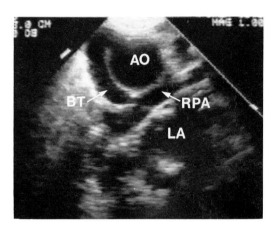

FIG 13–1.
Suprasternal short-axis view from a patient with a right Blalock-Taussig shunt (BT). The BT shunt is seen connecting the right subclavian artery to the right pulmonary artery (RPA). At its insertion into the RPA, the shunt becomes quite narrow. AO = aorta; LA = left atrium.

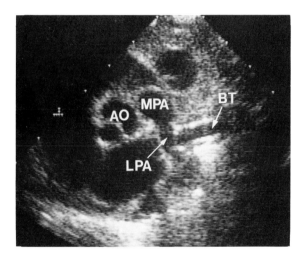

FIG 13–2.
Suprasternal view from a patient with a left Blalock-Taussig (BT) shunt. The transducer has been moved somewhat inferiorly and tilted to the far left to image the origin of the left pulmonary artery (LPA) from the main pulmonary artery (MPA). The BT shunt can be seen connecting to the LPA. AO = aorta.

this approach, good correlation has been found between Doppler estimates of pulmonary artery pressure and pulmonary artery pressure measured at cardiac catheterization. The Doppler estimate of the pressure drop across a long, narrow tubular shunt can be too low because of failure to take into account the pressure drop caused by viscous friction along the flow path. In this case, Doppler estimates of the pulmonary artery pressure will be too high. Doppler estimates of the pressure gradient will also be too low if the Doppler beam is not aligned parallel with the shunt flow. Thus, caution must be used when estimating

pulmonary artery pressure from the Doppler recording of flow velocities in a surgical shunt.

Because systemic vascular resistance exceeds pulmonary vascular resistance, surgical communications between the aorta and pulmonary artery cause a retrograde flow of blood in diastole from the descending aorta through the shunt and into the pulmonary artery. Retrograde diastolic flow can be detected on the Doppler examination of the descending aorta as a prominent holodiastolic M-shaped flow signal (Fig 13–4).[3, 4] Retrograde diastolic flow signals are of low velocity, therefore, their detection requires low wall filter settings on the Doppler instrument. On the color Doppler examination of the descending aorta from the suprasternal notch, retrograde flow is seen as a red flow area (toward the transducer) in diastole. The amount of retrograde diastolic flow is a useful indicator of the size of the left-to-right shunt through the surgical anastomosis. Quantitation of the shunt can be performed by measuring the ratio of the area under the retrograde portion of the flow to the area under the forward portion of the flow.[4]

The Doppler findings described above are identical to those for a patent ductus arteriosus or a stenotic bronchial collateral vessel.[2] Therefore, if a nonimaging continuous-wave Doppler transducer is used to evaluate a surgical shunt, one must be certain that the flow signals being evaluated arise from the shunt and not from a patent ductus arteriosus or collateral vessels.

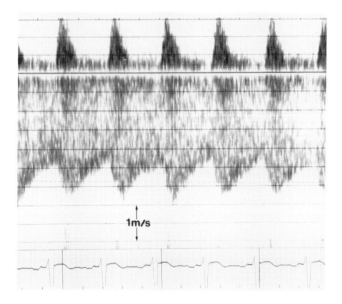

FIG 13–3.
Continuous-wave Doppler examination from the suprasternal view of an infant with a right Blalock-Taussig shunt. The flow signals displayed in systole above the baseline probably arise from flow in the aorta or aortic arch vessels directed toward the transducer. The high-velocity continuous-flow displayed below the baseline arises from flow through the Blalock-Taussig shunt into the right pulmonary artery. This flow has a peak velocity in late systole of 3.5 m/sec, indicating a large pressure gradient between the aorta and pulmonary artery.

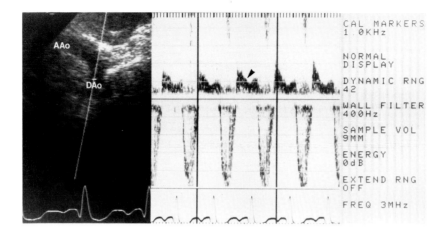

FIG 13–4.
Pulsed Doppler recording *(right)* from the descending aorta (DAo) of an infant with a Blalock-Taussig shunt. The freeze-frame image, *left,* shows the position of the sample volume in the DAO at the time of the Doppler recording. The Doppler tracing, *right,* shows flow signals in systole below the baseline that arise from antegrade flow down the descending aorta away from the transducer. In diastole, the signals above the baseline indicate flow up the DAO toward the transducer *(arrow).* These flow signals arise because of the retrograde flow of blood in diastole from the DAO through the shunt into the pulmonary artery. Retrograde diastolic flow signals characteristically are holodiastolic and have an M shape. AAo = ascending aorta. (From Snider AR: Doppler echocardiography in congenital heart disease, in Berger M (ed): *Doppler Echocardiography in Heart Disease.* New York, Marcel Dekker, 1987, p 297. Used by permission.)

PULMONARY ARTERY BAND

On the two-dimensional echocardiogram, a pulmonary artery band can be visualized as a bright, white echo across the main pulmonary artery. The position of the band can best be evaluated from parasternal, subcostal, and suprasternal views. The optimal position for placement of the pulmonary artery band is in the midportion of the main pulmonary artery (Fig 13–5); however, pulmonary artery bands can slip forward or backward after their initial placement. In the parasternal short-axis view, a band that has slipped forward will encroach on the pulmonary valve leaflets (Fig 13–6). In the suprasternal views, a band that has slipped backward will encroach on and distort the right pulmonary artery. Often, in patients with a very tight pulmonary band, the pulmonary valve leaflets appear echobright and thickened, and pulmonary valve prolapse is present. In patients with a tight pulmonary artery band, marked poststenotic dilatation of the main pulmonary artery distal to the band is often seen in the parasternal views. In patients who have had removal of a pulmonary artery band, an area of residual narrowing can be seen in the region previously occupied by the band. In addition, dense white echoes resembling a band can often be seen arising from scar tissue in the region of the previous pulmonary artery band.

Doppler echocardiography can be used to record the high-velocity systolic jet flow across the pulmonary artery band. The peak velocity of the jet can be used in the simplified Bernoulli equation to calculate the peak pressure gradient across the band.[5, 6] Doppler estimates of the pressure gradient across the band have correlated very well with those measured at catheterization[5] or in the animal laboratory.[6] Because most congenital defects that require a pulmonary artery band have a large nonrestrictive ventricular communication, the pulmonary artery systolic pressure can be estimated from the peak pressure gradient across the band and the systolic blood pressure. If there is

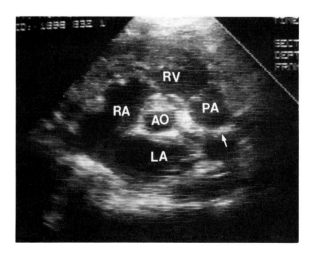

FIG 13–5.
Parasternal short-axis view from a child with a pulmonary artery band *(arrow)* in the proper location on the pulmonary artery (PA). The band is positioned midway in the PA and has not slipped toward the valve or the bifurcation. AO = aorta; LA = left atrium; RA = right atrium; RV = right ventricle.

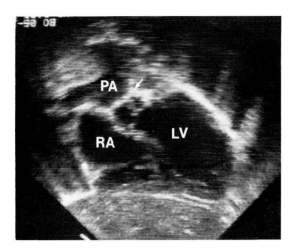

FIG 13–6.
Subcostal coronal view of the left ventricular (LV) outflow tract of a patient with *d*-transposition of the great arteries, a large ventricular septal defect, and a pulmonary artery (PA) band *(arrow)*. The PA band has slipped forward and is encroaching on the pulmonary valve leaflets. RA = right atrium.

no left ventricular outflow obstruction, the systolic blood pressure equals the right ventricular systolic pressure. Thus, pulmonary artery systolic pressure equals systolic blood pressure minus the pressure gradient.

On the color Doppler examination, the flow through the pulmonary artery band appears as a high-velocity, mosaic jet distal to the band. The spatial display of the jet on the color Doppler examination is useful for obtaining the best alignment between the continuous-wave Doppler beam and the jet flow.

CARDIAC PATCHES

Cardiac patches are often used in children with congenital heart defects to close septal defects or to reconstruct narrowed areas in the heart or great vessels (i.e., outflow tract patches, coarctation patch repair).

Pericardial patches often have the same reflecting properties as the surrounding cardiac walls and are difficult to visualize clearly on the two-dimensional echocardiogram. Patches constructed from synthetic materials (e.g., Dacron or Gore-tex) are easily visualized on the two-dimensional echocardiogram because they reflect more ultrasound than any of the surrounding tissues.

When a patch is used to close a septal defect, the position of the patch provides the echocardiographer with information about the anatomic type of defect that was repaired (Fig 13–7). For example, a patch located in the midportion of the atrial septum indicates that a secundum atrial septal defect was repaired (Fig 13–8). In the parasternal long-axis view, a patch on the ventricular septum that is oriented obliquely to reach the anterior aortic root indicates that an outlet ventricular septal defect associated with aortic override was repaired (Figs 13–9 and 13–10).

On the postoperative echocardiographic examination of the child who has had patch closure of a septal defect, a frequently asked question is whether or not there is residual shunting across the patch. Before the introduction of pulsed and color-flow Doppler techniques, peripheral

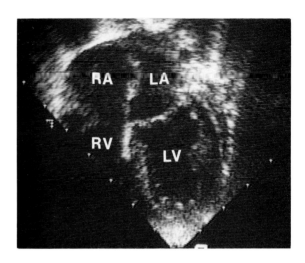

FIG 13–7.
Apical four-chamber view from a child who has undergone complete repair of an atrioventricular septal defect. The position of the patch in the midportion of the heart suggests that a previous atrioventricular septal defect was present. The patch extends from the lower one-third of the atrial septum through the common atrioventricular valve to the upper third of the ventricular septum. The atrial portion of the patch is less reflective because it is composed of pericardium. The ventricular portion of the patch is composed of synthetic material and therefore is more densely reflective. LA = left atrium; LV = left ventricle; RA = right atrium; RV = right ventricle.

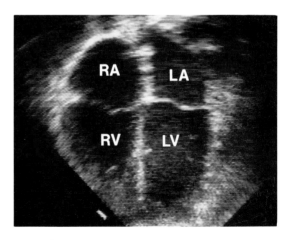

FIG 13–8.
Apical four-chamber view from a child who has undergone repair of a secundum atrial septal defect. The bright echoes from the patch are seen arising from the midportion of the atrial septum. The position of the patch suggests the diagnosis of a previous secundum atrial septal defect. LA = left atrium; LV = left ventricle; RA = right atrium; RV = right ventricle.

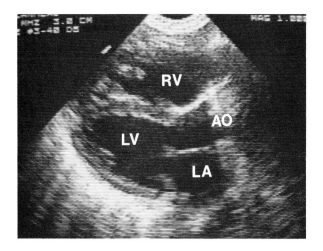

FIG 13–9.
Parasternal long-axis view from a patient who has undergone repair of tetralogy of Fallot. Bright echoes arising from the ventricular septal defect patch can be seen oriented obliquely from the ventricular septum to the anterior aortic (AO) root. The oblique course of the patch suggests that prior to closure of the ventricular septal defect, aortic override was present. LA = left atrium; LV = left ventricle; RV = right ventricle.

venous contrast echocardiography was used to detect residual right-to-left shunting across atrial or ventricular septal defect patches.[7, 8] With this technique, a contrast agent such as saline (see Chapter 3) is injected into a peripheral vein. If there is no intracardiac right-to-left shunt, echoes arising from the contrast material are seen only in the right heart chambers, as they are filtered in the pulmonary capillary bed and do not normally appear in the left heart chambers. Contrast echoes that are seen filling a left heart chamber immediately after their appearance in the corresponding right heart chamber indicate an intracardiac right-to-left shunt. The left heart chamber that fills first indicates the level of the right-to-left shunt.[7, 8] Peripheral venous contrast echocardiography is especially sensitive and can detect right-to-left shunts as small as 3% to 5% of systemic blood flow. Any significant left-to-right shunt will have this amount of right-to-left shunt and will, therefore, be detected by peripheral venous contrast injections. Alternatively, contrast echocardiography can be performed in the immediate postoperative period with injections into the left atrial line. Thus, if no left-to-right shunt is present, contrast echoes will appear only in the left heart chambers, as they are filtered by the systemic capillary bed and do not return to the right heart. The appearance of contrast echoes in a right heart chamber indicates a left-to-right intracardiac shunt. The left heart chamber that fills first indicates the level of the shunt.[7] Contrast echo studies in postoperative patients with septal patches have shown that temporary shunting across the patch in the first few days after surgery is extremely common. However, a temporary shunt cannot be distinguished from a true residual defect, so that follow-up echocardiographic examinations are necessary to make certain that residual shunts disappear.

For the detection of residual shunting across septal defect patches, pulsed and color-flow Doppler techniques have largely replaced contrast echocardiography. With pulsed Doppler echocardiography, the sample volume is moved along the right side of the septal patch in search of Doppler flow patterns that indicate an atrial or ventricular left-to-right shunt (see Chapter 5). For accurate diagnosis, the patch should be examined from multiple echocardiographic views. Even then, it is difficult to examine all the margins of a large patch with the small pulsed Doppler sample volume. The sensitivity for detection of residual shunting across septal patches has been greatly enhanced with the use of color-flow Doppler mapping techniques. With color-flow Doppler, sampling of flow velocities occurs over a very wide area so that even very tiny residual shunts are fairly easy to detect (Plates 47 and 48). If a residual shunt is detected, follow-up Doppler examinations are indicated to determine if the shunt will close by endotheliazation of the patch or if the shunt represents a true residual defect. The size of a residual shunt can be evaluated by two-dimensional and Doppler echocardiography using the techniques outlined in Chapters 4 and 5.

On the postoperative echocardiogram of the child who has had a patch placed to reconstruct a narrowed area in the heart or great vessels, a frequently asked question is whether or not there is residual narrowing or aneurysm formation in the region of the patch. Aneurysmal dilatation can occur with any type of patch; however, we have observed this complication more frequently when pericardial patches are used and when the patch is exposed to very high pressures. For example, aneurysmal dilatation of right ventricular outflow tract patches (placed to enlarge subpulmonic narrowing) frequently occurs when the patch is

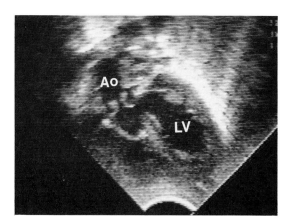

FIG 13–10.
Apical five-chamber view from an infant following repair of truncus arteriosus. The ventricular septal defect patch is seen stretching obliquely from the right side of the ventricular septum to the anterior aortic root. The oblique course of the patch suggests that aortic override was present prior to closure of the ventricular septal defect. This frame was taken during diastole and shows a large regurgitant orifice in the AO valve. In addition, the AO valve leaflets are rolled and thickened. LV = left ventricle.

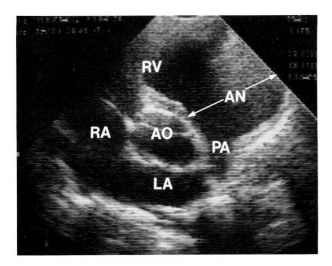

FIG 13–11.
Parasternal short-axis view from a patient following repair of tetralogy of Fallot. A large aneurysm (AN) has developed in the right ventricular (RV) outflow tract at the area of patch repair. AO = aorta; LA = left atrium; PA = pulmonary artery; RA = right atrium.

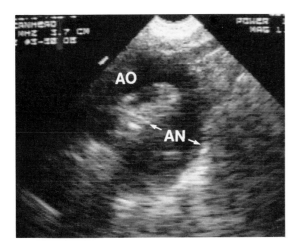

FIG 13–12.
Suprasternal long-axis view from a patient following patch repair of coarctation of the aorta (AO). The repair has been complicated by aneurysmal dilatation (AN) of the patch.

made of pericardium and when the right ventricular pressure is elevated because of a residual stenosis distal to the patch (Fig 13–11). Similarly, patch repair of coarctation of the aorta can be complicated by aneurysmal dilatation of the patch (Figs 13–12 and 13–13).

If residual stenosis occurs at the distal end of a patch (i.e., right ventricular outflow tract patch), the proximal portion of the patch is exposed to high pressures and becomes aneurysmal. In this situation, Doppler echocardiography can be used to detect high velocities distal to the stenosis and to calculate the peak gradient across the residual narrowing.

Frequently, echo-bright areas are seen within a patch or attached to a patch. These bright areas may be flattened against the patch surface or may protrude off the surface of the patch. Echo-bright areas attached to the patch can be areas of patch calcification, thrombus attached to the patch (Fig 13–14), vegetations attached to the patch, or irregularities in the surface contour of the patch. Often, it is not possible to distinguish these defects with echocardiography alone, and the clinical situation in which the echo-bright structure is observed may be useful in making this differential diagnosis.

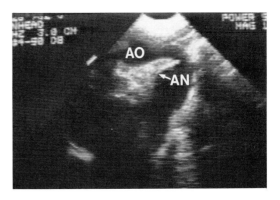

FIG 13–13.
Suprasternal long-axis view from a patient who has had patch repair of coarctation of the aorta (AO). Distal to the patch is an area of marked aneurysmal dilatation (AN) of the descending AO.

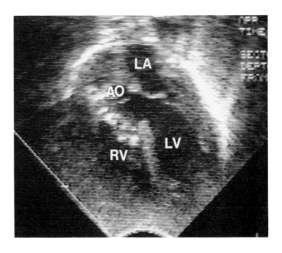

FIG 13–14.
Apical five-chamber view from a patient immediately after repair of truncus arteriosus. This patient developed evidence of peripheral emboli in the immediate postoperative period. The two-dimensional echocardiogram showed multiple thrombi (echo-bright areas) attached to the ventricular septal defect patch. AO = aorta; LA = left atrium; LV = left ventricle; RV = right ventricle.

VALVED AND NONVALVED CONDUITS

Right Ventricular to Pulmonary Artery Conduits

In infants and children with congenital heart disease, valved conduits are widely used for the repair of defects with right ventricular-pulmonary artery discontinuity (i.e., truncus arteriosus, pulmonary atresia with a ventricular septal defect, severe tetralogy of Fallot). In 1966, Ross and Somerville[9] introduced the use of fresh aortic homograft valved conduits; however, because of problems with limited availability and early calcification of these irradiated aortic homograft valved conduits, alternative valved conduits were sought.[10, 11] In 1973, the use of a porcine heterograft valve mounted in a woven Dacron tube was proposed;[12] and because of its ready availability, the heterograft porcine valved conduit soon became the most widely used conduit.[13, 14]

Long-term follow-up studies of children with heterograft porcine valved conduits showed a disappointing rate of development of obstruction at the porcine valve and in the Dacron conduit itself (neointimal proliferation).[15-18] As a result of these studies and because of the development of improved techniques for preparation and preservation of homograft valves, antibiotic-sterilized homograft valves are now being widely used in children and are favored by most surgeons because of their lower antigenicity compared to porcine valved conduits.[19-29] More recently, improved methods of controlled-rate liquid nitrogen freezing have made cryopreservation of both aortic and pulmonary homografts possible.

On the two-dimensional echocardiogram, heterograft and homograft valved conduits have nearly identical appearances. The artificial material of the conduit walls is highly reflective, whereas the tissue valve echoes are very faint. To image the valve leaflets, high-gain and low-reject settings are necessary. To image the conduit walls, low-gain and high-reject settings should be used. The synthetic material used to construct the conduit walls has a ribbed surface; and on the two-dimensional echocardiogram, the echoes reflected from the irregular surface give the conduit walls the appearance of corrugated cardboard. Right ventricular to pulmonary artery conduits are best imaged in the parasternal and subcostal views of the right ventricle (Fig 13–15). It is helpful to place the transducer directly over the area on the precordium that corresponds to the location of the valve ring on the chest x-ray. From this location, the transducer can be oriented in a long-axis view so that the entire conduit can be seen longitudinally or in a short-axis view so that the valve can be seen in cross-section. In some patients, the distal connections of the conduit to the branch pulmonary arteries are difficult to image clearly.[30] Calcification of the conduit walls is frequently seen on the two-dimensional echocardiogram and does not in itself indicate conduit stenosis.

Conduit function can be assessed with pulsed, continuous-wave, and color-flow Doppler examinations.[31] For example, conduit valve insufficiency can be detected on the Doppler examination as a diastolic flow of blood across

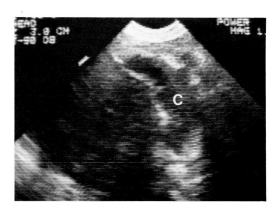

FIG 13–15.
Parasternal view of a heterograft valved conduit (C) placed between the right ventricle and pulmonary artery of a patient with pulmonary atresia and a ventricular septal defect. The walls of the conduit are made of a synthetic material with a ribbed surface which on the two-dimensional echocardiogram gives the appearance of corrugated cardboard. The heterograft valve is faintly seen in the conduit.

the valve from the conduit into the right ventricle (see Chapter 9). In 71 homograft valves that we examined in the immediate postoperative period with Doppler echocardiography, 35% had no insufficiency, 62% had mild insufficiency, and 3% had moderate insufficiency. On the intermediate follow-up examination of 38 of these conduit valves, 26% had no insufficiency, 66% had mild insufficiency, and 8% had moderate insufficiency. Progression of the amount of insufficiency occurred in 29% of patients; however, no patient developed severe insufficiency. Thus, the incidence and severity of conduit valve insufficiency is no different from that of normally functioning native pulmonary valves.[29]

In valved conduits, obstruction to forward flow can develop at the proximal conduit insertion, at the valve, or at the distal conduit insertions. With heterograft valved conduits, a thickened neointimal peel develops along the entire length of the conduit and contributes to conduit stenosis by decreasing the internal diameter of the conduit. The peel formation usually involves the heterograft valve leaflets so that they become thickened and immobile, often becoming fixed in an open or closed position. The neointimal peel is very difficult to image separately from the echo-bright conduit walls on the two-dimensional echocardiogram. Usually, the first hint of its existence is a decrease in the internal caliber of the conduit. When the valve is involved, it often appears echo-dense and immobile. In fact, if it is easy to visualize a heterograft valve on two-dimensional echocardiography, that valve is probably stenotic.

Obstruction in homograft valved conduits does not occur as a result of neointimal proliferation but instead develops at the proximal or distal conduit insertion, usually as a result of mechanical problems in the surgical placement of the conduit (Plate 49). In the 71 homograft valves we examined in the immediate postoperative period with Doppler echocardiography, the peak velocity of flow across the normally functioning homograft valve was 1.6 ± 0.3 m/sec. The majority of homograft valves (82%) had a peak flow velocity less than 1.3 m/sec and no homograft valve had a peak velocity greater than 2.6 m/sec. In the immediate postoperative period, no patient had Doppler echocardiographic evidence of proximal or distal conduit stenosis. At the intermediate term follow-up examination of 38 of the valved conduits, severe conduit stenosis developed in only 2 conduits (5%), both at the distal conduit insertion. No patient developed significant obstruction at the homograft valve itself. Thirty-four of the conduit valves had a peak velocity <1.4 m/sec at follow-up examination.[29]

If the distal insertion of the conduit is not accessible for Doppler examination, an indirect assessment of the severity of the obstruction can be obtained by estimating the right ventricular systolic pressure from the peak velocity of the tricuspid regurgitation jet (see Chapter 4). Thus, if continuous-wave Doppler examination predicts a very elevated right ventricular systolic pressure and Doppler examinations of the proximal conduit and conduit valve show no evidence of obstruction, significant distal conduit stenosis is probably present.

Apical Left Ventricular to Descending Aorta Conduit

In patients with severe aortic valvular stenosis, a small valve annulus, and a narrowed left ventricular outflow tract, left ventricular obstruction can be relieved with a valved conduit placed between the apex of the left ventricle and the descending aorta. In the early use of this conduit, the conduit was passed through the diaphragm and connected to the descending abdominal aorta. Because of complications such as erosion of the conduit into nearby

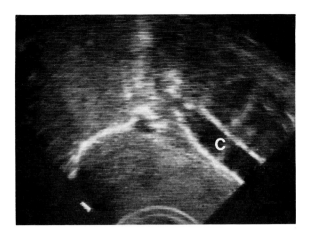

FIG 13–17.
Subcostal view from a patient with an apical left ventricular-descending aortic conduit. In this view, a longitudinal section of the conduit (C) is seen coursing from the region of the left ventricular apex to the descending thoracic aorta.

abdominal structures (i.e., the spleen), most of these conduits are now connected to the descending aorta above the diaphragm. The valve is generally positioned midway in the conduit and is usually a heterograft valve.

Because of the length and curvature of the conduit, it is usually not possible to image the entire conduit in one two-dimensional echocardiographic view. Instead, portions of the conduit can be imaged from multiple views. In the parasternal long-axis view and the subcostal four-chamber view of the left ventricular outflow tract, the metal stents that hold the conduit orifice open can be seen protruding into the left ventricular cavity in the region of the apex (Figs 13–16 and 13–17). These stents are highly reflective of ultrasound and, therefore, are very echodense. With patient growth, the proximal end of the conduit can migrate out of the left ventricular cavity. The parasternal and subcostal views are particularly useful for confirming proper proximal conduit position in the left ventricular cavity. In the apical views, the transducer can be tilted to the left to visualize a fair length of the conduit as it passes posterior to the left ventricle. The distal insertion of the conduit into the descending aorta can usually be imaged in subcostal sagittal views. These views are useful for detection of complications such as erosion of the conduit into adjacent lung tissue (Fig 13–18). Usually, the midportion of the conduit containing the heterograft valve is obscured from view by surrounding lung tissue.

In patients with a left ventricular to descending aorta conduit, pulsed and color Doppler techniques are useful for detecting conduit stenosis and conduit regurgitation into the left ventricle. In assessing conduit stenosis, the angle of the conduit valve and descending aorta usually prohibit direct examination of the conduit. If the pressure in the ascending aorta and descending aorta are the same (i.e., no coarctation), the pressure gradient across the native aortic valve must be the same as that across the conduit.

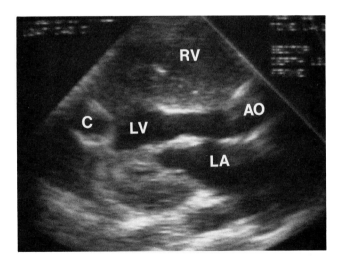

FIG 13–16.
Parasternal long-axis view from a patient with an apical left ventricular (LV) to descending aorta conduit (C). The conduit insertion is seen in the apex of the LV. AO = aorta; LA = left atrium; RV = right ventricle.

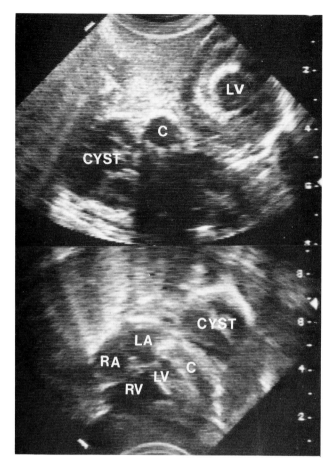

FIG 13–18.
Subcostal sagittal *(top)* and four-chamber *(bottom)* views from a
patient with an apical left ventricular (LV) to descending aorta
conduit (C). In this patient, the conduit inserted into the descending
thoracic aorta above the diaphragm. The echolucent area adjacent to the conduit represents a blood-filled cyst created by erosion
of the conduit into the adjacent lung tissue. LA = left atrium; RA = right
atrium; LV = left ventricle.

Hence, the peak velocity of the jet across the native aortic
valve can be used in the simplified Bernoulli equation to
estimate the peak gradient across the conduit.

In very small children, it may not be possible to fit a
large enough conduit between the left ventricle and the
descending aorta. We have examined a few infants in whom
heterograft valve conduits have been placed from the left
lateral wall of the left ventricle to the ascending aorta. This
type of conduit can be examined with two-dimensional
and Doppler echocardiography using the techniques discussed above.

Fontan Conduit

The Fontan anastomosis, a connection that allows systemic venous blood to reach the pulmonary arteries, can
be surgically created in a variety of ways. Often, a simple
direct anastomosis of the right atrial appendage to the pulmonary artery with pericardial augmentation is used. In

these patients, the Fontan conduit can be imaged directly
with high parasternal and subcostal views.[32] In some patients, a right atrial to right ventricular valved or nonvalved
conduit is used. Because of their retrosternal course, these
conduits usually cannot be imaged directly with two-dimensional echocardiography. More recently, intra-atrial
conduits (usually made of synthetic materials) have been
used to direct the inferior vena caval and/or hepatic venous
flow to the pulmonary artery, while the superior vena cava
is connected directly to the pulmonary artery branch. These
conduits can usually be visualized throughout most of their
course with parasternal and apical views (Fig 13–19).

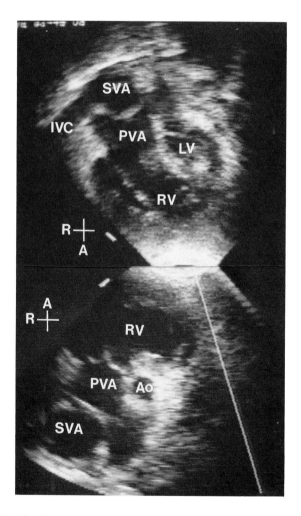

FIG 13–19.
Apical four-chamber *(top)* and parasternal short-axis *(bottom)* views
from a child with hypoplastic left ventricle (LV) following a Norwood
stage II or modified Fontan procedure. In this procedure, the superior vena cava is transected and anastamosed directly to the
surface of the right pulmonary artery branch. The inferior vena cava
(IVC) return is directed by way of the intra-atrial conduit (made of
synthetic material) along the lateral wall of the right atrium, through
the roof of the right atrium, to the undersurface of the right pulmonary artery branch. In effect, the intra-atrial conduit divides the
atrium into a systemic venous atrium (SVA) and a pulmonary venous
atrium (PVA). A = anterior; AO = aorta; R = right; RV = right ventricle.

Pulsed Doppler echocardiography has been used to interrogate flow in patients with right atrial to pulmonary artery conduits.[32] In the pulmonary artery in these patients, forward flow is biphasic with one peak velocity occurring in late systole to early diastole and a larger peak velocity occurring at atrial contraction. With inspiration, significant increases in both early diastolic and atrial waves occur. This predominantly diastolic pulmonary artery flow pattern is in contrast to the biphasic flow pattern in the normal superior vena cava where the predominant flow is systolic. Abnormal pulmonary artery flow patterns can be found in patients with a Fontan anastomosis and reduced systemic ventricular function. In this situation, pulmonary artery flow occurs predominantly in systole, and atrial waves are small or absent. The normal respiratory increase in flow velocity is absent or reduced in these patients.[32]

Prosthetic Valves

In pediatric patients, prosthetic valves are uncommonly used. Prosthetic valves can be entirely mechanical or composed partially or completely of biologic materials. Some of the more commonly encountered mechanical prosthetic valves that have been used in children are:

1. Ball and cage (Starr-Edwards valve).
2. Tilting disc and cage (Bjork-Shiley valve).
3. Bileaflet tilting hemidiscs (St. Jude valve).

Some of the more commonly encountered tissue valves in children are:

1. Porcine aortic (Hancock valve).
2. Bovine pericardial (Ionescu-Shiley).
3. Homograft aortic.

On the two-dimensional echocardiogram, the metal valve produces very bright echoes whose shape often helps identify the type of valve. For example, the Bjork-Shiley valve has a metal cage that is short (low-profile), while the Starr-Edwards valve has a long (high-profile) cage. The Hancock porcine valve is held in a sewing ring with three metal stents, which protrude forward in a characteristic shape (Fig 13–20).

In the Starr-Edwards, Bjork-Shiley, and St. Jude valves, the ball and the discs are strong reflectors of ultrasound. These structures often give rise to multiple reverberations that obscure visualization of the cardiac chamber behind the valve. These structures also prevent penetration of the ultrasound beam, making Doppler interrogation behind the metal valve virtually impossible.

When placed between the origin of the sound beam and the area being interrogated, prosthetic valves have different flow-masking properties. Starr-Edwards valves mask large areas and allow little penetration of the sound beam behind the valve. The Bjork-Shiley and St. Jude valves allow a reduced amount of sound through the central occluding discs; however, returning ultrasound signals are

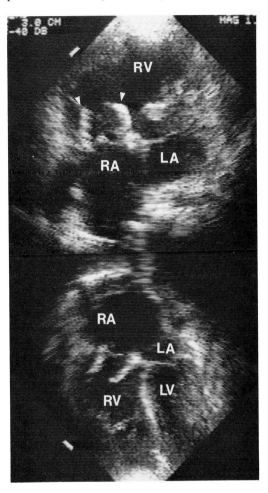

FIG 13–20.
Parasternal short-axis *(top)* and apical four-chamber *(bottom)* views from a patient with a Hancock porcine valve in the tricuspid position. The Hancock valve has three metal stents *(arrows)*, which protrude forward in a characteristic shape. The porcine valve leaflets are very visible in the valve. LA = left atrium; LV = left ventricle; RA = right atrium; RV = right ventricle.

extremely weak. Tissue valves allow proper transmission of sound waves, but flow masking occurs behind the sewing ring. Thus, when an abnormal flow is detected by a Doppler beam that does not traverse the prosthetic valve, the Doppler data is probably accurate. If the Doppler beam traverses the prosthetic valve on its way to an area of interest, the results may be unreliable. For example, high-velocity flows may be present but undetected.[33] To interrogate chambers behind a prosthetic valve, transducer positions and views should be used that prevent the Doppler beam from traversing the prosthetic valve (i.e., subcostal view to interrogate the right and left atria of patients with prosthetic tricuspid or mitral valves). Transesophageal echocardiography offers an alternative method of examining flow in chambers behind mechanical valves.

On the two-dimensional echocardiogram, the shape and movement of the echoes that arise from the ball or disc may help identify the type of valve. For example, the tilting disc of the Bjork-Shiley valve opens in a clamshell motion. The bileaflet hemidiscs of the St. Jude valve separate in the midline into two moving discs.

Bioprosthetic valves are easy to identify on the two-dimensional echocardiogram. The valve leaflets are thin and mobile and resemble normal human valve tissue on the echocardiogram. These valves do not produce multiple reverberations and do not prevent penetration of ultrasound to distant cardiac chambers. The Ionescu-Shiley valve contains a metal ring; the Hancock valve has metal stents as described previously; and the aortic homograft valve usually has no metal components.

To visualize the valve leaflets, high gain and low reject settings are often necessary. To visualize and measure the stent diameter of the Hancock valve, low gain and high reject settings are necessary. If the valve leaflets appear thickened and prominent on the two-dimensional echocardiogram, one should be suspicious that a thrombus, vegetation, or valve degeneration is present.

To diagnose prosthetic valve dysfunction, one must be aware of the flow characteristics of normally functioning prosthetic valves. These flow characteristics have been thoroughly investigated with pulsed and color-flow Doppler echocardiography in adult patients[34-43]; however, because of the small number of children with prosthetic valves, little information about the flow characteristics of prosthetic valves in children is available. Many pediatric patients have adult-sized prosthetic valves; therefore, the Doppler data derived from adult patients can probably be applied to these children in order to diagnose prosthetic valve dysfunction.

For the Hancock porcine valve in the aortic position, the peak flow velocity has been reported to be 2.0 ± 0.9 m/sec in one series[39] and 2.6 ± 0.6 in another series.[42] The peak velocity of the porcine valves ranged from 1.8 to 3.6 m/sec. For the St. Jude valve in the aortic position, peak velocities range from 1.0 to 3.9 m/sec (mean 2.3 ± 0.6 m/sec).[42] Comparable peak velocities have been reported for the Bjork-Shiley valve in the aortic position (peak velocity 2.6 ± 0.5 m/sec, range of 1.8 to 3.0 m/sec).[42] For the St. Jude valve in the mitral position, mean diastolic velocity has been reported to be 0.73 ± 0.16 m/sec and mean diastolic gradient averaged 2.3 ± 0.9 mm Hg.[43] For the Bjork-Shiley valve in the mitral position, mean diastolic gradients have ranged from 2 to 4 mm Hg (for sizes 27, 29, 31 mm valves). Hancock valves in the mitral position show a slightly higher mean diastolic gradient (5 to 7 mm Hg, valve size unspecified).[34, 36]

Trivial prosthetic valve regurgitation is common and, in most cases, is perfectly normal. For example, the disc and ball of a mechanical prosthesis do not fit tightly against the cage; otherwise, they might become stuck in the closed position. As a consequence, trivial amounts of regurgitation can occur between the disc or ball and the surrounding cage. With pulsed Doppler echocardiography, trivial regurgitation has been reported in 58% to 62% of aortic prosthetic valves of varying types and sizes.[36, 42] Regurgitation

has been found with pulsed Doppler echocardiography in 14% to 19% of various mitral prosthetic valves.[39] The lower incidence of mitral prosthetic valve regurgitation is probably the result of difficulty in examining the left atrium behind the valve with pulsed Doppler echocardiography. With pulsed Doppler echocardiography, it is extremely difficult to distinguish physiologic prosthetic valve insufficiency from pathologic paravalvular leaks.

With Doppler color-flow mapping, a better understanding of the characteristics of flow across prosthetic valves has been obtained.[44] With this technique, the flow characteristics of various prosthetic mitral valves have been defined.[44] Color Doppler studies have shown that all mechanical valve occluders are obstructing bodies in the valve flow field; hence, they cause whirling vortices or eddies (chaotic swirling flow with flow reversals). In the mitral position, these vortices are of low velocity; consequently, the flow region appears relatively uniform in color and velocity. For Starr-Edwards valves in the mitral position, color Doppler examinations show that flow through the valve occurs in the form of peripheral, turbulent circumferential jets with maximal velocities of 1.0 to 1.5 m/sec. Turbulence (mosaic colors) is detected along the edges of the forward flow jets. On the other hand, the Bjork-Shiley mitral valve produces two eccentric, high-velocity jets with maximal velocities of 1.0 to 1.5 m/sec in both the major and minor orifices. The St. Jude mitral prosthesis has a central flow field with three jets. The jets through the lateral two orifices have maximal velocities of 0.8 to 1.2 m/sec and are larger than the jet through the central orifice. In the mitral position, the Hancock bioprosthetic valve has a central flow field that occupies only 50% to 75% of the inflow area. These valves consequently have higher-velocity, more turbulent jets (peak velocities of 1.5 to 2.0 m/sec) which are nonaxisymmetric and often directed toward the septum. In the mitral position, the Ionescu-Shiley valve has a central flow area with a high-velocity turbulent jet (1.5 to 2.0 m/sec peak velocity) usually directed toward the apex.[44]

With color-flow mapping, it is possible to detect trivial valvular insufficiency in virtually all prosthetic valves. Color Doppler examination does provide a technique for distinguishing this normal insufficiency from pathologic insufficiency (e.g., paravalvular leaks, a valve stuck in the open position) (Plates 50 and 51).

CARDIAC TRANSPLANTATION

Two-dimensional and Doppler echocardiography are important techniques for evaluating the child who has undergone cardiac transplantation. Using the methods outlined in Chapter 4, left ventricular systolic and diastolic function can be assessed. Load-independent end-systolic indexes of left ventricular contractility measured by echocardiography and calibrated carotid pulse tracings show normal contractility and contractile reserve in the denervated, transplanted, nonrejecting left ventricle.[45] The left ventricular diastolic filling patterns measured by Doppler echocardiography are normal in 85% of transplant recipients, suggesting that most have normal diastolic function at rest.[46]

To date, no echocardiographic index of early acute rejection has been identified. Some investigators have suggested that an increase in left ventricular mass measured by M-mode echocardiography is an early sign of acute rejection.[47] Other investigators, however, have found increased left ventricular wall mass and end-diastolic wall thickness in transplant patients with no evidence of rejection on endomyocardial biopsy compared to normal subjects.[45] It is postulated that the increase in wall thickness and mass represents a physiologic response of the transplanted left ventricle to the increased systemic vascular resistance, peak systolic pressure, and peak systolic wall stress of the recipient. The high impedance state of the recipient may be caused by peripheral vasoconstriction associated with end-stage heart disease, immunosuppressive drugs such as cyclosporin A and prednisone, and the normal effects of aging.[45]

On the mitral valve inflow Doppler, approximately 15% of transplant recipients have findings that suggest restrictive myopathy (see Chapter 4). Compared to transplant recipients with normal mitral valve Doppler indexes, patients with the restrictive pattern of left ventricular diastolic filling had more rejection episodes, more extensive fibrosis on cardiac biopsy, and greater incidence of impaired systolic function. The restrictive pattern of diastolic filling was not related to acute rejection, but rather appeared to be related to chronic rejection.[46] Thus, echocardiographic indexes of diastolic function have not been useful for the detection of acute rejection. These indexes do, however, indicate a link between abnormal diastolic filling and chronic immune-mediated damage to the transplanted heart.

On the two-dimensional echocardiograms of children who have had cardiac transplantation, the atria usually appear very enlarged. The atria of the transplant patient is really composed of portions of the native and donor atria and, thus, appear dilated. Often, the suture lines between the two portions of the atrium can be visualized. Suture lines are also frequently visible at the great artery connections.

EFFUSIONS

Pericardial Effusions

In pediatric patients, pericardial effusions commonly occur after cardiac surgery but are also found in patients with infections, congestive heart failure, juvenile rheumatoid arthritis, renal disease, and hypothyroidism.[48] On the echocardiogram, a pericardial effusion appears as an echo-free space between the epicardium (visceral pericardium) and the parietal pericardium. The posterior pericardial echo is identified as the brightest echo in the far field and the last echo to disappear as the gains are de-

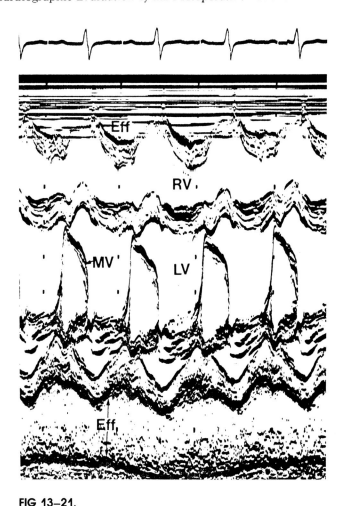

FIG 13–21.
M-mode echocardiogram of the left ventricle (LV) from a patient with a pericardial effusion (EFF). The effusion is seen as an echo-free space anterior to the right ventricle (RV) and posterior to the LV. MV = mitral valve.

creased. The anterior pericardial echo is difficult to visualize as a separate structure from the chest wall.[49, 50] Pericardial effusions can be detected by M-mode and two-dimensional echocardiography; however, two-dimensional echocardiography provides more information about the spatial distribution of the fluid and the presence of fluid loculations.[48]

On the echocardiogram, an echo-free space between the right ventricular anterior wall and the chest wall or between the left ventricular posterior wall and the pericardium indicates a pericardial effusion (Fig 13–21). Usually, the fluid first appears posteriorly in the dependent portion of the pericardial sac (Fig 13–22). The earliest manifestation of a tiny pericardial effusion is a small separation throughout systole and diastole of the epicardial surface of the left ventricular posterior wall and the parietal pericardium. A small separation of these two surfaces in systole only is normal and does not indicate a pathologic accumulation of pericardial fluid. The presence of a small

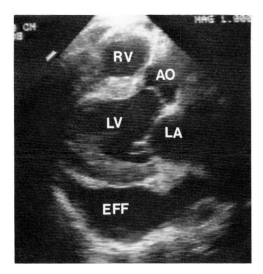

FIG 13–22.
Parasternal long-axis view from a patient with a posterior pericardial effusion (EFF). The EFF appears as a clear space posterior to the left ventricle (LV). AO = aorta; LA = left atrium; RV = right ventricle.

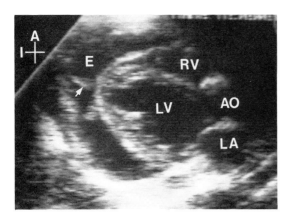

FIG 13–23.
Parasternal long-axis view from a patient with anterior and posterior pericardial effusions (E). The effusion is seen as a clear space surrounding the heart. In addition, fibrinous strands *(arrow)* are seen coursing through the pericardial fluid. A = anterior; AO = aorta; I = inferior; LA = left atrium; LV = left ventricle; RV = right ventricle.

posterior echo-free space and the absence of an anterior echo-free space suggests a small pericardial effusion. With further increases in the pericardial effusion, the posterior space widens; with large effusions, the fluid also appears anteriorly as an anterior echo-free space (Fig 13–23). With even larger accumulations of pericardial fluid, the anterior and posterior echo-free spaces increase even further in diameter.[50] Frequently, when a large anterior and posterior effusion is present, the heart can be seen swinging freely in the pericardial sac.[51] This swinging cardiac motion is responsible for electrical alternans on the electrocardi-

ogram and pulsus alternans on the physical examination.[52]

On the two-dimensional echocardiogram, pericardial effusions should be examined from all echocardiographic windows. In the parasternal and apical views, the patient lies in a left lateral decubitus position and, consequently, more fluid is distributed posteriorly. In the subcostal views, the patient lies supine, so that the fluid accumulates posteriorly and is distributed around the entire heart (Fig 13–24). This distribution of fluid often makes the effusion appear more sizeable than it actually is. With very large effusions, it is possible to image fluid around the great arteries (up to the level of the pericardial reflection) in the suprasternal views. Besides displaying the spatial distribution of the pericardial effusion, two-dimensional echocardiography provides information about the duration of the effusion. In patients with chronic pericardial effusions, fibrinous strands and other organized materials can be seen in the pericardial fluid (Fig 13–23). The formation of fibrinous strands may lead to fluid loculations that can be seen on the two-dimensional echocardiogram.

The exact volume of pericardial fluid cannot be determined with any degree of accuracy from the echocardiogram.[53] In general, effusions that are distributed anteriorly and posteriorly are large; patients with cardiac swinging motion have very large effusions. The total volume of fluid, however, is probably not as important hemodynamically as the rate at which it accumulates. There are several echocardiographic findings that suggest impending cardiac tamponade. On the M-mode echocardiogram of patients with cardiac tamponade, pronounced phasic variations in the end-diastolic dimensions of the right and left ventricle occur.[54] With inspiration, right ventricular dimension increases while left ventricular dimension decreases. Right ventricular compression occurs with expiration, and right ventricular end-diastolic dimensions

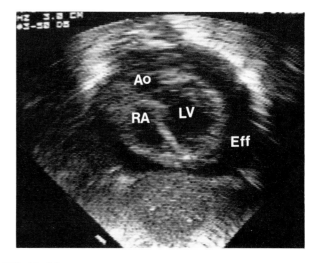

FIG 13–24.
Subcostal four-chamber view from a patient with a large pericardial effusion (Eff) surrounding the heart. The Eff is seen as an echo-free space around the heart. Ao = aorta; LV = left ventricle; RA = right atrium.

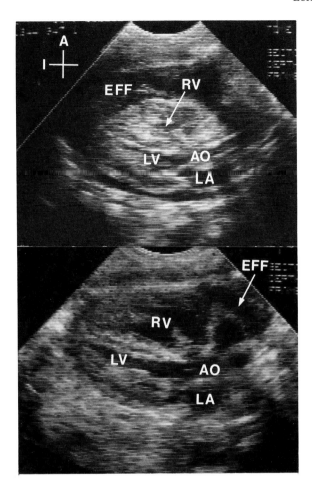

FIG 13–25.
Parasternal long-axis views from a patient with a large pericardial effusion (EFF) before *(top)* and after *(bottom)* pericardiocentesis. Before removal of the pericardial fluid *(top frame)*, the right ventricle (RV) is compressed by the pericardial fluid. This degree of RV compression is a sign· of cardiac tamponade. Following removal of a large majority of the pericardial effusion *(bottom frame)*, the RV cavity has re-expanded to its normal size. A = anterior; AO = aorta; I = inferior; LA = left atrium; LV = left ventricle.

of 4 mm or less have been found at end-expiration in adult patients with cardiac tamponade (Fig 13–25).[55] However, in patients with a hypertrophic, noncompliant right ventricle, cardiac tamponade can develop without echocardiographic evidence of right ventricular compression. On the two-dimensional echocardiogram, patients with cardiac tamponade have a striking late-diastolic inversion of the right atrial free wall.[56] In normal subjects, the right atrial wall is rounded and concave toward the center of the right atrium. This rounded configuration is maintained throughout the cardiac cycle, even as the atrium empties. In patients with cardiac tamponade, an abrupt buckling of the right atrial free wall toward the center of the right atrium begins at end-diastole and continues into systole. The more hemodynamically severe the tamponade, the longer the duration into systole of right atrial wall inver-

sion. Right atrial wall inversion occurs because the pressure within the pericardial sac exceeds the pressure in the right atrium at end-diastole when the atrium has emptied. As the right atrium fills during ventricular systole, right atrial pressure increases. When right atrial pressure exceeds the pressure within the pericardial sac, the free wall resumes its normal contour.

Doppler echocardiography is also useful for detecting cardiac tamponade.[57, 58] Patients with cardiac tamponade have a marked increase in the respiratory variation of transvalvular flow velocities, flow velocity time integrals, and left ventricular isovolumic relaxation time. In one study of patients with cardiac tamponade,[57] inspiration caused an 85% ±46% increase in the velocity time integral across the pulmonary valve, an 81% ±34% increase across the tricuspid valve, a 33% ±13% decrease across the aortic valve, and a 35% ±8% decrease across the mitral valve. With tamponade, there is an inspiratory increase in left ventricular isovolumic relaxation time of 85% ±14%, a decrease in mitral peak E velocity of 43% ±9%, and a decrease in mitral peak A of 25% ±12%.[58] As a result, the mitral E/A velocity ratio decreases with inspiration.[57]

Doppler echocardiography is also useful for detecting chronic constrictive pericardial disease. The Doppler findings in this disorder are included in Chapter 12.

In patients with large pericardial effusions, two-dimensional echocardiography can be used to guide the course of the needle during pericardiocentesis. When advancing the needle under ultrasound guidance, it is important that the plane of sound be tilted so that the tip of the needle can be imaged. If the tip of the needle passes out of the imaging plane, the echoes arising from the shaft of the needle may mislead the operator into believing that the needle can be safely advanced farther. If it is not possible to visualize the needle tip or if it is uncertain if the needle tip lies within the pericardial sac or the heart, a small amount of saline contrast material can be injected into the pericardiocentesis needle. If contrast echoes are seen filling the pericardial sac, then the needle tip is in good position within the pericardial cavity (Fig 13–26). If contrast echoes are seen filling the heart, the needle has punctured a cardiac wall. If contrast echoes are not seen, the needle has probably not been advanced far enough into the pericardial sac. We have found this technique particularly useful when the fluid withdrawn following pericardiocentesis is frankly bloody, and one is then uncertain if the needle has been advanced too far into the heart.

Pleural Effusions

In pediatric patients, pleural effusions commonly occur after cardiac surgery (i.e., Fontan procedure) but also occur in children with infections, congestive heart failure, and tumors. Pleural effusions appear as echo-free spaces, usually posterior to the left ventricle. In the parasternal long-axis view, pleural effusions do not produce a separation between the left ventricular posterior wall and the descending aorta, a factor that may help differentiate per-

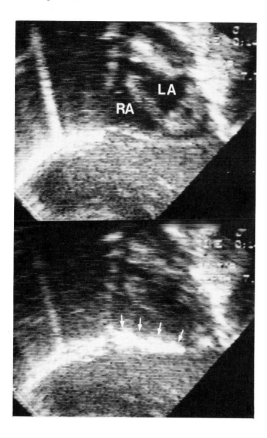

FIG 13–26.
Subcostal four-chamber views from an infant following removal of pericardial effusion with a pericardiocentesis catheter. On the echocardiogram, the tip of the catheter could not be clearly seen, and, because the pericardial fluid was bloody, concern existed that the catheter tip was in the atrium rather than the pericardial space. To confirm the location of the pericardial catheter, a small amount of saline was injected through the catheter. The *top frame* shows the right atrium (RA) and left atrium (LA) prior to injection of the contrast agent. In the *bottom frame,* contrast echoes *(arrows)* are seen in the pericardial sac, confirming the proper position of the catheter. No contrast echoes are seen in the atria.

icardial and pleural effusions.[59] When both pericardial and pleural effusions are present, the bright echo that arises from the parietal pericardium can be seen separating the two fluid layers.

In the subcostal views, even very small pleural effusions are easily imaged because the patient is lying supine and the fluid layers out posteriorly (Figs 13–27 and 13–28). Frequently, the tip of the collapsed lung can be seen as an echo-bright (air-filled) structure lying in the pleural effusion (Fig 13–29).

DIAPHRAGMATIC MOTION

The operative repair or palliation of congenital heart disease often involves surgery in the region of the aortic arch and damage to either phrenic nerve is common. Phrenic

nerve paralysis can be detected on the two-dimensional echocardiogram. For this diagnosis, the motion of both sides of the diaphragm is observed in the subcostal cross-sectional view of the abdomen as the patient breathes deeply. Normally, both halves of the diaphragm should move synchronously in an inferior direction with inspiration. Failure of one side of the diaphragm to move or movement of one side of the diaphragm in the opposite direction indicates a palsy or paralysis of the phrenic nerve to that half of the diaphragm. This diagnosis cannot be

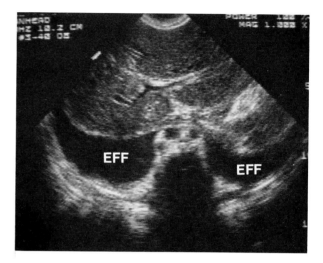

FIG 13–27.
Subcostal cross-sectional view in the abdomen from a patient with bilateral pleural effusions (EFF). The pleural effusion is seen as an echo-free space in the costophrenic angle.

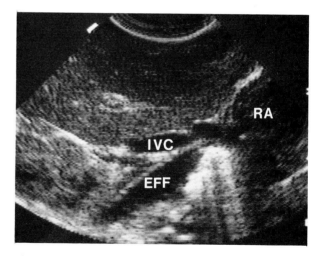

FIG 13–28.
Subcostal sagittal view through the inferior vena cava (IVC) and right atrium (RA) from a patient with a right-sided pleural effusion (EFF). The effusion is seen as an echo-free space in the costophrenic angle. The bright, white echoes represent air trapped in the collapsed tip of the right lung.

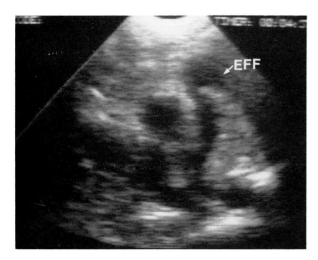

FIG 13–29.
Suprasternal short-axis view from an infant with an enormous right pleural effusion (EFF). The right lung, which is entirely collapsed, is seen outlined by the fluid.

made unless the child breathes spontaneously, without assistance from mechanical devices.

INTRAOPERATIVE ECHOCARDIOGRAPHY

Intraoperative echocardiography is a relatively new procedure in which ultrasound techniques are used to assess the adequacy of an operation while the patient is still in the operating room. Intraoperative echocardiography can be used to assess the adequacy of valve repair and the presence of residual shunts.[60–62] The technique usually involves a combination of two-dimensional imaging and Doppler color-flow mapping and can be performed with the transducer applied directly to the epicardial surface of the heart or with a transesophageal transducer. In children, intraoperative echocardiography has largely been performed using an epicardial approach because of the lack of commercially available transesophageal probes whose diameters are suitable for examining small children.

For the intraoperative epicardial examination, the cleaned transducer and cable are inserted into a commercially available sterile plastic bag. To ensure good ultrasound coupling, a large quantity of sterile gel is placed into the plastic bag and warm saline is poured over the heart. The transducer and its sterile covering are then placed directly on the anterior surface of the heart and multiple long- and short-axis cuts are obtained. True apical views cannot be obtained with the heart lying in the open thoracic cage; however, foreshortened apical views can be obtained.

This technique has been extremely valuable for detecting residual defects such as residual ventricular septal defects or tiny patent ductus arteriosus.[62] The technique has also been extremely useful for detecting residual valvular insufficiency following valvuloplasty procedures or following repair of atrioventricular septal defect.[60, 61] In the

evaluation of valvular regurgitation, the patient's heart rate and blood pressure must be in the normal physiologic range before any conclusions can be made from the color Doppler display of the insufficiency jet. In some cases, this may require administration in the operating room of drugs such as phenylephrine to raise the patient's blood pressure. An intraoperative color Doppler examination obtained prior to opening the pericardium and beginning cardiopulmonary bypass can be an important standard of comparison for the postoperative examination.

REFERENCES

1. Allen HD, Sahn DJ, Lange L, et al: Noninvasive assessment of surgical systemic to pulmonary artery shunts by range-gated pulsed Doppler echocardiography. *J Pediatr* 1979; 94:395–402.
2. Stevenson JG, Kawabori I, Bailey WW: Noninvasive evaluation of Blalock-Taussig shunts: Determination of patency and differentiation from patent ductus arteriosus by Doppler echocardiography. *Am Heart J* 1983; 106:1121–1132.
3. Serwer GA, Armstrong BE, Sterba RJ, et al: Alterations in carotid-arterial velocity-time profile produced by the Blalock-Taussig shunt. *Circulation* 1981; 63:1115–1120.
4. Serwer GA, Armstrong BE, Anderson PAW: Noninvasive detection of retrograde descending aortic flow in infants using continuous wave Doppler ultrasonography. *J Pediatr* 1980; 97:394–400.
5. Fyfe DA, Currie PJ, Seward JB, et al: Continuous-wave Doppler determination of the pressure gradient across pulmonary artery bands: Hemodynamic correlation in 20 patients. *Mayo Clin Proc* 1984; 59:744–750.
6. Valdes-Cruz LM, Horowitz S, Sahn DJ, et al: Validation of a Doppler echocardiographic method for calculating severity of discrete stenotic obstruction in a canine preparation with a pulmonary arterial band. *Circulation* 1984; 69:1177–1181.
7. Valdes-Cruz LM, Pieroni DR, Roland J-MA, et al: Recognition of residual postoperative shunts by contrast echocardiographic techniques. *Circulation* 1977; 55:148–152.
8. Duff DF, Gutgesell HP: The use of saline or blood for ultrasonic detection of a right-to-left intracardiac shunt in the early postoperative patient. *Am Heart J* 1977; 94:402–406.
9. Ross DN, Somerville J: Correction of pulmonary atresia with a homograft aortic valve. *Lancet* 1966; 2:1446–1447.
10. Park SC, Neeches WH, Lenox CC, et al: Massive calcification and obstruction in a homograft after the Rastelli procedure for transposition of the great arteries. *Am J Cardiol* 1973; 32:860–864.
11. Moodie DS, Mair DD, Fulton RE, et al: Aortic homograft obstruction. *J Thorac Cardiovasc Surg* 1976; 72:553–561.
12. Bowman FO, Jr, Hancock WD, Malm JR: A valve-containing Dacron prosthesis: Its use in restoring pulmonary artery-right ventricular continuity. *Arch Surg* 1973; 107:724–728.

13. Bailey WW, Kirklin JW, Bargeron LM, Jr, et al: Late results with synthetic valved external conduits from venous ventricle to pulmonary arteries. *Circulation* 1977; 56(suppl II):73–79.

14. Ciaravella JM Jr, McGoon DC, Danielson GK, et al: Experience with the extracardiac conduit. *J Thorac Cardiovasc Surg* 1979; 78:920–930.

15. Norwood WI, Freed MD, Rocchini AP, et al: Experience with valved conduits for repair of congenital cardiac lesions. *Ann Thorac Surg* 1977; 24:223–232.

16. Bissett GS III, Schwartz DC, Benzing G III, et al: Late results of reconstruction of right ventricular outflow tract with porcine xenografts in children. *Ann Thorac Surg* 1981; 31:437–443.

17. Agarwal KC, Edwards WD, Feldt RH, et al: Clinicopathological correlates of obstructed right-sided porcine valved extracardiac conduits. *J Thorac Cardiovasc Surg* 1981; 81:591–601.

18. Schaff HV, DiDonato RM, Danielson GK: Reoperation for obstructed pulmonary ventricle-pulmonary artery conduits: Early and late results. *J Thorac Cardiovasc Surg* 1984; 88:334–343.

19. Moore CH, Martelli B, Ross DN: Reconstruction of right ventricular outflow tract with a valved conduit in 75 cases of congenital heart disease. *J Thorac Cardiovasc Surg* 1976; 71:11–19.

20. Shabbo FP, Wain WH, Ross DN: Right ventricular outflow reconstruction with aortic homograft conduit: Analysis of the long-term results. *Thorac Cardiovasc Surg* 1980; 28:21–25.

21. Al-Janabi N, Ross DN: Enhanced viability of fresh aortic homografts stored in nutrient medium. *Cardiovasc Res* 1973; 7:817–822.

22. Yacoub M, Kittle CF: Sterilization of valve homografts by antibiotic solution. *Circulation* 1970; 41(suppl II):29–31.

23. DiCarlo D, de Leval MR, Stark J: "Fresh," antibiotic sterilized aortic homografts in extracardiac valved conduits: Long-term results. *Thorac Cardiovasc Surg* 1984; 32:10–14.

24. Fontan F, Choussat A, Deville C, et al: Aortic valve homografts in the surgical treatment of complex cardiac malformations. *J Thorac Cardiovasc Surg* 1984; 87:649–657.

25. Kay PH, Ross DN: Fifteen years' experience with the aortic homograft: The conduit of choice for right ventricular outflow reconstruction. *Ann Thorac Surg* 1985; 40:360–364.

26. Kirklin JW, Barratt-Boyes BG: *Cardiac Surgery.* New York, Wiley, 1986, p 800.

27. Kirklin JW, Blackstone EH, Maehara T, et al: Intermediate-term fate of cryopreserved allograft and xenograft valved conduits. *Ann Thorac Surg* 1987; 44:598–606.

28. Lamberti JJ, Angell WW, Waldman JD, et al: The cryopreserved homograft valve in the pulmonary position: Early results and technical considerations. *J Cardiac Surg* 1988; 3:247–251.

29. Meliones JN, Snider AR, Bove EL, et al: Doppler evaluation of homograft valves in children. *Am J Cardiol* 1989; 64:354–358.

30. Silverman NH, Snider AR: *Two-dimensional Echocardiography in Congenital Heart Disease.* Norwalk, Appleton-Century-Crofts, 1982, pp 222–223.

31. Canale JM, Sahn DJ, Copeland JG, et al: Two-dimensional Doppler echocardiographic/M-mode echocardiographic and phonocardiographic method for study of extracardiac heterograft valved conduits in the right ventricular outflow position. *Am J Cardiol* 1982; 49:100–107.

32. Hagler DJ, Seward JB, Tajik AJ, et al: Functional assessment of the Fontan operation: Combined M-mode, two-dimensional and Doppler echocardiographic studies. *J Am Coll Cardiol* 1984; 4:756–764.

33. Sprecher DL, Adamick R, Adams D, et al: In vitro color flow, pulsed and continuous wave Doppler ultrasound masking of flow by prosthetic valves. *J Am Coll Cardiol* 1987; 9:1306–1310.

34. Holen J, Simonson S, Frysaker T: An ultrasound Doppler technique for the non-invasive determination of the pressure gradient in the Bjork-Shiley mitral valve. *Circulation* 1979; 59:436–442.

35. Ramirez ML, Wong M, Sadler N, et al: Doppler evaluation of 106 bioprosthetic and mechanical aortic valves. *J Am Coll Cardiol* 1985; 5:527.

36. Hatle L, Angelsen B: *Doppler Ultrasound in Cardiology: Physical Principles and Clinical Applications.* ed 2. Philadelphia, Lea and Febiger, 1985, pp 188–196.

37. Gross CM, Wann LS: Doppler echocardiographic diagnosis of porcine bioprosthetic cardiac valve malfunction. *Am J Cardiol* 1984; 53:1203–1205.

38. Kotler MN, Mintz GS, Panidis IP, et al: Noninvasive evaluation of normal and abnormal prosthetic valve function. *J Am Coll Cardiol* 1983; 2:151–173.

39. Sagar KB, Wann LS, Paulsen WHJ, et al: Doppler echocardiographic evaluation of Hancock and Bjork-Shiley prosthetic valves. *J Am Coll Cardiol* 1986; 7:681–687.

40. Ferrara RP, Labovitz AJ, Wiens RD, et al: Prosthetic mitral regurgitation detected by Doppler echocardiography. *Am J Cardiol* 1985; 55:229–230.

41. Williams GA, Labovitz AJ: Doppler hemodynamic evaluation of prosthetic (Starr-Edwards and Bjork-Shiley) and bioprosthetic (Hancock and Carpentier-Edwards) cardiac valves. *Am J Cardiol* 1985; 56:325–332.

42. Panidis IP, Ross J, Mintz GS: Normal and abnormal prosthetic valve function as assessed by Doppler echocardiography. *J Am Coll Cardiol* 1986; 8:317–326.

43. Weinstein IR, Marbarger JP, Perez JE: Ultrasonic assessment of the St. Jude prosthetic valve: M-mode, two-dimensional, and Doppler echocardiography. *Circulation* 1983; 68:897–905.

44. Jones M, Eidbo EE: Doppler color flow evaluation of prosthetic mitral valves: Experimental epicardial studies. *J Am Coll Cardiol* 1989; 13:234–240.

45. Borow KM, Neumann A, Arensman FW, et al: Left ventricular contractility and contractile reserve in humans after cardiac transplantation. *Circulation* 1985; 71:866–872.

46. Valantine HA, Appleton CP, Hatle LK, et al: A hemodynamic and Doppler echocardiographic study of ventricular function in long-term cardiac allograft recipients: Etiology and prognosis of restrictive-constrictive physiology. *Circulation* 1989; 79:66–75.

47. Sagar KB, Hastillo A, Wolfgang TC, et al: Left ven-

tricular mass by M-mode echocardiography in cardiac transplant patients with acute rejection. *Circulation* 1981; 64(suppl 2):216.

48. Silverman NH, Snider AR: In Ref 30, pp 215–217.
49. Feigenbaum H, Waldhausen JA, Hyde LP: Ultrasound diagnosis of pericardial effusion. *JAMA* 1965; 191:711–717.
50. Tajik AJ: Echocardiography in pericardial effusion. *Am J Med* 1977; 63:29–40.
51. Feigenbaum J, Zaky A, Grabhorn LL: Cardiac motion in patients with pericardial effusion: A study using reflected ultrasound. *Circulation* 1966; 34:611–616.
52. Usher BW, Popp RL: Electrical alternans: Mechanism in pericardial effusion. *Am Heart J* 1972; 83:459–465.
53. Horowitz MS, Schultz CS, Stinson EB, et al: Sensitivity and specificity of echocardiographic diagnosis of pericardial effusion. *Circulation* 1974; 50:239–245.
54. D'Cruz IA, Cohen HC, Prabhu R, et al: Diagnosis of cardiac tamponade by echocardiography: Changes in mitral valve motion and ventricular dimensions, with special reference to paradoxical pulse. *Circulation* 1975; 52:460–465.
55. Schiller NB, Botvinick EH: Right ventricular compression as a sign of cardiac tamponade: An analysis of echocardiographic ventricular dimensions and their clinical implications. *Circulation* 1977; 56:774–779.
56. Gillam LD, Guyer DE, Gibson TC, et al: Hydrodynamic compression of the right atrium: A new echocardiographic sign of cardiac tamponade. *Circulation* 1983; 68:294–301.
57. Leeman DE, Levine MJ, Come PC: Doppler echocardiography in cardiac tamponade: Exaggerated respiratory variation on transvalvular blood flow velocity integrals. *J Am Coll Cardiol* 1988; 11:572–578.
58. Appleton CP, Hatle LK, Popp RL: Cardiac tamponade and pericardial effusion: Respiratory variation in transvalvular flow velocities studied by Doppler echocardiography. *J Am Coll Cardiol* 1988; 11:1020–1030.
59. Haaz WS, Mintz GS, Kotler MN, et al: Two-dimensional echocardiographic recognition of the descending thoracic aorta: Value in differentiating pericardial from pleural effusions. *Am J Cardiol* 1980; 45:401.
60. Gussenhoven EJ, Van Herwerden LA, Roelandt J, et al: Intra-operative two-dimensional echocardiography in congenital heart disease. *J Am Coll Cardiol* 1987; 9:565–572.
61. Maurer G, Czer LSC, Chaux A, et al: Intraoperative Doppler color flow mapping for assessment of valve repair for mitral regurgitation. *Am J Cardiol* 1987; 60:333–337.
62. Hagler DJ, Tajik AJ, Seward JB, et al: Intra-operative two-dimensional Doppler echocardiography. A preliminary study for congenital heart disease. *J Thorac Cardiovasc Surg* 1988; 95:516–522.

14

Diagnostic Approach to Complex Congenital Heart Disease

Two-dimensional echocardiography has had a major impact on the ability to diagnose complex congenital heart defects. With this technique, it is possible to image detailed structural anatomy even more precisely than with cardiac catheterization in the majority of patients. The echocardiographic approach to the diagnosis of complex congenital heart disease is a logical and systematic approach that requires a basic knowledge of how cardiac chambers are identified on the two-dimensional echocardiogram. This chapter will review (1) the echocardiographic approach to the segmental analysis of the heart, (2) the examination techniques used to evaluate the child with dextrocardia, and (3) the echocardiographic features of the more frequently encountered forms of complex congenital heart disease.

ECHOCARDIOGRAPHIC APPROACH TO THE SEGMENTAL ANALYSIS OF THE HEART

General Considerations

The echocardiographic approach to the diagnosis of complex congenital heart disease involves a segmental analysis of the heart.[1-6] In this type of analysis, the heart can be thought of as being much like a house. To describe a house completely, it is first necessary to describe where the rooms or chambers are located on each floor. In the cardiac house, this includes describing each atrium on the ground floor, the ventricles on the second story, and the position of each great artery at the top of the house. In addition, a complete description of a house would include the location of the staircases that connect the floors. For the ''cardiac house,'' this includes a description of the atrioventricular connections and the ventriculoarterial connections. Thus, if the atria are not correctly identified, the entire ''house'' comes tumbling down.[7]

Therefore, the approach to the echocardiographic diagnosis of the child with complex congenital heart disease begins with a determination of the atrial situs. In atrial situs solitus, the morphologic right atrium is on the right; and the morphologic left atrium is on the left. In situs inversus, the morphologic left atrium is on the right and the morphologic right atrium is on the left. In situs ambiguus, the atria are not differentiated as right and left atria. Instead, both atria can have features of a morphologic right atrium, a condition called asplenia, or both atria can have the features of a morphologic left atrium, a condition called polysplenia.[2,6,8] The echocardiographic findings used to identify the morphology of the atria will be discussed below.

The next step in the diagnosis of complex congenital heart disease is determination of the bulboventricular loop. The bulboventricular loop describes the locations of the ventricles. In a d-loop (dextro loop), the morphologic right ventricle is on the right and the morphologic left ventricle is on the left. In an l-loop (levo loop), the morphologic right ventricle is on the left and the morphologic left ventricle is on the right. These definitions of d- and l-loop apply regardless of what the atrial situs is. Thus, concordant or normal connections between the atria and ventricles (morphologic right atrium to morphologic right ventricle; morphologic left atrium to morphologic left ventricle) occur when there is situs solitus with a d-loop or situs inversus with an l-loop. Discordant or abnormal connections between the atria and ventricles (morphologic right atrium to morphologic left ventricle; morphologic left atrium to morphologic right ventricle) occur when there is situs solitus with an l-loop or situs inversus with a d-loop.[1,2,5]

The final step in the diagnosis of complex congenital heart disease is a description of the great artery connections. In normal or concordant connections, the pulmonary artery arises from the morphologic right ventricle and the

348

aorta arises from the morphologic left ventricle. Transposition is the situation where the aorta arises from the morphologic right ventricle and the pulmonary artery arises from the morphologic left ventricle. Transposition is a discordant ventriculoarterial connection. Other types of great artery connections include double-outlet right ventricle, double-outlet left ventricle, and single outlet from the heart. Three common forms of single outlet from the heart include truncus arteriosus, aortic atresia, and pulmonary atresia.[2, 4, 9]

Before reviewing how cardiac chambers are identified on the two-dimensional echocardiogram, it is necessary to review the rule of 50%. This rule states that a chamber is a ventricle if it receives 50% or more of an inlet. The inlet consists of the fibrous ring of the atrioventricular valve and need not always include a patent atrioventricular valve with well-formed valve leaflets. For example, in hypoplastic left heart with aortic and mitral atresia, the fibrous ring of the mitral valve contains an imperforate membrane and is situated over the small left ventricle. Thus, this small left-sided chamber is a ventricle because it receives 100% of an inlet (even though there is no antegrade flow across the inlet). It is important to note that a chamber need not have an outlet to be a ventricle. For example, the left ventricle in double-outlet right ventricle is a ventricle because it receives the mitral valve even though it does not have an outlet. The rule of 50% also states that if 50% or more of a great artery arises above a chamber, the great artery is defined as being connected to that chamber.[6, 10] As will be discussed below, multiple echocardiographic views are necessary to determine if an atrioventricular valve or great artery is committed by 50% or more to a chamber. In most cases, this determination can be made easily from the two-dimensional echocardiogram; in some cases, however, the atrioventricular valve or great artery appears to be equally committed to both ventricular chambers. In these cases, additional information, such as the orientation of the trabecular septum relative to the crux of the heart (see the section on single ventricle), may be helpful in deciding to which chamber an atrioventricular valve or great artery is connected. In the rare cases where the connections are not readily apparent from the two-dimensional echocardiogram, there is usually controversy about the connections even at the pathologic examination.

Application of the rule of 50% requires definitions for chambers that are not ventricles. Rudimentary chambers are chambers that receive less than 50% of an inlet and, therefore, do not qualify as ventricles. Rudimentary chambers are of two types. An outlet chamber is a chamber that has less than 50% of an inlet but has 50% or more of an outlet or great artery. A trabecular pouch is a chamber that has less than 50% of an inlet and less than 50% of an outlet.[10]

Definition of Cardiac Chambers From the Two-Dimensional Echocardiogram

Anatomic Landmarks on the Septal Surfaces
To diagnose complex congenital heart disease, one must

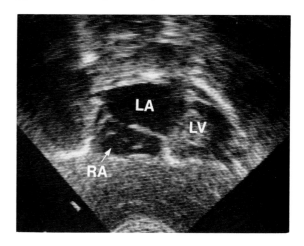

FIG 14–1.
Subcostal four-chamber view from a normal patient showing the anatomic features of the morphologic right atrium (RA). The morphologic RA has a septal surface that receives the tendonous insertion of the eustachian valve. In this view, the eustachian valve can be seen crossing the floor of the RA from the orifice of the inferior vena cava to its insertion into the septum primum. LA = left atrium; LV = left ventricle.

know how cardiac chambers are identified on the two-dimensional echocardiogram. The cardiac chambers are largely defined by the anatomic landmarks on their septal surfaces.[11] The morphologic right atrium has a septal surface that receives the tendonous insertion of the eustachian valve and has the limbus of the fossa ovalis. The eustachian valve crosses the floor of the right atrium from the orifice of the inferior vena cava and inserts into the septum primum (the lower portion of the atrial septum adjacent to the atrioventricular valves). This tendonous insertion is located along the lower border of the fossa ovalis and is called the inferior limbic band (Fig 14–1).[3, 4, 11] In real time, the eustachian valve moves rapidly back and forth in the right atrium and can be visualized in virtually all infants and in many older children and adults. The subcostal four-chamber and sagittal views are particularly useful for visualizing the eustachian valve.

The left atrial septal surface has the flap valve of the fossa ovalis. This is the septum primum tissue that covers the foramen ovale and seals it closed after birth.[11] On the two-dimensional echocardiogram, the flap valve can be seen protruding into the left atrium in the fetus when the foramen ovale is open; after birth, however, the flap valve cannot usually be identified on the two-dimensional echocardiogram. In congenital heart defects associated with high right atrial pressure (i.e., tricuspid atresia, severe pulmonary stenosis), the foramen ovale remains open and the flap valve can be seen protruding into the left atrium (Fig 14–2). In cases where the flap valve is tightly adherent to the left atrial septal surface and therefore cannot be visualized as a separate structure on the two-dimensional echocardiogram, other methods of identifying the left atrium must be used.

The morphologic right ventricle is the chamber whose

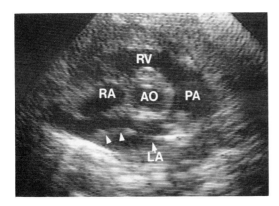

FIG 14-2.
Parasternal short-axis view from a newborn with severe primary pulmonary artery hypertension. Because of the elevated right atrial (RA) and right ventricular (RV) pressures in this infant, the flap valve *(arrows)* of the foramen ovale remains open and is seen protruding into the left atrium (LA). The flap valve of the foramen ovale is an anatomic marker of the morphologic LA. AO = aorta; PA = pulmonary artery.

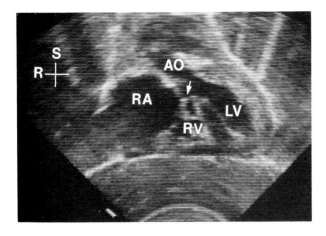

FIG 14-3.
Subcostal four-chamber view through the left ventricular (LV) outflow tract from a patient with a ventricular septal defect. Chordal attachments of the tricuspid valve to the crest of the ventricular septum *(arrow)* can be seen. The chordal attachments are an anatomic feature of the morphologic right ventricle (RV). AO = aorta; R = right; RA = right atrium; S = superior.

septal surface has prominent muscle bundles that cross from the septum to the parietal free wall (see Fig 3–15). The largest of these septoparietal muscle bundles is the moderator band. In addition, the septal surface of the right ventricle receives chordal insertions from the tricuspid valve septal leaflet (Fig 14–3).[3, 4, 11]

The morphologic left ventricle is the chamber whose septal surface is smooth. There are no septoparietal free wall muscle bundles, and the mitral valve normally has no chordal insertions into the septum (see Fig 3–15).[3, 4, 11]

Atrioventricular Valve Morphology

Another anatomic feature that is useful in identifying the cardiac chambers is that the atrioventricular valve always belongs to the appropriate ventricle. Thus, the tricuspid valve is always found in the morphologic right ventricle and the mitral valve is always found in the morphologic left ventricle. The tricuspid valve is closer to the cardiac apex (see Fig 3–15), has three leaflets, and has chordal insertions into the ventricular septum (Fig 14–3). The mitral valve is farther from the cardiac apex, is a fish-mouth bicuspid valve, and has chordal insertions into only two papillary muscles in the left ventricle (see Figs 3–12 and 3–13).[11] The apical and subcostal four-chamber views are especially useful for determining the relative distances of the atrioventricular valves from the cardiac apex. The parasternal and subcostal short-axis views are particularly useful for identifying which of the ventricles has the fish-mouthed atrioventricular valve and two papillary muscles and is, therefore, the morphologic left ventricle.

Systemic and Pulmonary Venous Return

Systemic and pulmonary venous return can be helpful in identifying the atria. The pulmonary veins usually drain to the morphologic left atrium; however, because the pulmonary veins can drain anomalously, this is not a constant feature of the left atrium. If three or more pulmonary veins are seen draining by separate orifices into a chamber and there is no evidence of a pulmonary venous confluence, that chamber is most likely a morphologic left atrium (Fig 14–4). The inferior vena cava usually drains to the morphologic right atrium. This relationship is constant in the majority of cases except in patients with situs ambiguus, as will be discussed below. The superior vena cava usually drains to the morphologic right atrium; however, this re-

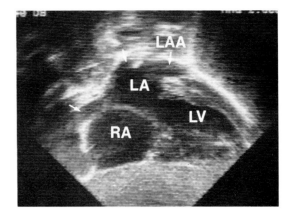

FIG 14-4.
Subcostal four-chamber view from a normal patient. The pulmonary veins *(arrows)* are seen draining to the left-sided atrium by way of two separate orifices. This type of pulmonary venous drainage usually indicates that the chamber receiving the pulmonary veins is a morphologic left atrium (LA). LAA = left atrial appendage; LV = left ventricle; RA = right atrium.

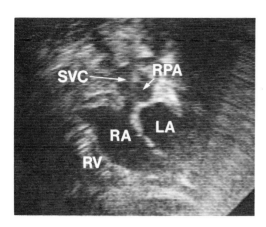

FIG 14–5.
Subcostal short-axis view of the right atrium (RA) of a normal patient. The right atrial appendage is short and stout and resembles "Snoopy's" nose. LA = left atrium; RPA = right pulmonary artery; RV = right ventricle; SVC = superior vena cava.

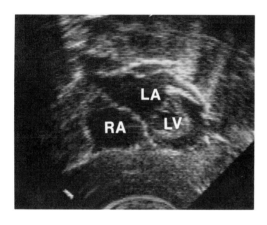

FIG 14–6.
Subcostal four-chamber view from a normal patient. Note the long fingerlike appearance of the left atrial appendage. The left atrial appendage resembles "Snoopy's" ear. LA = left atrium; LV = left ventricle; RA = right atrium.

lationship is not constant as the superior vena cava can drain to either or both atria (see Chapter 10).[3, 4, 10]

Atrial Appendage Morphology

The morphology of the atrial appendages can be helpful in identifying the atria.[3] The right atrial appendage is short and stout (resembling "Snoopy's" nose) and is well visualized in the parasternal long-axis view through the right ventricular inflow tract and the subcostal sagittal view (Fig 14–5). The left atrial appendage is long and fingerlike (resembling "Snoopy's" ear) and is well seen in the parasternal short-axis view and the subcostal four-chamber view (Fig 14–6).

Abdominal Situs

The abdominal situs can provide information that is

helpful in determining the atrial situs.[3, 4, 11] For example, in the majority of patients with atrial situs solitus, abdominal situs solitus will also be found. Thus, subcostal views of the abdomen show that the inferior vena cava is to the right of the spine, the descending aorta is to the left of the spine, the stomach bubble is on the left, and the liver is on the right (Fig 14–7). Likewise, in the majority of patients with atrial situs inversus, there is also abdominal situs inversus. Subcostal views of the abdomen show that the inferior vena cava is usually to the left of the spine and the descending aorta is usually to the right of the spine. The stomach bubble is on the right and the liver is on the left (Fig 14–8). In atrial situs ambiguus, the liver may be

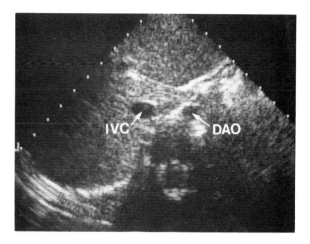

FIG 14–7.
Subcostal short-axis view from a patient with atrial and abdominal situs solitus. The liver is on the patient's right. The inferior vena cava (IVC) is to the right of the spine, and the descending aorta (DAO) is to the left.

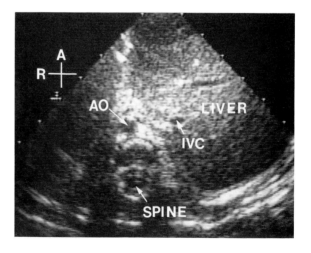

FIG 14–8.
Subcostal short-axis view in the abdomen from a patient with atrial and abdominal situs inversus. The patient's liver is on the left. The inferior vena cava (IVC) is seen to the left of the spine and the descending aorta (AO) is seen to the right. A = anterior; R = right.

to the right, to the left, or transverse. The stomach bubble can be on either side or in the midline. Several types of anomalies of systemic venous drainage are often present and suggest the diagnosis of situs ambiguus. These anomalies will be discussed in detail and illustrated below.

When the atrial and abdominal situs are discordant (atrial situs solitus with abdominal situs inversus or vice versa), the incidence of severe, complex congenital heart disease is high. Defects with atrioventricular and ventriculoarterial discordance are especially frequent in this situation.[4]

TECHNIQUES FOR EVALUATION OF THE CHILD WITH DEXTROCARDIA

The term dextrocardia indicates that the heart is located primarily in the right chest and implies that one of three conditions is present.[12, 13] First, dextrocardia can occur because the heart is displaced into the right chest, either because of a space-occupying mass in the left chest or the absence of normal lung volume filling the right chest. This form of dextrocardia is commonly called dextroposition. Second, dextrocardia can occur because the cardiac apex fails to pivot to the left. This condition, known as dextroversion, is frequently associated with atrioventricular discordance.[4] Third, dextrocardia can occur in association with abnormal atrial situs (i.e., situs inversus or situs ambiguus). The most common condition in this category is situs inversus totalis in which the heart is located in the mirror-image position of normal.

In our laboratory, if a child is referred with a diagnosis of dextrocardia, the echocardiographic examination is begun from the subcostal position rather than from the parasternal window, which is the routine starting location. This approach allows us to determine immediately whether (1) the child has dextroposition, dextroversion, or dextrocardia with abnormal atrial situs and (2) the direction along which the major axis of the heart is aligned. For example, from the subcostal four-chamber view, patients with dextroposition have the morphologic right atrium and right ventricle to the right of the morphologic left atrium and left ventricle. Usually, the alignment of the major axis of the heart is normal (pointed to the left) or rotated slightly vertically; however, the entire heart is shifted to the right of midline or to the retrosternal area. In patients with dextroversion, the morphologic right atrium is to the right of the morphologic left atrium; however, the major axis of the heart is aligned from the left shoulder toward the right hip.[13] In this condition, the cardiac apex is to the right of midline and the atria are usually in their normal positions or shifted slightly to the right (Figs 14–9 and 14–10). In dextrocardia with atrial situs inversus, the morphologic left atrium is to the right of the morphologic right atrium and both atria are usually located entirely to the right of the sternum. The cardiac apex is usually located in the right fifth or sixth intercostal space at the anterior axillary line; hence, the major axis of the heart is aligned between

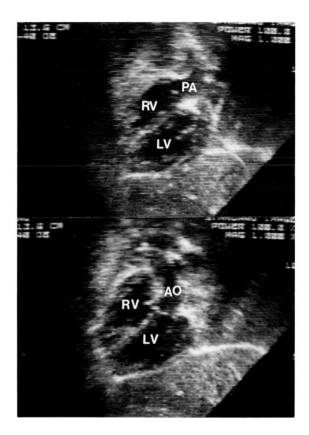

FIG 14–9.
Subcostal four-chamber views from a patient with dextroversion of the cardiac apex. In the *top frame,* the plane of sound has been tilted far anteriorly. The right-sided ventricle has a prominent moderator band in its apical portion and is, therefore, a morphologic right ventricle (RV). The RV gives rise to a vessel that bifurcates and is therefore a pulmonary artery (PA). The *bottom frame* was obtained by tilting the transducer in the subcostal coronal view slightly posteriorly. The smooth-walled, left-sided ventricle, which is the morphologic left ventricle (LV), gives rise to a vessel that arches and is, therefore, the aorta (AO). Other echocardiographic views showed that this patient had atrial situs solitus. Therefore, the atrioventricular and ventriculoarterial connections are normal. The only abnormality in this heart is the failure of the cardiac apex to pivot to the left.

the left shoulder and the right hip.[13] Compared to the major axis alignment in dextroversion, the alignment of the major axis of the heart in dextrocardia with situs inversus is similar in direction and angle but is shifted more to the right. Major axis alignment in dextrocardia with situs ambiguus is about the same as that found in dextrocardia with situs solitus.

After visualizing the alignment of the heart from the base to the apex and imaging the position of the atria relative to the midline, the examiner is better informed about how to position the transducer to obtain the parasternal and apical views. For example, with dextroposition, the parasternal long- and short-axis views are obtained with the usual orientation of the plane of sound but with the transducer positioned just to the right of the sternum. The apical views are also obtained with the usual orientation of the plane of sound but with the transducer positioned just to the right of the lower sternal border. With dextroversion, the parasternal long-axis view is obtained with the plane of sound oriented in the mirror-image direction of normal. Depending on the location of the base of the heart, the transducer position may be just to the right or left of the sternum. Because the atria are usually positioned normally and the great arteries arise normally from the ventricles, the parasternal short-axis view is obtained with the normal orientation of the plane of sound. In dextroversion, the apical views are obtained by placing the transducer directly over the location where the cardiac apex was imaged from the subcostal views (usually just at the right lower sternal border). With dextrocardia and atrial situs inversus, the parasternal long-axis view is obtained from the right second or third intercostal space with the plane of sound oriented in a mirror-image of normal (from the left shoulder to the right hip). The parasternal long-axis view has only anterior-posterior and superior-inferior directions and does not display the right-left orientation of cardiac structures. Thus, on the video monitor, cardiac structures appear to be oriented in a normal fashion, and only the examiner knows that the images were obtained in a mirror-image plane. The parasternal short-axis views are obtained from the same transducer location, with the plane of sound also oriented in the mirror-image direction of normal (from the right shoulder to the left hip). Unlike the parasternal long-axis view, the parasternal short-axis views display the right-left orientation of the cardiac structures. Thus, on the video monitor, in patients with dextrocardia and situs inversus, the parasternal short-axis view will

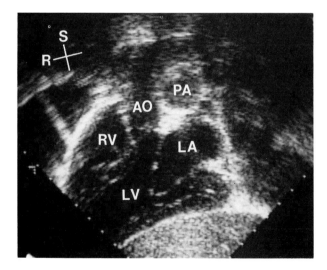

FIG 14–10.
Subcostal coronal view through the left ventricular (LV) outflow tract from a patient with dextroversion of the cardiac apex. The cardiac apex is oriented toward the patient's right. The aorta (AO) arises normally from the LV. In this case, the structural abnormality is failure of the cardiac apex to pivot to the left. LA = left atrium; PA = pulmonary artery; R = right; RV = right ventricle; S = superior.

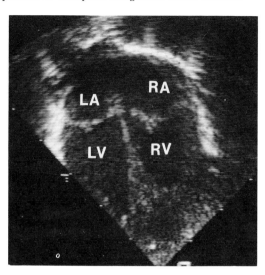

FIG 14–11.
Apical four-chamber view from a patient with mirror-image dextrocardia. In this patient, the right-sided atrium received all of the pulmonary veins and was the morphologic left atrium (LA); therefore, the patient had atrial situs inversus. The left-sided ventricle had a prominent moderator band and was, therefore, the morphologic right ventricle (RV). Thus, this patient has an *l*-bulboventricular loop. In this patient, the apical four-chamber view appears inverted from that of a patient with atrial situs solitus. LV = left ventricle; RA = right atrium.

appear to be a backward version of normal. It is important that the examiner not "correct" the image by using the left-right invert button. Inverting the images to make the views appear "normal" is contrary to the accepted guidelines for two-dimensional image orientation and will only lead to confusion in understanding the cardiac spatial anatomy. In dextrocardia with situs inversus, the apical views are obtained with the transducer positioned in the right fifth or sixth intercostal space in the anterior axillary line and with the plane of sound oriented in a mirror-image direction of normal. Like the parasternal short-axis view, the apical view displays the right-left orientation of the cardiac structures. When properly displayed on the video monitor, the apical four-chamber view in dextrocardia with situs inversus will appear to be backward (Fig 14–11).

If for some reason a patient is referred to our laboratory without a prior diagnosis of dextrocardia and the echocardiographic examination is begun, as is our routine, from the parasternal window as is our routine, we use the following approach to the examination. First, attempts are made to obtain the parasternal long-axis view from the left upper sternal border, with a normal orientation of the plane of sound (from the right shoulder to the left hip). After rotating or tilting the transducer slightly, if no image resembling a parasternal long-axis view is found, the transducer is slid to the right of the sternum and the orientation of the plane of sound is kept unchanged. If this maneuver results in imaging of the parasternal long-axis view, the patient most likely has dextroposition. This suspicion is confirmed by imaging the parasternal short-axis view from the right sternal border with a normal orientation of the plane of sound. If this maneuver results in no image that resembles a parasternal long-axis view, the transducer position is held constant and the plane of sound is rotated into the mirror-image of a normal long-axis plane (from left shoulder to right hip). If this maneuver results in imaging of the parasternal long-axis view, the patient probably has dextroversion or dextrocardia with situs inversus. The plane of the parasternal short-axis view helps distinguish these latter two defects (the plane is the mirror-image of normal in situs inversus and is usually normal in dextroversion).

ECHOCARDIOGRAPHIC FEATURES OF FREQUENTLY ENCOUNTERED COMPLEX CONGENITAL CARDIAC DEFECTS

This section will review the echocardiographic features of some of the more frequently encountered complex congenital defects. This discussion includes not only the anatomy of the defect but also the associated lesions that should alert the examiner to the diagnosis.

Juxtaposition of the Atrial Appendages

Juxtaposition of the atrial appendages is frequently associated with complex cyanotic congenital heart disease, especially defects in which there is transposition of the great arteries and/or malposition of the ventricles relative to the atria.[14] Recognition of this defect is important because of the implications its presence has for the diagnosis and surgical management of complex heart disease in children. The two-dimensional echocardiographic features of left juxtaposition of the right atrial appendage have been well described.[15] In general, the noninvasive diagnosis of left juxtaposition of the atrial appendages is based on (1) direct visualization of the juxtaposed right atrial appendage and (2) visualization of an unusual configuration of the posterior atrial septum. These two echocardiographic features can be appreciated from several different imaging planes.

On the two-dimensional echocardiographic examination, the presence of left juxtaposition of the right atrial appendage is often first suspected in the parasternal long-axis view. Because of the abnormal orientation of the anterior portion of the atrial septum in patients with left juxtaposition of the right atrial appendage (orientation is horizontal from right to left), a portion of the atrial septum can be seen in the parasternal long-axis view aligned vertically from the posterior aortic root to the left atrial posterior wall. Normally, the atrial septum cannot be imaged in the parasternal long-axis view; therefore, visualization of the atrial septum in this view should alert the examiner to the possible presence of left juxtaposition. This finding, however, is not specific for left juxtaposition as other car-

diac defects may result in abnormal rotation of the atrial septum.

In the parasternal short-axis view at the base of the heart, the juxtaposed right atrial appendage can be visualized directly. Normally, the right atrial appendage cannot be visualized in this view and the atrial septum is oriented anteroposteriorly (vertically on the two-dimensional image) from the posterior great artery to the posterior cardiac wall. In patients with left juxtaposition of the right atrial appendage, the posterior one-third of the atrial septum is oriented normally; however, the anterior portion of the atrial septum is transverse (oriented horizontally from right to left on the two-dimensional image) (Fig 14–12). The horizontal portion of the atrial septum is the floor of the juxtaposed right atrial appendage. The right atrial appendage is visualized to the patient's left, interposed between the great arteries anteriorly and the left atrium and left atrial appendage posteriorly.[15]

In the apical and subcostal four-chamber views, the abnormal orientation of the atrial septum can be seen. Normally in these views, the atrial septum curves and has its convexity to the right. In left juxtaposition (Fig 14–13), the atrial septum has a curvature with the convexity to the left. Superiorly, the atrial septum appears to wrap around the right atrium. This makes the right atrium appear smaller than the left atrium. Inferiorly, the atrial septum is aligned normally with the ventricular crest. This abnormal curvature of the atrial septum and the appearance of a small right atrium is quite distinct from the curvature of the atrial septum and the right atrial size found in patients with right atrial hypertension. However, the abnormal septal curva-

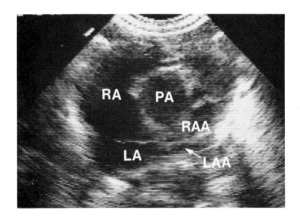

FIG 14–12.
Parasternal short-axis view from a patient with d-transposition of the great arteries and left juxtaposition of the right atrial appendage. In this view, the anterior portion of the atrial septum is oriented horizontally from right to left instead of vertically. The horizontal portion of the atrial septum is the floor of the juxtaposed right atrial appendage (RAA). The RAA is seen on the left heart border, interposed between the posterior pulmonary artery (PA) and the left atrium (LA) and left atrial appendage (LAA) posteriorly. RA = right atrium.

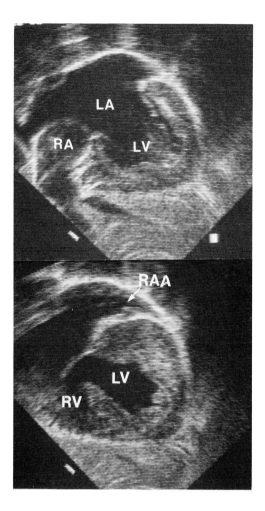

FIG 14–13.
Subcostal four-chamber views from a patient with tricuspid atresia, *d*-transposition of the great arteries, and left juxtaposition of the right atrial appendage (RAA). The *top frame* was obtained with the plane of sound tilted posteriorly to image the atrial septum. In this view, the atrial septum has an abnormal curvature with its convexity to the left. Superiorly, the atrial septum appears to wrap around the right atrium (RA), which makes the RA appear smaller than the left atrium (LA). Inferiorly, the atrial septum is aligned normally with the ventricular crest. Note the posterior left atrial appendage. In the *bottom frame,* the plane of sound has been tilted anteriorly. The left juxtaposed RAA can be imaged directly as it courses from right to left posterior to the great arteries and superior to the LA. LV = left ventricle; RV = right ventricle.

ture is not specific for the diagnosis of left juxtaposition of the atrial appendage.[15]

When the plane of sound is tilted anteriorly from the standard apical and subcostal four-chamber views, the left juxtaposed right atrial appendage can be imaged directly as it courses from right to left posterior to the great arteries and superior to the left atrium (Fig 14–13). In this projection, care must be taken not to mistake the connection between the body of the right atrium and the right atrial appendage for an atrial septal defect (Fig 14–14).

In the subcostal sagittal views, the abnormal transverse

orientation of the atrial septum can again be seen (Fig 14–15). The subcostal view through the right atrium and vena cava shows an abnormal contour of the anterior border of the right atrium. This contour is caused by the absence of the right atrial appendage anteriorly and to the right (Fig 14–16).

Univentricular Heart

Definitions
Considerable controversy exists surrounding the def-

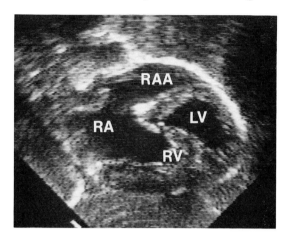

FIG 14–14.
Subcostal four-chamber view from a patient with double-outlet right ventricle, pulmonary atresia, and left juxtaposition of the right atrial appendage (RAA). In this view, the juxtaposed RAA can be visualized directly as it courses from right to left. LV = left ventricle; RA = right atrium; RV = right ventricle.

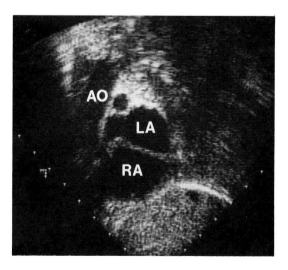

FIG 14–15.
Subcostal sagittal view through the aortic arch of a patient with left juxtaposition of the right atrial appendage. The abnormal transverse orientation of the atrial septum can be seen. AO = aorta; LA = left atrium; RA = right atrium.

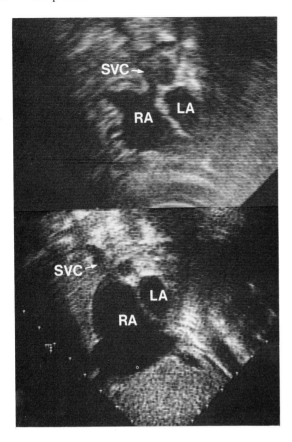

FIG 14–16.
Subcostal sagittal view through the right atrium (RA) of a normal patient is shown in the *top frame.* In this view, the right atrial appendage can be seen on the upper border of the RA. Subcostal sagittal view through the RA of a patient with left juxtaposition of the right atrial appendage is shown in the *bottom frame.* In this view, the anterior border of the RA has an abnormal appearance because of the absence of the right atrial appendage on the right border of the heart. LA = left atrium; SVC = superior vena cava.

inition, classification, and nomenclature for the various forms of univentricular heart. Our approach to the echocardiographic diagnosis of univentricular heart is based on the definitions and classification proposed by Anderson and colleagues.[16–18]

To understand what constitutes a single ventricle or univentricular heart, one must have a clear definition of what constitutes a ventricle. The ventricles of the normal heart possess inlet, trabecular, and outlet portions.[18] The inlet portion extends from the atrioventricular annulus to the insertions of the papillary muscles and, as stated earlier, need not contain a perforate atrioventricular valve. The outlet portion supports the semilunar valve, and the trabecular portion extends from the inlet and outlet portions to the ventricular apex. In the normal heart, the inlet and outlet portions of the morphologic left ventricle are in fibrous continuity. In the morphologic right ventricle, these two portions are separated from one another by the crista supraventricularis. In the normal heart, each trabecular

zone receives its own inlet; however, all the atrioventricular inlets can be committed to one trabecular portion, which is the generally accepted definition of single ventricle.[16, 18] Thus, to be classified as a ventricle, a chamber must have 50% or more of an inlet portion. A chamber need not have an outlet portion to be a ventricle (i.e., the left ventricle in double-outlet right ventricle has only inlet and trabecular portions). Chambers that receive less than 50% of an inlet are called rudimentary chambers. Rudimentary chambers possessing an outlet portion are called outlet chambers, while those possessing only a trabecular zone are known as trabecular pouches.

In the most common situation, all atrioventricular connections are committed to a chamber with a left ventricular trabecular zone. In this case, the rudimentary chamber will have a right ventricular trabecular pattern and will be located anterosuperiorly in the ventricular mass. This defect has been called double-inlet left ventricle, single ventricle of the left ventricular type, and univentricular heart of the left ventricular type. Conversely, when all atrioventricular connections are committed to a chamber with a right ventricular trabecular pattern, the rudimentary chamber contains a left ventricular trabecular portion. This defect is known as univentricular heart of the right ventricular type. When neither right nor left ventricular trabecular portions are well formed and a single chamber is present with indeterminate trabecular pattern, the defect is called univentricular heart of the indeterminate type without rudimentary chamber.[17, 18]

Another important point in the morphology and echocardiographic diagnosis of univentricular heart is the nature of the septum that separates the main ventricle from the rudimentary chamber. Since the ventricles are considered to possess inlet, trabecular, and outlet portions, the septum that separates them can be considered to possess inlet, trabecular, and outlet portions. Both inlets are committed to only one chamber; hence, by definition, the inlet septum is absent in the univentricular heart. This means that the septum that separates the ventricle from the rudimentary chamber must be the trabecular septum. The position and orientation of the trabecular septum in the ventricular mass is a key feature in the echocardiographic diagnosis of the univentricular heart.[18]

Echocardiographic Diagnosis of the Type of Univentricular Heart

In univentricular heart of the left ventricular type, the rudimentary chamber is located anterior to the main ventricle and is separated from it by an anterior trabecular septum. Because the trabecular septum is an anterior structure, it is well visualized in the parasternal long- and short-axis views.[19–21] In the parasternal long-axis view (Fig 14–17), the rudimentary chamber is seen anteriorly and separated from the main chamber by the trabecular septum. The outlet foramen is seen connecting the main ventricle and the rudimentary chamber. With this view alone, it is not possible to distinguish a univentricular heart of the left ventricular type from a ventricular septal defect with a large left ventricle. This distinction is not possible because the parasternal long-axis view allows visualization of only one atrioventricular connection. Also, because the parasternal long-axis view has only anterior-posterior and inferior-superior orientations, it is not possible to determine if the rudimentary chamber is located at the right or left basal aspect of the heart.

When the transducer is rotated into the parasternal short-axis view, the distinction between univentricular heart of the left ventricular type and ventricular septal defect with a large left ventricle is immediately apparent. In univentricular heart of the left ventricular type, both atrioventricular valves lie posterior to the trabecular septum (Fig 14–18). These valves usually do not have the anatomic features of the normal tricuspid and mitral valves; therefore, we will refer to them as the right and left atrioventricular valves. Because no inlet septum intervenes between the two atrioventricular valves, they may actually touch one another when they open in diastole (so-called kissing atrioventricular valves) (Fig 14–19). In addition, both atrioventricular valves are in fibrous continuity with the posterior great artery.

From the parasternal short-axis view, one can determine if the rudimentary chamber lies to the right or left basal aspect of the heart. Most commonly, the rudimentary chamber lies to the left, and the trabecular septum courses obliquely and somewhat posteriorly from the right and anterior cardiac border to the acute margin of the heart (Fig 14–18). When the rudimentary chamber lies to the right, the trabecular septum courses obliquely and somewhat

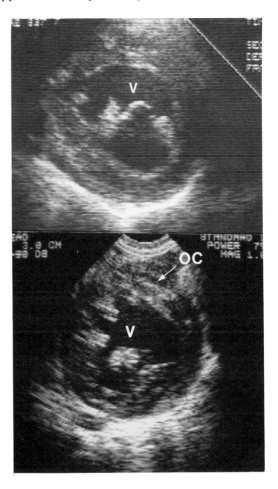

FIG 14–18.
Parasternal short-axis views from a patient with a univentricular heart of the left ventricular type and ventriculoarterial discordance. In the *top frame*, the right and left atrioventricular valves are both committed to the main ventricle (V). No septum intervenes between the valves. In the *bottom frame*, the plane of sound has been tilted slightly inferiorly to image the anterior and leftward outlet chamber (OC). Both atrioventricular valves are posterior to the trabecular septum, which lies between the OC and the V. In this patient, the trabecular septum is oriented toward the acute margin of the heart.

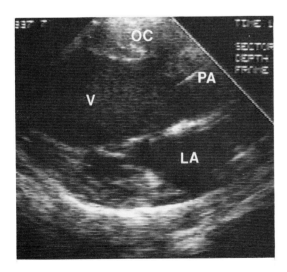

FIG 14–17.
Parasternal long-axis view from a patient with a univentricular heart of the left ventricular type and discordant ventriculoarterial connections. In this view, the small outlet chamber (OC) can be seen anterior to the main ventricle (V). In this patient, the pulmonary artery (PA) arose from the main V and the aorta arose from the OC. Note the communication between the V and OC. LA = left atrium.

posteriorly from the left anterior cardiac border to the obtuse margin of the heart (Fig 14–20). From the parasternal short-axis views, one can easily understand why the rudimentary chamber and trabecular septum cannot be seen in the four-chamber views in patients with univentricular heart of the left ventricular type. The apical and subcostal four-chamber views are posterior planes that pass through both atrioventricular valve inlets and the crux of the heart; therefore, these planes lie posterior to the trabecular septum and the rudimentary chamber (Fig 14–21).

In univentricular heart of the right ventricular type, the rudimentary chamber possesses the left ventricular trabecular portion and is, thus, located posteriorly. Likewise, the trabecular septum runs posteriorly to the crux of the heart. In the parasternal long- and short-axis views, visu-

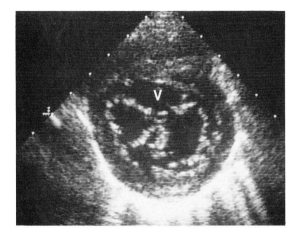

FIG 14–19.
Parasternal short-axis view from a patient with univentricular heart of the left ventricular type. Both atrioventricular valves lie posterior to the trabecular septum. Because no inlet septum intervenes between the two atrioventricular valves, the valves may actually touch one another when they open in diastole. V = ventricle.

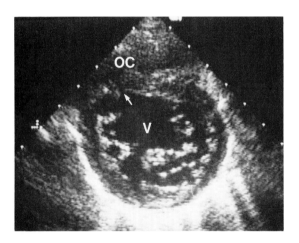

FIG 14–20.
Parasternal short-axis view from a patient with univentricular heart of the left ventricular type and a small outlet chamber (OC) located at the right basal aspect of the heart. In this patient, the main ventricle (V) communicated with the OC by way of a restrictive outlet foramen *(arrow)*. The OC gave rise to a rightward and anterior aorta and the main V gave rise to a posterior and leftward pulmonary artery.

alization of the atrioventricular connections anterior to the trabecular septum is diagnostic of univentricular heart of the right ventricular type (Figs 14–22,A and B). The rudimentary chamber can be located posteriorly and to the right or posteriorly and to the left. Because the rudimentary chamber is posterior and the trabecular septum extends to the crux of the heart, portions of these two structures can normally be seen in the apical and subcostal four-chamber views.

If a single chamber is present in the heart with no evidence of a trabecular septum or rudimentary chamber in any echocardiographic view, the diagnosis of univentricular heart of indeterminate type can be made.

Echocardiographic Evaluation of the Ventriculoarterial Connections

With the univentricular heart, any ventriculoarterial connection can occur, including concordant connections, discordant connections, double outlet from the main or outlet chambers, and single outlet from the heart. However, certain combinations of univentricular heart and ventriculoarterial connections are commonly associated with one another and, therefore, should be mentioned. A high percentage of patients with univentricular heart of the left ventricular type have discordant ventriculoarterial connections. That is, the aorta arises from the outlet chamber

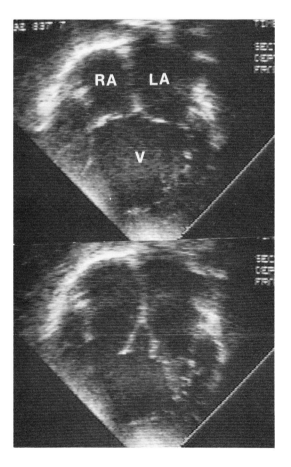

FIG 14–21.
Apical four-chamber views in systole *(above)* and diastole *(below)* from a patient with univentricular heart of the left ventricular type. The apical four-chamber view is a posterior plane that passes through both atrioventricular valve inlets and the crux of the heart; therefore, this plane lies posterior to the trabecular septum and rudimentary chamber. RA = right atrium; LA = left atrium; V = ventricle.

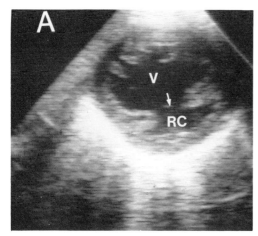

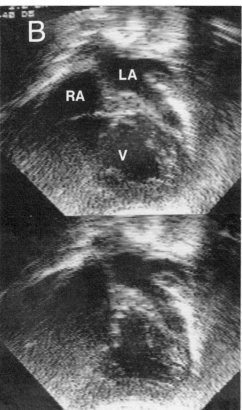

and the pulmonary artery arises from the main ventricle. Because there are not two separate ventricles, it is not entirely correct to refer to these connections as *d-* or *l-*transposition. Instead, the term discordant connections is used. Nevertheless, the great vessels are aligned parallel and exhibit many of the echocardiographic features of transposition (parallel alignment of the great arteries in long-axis views, posterior sweep of the posterior pulmonary artery in long-axis views, double circles in short-axis views) (Fig 14–23). In univentricular heart of the left ventricular type with absent right atrioventricular connection, the ventriculoarterial connections are most often concordant.[16–18]

In univentricular heart of the right ventricular type, the ventriculoarterial connections are usually double out-

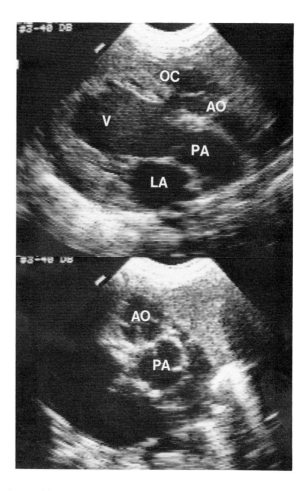

FIG 14–22.

A, parasternal short-axis view from a patient with univentricular heart of the right ventricular type. In this patient, the main ventricle (V) is located anterior to a small rudimentary chamber (RC). Parasternal short-axis views obtained slightly superior to the level of this view showed that both atrioventricular valves emptied into the main V anterior to the trabecular septum. Note that the RC communicates with the V by way of a large foramen. **B,** apical four-chamber views in systole *(above)* and diastole *(below)* from a patient with univentricular heart of the right ventricular type, absent left atrioventricular connection, and double outlet from the main ventricle (V). The floor of the left atrium (LA) is located above the V. Thus, both atrioventricular inlets are connected to the main V even though the left atrioventricular valve inlet is not perforate. In this patient, a small trabecular pouch was seen in a plane posterior to the standard apical four-chamber view. RA = right atrium.

FIG 14–23.

Parasternal long-axis *(top)* and short-axis *(bottom)* views from a patient with univentricular heart of the left ventricular type and discordant ventriculoarterial connections. In this patient, the main ventricle (V) was connected to a posterior pulmonary artery (PA). A small rightward and anterior outlet chamber (OC) gave rise to an anterior and rightward aorta (AO). Many of the echocardiographic features of transposition of the great vessels can be seen. In the parasternal long-axis view, the great vessels are in parallel alignment and the posterior PA has a posterior sweep; in the parasternal short-axis view, both great vessels appear in cross-section as double circles. LA = left atrium.

let from the main chamber or single outlet from the heart with pulmonary atresia. In univentricular heart of indeterminate type and no outlet chamber, there can only be double outlet or single outlet from the main chamber.[18]

Echocardiographic Evaluation of the Atrioventricular Connections

Double-Inlet Connections.—In the most common situation, univentricular heart of the left ventricular type exists with double inlet connection. In short-axis and four-chamber views, the two atrioventricular valves can both be seen situated posterior to the trabecular septum (see Figs 14–18 and 14–21). There is no intervening inlet septum and both valves are in continuity with the posterior great artery. Univentricular hearts of the right ventricular type can also have double inlet connection. Usually the valves lie side by side and anterior to the trabecular septum.[18] Univentricular hearts of indeterminate type usually have a double inlet connection; however, this connection is generally through a common atrioventricular valve rather than through separate right and left atrioventricular valves.

Absence of an Atrioventricular Connection.—Many hearts with atresia of an atrioventricular valve have absence of the connection rather than an imperforate valve. In absent connection, the floor of the atrium is entirely muscular and is separated from the main ventricle by the atrioventricular sulcus.[18] This is quite distinct from situations in which an imperforate membrane or connection sits above a tiny ventricular chamber. For example, in patients with univentricular heart of the left ventricular type and right atrioventricular valve atresia, the apical and subcostal four-chamber views show the right and left atria above the main ventricle. There is no small chamber situated beneath the atretic right connection and no evidence of a septum oriented to the crux of the heart. The rudimentary chamber and trabecular septum are located anteriorly and have no connection to the blind-ending right atrium.[17, 18] In tricuspid atresia with an imperforate membrane and two separate ventricles, the blind-ending right atrium can be seen in the four-chamber views situated directly above and connected to a small right ventricular chamber. The ventricular septum courses to the crux of the heart between the right and left ventricles. The same diagnostic approach applies to the distinction between hypoplastic left heart with mitral atresia and univentricular hearts of the right ventricular type with absent left atrioventricular connection (see Fig 14–22,B).

Straddling Valves.—In univentricular hearts, an inlet portion can override or straddle the trabecular septum, whether it is located anteriorly or posteriorly. The degree of commitment of the straddling valve to its own trabecular zone or to the trabecular zone of a chamber already receiving an inlet determines if the heart is classified as biventricular or univentricular.[18] In some cases, the straddling inlet appears equally committed to both chambers on the two-dimensional echocardiogram and a definite di-

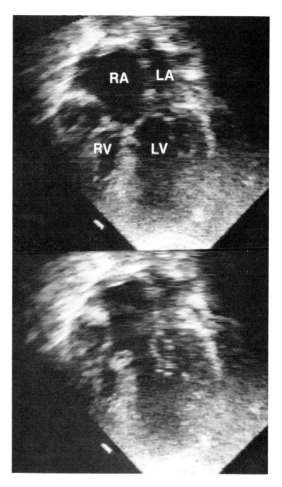

FIG 14–24.
Apical four-chamber views in systole *(above)* and diastole *(below)* from a patient with an overriding and straddling right atrioventricular valve. In this patient, the right atrioventricular valve appears to be nearly equally committed to both the right- and left-sided chambers. Other views in this patient showed an anterior and rightward aorta arising from the small right-sided chamber and a posterior and leftward pulmonary artery arising from the main chamber. Possible diagnoses in this patient include (1) *d*-transposition with an inlet ventricular septal defect, straddling tricuspid valve, and a small right ventricle (RV), and (2) univentricular heart of the right ventricular type with an outlet chamber giving rise to the aorta (concordant connections). Because of the orientation of the trabecular septum to the crux of the heart, this patient was interpreted as having *d*-transposition of the great arteries with a small RV and straddling tricuspid valve. LA = left atrium; LV = left ventricle; RA = right atrium.

agnosis cannot be made. In these situations, the position of the small chamber and septum may suggest the most likely diagnosis. For example, in Figure 14–24, the right atrioventricular valve straddles a posterior septum and is nearly equally committed to both chambers. Other echocardiographic views showed an anterior and rightward aorta arising from the small right-sided chamber and a posterior and leftward pulmonary artery arising from the main chamber. Possible diagnoses include (1) *d*-transposition with an inlet ventricular septal defect, straddling tricuspid valve, and small right ventricle and (2) univentricular heart of the right ventricular type with an outlet chamber giving rise to the aorta (concordant connections). This heart cannot represent univentricular heart of the left ventricular type because both atrioventricular valves, if considered to arise from the main chamber, would be located anterior to the trabecular septum. The finding of an anterior and rightward aorta arising from the small chamber is strong supporting evidence for the first diagnosis, as the majority of univentricular hearts of the right ventricular type have a double-outlet connection of the great arteries from the main ventricle. Nevertheless, any variation is possible, and an exact diagnosis cannot be made with certainty in cases where the straddling inlet appears equally committed to both chambers.

Echocardiographic Evaluation of Associated Abnormalities

Two-dimensional and Doppler echocardiography are especially useful for evaluating abnormalities frequently associated with the univentricular heart. For example, the size of the outlet foramen can be assessed from the parasternal long- and short-axis views. The pressure gradient across a restrictive outlet foramen can be estimated from these views using Doppler echocardiography. The presence of muscular or membranous outflow obstruction in the main ventricle or the rudimentary chamber can be assessed from parasternal long-axis, apical four-chamber, and subcostal four-chamber views. Stenoses of the atrioventricular valves are readily apparent in the four-chamber views.

Situs Ambiguus

Although the diagnosis of asplenia or polysplenia is largely determined from the radiographic appearance of the tracheobronchial tree,[22] there are several associated anomalies whose presence may suggest one or the other diagnosis.[23–26] For example, in situs ambiguus, anomalies of systemic venous drainage are common. Bilateral superior venae cavae, each draining to the ipsilateral atrial cavity, are commonly found in both asplenia and polysplenia; however, drainage of the left-sided superior vena cava to the coronary sinus is encountered only in patients with polysplenia. The echocardiographic techniques used to visualize a persistent left superior vena cava were described in Chapter 10.

Anomalies of the systemic veins that drain the abdomen are also frequent. In asplenia syndrome, the inferior vena cava and aorta tend to be on the same side of the spine, either to the right or to the left. The frequency of this finding makes it an extremely valuable diagnostic sign.[23] The subcostal views in the abdomen show the inferior vena cava positioned alongside and anterior to the descending aorta (Fig 14–25). In polysplenia syndrome, the inferior vena cava is frequently interrupted (see Chapter 10). In these cases, lower systemic venous return is by way of the azygous or hemiazygous vein and the hepatic veins drain directly into one or both atria (Fig 14–26).[23] In the subcostal

views in the abdomen, the azygous or hemiazygous vein can sometimes be seen on the same side of the spine as the aorta; however, in this situation, the systemic vein is posterior rather than anterior to the aorta. In asplenia or polysplenia syndrome, the inferior vena cava, when present, can drain to either atria. The subcostal sagittal views in the abdomen are particularly useful for tracing the inferior vena cava to its drainage site (Fig 14–27).

Anomalous pulmonary venous return is also common in situs ambiguus. In asplenia syndrome, total anomalous pulmonary venous return is nearly always present (in more than 80% of cases) and can be of any type. When the veins enter the cardiac atrium directly (rather than by way of a pulmonary venous confluence and common pulmonary vein), they tend to drain to the smooth intercaval portion of the atria (Fig 14–28). In polysplenia syndrome, the pulmonary veins enter one atrium in a normal fashion in one-

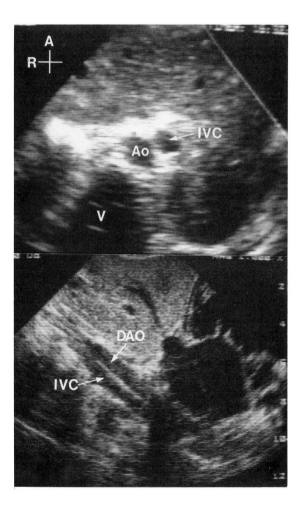

FIG 14–25.
Subcostal short-axis *(top)* and sagittal *(bottom)* views from a patient with asplenia syndrome. In this patient, the inferior vena cava (IVC) is on the same side of the spine as the descending aorta (DAO). Note that the IVC is anterior to the DAO. This abnormality of systemic venous drainage is commonly present in patients with asplenia syndrome. A = anterior; R = right; V = vertebral body.

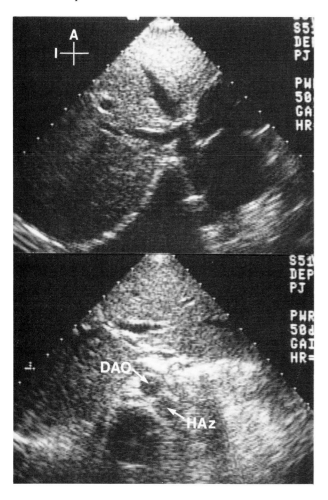

FIG 14–26.
Subcostal long-axis *(top)* and short-axis *(bottom)* views from a patient with polysplenia syndrome and interrupted inferior vena cava. In the subcostal long-axis view, *top,* the hepatic veins are seen draining to the right side of the common atrium. There is no evidence of an inferior vena cava below the hepatic veins. In the subcostal short-axis view, *bottom,* a large venous structure is seen posterior to the descending aorta (DAO) in the abdomen. This posterior structure represents a large hemiazygous (HAz) vein through which the lower body systemic venous drainage returned to a left-sided superior vena cava. A = anterior; I = inferior.

third of cases. In more than 50% of cases, however, the right veins enter the right-sided atrium and the left veins enter the left-sided atrium.[23]

The anatomy of the cardiac chambers and great vessels is extremely variable in situs ambiguus; however, a few common associations deserve mention. In asplenia syndrome, atrioventricular septal defects and univentricular heart are common (Fig 14–28). The great arteries are frequently transposed and there is a high incidence of severe pulmonary stenosis or atresia. In polysplenia syndrome, atrial septal defects, ventricular septal defects, and double-outlet right ventricle are frequently encountered. Transposition of the great arteries and severe pulmonary stenosis are uncommon in polysplenia syndrome.[23, 26]

Situs Inversus

A variety of cardiac abnormalities can occur in the context of atrial situs inversus. Figures 14–29 to 14–31 illustrate how the two-dimensional echocardiogram can be used to diagnose cardiac defects associated with situs inversus. Figures 14–29 and 14–30 are subcostal coronal views from a patient with dextrocardia (note the cardiac apex pointing to the patient's right). In Figure 14–29 *(top),* the plane of sound is aimed far posteriorly so that the orifice of the coronary sinus can be seen emptying into the left-sided atrium. Thus, the left-sided atrium is a morphologic right atrium and there is atrial situs inversus. In Fig 14–29 *(bottom),* the plane of sound is tilted anteriorly so

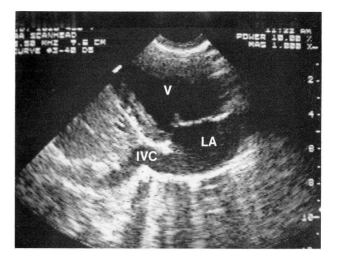

FIG 14–27.
Parasternal long-axis view from a patient with asplenia syndrome and a left-sided inferior vena cava (IVC) draining to the left-sided atrium (LA). In this patient, the plane of sound has been tilted to the patient's left to image the connection of the left IVC to the left-sided atrium. V = ventricle.

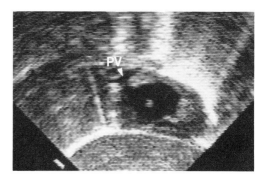

FIG 14–28.
Subcostal four-chamber view from a patient with asplenia syndrome, an atrioventricular septal defect, and total anomalous pulmonary venous drainage directly to the right-sided atrium. In this view, several of the pulmonary veins (PV) can be seen draining to the smooth, intercaval portion of the atrium.

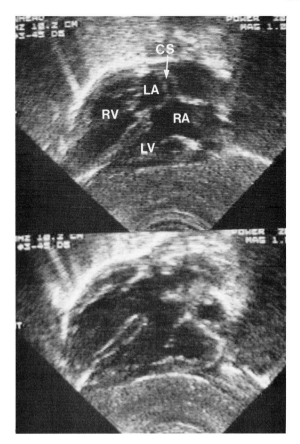

FIG 14–29.
Subcostal four-chamber views from a patient with dextrocardia. Note that the cardiac apex points to the patient's right. In the *top frame*, the plane of sound has been tilted far posteriorly. The coronary sinus (CS) can be seen emptying into the left-sided atrium. This anatomical feature suggests that the left-sided atrium is a morphologic right atrium (RA) and that there is atrial situs inversus. In the *bottom frame*, the plane of sound has been tilted anteriorly so that an atrioventricular septal defect is seen. LA = left atrium; LV = left ventricle; RV = right ventricle.

that an atrioventricular septal defect is seen. Figure 14–30 was obtained from the same patient by tilting the transducer even more anteriorly. As can be seen in this frame, both great arteries arise from the right-sided ventricle (double outlet connection) with the pulmonary artery bifurcation seen to the patient's right. The right-sided ventricle is triangular, and, in other views, had coarse septoparietal muscle bundles. Hence, this ventricle is a morphologic right ventricle and there is d-looping. The complete diagnosis after segmental analysis is situs inversus, d-loop, double-outlet right ventricle with an atrioventricular septal defect and dextrocardia. Figure 14–31 is an apical four-chamber view from another patient with situs inversus, d-loop, and a large inlet ventricular septal defect. The right-sided ventricle has chordal attachments of its atrioventricular valve to the crest of the septum and has prominent septoparietal muscle bundles. Thus, this chamber is a morphologic right ventricle and there is a d-bulboventricular loop.

Criss-Cross Hearts

The term criss-cross heart has been used to describe the rare abnormality in which the systemic and pulmonary venous streams cross at the atrioventricular level without mixing. The right-sided atrium connects to the left-sided ventricle and the left-sided atrium connects to the right-sided ventricle. The ventricles are usually arranged in a superoinferior manner and the defect can be found with concordant or discordant atrioventricular connections. A ventricular septal defect is invariably present, and discordant ventriculoarterial connections are common. Associated defects can be expected.[27]

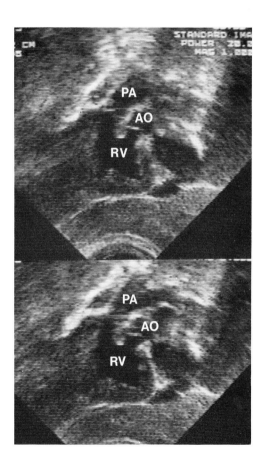

FIG 14–30.
Subcostal coronal view from the same patient as in Figure 14–29, with the plane of sound tilted far anteriorly. As can be seen in this view, both great arteries arise from the right-sided anterior ventricle (double outlet connection). The vessel on the patient's right bifurcates and is, therefore, the pulmonary artery (PA). The vessel on the patient's left is, therefore, the aorta (AO). The right-sided and anterior ventricle is triangular, suggesting that it is a morphologic right ventricle (RV). Thus, from the information in these views and in Figure 14–29, this patient's complete diagnosis is situs inversus, d-loop, double-outlet right ventricle with atrioventricular septal defect and dextrocardia.

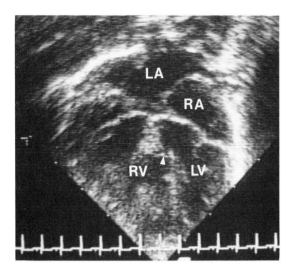

FIG 14-31.
Apical four-chamber view from another patient with atrial situs inversus. In this patient, the right-sided atrium receives the pulmonary veins, suggesting that this atrium is a morphologic left atrium (LA). The left-sided atrium is, therefore, a morphologic right atrium (RA) and there is atrial situs inversus. The right-sided ventricle has coarse septal parietal muscle bundles and attachments of its atrioventricular valve to the crest of the ventricular septum. These anatomic features suggest that the right-sided ventricle is a morphologic right ventricle (RV). The left-sided ventricle is, therefore, a morphologic left ventricle (LV). This patient's diagnosis is atrial situs inversus with *d*-loop. Note the large inlet ventricular septal defect.

The two-dimensional echocardiographic features of criss-cross heart have been well described.[27-30] In this defect, the subcostal views provide the best imaging of the connections and spatial relations of the cardiac chambers and great arteries.[27, 28] The diagnosis of criss-cross heart should be suspected when a parallel arrangement of the atrioventricular valves and ventricular inflow regions cannot be found in the standard subcostal (and apical) four-chamber views. In the most posterior subcostal four-chamber view, the left-sided atrium can be seen communicating by way of an atrioventricular valve to the right-sided ventricle. In the usual situation, the left-sided atrium is a morphologic left atrium which is connected to a right-sided morphologic left ventricle. The left ventricle is posterior, inferior, and rightward. The posterior mitral valve is oriented from posterior-superior to anterior-inferior (Fig 14-32).[29] As the plane of sound is tilted farther anteriorly, the connection from the right-sided atrium to the left-sided ventricle can be seen (Fig 14-33). In the usual situation, the right-sided morphologic right atrium is connected to a morphologic right ventricle which is anterior, superior, and leftward. The anterior and superior tricuspid valve is oriented from right to left and from posterior to anterior. Frequently in this plane, a distal portion of the mitral valve leaflets can be seen in cross-section, inferior to the longitudinal section through the tricuspid leaflets (Fig 14-33). With even further tilting of the plane of sound anteriorly,

the entire anterior ventricle and its outflow portion can be visualized (Fig 14-34). In the usual situation, this anterior and superior ventricle is a morphologic right ventricle that gives rise to a transposed aorta.

From the above description, it is apparent that the atrioventricular valves are not seen together in the subcostal four-chamber view.[28] It is important, therefore, to perform a careful sweep of the heart from posterior to anterior to avoid the false impression of an absent right atrioventricular connection created by the standard subcostal four-chamber view alone (see Fig 14-32).[30] It is possible, in both subcostal four-chamber and sagittal views (Fig 14-35) to see portions of both atrioventricular valves simultaneously. However, instead of being aligned in their normal parallel arrangement, the atrioventricular valves are nearly perpendicular to one another so that a longitudinal section through one valve is usually imaged simultaneously with a cross-section of the other valve.

Associated defects are common in criss-cross hearts.

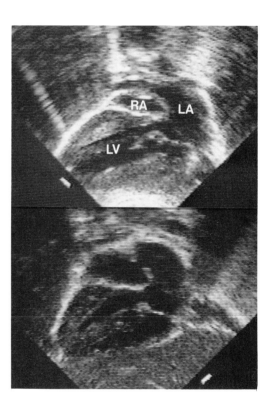

FIG 14-32.
Subcostal four-chamber views from a patient with a criss-cross heart and dextrocardia. In the *top frame*, the plane of sound is tilted far posteriorly. The pulmonary veins drain to the left-sided atrium, suggesting that this is a morphologic left atrium (LA). The morphologic LA is connected to a smooth-walled ventricle that has the anatomic features of a morphologic left ventricle (LV). The LV is located posteriorly, inferiorly, and rightward. The posterior mitral valve is oriented from posterior-superior to anterior-inferior. In the *bottom frame*, the plane of sound has been tilted slightly anteriorly so that a secundum atrial septal defect can be seen. Note that the outlet of the right atrium (RA) cannot be seen in this view.

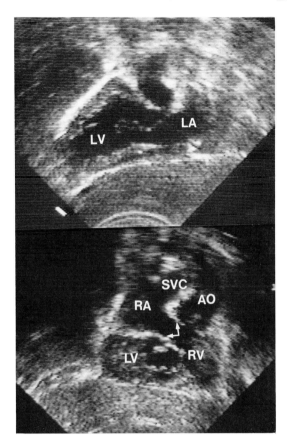

FIG 14–33.
Subcostal coronal views from the same patient as in Figure 14–32. In the *top frame,* the connection from the left-sided morphologic left atrium (LA) to the right-sided morphologic left ventricle (LV) is again seen. As the plane of sound is tilted anteriorly *(bottom frame),* the connections from the right-sided atrium to the left-sided ventricle can be seen. The right-sided atrium received the drainage of the superior vena cava (SVC) and had other features suggesting that this chamber was a morphologic right atrium (RA). Subsequent views showed that the left-sided ventricle had the features of a morphologic right ventricle (RV) and gave rise to the leftward and anterior aorta (AO). Note that the morphologic RV is anterior, superior, and leftward. The anterior and superior tricuspid valve *(arrows)* is oriented from right to left and from posterior to anterior. A cross-section of the distal portion of the mitral valve leaflets can be seen inferior to the longitudinal section through the tricuspid valve leaflets. This view provides direct visualization of the criss-cross arrangement of the atrioventricular valves.

Ventricular septal defects are invariably present and usually occur in the inlet septum. When the pulmonary valve is posterior and the ventriculoarterial connections are discordant, the pulmonary valve is wedged between the tricuspid and mitral valves. In this situation, subvalvular and valvular pulmonary stenosis commonly occur (Fig 14–35). Finally, straddling atrioventricular valves are also frequently encountered in criss-cross relations.

Criss-cross heart is one of the few congenital defects in which the loop may not predict the atrioventricular connections or alignments properly. The loop indicates the

situs or position of the ventricles which, in turn, usually corresponds to the atrioventricular connections. Thus, the usual form of criss-cross heart (right-sided morphologic right atrium to left-sided morphologic right ventricle to left-sided aorta) can be described as atrial situs solitus, *l*-loop, and *l*-transposition of the great arteries. Without further explanation, one would assume from this nomenclature that the atrioventricular alignments are discordant. It is suggested, therefore, that in the rare instances where the loop alone (or ventricular situs) does not indicate the ventricular alignments, both alignments and ventricular situs be stated. The previously mentioned heart would then be referred to as atrial situs solitus, concordant alignments, *l*-loop ventricles, and *l*-transposition of the great arteries.[31]

Atrioventricular Discordance with Ventriculoarterial Concordance

Isolated Ventricular Inversion
Isolated ventricular inversion is a term first used by

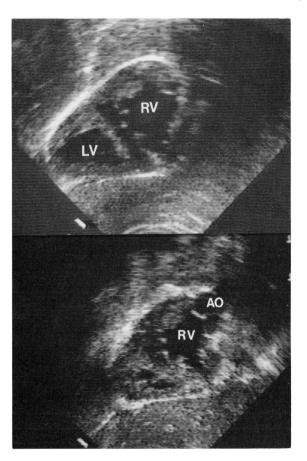

FIG 14–34.
Subcostal four-chamber views from the same patient as in Figure 14–33. The plane of sound has been tilted even more anteriorly. A triangular, heavily trabeculated morphologic right ventricle (RV) can be seen located anterior, superior, and leftward. In the *bottom frame,* the aorta (AO) can be seen arising from the RV. LV=left ventricle.

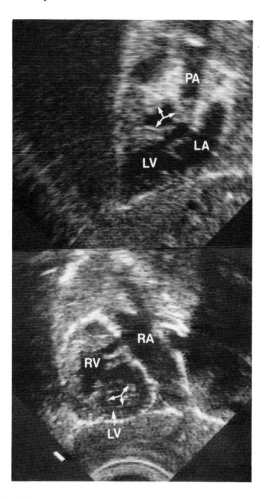

FIG 14–35.
Subcostal sagittal views from a patient with a criss-cross heart. In the *top frame,* a longitudinal section through the mitral valve is seen. The left atrium (LA) communicates with a rightward, posterior, and inferior left ventricle (LV). The tricuspid valve can be seen in cross-section *(arrows)* superior to the mitral valve. The pulmonary artery (PA) is wedged between the tricuspid and mitral valves. There is severe valvular and subvalvular pulmonary stenosis. In the *bottom frame,* the plane of sound has been tilted slightly to the right to obtain a subcostal sagittal view through the right atrium (RA). The tricuspid valve can be seen superiorly in longitudinal section. Inferiorly, a portion of the mitral valve can be seen in cross-section *(arrows).* This view shows that the atrioventricular valves are aligned perpendicular rather than parallel to one another. RV = right ventricle.

Van Praagh and Van Praagh[32] in 1966 to describe the rare congenital cardiac malformation of ventricular inversion without transposition of the great arteries (i.e., atrioventricular discordance and ventriculoarterial concordance). Because isolated ventricular inversion causes a physiologic state identical to that of complete transposition of the great arteries, most patients with this defect are symptomatic in infancy with cyanosis and congestive heart failure. The two-dimensional echocardiographic features of this defect

were first reported by us in 1984.[33] Because we have not examined another child with this defect since that time, the two-dimensional echocardiograms from the original case are used to illustrate this defect. These echocardiograms were obtained prior to the current practice of anatomic orientation of the image and are, therefore, upside down.

On the two-dimensional echocardiogram, patients with isolated ventricular inversion have atrioventricular discordance. The echocardiographic features of atrioventricular discordance have been described above. In the usual situation, there is atrial situs solitus and *l*-bulboventricular loop (Fig 14–36). The ventriculoarterial connections are normal. Thus, a posterior aorta usually arises from a right-sided morphologic left ventricle (Fig 14–37) and is in fibrous continuity with the right-sided mitral valve (Fig 14–38). An anterior pulmonary artery arises from the left-sided morphologic right ventricle and is separated from the left atrioventricular valve by a persistent subpulmonary conus. The normal relationships of the great arteries to one another (aortic valve rightward, posterior, and inferior to the pulmonary valve; great arteries coiled around each other) create a circle-sausage appearance in the parasternal and subcostal short-axis views (Fig 14–37).

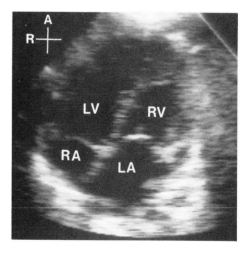

FIG 14–36.
Apical four-chamber view showing normal atrial situs and discordant atrioventricular connections in a patient with isolated ventricular inversion. The pulmonary veins can be seen draining to the left-sided atrium, suggesting that this chamber is the morphologic left atrium (LA); therefore, there is atrial situs solitus. The left-sided ventricle has a prominent septoparietal muscle bundle and an atrioventricular valve closer to the cardiac apex. These features show that this chamber is the morphologic right ventricle (RV); therefore, there is ventricular inversion. The right-sided morphologic left ventricle (LV) has no septoparietal muscle bundles and has an atrioventricular valve farther from the cardiac apex. A = apex; R = right; RA = right atrium. (From Snider AR, Enderlein MA, Teitel DR, et al: *Pediatr Cardiol* 1984; 5:28. Used by permission.)

Anatomically Corrected Malposition

Another rare defect with atrioventricular discordance and ventriculoarterial concordance is anatomically corrected malposition.[5] The echocardiographic techniques described above are used to diagnose atrioventricular discordance (morphologic right atrium connected to the morphologic left ventricle) and ventriculoarterial concordance (aorta arising from the morphologic left ventricle).[34] In anatomically corrected malpositions, however, there is an abnormal relationship between the aorta and the atrio-

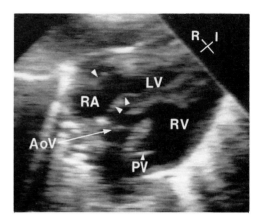

FIG 14–38.
Subcostal view from a patient with isolated ventricular inversion showing the characteristic features of ventricular inversion with a normal relationship between the great vessels and the atrioventricular canal. The right atrium (RA) is connected to the right-sided morphologic left ventricle (LV). The morphologic right ventricle (RV) with its moderator band can be seen on the left. The aorta arises from the LV and there is fibrous continuity between the aortic valve (AoV) and the right-sided (mitral) atrioventricular valve *(white arrows)*. The pulmonary valve (PV) is superior to the AoV because of the persistence of a well-developed, subpulmonic conus. The AoV is also to the right and posterior to the PV. I = inferior; R = right. (From Snider AR, Enderlein MA, Teitel DR, et al: *Pediatr Cardiol* 1984; 5:29. Used by permission.)

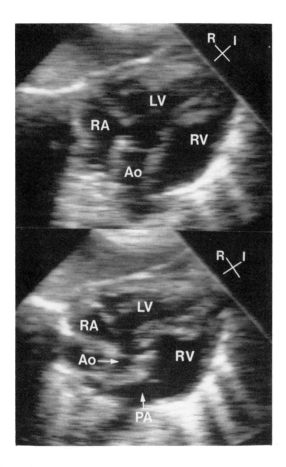

FIG 14–37.
Subcostal views obtained by tilting the transducer anteriorly from the standard subcostal four-chamber view. These views show discordant atrioventricular connections and normal relationships between the great arteries and the ventricles in a patient with isolated ventricular inversion. With a slight anterior tilt of the transducer from the standard subcostal four-chamber view *(top)*, the aorta (Ao) and aortic arch can be seen arising from the right-sided ventricle which the four-chamber view in Figure 14–36 has shown to be the morphologic left ventricle (LV). With even more anterior tilt of the transducer *(bottom)*, the anteriorly positioned pulmonary artery (PA) and its bifurcation can be seen arising from the left-sided morphologic right ventricle (RV). In addition, the great vessels are normally coiled around each other in a circle-sausage appearance. A subaortic ventricular septal defect can also be seen. I = inferior; R = right; RA = right atrium. (From Snider AR, Enderlein MA, Teitel DR, et al: *Pediatr Cardiol* 1984; 5:28. Used by permission.)

ventricular canal such that mitral-aortic fibrous continuity does not occur (there is usually bilateral conus). In addition, although the great vessels arise above the correct chamber, the aortic valve is anterior to the pulmonary valve and the great vessels exit the heart in a parallel fashion (double circles in the short-axis views).

REFERENCES

1. Van Praagh R, Ongley PA, Swan HJC: Anatomic types of single or common ventricle in man: Morphologic and geometric aspects of 60 necropsied cases. *Am J Cardiol* 1964; 13:367–386.
2. Van Praagh R: The segmental approach to diagnosis in congenital heart disease, in Bergsma D (ed): *Birth Defects: Original Article Series.* Baltimore, Williams and Wilkins, 1972, pp 4–23.
3. Shinebourne EA, Macartney FJ, Anderson RH: Sequential chamber localization: Logical approach to diagnosis in congenital heart disease. *Br Heart J* 1976; 38:327–340.
4. Stanger P, Rudolph AM, Edwards JE: Cardiac malpositions: An overview based on study of sixty-five necropsy specimens. *Circulation* 1977; 56:159–172.
5. Van Praagh R: Terminology of congenital heart disease: Glossary and commentary. *Circulation* 1977; 56:139–143.
6. Tynan MG, Becker AE, Macartney FJ, et al: Nomenclature and classification of congenital heart disease. *Br Heart J* 1979; 41:544–553.

7. Macartney FJ, Partridge JB, Shinebourne EA, et al: Identification of atrial situs, in Anderson RH, Shinebourne EA (eds): *Paediatric Cardiology 1977.* Edinburgh, Churchill Livingstone, 1978, pp 16–26.

8. de la Cruz MV, Berrazueta JR, Arteaga M, et al: Rules for diagnosis of arterioventricular discordances and spatial identification of ventricles. Crossed great arteries and transposition of the great arteries. *Br Heart J* 1976; 38:341–354.

9. Kirklin JW, Pacifico AD, Bargeron LM, et al: Cardiac repair in anatomically corrected malposition of the great arteries. *Circulation* 1973; 48:153–159.

10. Anderson RH, Macartney FJ, Shinebourne EA, et al: Definitions of cardiac chambers, in Anderson RH, Shinebourne EA (eds): *Paediatric Cardiology 1977.* Edinburgh, Churchill Livingstone, 1978, pp 5–15.

11. Goor DA, Lillehei CW: *Congenital Malformations of the Heart.* New York, Grune and Stratton, 1975, pp 1–37.

12. Van Praagh R, Van Praagh S, Vlad P, et al: Anatomic types of congenital dextrocardia: Diagnostic and embryologic implications. *Am J Cardiol* 1964; 13:510–531.

13. Calcaterra G, Anderson RH, Lau KC, et al: Dextrocardia: Value of segmental analysis in its categorisation. *Br Heart J* 1979; 42:497–507.

14. Melhuish BPP, Van Praagh R: Juxtaposition of the atrial appendages: A sign of severe cyanotic congenital heart disease. *Br Heart J* 1968; 30:269–284.

15. Rice MJ, Seward JB, Hagler DJ, et al: Left juxtaposed atrial appendages: Diagnostic two-dimensional echocardiographic features. *J Am Coll Cardiol* 1983; 1:1330–1336.

16. Anderson RH, Tynan M, Freedom RM, et al: Ventricular morphology in univentricular heart. *Herz* 1979; 4:184–197.

17. Anderson RH, Becker AE, Freedom RM, et al: Problems in the nomenclature of the univentricular heart. *Herz* 1979; 4:97–106.

18. Anderson RH, Tynan M, Becker AE: Echocardiography of the univentricular heart, in Lundstrom N-R (ed): *Pediatric Echocardiography-Cross Sectional, M-mode, and Doppler.* Amsterdam, Elsevier/North-Holland Biomedical Press, 1980, pp 129–146.

19. Rigby ML, Anderson RH, Gibson D, et al: Two-dimensional echocardiographic categorization of the univentricular heart. Ventricular morphology, type, and mode of atrioventricular connection. *Br Heart J* 1981; 46:603–612.

20. Freedom RM, Picchio F, Duncan WJ, et al: The atrioventricular junction in the univentricular heart: A two-dimensional echocardiographic analysis. *Ped Cardiol* 1982; 3:105–117.

21. Huhta JC, Seward JB, Tajik AJ, et al: Two-dimensional echocardiographic spectrum of univentricular atrioventricular connection. *J Am Coll Cardiol* 1985; 5:149–157.

22. Van Mierop LHS, Eisen S, Schiebler GL: The radiographic appearance of the tracheobronchial tree as an indicator of visceral situs. *Am J Cardiol* 1970; 26:432–435.

23. Van Mierop LHS, Gessner IH, Schiebler GL: Asplenia and polysplenia syndromes, in Bergsma D (ed): *Birth Defects: Original Article Series.* Baltimore, Williams and Wilkins, 1972, pp 36–44.

24. Van Mierop LHS, Wiglesworth FW: Isomerism of the cardiac atria in the asplenia syndrome. *Laboratory Invest* 1962; 11:1303–1315.

25. Moller JH, Nakib A, Anderson RC, et al: Congenital cardiac disease associated with polysplenia: A developmental complex of bilateral "left-sidedness." *Circulation* 1967; 36:789–799.

26. Stewart PA, Becker AE, Wladimiroff JW, et al: Left atrial isomerism associated with asplenia: Prenatal echocardiographic detection of complex congenital cardiac malformations. *J Am Coll Cardiol* 1984; 4:1015–1020.

27. Robinson PJ, Kumpeng V, Macartney FJ: Cross sectional echocardiographic and angiographic correlation in criss cross hearts. *Br Heart J* 1985; 54:61–67.

28. van Mill G, Moulaert A, Harinck E, et al: Subcostal two-dimensional echocardiographic recognition of a criss-cross heart with discordant ventriculoarterial connections. *Pediatr Cardiol* 1982; 3:319–323.

29. Marino B, Sanders SP, Pasquini L, et al: Two-dimensional echocardiographic anatomy in crisscross heart. *Am J Cardiol* 1986; 58:325–333.

30. Carminati M, Valsecchi O, Borghi A, et al: Cross-sectional echocardiographic study of criss-cross hearts and superoinferior ventricles. *Am J Cardiol* 1987; 59:114–118.

31. Van Praagh R: When concordant or discordant atrioventricular alignments predict the ventricular situs wrongly. I. Solitus atria, concordant alignments, and l-loop ventricles. II. Solitus atria, discordant alignments, and d-loop ventricles. *J Am Coll Cardiol* 1987; 10:1278–1279.

32. Van Praagh R, Van Praagh S: Isolated ventricular inversion: A consideration of the morphogenesis, definition and diagnosis of nontransposed and transposed great arteries. *Am J Cardiol* 1966; 17:395–406.

33. Snider AR, Enderlein MA, Teitel DF, et al: Isolated ventricular inversion: Two-dimensional echocardiographic findings and a review of the literature. *Pediatr Cardiol* 1984; 5:27–33.

34. Pasquini L, Sanders SP, Parness I, et al: Echocardiographic and anatomic findings in atrioventricular discordance with ventriculoarterial concordance. *Am J Cardiol* 1988; 62:1256–1262.

Index